Practical Haematology

Practical Haematology

Sir John V. Dacie
MD(Lond) FRCP(Lond) FRCPath FRS
Emeritus Professor of Haematology, University of London,
Royal Postgraduate Medical School, London

S. M. Lewis
BSc MD(Cape Town) DCP(Lond) FRCPath
Reader in Haematology, University of London, Royal
Postgraduate Medical School and Consultant Haematologist,
Hammersmith Hospital, London

SIXTH EDITION

CHURCHILL LIVINGSTONE
EDINBURGH LONDON MELBOURNE AND NEW YORK 1984

CHURCHILL LIVINGSTONE
Medical Division of Longman Group UK Limited

Distributed in the United States of America by
Churchill Livingstone Inc., 1560 Broadway, New York,
N.Y. 10036, and by associated companies, branches
and representatives throughout the world.

First Edition 1950
Second Edition 1956
    Italian Edition 1957
Third Edition 1963
    Spanish Edition 1963
Fourth Edition 1968
    Spanish Edition 1970
    Italian Edition 1972
Fifth Edition 1975
    Japanese Edition 1980
Sixth Edition 1984
    Reprinted 1985 (twice)
    Reprinted 1986

ISBN 0 443 01981 9

British Library Cataloguing in Publication Data

Dacie, J.V.
    Practical haematology. — 6th ed.
    1. Blood — Examination
    I. Title   II. Lewis, S.M.
    616.1'507'5   RB45

Library of Congress Cataloging in Publication Data

Dacie, John V. (John Vivian)
    Practical haematology.

    Includes index.
    1. Blood — Examination.   2. Hematology — Technique.
I. Lewis, S.M. (Shirley Mitchell)   II. Title.
[DNLM: 1. Blood.   2. Diagnosis, Laboratory.
3. Hematologic diseases — Diagnosis, QY 400 D118p]
RB45,D24   1984   616.07'561   83-14387

Produced by Longman Singapore Publishers Pte Ltd
Printed in Singapore

Preface to the Sixth Edition

Much has happened in the field of haematology since the publication of the 5th edition of this book in 1975, and in this new edition, as in the past editions, we describe how the laboratory aspects of haematology are currently practised and taught at Hammersmith Hospital and the Royal Postgraduate Medical School in London. Every page of the previous edition has been closely scrutinized; every existing chapter has been revised, and four new chapters have been added. There have been, too, some rearrangements. Quality Assurance, of increasing importance in laboratory work, has been given a chapter of its own; the Investigation of the Haemorrhagic Disorders is now dealt with in three chapters instead of in one; the Blood Groups and the Laboratory Aspects of Blood Transfusion are dealt with in separate chapters and the chapter on the Investigation of the Auto-Immune Haemolytic Anaemias follows that on the Laboratory Aspects of Blood Transfusion. Descriptions of some obsolete techniques have been omitted but the amount of new material added has meant that the size of the book has inevitably had to be still further increased. It is a sobering thought to recollect that the first edition of the book, published in 1950, ran to only 172 pages and cost but 10 shillings (50 p.)!

It is sad to report that one of our valued collaborators, Dr Sheila Worlledge, died in January 1980 and that we have not had the benefit of her knowledge and expertise in revising the chapters she helped us with in the past. Dr Patricia Chipping and Miss Eleanor Lloyd have, however, given us valuable help in her place (in Chapters 21, 22 and 23). We warmly welcome, too, Miss Beverley A. Frost (Chapter 11) and Dr Milica Brozovic (Chapters 13, 14, 15 and 16) as new contributors. As before, we are much indebted to Dr D. Catovs-ky, Dr E. C. Gordon-Smith, Professor A. V. Hoffbrand, Professor Sylvia Lawler, Professor W. R. Pitney and Professor J. M. White for their valued contributions to the chapters which deal with aspects of practical haematology in which they have special knowledge and experience.

We are also indebted to past and present colleagues who have read parts of the text and have given us valuable advice. For this we thank particularly Drs H. I. Glass, M. Myers, A. M. Peters and Professor L. Luzzatto.

In referring to special reagents and apparatus, we have thought it useful to state the sources (generally in the UK) from which our supplies have been obtained. This does not mean that equivalent material cannot be used or that it cannot be obtained from other sources.

The photomicrographs of blood films, new to this edition, have been taken for us by Mr W. F. Hinkes. We greatly appreciate his skill. Finally, we should like to thank Mrs Eleanor Panayi for secretarial assistance and Mr Andrew Stevenson and his staff at Churchill Livingstone for their help at every stage in the preparation of this book.

1984
John Dacie
Mitchell Lewis

UNITS OF MEASUREMENT

In keeping with current practice, we have used the Systéme International (SI) for expressing quantities and units. In this system the basic unit of volume is the litre. The World Health Organization, the International Committee for Standardization in Haematology and other international authorities have recently recommended that haemoglobin, too, should be expressed in g/l in preference to g/dl. This convention has been adopted in the present edition.

Contributors

Milica Brozovic, FRCPath
Consultant Haematologist, Central Middlesex Hospital, London.

D. Catovsky, MD, MRCPath
Senior Lecturer in Haematology and Medicine, MRC Leukaemia Unit, Royal Postgraduate Medical School, and Consultant Physician, Hammersmith Hospital, London.

Patricia M. Chipping, BSc, MB, MRCP, MRCPath
Consultant Haematologist, North Staffordshire Hospital Centre, Stoke-on-Trent.

Beverley A. Frost, FIMLS
Chief Medical Laboratory Scientific Officer, Department of Haematology, King's College Hospital Medical School, London.

E. C. Gordon-Smith, MA, BM, BSc(Oxon), MSc(Lond), FRCP(Lond)
Senior Lecturer in Haematology and Medicine, Royal Postgraduate Medical School, and Consultant Physician, Hammersmith Hospital, London.

A. V. Hoffbrand, MA, DM(Oxon), FRCP(Lond), FRCPath, DCP(Lond)
Professor of Haematology, University of London, Royal Free Hospital Medical School, and Consultant Haematologist, Royal Free Hospital, London.

Sylvia D. Lawler, MD(Lond), MRCP(Lond), FRCPath
Professor of Human Genetics, Institute of Cancer Research, and Consultant in Cytogenetics and Immunology to Royal Marsden Hospital, London.

Eleanor E. Lloyd, FIMLS
Principal Medical Laboratory Scientific Officer, Department of Haematology, Royal Postgraduate Medical School, London.

W. R. Pitney, MD(Melbourne), FRACP, FRCPA
Professor of Medicine in the University of New South Wales, and Consultant Physician, St. George's Hospital, Kogarah, NSW, Australia.

J. M. White, MD(Sheffield), MRCPath
Director of Pathology, Corniche Hospital, Abu Dhabi; formerly Professor of Haematology, University of London, King's College Hospital Medical School, and Consultant Haematologist, King's College Hospital, Denmark Hill, London.

Contents

1

Collection of blood and haematological values in health

COLLECTION OF BLOOD FROM PATIENTS

Venous blood is preferred for most haematological examinations, but peripheral samples can be almost as satisfactory for some purposes if a free flow of blood is obtained.

VENOUS BLOOD

This is best withdrawn from an antecubital vein by means of a dry glass or plastic syringe. The needles should not be too fine or too long; those of 19 or 20 SWG★ are suitable, and short needles with shafts about 15 mm long are particularly valuable for use with children. A method for collection of blood which obviates the need for a syringe is by means of an evacuated specimen tube and needle[†].

When a series of samples are required or when the blood sampling is to be followed by a transfusion, it is convenient to collect the blood by means of a length of plastic tubing attached to the patient's arm. If a large volume of blood is required, and a large syringe is not available, a needle of larger bore, e.g. 16 SWG★, provided with a short length of plastic tubing should be used; with this equipment 100 ml of blood or more can be easily withdrawn.

Except in the case of very young children it should be possible with practice to obtain venous blood even from patients with difficult veins. Successful venepuncture may be facilitated by keeping the subject's arm warm, applying to the upper arm a sphygmomanometer cuff kept at approxi-

mately diastolic pressure and smacking the skin over the site of the vein. In obese patients it may be easier to use a vein on the dorsum of the hand, which is warmed by immersion in warm water. When the hand is dried and the fist clenched, veins suitable for puncture will usually become apparent. If the veins are very small, a 23 SWG★ needle should be used and this should enable at least 2 ml of blood to be obtained satisfactorily. Vein punctures in the dorsum of the hand tend to bleed more readily than at other sites. The arm should be elevated after withdrawal of the needle and pressure should be applied for several minutes before an adhesive dressing is placed over the puncture site.

If possible, congestion should be completely avoided so as to prevent haemoconcentration. In practice, it is usually necessary to use a tourniquet. Ideally this should be loosened once the needle has been inserted into the vein. The piston of the syringe should be withdrawn slowly and no attempt made to withdraw blood faster than the vein is filling. After detaching the needle, the blood should be delivered carefully from the syringe into a container, and if it is desired to prevent coagulation it should be promptly and thoroughly but gently mixed with anticoagulant.

Patients with Australia antigen in their blood (HB$_s$Ag positive) are a potential source of infection. When blood is collected from such patients, special precautions must be taken to avoid contamination, e.g. by the wearing of rubber gloves, the prompt disposal of syringe, needle, dressings, etc. and decontamination of any spillage which may occur.

★ The nearest equivalent American gauges and diameters are as follows: 16 SWG = 14 (1.625 mm); 19 SWG = 18 (1.016 mm); 20 SWG = 19 (0.914 mm); 23 SWG = 22 (0.610 mm).

[†] e.g. 'Vacutainer' (Becton Dickinson Ltd.).

1

Other high risk patients, for whom similar precautions should be instituted, are those with Australia-antigen-negative hepatitis or a recent history suggestive of hepatitis. The same technique should be employed in the collection of blood from patients who for any reason have received blood or blood products from five or more donors or who are on renal dialysis or who have defective immunological competence. The above careful technique is all the more important if such patients are also receiving immunosuppressive drugs.

Ideally, blood films should be made immediately the blood has been withdrawn. It is convenient to deliver a small volume of blood on to a glass slide and to take from this blood without delay small sub-samples sufficient for a single film, using a short length of glass tubing into which the blood will run by capillarity. In practice, blood samples are often collected by the clinical staff and sent to the laboratory after a variable delay. Films should be made in the laboratory from such blood as soon as is practicable. Again, a glass capillary can be used to sample the blood and to deliver a drop of the right size on to a slide so that films can be made.

The differences between films made of fresh blood (no anticoagulant) and anticoagulated blood are dealt with on p. 4.

It is convenient to use as containers for blood samples disposable glass or plastic flat-bottomed tubes fitted with caps. Because of the possibility of infection of personnel when there is leakage of the blood from the container or when removal of the cap causes an aerosol discharge of the contents, it is essential to use containers designed to minimize the risks.[35] Design requirements for this and other specifications for both evacuated and non-evacuated containers have been described in a number of national and international standards, e.g. those of the *British Standards Institution* (BS 4851) and the *International Organization for Standardization* (ISO 4822) for non-evacuated containers; and of the US *National Committee for Clinical Laboratory Standards* (NCCLS–ASH 1) for evacuated tubes.

Except for coagulation studies, the choice between glass and plastic is a matter of personal preference; evacuated containers, however, are invariably made of glass as they must maintain an adequate vacuum during storage before use. The most common disposable containers available from commercial sources contain dipotassium or tripotassium or disodium EDTA as anticoagulant and are marked at the 2.5 or 5 ml level to indicate the correct amount of blood to be added (see p. 3).

Haemolysis can be avoided or minimized by using clean apparatus, withdrawing the blood slowly, not using too fine a needle, delivering the blood gently into the receiver and avoiding frothing during the withdrawal of the blood and subsequent mixing with the anticoagulant.

Serum

Blood collected in order to obtain serum should be delivered into sterile tubes or screw-capped bottles and allowed to clot undisturbed for 1–2 h at 37°C. When the blood has firmly clotted and the clot has started to retract, the sample may be left in a refrigerator overnight at 4°C, so that clot retraction may become complete under conditions unfavourable for the growth of bacteria. If the clot fails to retract, it may be gently detached from the wall of the container by means of a platinum wire or sealed Pasteur pipette. If it is roughly treated, lysis is certain to follow. However, exactly how serum should be obtained depends also on what it is required for. For instance, if complement is to be estimated, the serum should be separated and then frozen at −20°C or below with the minimum of delay.

When serum is required urgently or when both serum and cells are required, as in the investigation of certain types of haemolytic anaemia, the sample can be defibrinated. This is simply performed by placing the blood in a receiver such as a conical flask containing a central glass rod on to which small pieces of glass capillary have been fused (Fig. 1.1). The blood is whisked around the central rod by moderately rapid rotation of the flask. Coagulation is usually complete within 5 min, most of the fibrin collecting upon the central rod. When fibrin formation seems complete, the defibrinated blood may be centrifuged and serum obtained quickly and in relatively large volumes. Blood defibrinated in this way should not undergo any visible degree of lysis. The morphology of the red cells and the leucocytes is well preserved.

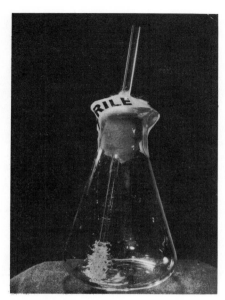

Fig. 1.1 Flask for defibrinating 10–50 ml of blood. The central glass rod has had some small pieces of drawn-out glass capillary fused to its lower end.

If cold agglutinins are to be titrated, the blood must be kept at 37°C until the serum has separated, and if cold agglutinins are known to be present in high concentration it is best to bring the patient to the laboratory and, using a needle connected to a length of plastic tubing, to collect blood into containers previously warmed to 37°C. When filled they should be promptly replaced in the 37°C water-bath. In this way it is possible to obtain serum free from haemolysis even when cold antibodies are present capable of causing agglutination at temperatures as high as 30°C. Alternatively, the blood may be collected in a warmed syringe. A practical way of achieving this is to place the syringe in its container for 10 min in an oven at approximately 50°C. When the clot has retracted and clear serum has been expressed, the serum is removed by a Pasteur pipette and transferred to a tube which has been warmed by being allowed to stand in a water-bath. It is then rapidly centrifuged so as to rid it of any suspended red cells.

ANTICOAGULANTS

For various purposes a number of different anticoagulants are available.

Ethylenediamine tetra-acetic acid (EDTA)

The sodium and potassium salts of EDTA are powerful anticoagulants and they are the anticoagulant of choice for routine haematological work. EDTA acts by its chelating effect on the calcium molecules in blood. To achieve this requires a concentration of 1.2 mg (approximately 4 μmol) of the anhydrous salt per ml of blood. The recommended concentration of the dipotassium salt is 1.50 ± 0.25 mg/ml of blood.

Excess of EDTA affects both red cells and leucocytes, causing shrinkage and degenerative changes. EDTA in excess of 2 mg/ml of blood may result in significant decrease in packed cell volume (PCV) and increase in mean cell haemoglobin concentration (MCHC).[31,46] The platelets are also affected; excess of EDTA causes them to swell and then disintegrate, causing an artificially high platelet count as the fragments are large enough to be counted as morphologically normal platelets. Care must therefore be taken to ensure that the correct amount of blood is added, and that by repeated inversions of the container the anticoagulant is thoroughly mixed in the blood added to it. The dipotassium salt is very soluble (1650 g/l) and is to be preferred on this account to the disodium salt which is considerably less soluble (108 g/l).[24] Rapid solution of the EDTA can be ensured by coating the container with a thin film of the salt.

The dilithium salt of EDTA is equally effective as an anticoagulant,[47] and its use has the advantage that the same sample of blood can be used for chemical investigation. However, it is less soluble than the dipotassium salt (160 g/l).

EDTA is not suitable for use in the investigation of coagulation problems and should not be used in the estimation of prothrombin time.

Trisodium citrate

0.109 mol/l trisodium citrate (32 g/l $Na_3C_6H_5O_7 . 2H_2O$)⋆ is the anticoagulant of choice in coagulation studies. Nine volumes of blood are added to 1 volume of the sodium citrate solution and immediately well mixed with it. Sodium citrate is also the anticoagulant most widely used in the

⋆ Formerly available as $2Na_3C_6H_5O_7 . 11H_2O$; the equivalent concentration of this salt is 38 g/l.

estimation of the sedimentation rate (ESR); for this 4 volumes of venous blood are diluted with 1 volume of the sodium citrate solution.

Heparin

This may be used at a concentration of 15 ± 2.5 iu per ml of blood. Heparin is an effective anticoagulant and does not alter the size of the red cells; it is a good dry anticoagulant when it is important to reduce to a minimum the chance of lysis occurring after blood has been withdrawn. However, heparinized blood should not be used for making blood films as it gives a faint blue colouration to the background when the films are stained by Romanowsky dyes. This is especially marked in the presence of abnormal proteins. Heparin is the best anticoagulant to use for osmotic fragility tests; otherwise it is inferior to EDTA for general use and should not be used for leucocyte counts as it tends to cause the leucocytes to clump.

EFFECTS OF ANTICOAGULANTS ON BLOOD-CELL MORPHOLOGY

If blood is allowed to stand in the laboratory before films are made, degenerative changes occur. The changes are not solely due to the presence of an anticoagulant for they also occur in defibrinated blood.

Irrespective of anticoagulant, films made from blood which has been standing for not more than 1 h at room temperature (18–25°C) are not easily distinguished from films made immediately after collection of the blood. By 3 h changes may be discernible and by 12–18 h these become striking. Some but not all neutrophils are affected: their nuclei may stain more homogeneously than in fresh blood, the nuclear lobes may become separated and the cytoplasmic margin may appear ragged or less well defined; small vacuoles appear in the cytoplasm (Fig. 1.2). Some or many of the large mononuclears develop marked changes; small vacuoles appear in the cytoplasm and the nucleus undergoes irregular lobulation which may almost amount to disintegration (Fig. 1.3). Some of the lymphocytes, too, undergo a similar types of change: a few vacuoles may be seen in the cytoplasm and the nucleus may undergo major budding

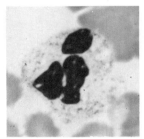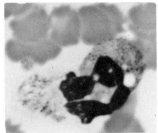

Fig. 1.2 Effect of storage on leucocyte morphology. Photomicrographs of polymorphonuclear neutrophils in a film made from EDTA-blood after 18 h at 20°C. ×1200.

so as to give rise to nuclei with two or three lobes (Fig. 1.4). Other lymphocyte nuclei may stain more homogeneously than usual.[45]

The red cells (of normal blood at least) are little affected by standing for up to 6 h at room temperature (18–25°C). Longer periods lead to progressive crenation and sphering (see Fig. 5.41, p. 74).

The cells in defibrinated blood undergo degenerative changes at about the same rate as those in EDTA blood.

All the above changes are retarded but not abolished in blood kept at 4°C. Their occurrence

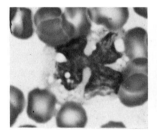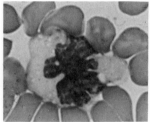

Fig. 1.3 Effect of storage on leucocyte morphology. Photomicrographs of monocytes in a film made from EDTA-blood after 18 h at 20°C. ×1200.

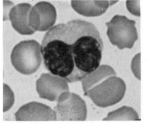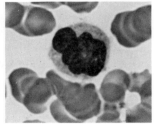

Fig. 1.4 Effect of storage on leucocyte morphology. Photomicrographs of lymphocytes in a film made from EDTA-blood after 18 h at 20°C. ×1200.

underlines the importance of making films as soon as possible after withdrawal. But delay of up to 1–3 h or so is certainly permissible.

The practice of making films of blood before it is added to the anticoagulant (e.g. at the bedside) is to be commended, especially when screening for lead toxicity, as the granules of punctate basophilia may not stain in anticoagulated blood. In fresh blood films, however, the platelets usually clump and it is less easy to estimate the platelet count from inspection of the film. Such films are nevertheless of particular value in investigating patients suspected of suffering from purpura, as in certain rare conditions, the absence of platelet clumping is a useful pointer to the diagnosis (see p. 82).

MODE OF ACTION OF ANTICOAGULANTS

EDTA and sodium citrate remove calcium which is essential for coagulation. Calcium is either precipitated as insoluble oxalate (crystals of which may be seen in oxalated blood) or bound in a non-ionized form. Heparin works in a different way; it neutralizes thrombin by inhibiting the interaction of several clotting factors in the presence of a plasma co-factor, antithrombin III. Sodium citrate or heparin can be used to render blood incoagulable before transfusion. For better long-term preservation of red cells for certain tests and for transfusion purposes citrate is used in combination with dextrose in the form of acid-citrate-dextrose (ACD), citrate-phosphate-dextrose (CPD) or Alsever's solution (see p. 432).

STORAGE OF BLOOD BEFORE QUANTITATIVE ESTIMATIONS ARE PERFORMED

Regardless of the anticoagulant, certain changes take place when blood is allowed to stand in vitro at room temperature (18–25°C), although they are less marked in blood in ACD, CPD or Alsever's solution than in EDTA blood. The red cells start to swell, with the result that the MCV increases, osmotic fragility and prothrombin time slowly increase and the sedimentation rate decreases; the leucocyte and platelet counts gradually fall.[5] There

is no significant change in MCV if the blood is kept overnight at 4°C.[5,32] Other changes, too, take place more slowly at this temperature, so that for many purposes blood may safely be allowed to stand overnight in the refrigerator if precautions against freezing are taken. Nevertheless, it is best to count leucocytes and especially platelets within 2 h. The reticulocyte count decreases as early as 6 h at 20°C and nucleated red cells disappear from the blood specimen within 1–2 days.[2] The advisability of making films at once has already been stressed.

Haemoglobin remains unchanged for days, provided that the blood does not become infected.

The importance of effectively mixing blood after collection, particularly if it has been stored and is cold and viscid, cannot be over-emphasized. If cold, the blood should first be allowed to warm up to room temperature, then mixed, preferably by rotation, for at least 2 min. The difficulty of mixing stored blood is a strong point in favour of performing blood counts without delay.

'CAPILLARY' (PERIPHERAL) BLOOD

Capillary blood is liable to give discrepant results, and should be used only when it is not possible to obtain venous blood. It can be obtained from an ear-lobe or finger of an adult or from the heel of an infant. A free flow of blood is essential, and only the very gentlest squeezing is permissible; ideally, large drops of blood should exude slowly but spontaneously. If it is necessary to squeeze firmly in order to obtain blood, the results are unreliable. If the poor flow is due to the part being cold and cyanosed, too high figures for red-cell count, Hb content and leucocyte count are usually obtained.

The discrepancies between peripheral and venous samples are more marked if the ear-lobe rather than the finger is chosen as the site for puncture.[7,36] However, if the ear is rubbed well with a square of lint until it is pink and warm, a good spontaneous flow of blood is obtained from most patients if sterile lancets are used as prickers. Under these circumstances the figures for red-cell count, Hb content and leucocyte count approximate closely to those of venous blood.

Ear-lobe puncture is carried out as follows. Rub the ear with lint until warm. Then prick it to a depth of 2–3 mm with a sterile steel lancet, thrusting the lancet into the ear-lobe by a single stabbing action. Wipe away the first few drops and collect the sample when the blood is flowing spontaneously, usually in about 30 s. A separate lancet must be used for each patient.

Heel blood

Satisfactory samples can be obtained in infants by a deep puncture using a steel lancet, but only if the heel is really warm—it may be necessary to bathe it in hot water.

COLLECTION OF CAPILLARY BLOOD FOR QUANTITATIVE STUDIES

The usual procedure is to use a micropipette to draw up the correct amount of blood (usually 20 μl). An alternative method is to use disposable capillary tubes cut to size so as to contain the exact volume of blood when completely filled. Fill the capillary tube by capillarity and then drop it into a tube containing the appropriate amount of diluent solution. A potential disadvantage is the presence of contaminating blood on the outside of the capillary where it has been in contact with the source. Such blood is difficult to wipe off without causing the loss of a portion of the blood contained within the capillary. However, by providing a length of tubing greater than that necessary for the required volume, and a break-off point at the correct length, it is possible to fill the capillary from the non-calibrated end, which is discarded.[34] This method avoids contaminating the diluent with the exterior portion of the capillary which has been in contact with the blood. In another system (Unopette) the calibrated capillary, which is completely filled, is attached by a special holder directly to a reservoir containing the premeasured volume of diluent*.[20]

As an alternative method the capillary can be connected to a rubber teat and its contents can then be discharged into the diluent by squeezing the teat†. These methods are particularly suitable for use by the bedside or in the 'field', as less technical skill is required to draw up the correct amount of blood than in the micropipette method.

DIFFERENCES BETWEEN 'CAPILLARY' AND VENOUS BLOOD

It is probable that the PCV, red-cell count and Hb content of venous blood and capillary blood are not quite the same, even if the latter is freely flowing.

It is likely that freely flowing blood obtained by skin puncture is more nearly arteriolar in composition than capillary. Indeed, the PCV, red-cell count and Hb content of true capillary blood are significantly less than those of venous blood.[22] This results in the venous PCV being significantly greater than the 'whole body' PCV, a difference which is of significance in the calculation of total blood volume from an estimation of plasma or red-cell volume (see p. 285).

The platelet count appears to be higher in venous than in capillary blood—this may be due to adhesion of platelets to the site of the skin puncture. Leucocyte counts are probably identical, but only if the peripheral blood is freely flowing—if the ear is cold, the capillary count may be much higher than the venous count.[36]

REFERENCE VALUES IN HAEMATOLOGY

There is no reliable method of defining 'normal values' or the 'normal range' for the results of laboratory tests; hence it is extremely difficult to state the limits of haematological values in health. A number of factors determine important differences. These include:

1. The sex, age, occupation, body build, genetic and ethnic background and geographical location, especially altitude.

2. The environmental and physiological conditions under which the specimens are obtained, including the subject's diet, his posture when the sample was taken, whether he has recently exercised and whether hospitalized.

3. The technique and timing of specimen collection, transport and storage.

4. Variation in the analytical methods used.

* Becton Dickinson Ltd.
† e.g. Drummond Microcaps or 'Volupettes', Scientific Supplies Co. Ltd.

Furthermore, it is difficult to be certain in any survey of a population for the purposes of obtaining data from which a reference range may be constructed that the 'normal' subjects are completely healthy and do not have mild chronic infections, parasitic infestations or nutritional deficiencies.

The borderline between health and ill-health is indefinite; so it is with haematological values, for the normal and abnormal undoubtedly overlap. For instance, a value well within the recognised normal range may be definitely pathological in a particular subject, e.g. a total leucocyte count of $10.0 \times 10^9/l$ is abnormal for a man whose count usually ranges between 4.0 and $6.0 \times 10^9/l$. For these reasons the concept of 'normal values' and 'normal range' is slowly being replaced by 'reference values' and 'reference limits' in which the variables are defined when establishing the values for the reference population in a particular test.[23,28] Thus, for each test several reference ranges may be necessary as a guide to the significance of an individual measurement. The ultimate goal is to have a data bank of reference values which take account of the physiological variables mentioned above, so that an individual's result can be expressed and interpreted relative to a comparable normal. Such data are at present available for only a limited number of haematological tests, mainly for red-cell indices.[30]

A reference range for a population can be established from measurements on a relatively small number of subjects if they are assumed to be representative of the population as a whole.[21,28,56] A frequency histogram is plotted (Fig. 1.5). Taking the modal value and the calculated SD as reference points, a Gaussian curve is superimposed. From this curve a mean reference value can be estimated and the ± 2 SD limits can be determined even if the original histogram included results from some subjects not belonging to the normal population. When there is a skew distribution of measurements, the range to -2 SD may extend below zero. To avoid this anomaly the data should be transformed to their logarithms, and the mean and SD then calculated; this is known as a 'log-normal' distribution.

The data given in Table 1.1 provide a rough guide to so-called normal values which are applicable to many but not all healthy individuals. The

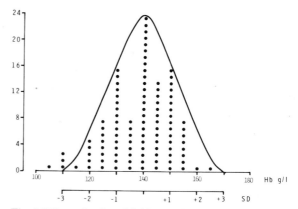

Fig. 1.5 Example of establishing a reference range. Data of haemoglobin measurements in a population, with Gaussian curve superimposed.

data have been derived from various sources, including observations from the authors' own laboratory and personal communications. The range of ± 2 SD from the mean indicates the limits which should cover 95% of normal subjects; 99% of normal subjects will be included in a range of ± 3 SD.

A 'normal range' has been given without SD, when the distribution of data is too skew to provide a Gaussian curve or when the data are too scanty for analysis.

PHYSIOLOGICAL VARIATION

Physiological variation in Hb content, PCV and red-cell counts

It is well known that there is considerable variation in the red-cell count and Hb content at different periods of life. At birth the Hb is higher than at any period subsequently (Table 1.1). The red-cell count is high immediately after birth,[8,14,37] and values for Hb greater than 200 g/l and red-cell count higher than $6.0 \times 10^{12}/l$ are encountered frequently when the cord is tied late after delivery. Probably it is the cessation of pulsation of the cord as well as the uterine contractions which permit the blood contained in the placenta to re-enter the infant's circulation. After the immediate post-natal period the Hb falls fairly steeply to a minimum of about 100 g/l or even less at about the 2nd or 3rd month.[8,14,37] The red-cell count and PCV also fall,

Table 1.1 Normal haematological values expressed as mean ± 2 SD (95% range)

Red-cell count
Men	$5.5 \pm 1.0 \times 10^{12}/l$
Women	$4.8 \pm 1.0 \times 10^{12}/l$
Infants (full-term, cord blood)	$5.0 \pm 1.0 \times 10^{12}/l$
Children, 3 months	$4.0 \pm 0.8 \times 10^{12}/l$
Children, 1 yr	$4.4 \pm 0.8 \times 10^{12}/l$
Children, 3–6 yr	$4.8 \pm 0.7 \times 10^{12}/l$
Children, 10–12 yr	$4.7 \pm 0.7 \times 10^{12}/l$

Haemoglobin
Men	155 ± 25 g/l*
Women	140 ± 25 g/l
Infants (full-term, cord blood)	165 ± 30 g/l
Children, 3 months	115 ± 20 g/l
Children, 1 yr	120 ± 15 g/l
Children, 3–6 yr	130 ± 10 g/l
Children, 10–12 yr	130 ± 15 g/l

Packed cell volume (PCV; haematocrit value)
Men	0.47 ± 0.07 (1/l)
Women	0.42 ± 0.05 (1/l)
Infants (full-term, cord blood)	0.54 ± 0.10 (1/l)
Children, 3 months	0.38 ± 0.06 (1/l)
Children, 3–6 yr	0.40 ± 0.04 (1/l)
Children 10–12 yr	0.41 ± 0.04 (1/l)

Mean cell volume (MCV)
Adults	86 ± 10 fl
Infants (full-term, cord blood)	106 fl (mean)
Children, 3 months	95 fl (mean)
Children, 1 yr	78 ± 8 fl
Children, 3–6 yr	81 ± 8 fl
Children, 10–12 yr	84 ± 7 fl

Mean cell haemoglobin (MCH)
Adults	29.5 ± 2.5 pg
Children, 3 months	29 ± 5 pg
Children, 1 yr	27 ± 4 pg
Children, 3–6 yr	27 ± 3 pg
Children, 10–12 yr	27 ± 3 pg

Mean cell haemoglobin concentration (MCHC)
Adults and children	325 ± 25 g/l

Red-cell diameter (mean values)
Adults (dry films)	6.7–7.7 μm

Red-cell density
1092–1100 g/l

Reticulocytes
Adults and children	0.2–2.0% (c 25–85 $\times 10^9/l$)
Infants (full-term, cord blood)	2–6% (mean 150 $\times 10^9/l$)

Blood volume
Red-cell volume, men	30 ± 5 ml/kg
women	25 ± 5 ml/kg
Plasma volume	45 ± 5 ml/kg
Total blood volume	70 ± 10 ml/kg

* Throughout the book Hb is expressed in g/l, i.e. g/dl $\times$ 10; see p 29.

Table 1.1 (*Contd.*)

Red-cell life-span 120 ± 30 days

Leucocyte count

Adults	$7.5 \pm 3.5 \times 10^9/l$
Infants (full-term, 1st day)	$18 \quad \pm 8 \quad \times 10^9/l$
Infants, 1 yr	$12 \quad \pm 6 \quad \times 10^9/l$
Children 4–7 yr	$10 \quad \pm 5 \quad \times 10^9/l$
Children, 8–12 yr	$9 \quad \pm 4.5 \times 10^9/l$

Differential leucocyte count

Adults: Neutrophils	$2.0 -7.5 \times 10^9/l$ (40–75%)
Lymphocytes	$1.5 -4.0 \times 10^9/l$ (20–45%)
Monocytes	$0.2 -0.8 \times 10^9/l$ (2–10%)
Eosinophils	$0.04-0.4 \times 10^9/l$ (1–6%)
Basophils	$<0.01-0.1 \times 10^9/l$ (<1%)
Infants (1st day):	
Neutrophils	$5.0 -13.0 \times 10^9/l$
Lymphocytes	$3.5 - 8.5 \times 10^9/l$
Monocytes	$0.5 - 1.5 \times 10^9/l$
Eosinophils	$0.1 - 2.5 \times 10^9/l$
Basophils	$<0.01- 0.1 \times 10^9/l$
Infants (3 days):	
Neutrophils	$1.5 -7.0 \times 10^9/l$
Lymphocytes	$2.0 -5.0 \times 10^9/l$
Monocytes	$0.3 -1.1 \times 10^9/l$
Eosinophils	$0.2 -2.0 \times 10^9/l$
Basophils	$<0.01-0.1 \times 10^9/l$
Children (6 yr):	
Neutrophils	$2.0 -6.0 \times 10^9/l$
Lymphocytes	$5.5 -8.5 \times 10^9/l$
Monocytes	$0.7 -1.5 \times 10^9/l$
Eosinophils	$0.3 -0.8 \times 10^9/l$
Basophils	$<0.01-0.1 \times 10^9/l$

Platelet count	$150–400 \times 10^9/l$
Bleeding time (Ivy's method)	2–7 min
(Template method)	2.5–9.5 min
Coagulation time (Lee and White's method, 37°C)	5–11 min
Prothrombin time (brain-thromboplastin time, 1-stage (Quick)	10–14 s
Partial thromboplastin time (PTTK)	35–43 s
Prothrombin-consumption index	0–30%
Plasma fibrinogen	2.0–4.0 g/l

Osmotic fragility (at 20°C and pH 7.4)

NaCl (g/l)	Before incubation % lysis	After incubation for 24 h at 37°C % lysis
2.0	100	95–100
3.0	97–100	85–100
3.5	90–99	75–100
4.0	50–95	65–100
4.5	5–45	55–95
5.0	0–6	40–85
5.5	0	15–70
6.0	0	0–40
6.5	0	0–10
7.0	0	0–5
7.5	0	0
8.0	0	0
8.5	0	0

Median corpuscular fragility (MCF) (g/l NaCl)

4.0–4.45	4.65–5.9

Table 1.1 (*Contd.*)

Autohaemolysis (*37°C*)	
48 h, without added glucose	0.2–4.0%
48 h, with added glucose	0–0.5%
Cold-agglutinin titre (*4°C*)	<64
Serum iron	13–32 μmol/l
	(0.7–1.8 mg/l)
Total iron-binding capacity	45–70 μmol/l
	(2.5–4.0 mg/l)
Transferrin	1.2–2.0 g/l
Serum vitamin B$_{12}$ (*as cyanocobalamin*)	160–925 ng/l
Serum folate	3–20 μg/l
Red-cell folate	160–640 μg/l
Plasma haemoglobin	10–40 mg/l
Serum haptoglobin (*Hb-binding*)	0.3–2.0 g/l
Sedimentation rate (*Westergren, 1 h*) (*at 20 ± 3°C*)	
Men 17–50 yr	1–7 mm
> 50 yr	2–10 mm
Women 17–50 yr	3–9 mm
> 50 yr	5–15 mm
Plasma viscosity (*at 25°C*)	1.61 ± 0.05 cP
Heterophile (*anti-sheep red-cell*) *agglutinin titre*	<80
After absorption with guinea-pig kidney	<10

though less steeply and the cells become hypochromic with the development of 'physiological' iron-deficiency anaemia.

The Hb remains at about the same level up to the age of 3 yr. The mean MCHC is 300 g/l with a SD of 27 g/l on the 2nd day of life; it does not alter significantly during the first 3 yr but the SD diminishes. The mean MCV is 122 fl at 2 days, 101 at 2 months, and within the adult range by 3 yr.

The Hb content and red-cell count normally rise gradually to almost adult levels by the time of puberty; thereafter the levels in women tend to be significantly lower than those of men.[26,30] Factors influencing the difference between men and women include the hormonal influence on haemopoiesis and menstrual blood loss; the extent to which the latter is a significant factor is not clear, as a loss of up to 100 ml of blood with each period does not appear to cause a fall in Hb although it results in lower levels of serum iron.[13,25] Moreover, arrest of menstruation by oral contraceptives causes an increase in serum iron without affecting the haemoglobin level.[9]

In old age the Hb is reported to fall; in one study this was found to be, in men, to a mean level of 134 g/l at 65, 129 g/l at 75 and 122 g/l at over the age of 85.[51] Lesser differences have been recorded by others.[26,30] By contrast, in older women the level tends to rise, so that a sex difference of 20 g/l

in younger age groups is reduced to 10 g/l or less in old age.[13,42] The MCHC remains remarkably constant at all ages, in both men and women.

In addition to the permanent effects of age and sex, there seem to be transient fluctuations, the significance of which is often difficult to assess. Muscular activity, if at all strenuous, unquestionably raises the red-cell count and Hb, presumably largely due to the re-entry into the circulation of cells previously sequestered in shut-down capillaries or to the loss of circulating plasma; increases in red cells amounting to 0.5×10^{12}/l and in Hb of 15 g/l may be observed. Posture, too, appears to cause transient alterations in the Hb and PCV. There is a small but significant increase as the posture changes from lying to sitting,[19] and conversely change from the upright to the recumbent position results in up to a 5% fall in Hb content; this occurs within 20 min, after which time, the Hb is stabilized at the lower level.[16,38] Consistently similar findings have also been reported by Eisenberg in a study of 25 subjects.[15] He also showed that the position of the arm during venous sampling affected the magnitude of the increase in PCV; it was 2–4% lower when the arm was held at the atrial level instead of being dependent.

It is not clear whether emotion or light exercise raises the red-cell count or Hb significantly above the base line observed with the subject at rest; the effects may be small enough to be submerged in the technical errors of estimation.[52] Athletes tend to have slightly lower Hb levels than non-athletes, with significantly higher total red-cell volume which is partly obscured by a concomitant increase in plasma volume.[6] Diurnal variation is usually slight[17] but fluctuations as much as 15% have been reported;[53] in most cases the Hb was highest in the morning and lowest in the evening, the mean difference being about 8%.

It has been suggested that seasonal variations also occur, but the evidence for this is conflicting.[44,48]

The effect of altitude is to raise the Hb and increase the number of circulating red cells; the magnitude of the polycythaemia depends on the degree of anoxaemia.[27] At an altitude of 2 km (c 6500 ft) the Hb is c 10 g/l higher than at sea level; at 3 km (c 10 000 ft) it is c 20 g/l higher. Corresponding increases occur at intermediate altitudes. These increases appear to be due both to increased erythropoiesis as a result of the anoxic stimulus and to the decrease in plasma volume which occurs at high altitudes.[33,43] Erythropoiesis is affected by cigarette smoking, probably in consequence of the accumulation of carboxyhaemoglobin in the blood, as slightly higher Hb values and PCV are found in smokers.[26,29] There may even be frank polycythaemia.[50]

Physiological variations in the total leucocyte count[3,26,52]

The effect of age is indicated in Table 1.1; at birth the neutrophil polymorphonuclears predominate, reaching a peak of c 13.0 × 10^9/l at 12 h and then falling to c 4.0 × 10^9/l over the next 2–3 days, at which level the count remains steady. The lymphocytes, which are about 5.5 × 10^9/l at birth, fall during the first 3 days of life to a low level of c 3.0 × 10^9/l and then rise up to the 10th day;[58] after this time they are the predominant cell (up to about 60%) until the 5th–7th yr when they give way to the neutrophils. There are slight sex differences in the neutrophil count, which is about 0.6 × 10^9/l higher in women than men.[3] Sex differences are insignificant in the total leucocyte count until after the age of 50 yr when the count becomes less in women than in men.[1,12]

People differ considerably in their leucocyte counts. Some tend to maintain a relatively constant level over long periods of time;[4] others have counts which may vary by as much as 100% at different times. In some subjects there appears to be a rhythm, occurring in cycles of 14–23 days, and in women this may be related to some extent to the menstrual cycle.[39,41] Some forms of oral contraception have been reported to raise the leucocyte count.[18] There is also diurnal variation which differs on an hour-to-hour basis as well as from day to day;[52] it affects the total leucocyte count as well as all the individual cell types. The minimum count is found in the morning with the subject at rest; the maximum in the afternoon. Random activity may raise the count slightly; strenuous exercise causes rises of up to 30 × 10^9/l, chiefly due, it is thought, to liberation into the blood stream of neutrophils formerly sequestered in shut-down capillaries. Large numbers of lymphocytes from lymphatic channels also probably enter the blood stream during strenuous exercise.

Adrenaline injection causes an increase in the leucocyte count; here, too, increases in the numbers of all major types of leucocytes (and platelets) occur.[10] The rise has been thought to be a reflection of the extent of the reservoir of mature blood cells present not only in the bone marrow and spleen but also in other tissues and organs of the body. Emotion may possibly cause an increase in the leucocyte count in a similar way. The effect of ingestion of food is uncertain. Cigarette smoking causes a significant increase in the leucocyte count.[11,26,55] A moderate leucocytosis of up to 15 × 10^9/l is common during pregnancy, with the peak about 8 weeks before parturition. The count returns to normal levels a week or so after delivery.[12] The rise in leucocytes is due to neutrophilia; the lymphocyte count falls in the first trimester and then remains steady throughout pregnancy.

Diurnal variation of the eosinophil count is especially marked.[52] The height of the count is controlled at least in part by the adrenal cortex, increased adrenocortical activity leading to a fall in the number of circulating eosinophils; diurnal fluctuations parallel diurnal glucocorticoid fluctuation.

It is clear that the environment may influence the leucocyte count. Thus in tropical Africa there is a tendency for a reversal of the neutrophil: lymphocyte ratio, with low total leucocyte counts.[49,57] This may be due to endemic parasitic and protozoal disease, and in some areas reactive eosinophilia or monocytosis is sufficiently common to be regarded as 'normal', or at least as a reference value.

Physiological variation in the platelet count

There may be a sex difference; thus, in women the count has been reported to be about 20% higher than in men.[54] A fall in the platelet count may occur in women at about the time of menstruation and there is some evidence of a cycle with a 21–35 day rhythm.[40] There is no evidence that oral contraceptives affect the platelet count. There is a diurnal variation which is more marked on a day-to-day basis than during the course of a day.[52] Within the wide normal range there are no obvious age differences; at birth and in the first few weeks of infancy, however, the platelet count tends to be at the lower level of the adult normal range, rising to adult values at about 6 months.

Refinement of present day blood counting systems has produced remarkably increased precision, so that even small differences in successive measurements may be significant. It is thus most important to establish and understand the limits of physiological variation etc. for the various tests. With this proviso, present day blood count data can now provide sensitive indications of minor abnormalities which may be important in clinical interpretation and health screening.

REFERENCES

[1] ALLAN, R. S. and ALEXANDER, M. K. (1968). A sex difference in the leucocyte count. *Journal of Clinical Pathology*, **21**, 691.

[2] BAER, D. M. and KRAUSE, R. B. (1968). Spurious laboratory values resulting from simulated mailing conditions. *American Journal of Clinical Pathology*, **50**, 111.

[3] BAIN, B. J. and ENGLAND, J. M. (1975).Normal haematological values: sex differences in neutrophil count. *British Medical Journal*, **i**, 306.

[4] BOOTH, K. and HANCOCK, R. E. T. (1961). A study of the total and differential leucocyte counts and haemoglobin levels in a group of normal adults over a period of two years. *British Journal of Haematology*, **7**, 9.

[5] BRITTIN, G. M., BRECHER, G., JOHNSON, C. A. and ELASHOFF, R. M. (1969). Stability of blood in commonly used anticoagulants. *American Journal of Clinical Pathology*, **52**, 690.

[6] BROTHERHOOD, J., BROZOVIC, B. and PUGH, L. G. C. (1975). Haematological status of middle and long distance runners. *Clinical Science and Molecular Medicine*, **48**, 139.

[7] BRÜCKMANN, G. (1942). Blood from the ear lobe: preliminary report. *Journal of Laboratory and Clinical Medicine*, **27**, 487.

[8] BURMAN, D. (1972). Haemoglobin levels in normal infants aged 3 to 24 months and the effect of iron. *Archives of Diseases in Childhood*, **47**, 261.

[9] BURTON, J. L. (1967). Effect of oral contraceptives on haemoglobin, packed cell volume, serum-iron and total iron-binding capacity in healthy women. *Lancet*, **i**, 978.

[10] CHATTERJEA, J. B., DAMESHEK, W. and STEFANINI, M. (1953). The adrenalin (epinephrin) test as applied to hematologic disorders. *Blood*, **8**, 211.

[11] CORRE, F., LELLOUCH, J. and SCHWARTZ, D. (1971). Smoking and leucocyte counts: results of an epidemiological survey. *Lancet*, **ii**, 632.

[12] CRUICKSHANK, J. M. (1970). The effects of parity on the leucocyte count in pregnant and non-pregnant women. *British Journal of Haematology*, **18**, 531.

[13] CRUICKSHANK, J. M. and ALEXANDER, M. K. (1970). The effect of age, parity, haemoglobin level and oral contraceptive preparations on the normal leucocyte count. *British Journal of Haematology*, **18**, 541.

[14] DeMARSH, Q. B., ALT, H. L., WINDLE, W. F. and HILLIS, D. S. (1941). The effect of depriving the infant of its placental blood. *Journal of American Medical Association*, **116**, 2568.

[15] EISENBERG, S. (1963). The effect of posture and position of the venous sampling site on the hematocrit and serum protein concentration. *Journal of Laboratory and Clinical Medicine*, **51**, 755.

[16] EKELUND, L. G., EKLUND, B. and KAIJSER, L. (1971). Time course for the change in hemoglobin concentration with change in posture. *Acta Medica Scandinavica*, **190**, 335.

[17] ELWOOD, P. C. (1962). Diurnal haemoglobin variation in normal male subjects. *Clinical Science*, **23**, 379.

[18] ENGLAND, J. M. and BAIN, B. J. (1976). Total and differential leucocyte count. *British Journal of Haematology*, **33**, 1.

[19] FELDING, P., TRYDING, N., HYLTOFT PETERSEN, P. and HØRDER, M. (1980). Effects of posture on concentration of blood constituents in healthy adults: practical application of blood specimen collection procedures recommended by the Scandinavian Committee on Reference Values. *Scandinavian Journal of Clinical Laboratory Investigation*, **40**, 615.

[20] FREUNDLICH, M. H. and GERARDE, H. W. (1963). A new, automatic, disposable system for blood counts and hemoglobin. *Blood*, **21**, 648.

[21] GARBY, L. (1970). The normal haemoglobin level (Annotation). *British Journal of Haematology*, **19**, 429.

[22] GIBSON, J. G. 2nd, SELIGMAN, A. M., PEACOCK, W. C., AUB, J. C., FINE, J. and EVANS, R. D. (1964). The distribution of red cells and plasma in large and minute vessels of the normal dog, determined by radioactive isotopes of iron and iodine. *Journal of Clinical Investigation*, **25**, 848.

[23] GRÄSBECK, R. and SARIS, N. E. (1969). Establishment and use of normal values. *Scandinavian Journal of Clinical and Laboratory Investigation*, **24** Suppl., 110.

[24] HADLEY, G. G and WEISS, S. P. (1955). Further notes on use of salts of ethylenediamine tetraacetic acid (EDTA) as anticoagulants. *American Journal of Clinical Pathology*, **25**, 1090.

[25] HALLBERG, L., HÖGDAHL, A-M, NILSSON, L. and RYBO, G. (1966). Menstrual blood loss and iron deficiency. *Acta Medica Scandinavica*, **180**, 639.

[26] HELMAN, N. and RUBENSTEIN, L. S. (1975). The effects of age, sex and smoking on erythrocytes and leukocytes. *American Journal of Clinical Pathology*, **63**, 35.

[27] HURTADO, A., MERINO, C. and DELGADO, E. (1945).

Influence of anoxemia on the hemopoietic activity. *Archives of Internal Medicine*, **75**, 284.

[28] International committee for standardization in haematology. (1981). The theory of reference values. *Clinical and Laboratory Haematology*, **3**, 369.

[29] ISAGER, H. and HAGERUP, L. (1971). Relationship between cigarette smoking and high packed cell volume and haemoglobin levels. *Scandinavian Journal of Haematology*, **8**, 241.

[30] KELLY, A. and MUNAN, L. (1977). Haematologic profile of natural populations: red cell parameters. *British Journal of Haematology*, **35**, 153.

[31] LAMPASSO, J. A. (1965). Error in hematocrit value produced by excessive ethylenediaminetetraacetate. *American Journal of Clinical Pathology*, **44**, 109.

[32] LAWRENCE, A. C. K., BEVINGTON, J. M. and YOUNG, M. (1975). Storage of blood and the mean corpuscular volume. *Journal of Clinical Pathology*, **28**, 345.

[33] LEVIN, N. W., METZ. J., HART, D., VAN HEERDEN D. R., BOARDMAN, R. G. and FARBER, S. A. (1960). The blood volume of healthy adult males resident in Johannesburg (altitude 5740 feet). *South African Journal of Medical Sciences*, **28**, 132.

[34] LEWIS, S. M. and BENJAMIN, H. (1965). Break-off capillary tube method for blood counts. *Journal of Clinical Pathology*, **18**, 689.

[35] LEWIS, S. M. and WARDLE, J. M. (1978). An analysis of blood specimen container leakage. *Journal of Clinical Pathology*, **31**, 888.

[36] LUCEY, H. C. (1950). Fortuitous factors affecting the leucocyte count in blood from the ear. *Journal of Clinical Pathology*, **3**, 146.

[37] MATOTH, Y., ZAIZON, R. and VARSANO, I. (1971). Post-natal changes in some red cell parameters. *Acta Paediatrica Scandinavica*, **60**, 317.

[38] MOLLISON, P. L. (1979). *Blood Transfusion in Clinical Medicine*, 5th edn., p. 128. Blackwell Scientific Publications, Oxford.

[39] MORLEY, A. A. (1966). A neutrophil cycle in healthy individuals. *Lancet*, **ii**, 1220.

[40] MORLEY, A. (1969). A platelet cycle in normal individuals. *Australasian Annals of Medicine*, **18**, 127.

[41] MORLEY, A. (1973). Correspondence. *Blood*, **41**, 329.

[42] MYERS, A. M., SAUNDERS, C. R. G and CHALMERS, D. G. (1968). The haemoglobin level of fit elderly people. *Lancet*, **ii**, 261.

[43] MYHRE, L. D., DILL, D. B., HALL, F. G. and BROWN, D. K. (1970). Blood volume changes during three-week residence at high altitude. *Clinical Chemistry*, **16**, 7.

[44] NATVIG, H., BJERKEDAL, T. and JONASSEN, O. (1963). Studies on hemoglobin values in Norway. III. Seasonal variations. *Acta Medica Scandinavica*, **174**, 351.

[45] NORBERG, B. and SÖDERSTRÖM, N. (1967). 'Radial segmentation' of the nuclei in lymphocytes and other blood cells induced by some anticoagulants. *Scandinavian Journal of Haematology*, **4**, 68.

[46] PENNOCK, C. A. and JONES, K. W. (1966). Effect of ethylene-diamine-tetraacetic acid (dipotassium salt) and heparin on the estimation of packed cell volume. *Journal of Clinical Pathology*, **19**, 196.

[47] SACKER, L. S., SAUNDERS, K. E., PAGE, B. and GOODFELLOW, M. (1959). Dilithium sequestrene as an anticoagulant. *Journal of Clinical Pathology*, **12**, 254.

[48] SAUNDERS, C. (1965). Some erythrocyte parameters on a cross section of U.K.A.E.A. employees. *Laboratory Practice*, **14**, 1390.

[49] SHAPER, A. G. and LEWIS, P. (1971). Genetic neutropenia in people of African origin. *Lancet*, **ii**, 1021.

[50] SMITH, J. R. and LANDOW, S. A. (1978). Smokers' polycythaemia. *New England Journal of Medicine*, **298**, 6.

[51] SMITH, J. S. and WHITELAW, D. M. (1971). Hemoglobin values in aged men. *Canadian Medical Association Journal*, **105**, 816.

[52] STATLAND, B. E., WINKEL, P., HARRIS, S. C., BURDSALL, M. J. and SAUNDERS, A. M. (1978). Evaluation of biologic sources of variation of leukocyte counts and other hematologic quantities using very precise automated analyzers. *American Journal of Clinical Pathology*, **69**, 48.

[53] STENGLE, J. M. and SCHADE, A. L. (1957). Diurnal-nocturnal variations of certain blood constituents in normal human subjects: plasma iron, siderophilin, bilirubin, copper, total serum protein and albumin, haemoglobin and haematocrit. *British Journal of Haematology*, **3**, 117.

[54] STEVENS, R. F. and ALEXANDER, M. K. (1977). A sex difference in the platelet count. *British Journal of Haematology*, **37**, 295.

[55] TIBBLIN, E., BENGTSSON, C., HALLBERG, L. and LENNARTSSON, J. (1979). Haemoglobin concentration and peripheral blood cell counts in women. The population study of women in Göteborg, 1968–1969. *Scandinavian Journal of Haematology*, **22**, 5.

[56] VITERI, F. E., DE TUNA, V. and GUZMAN, M. A. (1972). Normal haematological values in the Central American population. *British Journal of Haematology*, **23**, 189.

[57] WOODLIFF, H. J., KATAAHA, P. K., TIBALEKA, A. K. and NZARO, E. (1972). Total leucocyte count in Africans. *Lancet*, **ii**, 875.

[58] XANTHOU, M. (1970). Leucocyte blood picture in healthy full-term and premature babies during neonatal period. *Archives of Disease in Childhood*, **45**, 242.

2

Quality assurance

Quality assurance in the haematology laboratory is intended to ensure the reliability of the laboratory tests. The laboratory director should, however, in this context, take account not only of test results but also of the general organization within the laboratory, including proficiency in the collection, labelling, delivery and storage of specimens before the tests are performed, efficiency of recording and reporting of results, and the protection of laboratory staff against health risks and hazards when handling specimens and equipment.

A quality assurance programme has two separate aspects, namely, internal quality control and external quality assessment. Internal quality control is based on monitoring various aspects of the haematology test procedures which are performed in the laboratory. In includes measurements on specially prepared materials, and repeated measurements on routine specimens, as well as statistical analysis, day by day, of data obtained from the tests which have been routinely carried out. External quality assessment is the objective evaluation by an outside agency of performance by a number of laboratories on material which is supplied specially for the purpose; this is usually organized on a national or regional basis. The objective of a quality assurance programme is to achieve precision and accuracy.

Accuracy refers to the closeness of the estimated value to that considered to be true. Precision refers to the reproducibility of a result, accurate or inaccurate. Inaccuracy and/or imprecision occur as a result of improper standards or reagents, incorrect instrument calibration, or poor technique, e.g. consistently faulty dilution or the use of a method giving a reaction that is incomplete or not specific for the test. Precision can be controlled by replicate tests, check tests on previously measured speci-

mens and statistical evaluation of results. Accuracy can, as a rule, be checked only by the use of reference materials which have been assayed by independent methods of known precision. In general, reference materials are either assayed samples which can be measured alongside each batch of routine specimens without being identifiable during the test or standard preparations handled in a special way. It is important to distinguish between reference standards that are used for instrument calibration and fresh or preserved blood used for quality control. In some cases the same material may serve both functions, but it is important that their different purposes are appreciated.

REFERENCE MATERIAL

Haemoglobin

The availability of an international reference preparation[8] has contributed to improved accuracy of Hb measurement. In several countries working standards are prepared which conform to the international reference preparation and the appropriate national authority certifies that this is so.

For quality assurance, blood of attested Hb content is valuable. Because such blood can be kept only for a short time, it cannot be used as an alternative to a HiCN standard. Both whole blood and lysates are of use, as differences in results obtained with these preparations help to distinguish errors due to incorrect dilution from those due to inadequate mixing or failure of a reagent to bring about complete lysis. Whole-blood reference samples should be introduced into a batch of blood samples and all the samples assayed together.

Blood-cell standards

Reference preparations for the blood count are essential for the calibration of electronic particle counters, especially automated systems which can be adjusted arbitrarily. This means that to obtain a true result the machine has to be calibrated using a reference preparation with assigned values of known accuracy.

Natural blood, collected into EDTA, because of its short life in the laboratory, is of no value as a reference preparation. Blood will keep for a few weeks at 4°C if acid citrate dextrose (ACD) or citrate phosphate dextrose (CPD) has been added to it. Even so, there is a slow increase in the MCV and some of the red cells are slowly lost, with the result that the blood cannot be regarded as a reference material, although it can be used as a control to check the precision and reliable functioning of a cell counting system over relatively short periods of time.[12]

Attempts have been made to provide suitably sized particles in stable suspension as substitutes for normal blood cells, e.g. by the use of pollens, yeasts, polystyrene latex, tanned red cells and glutaraldehyde-fixed red cells.[14] Blood cells can be permanently stabilized by fixation, especially in glutaraldehyde solution. The fixed red cells shrink in size immediately and the shrinking process continues for 3–4 days. Thereafter, the cells remain constant in size and shape, and the results of cell counts and cell size distribution remain consistently the same for months or even years. Unfortunately, there are major disadvantages in using these cells as a red-cell reference preparation: in most counting systems, natural (fresh) red blood cells become spherical when diluted, whereas the fixed red cells remain biconcave discs, are inflexible and have different flow properties so that they cannot be used to calibrate an instrument for subsequent measurement of natural blood.[18] Moreover, blood cells whether fixed or unfixed, are unsuitable for calibrating instruments for cell sizing, as their size distribution is usually too wide for this purpose. Latex spheres have recently become available in a series of defined sizes between 2 and 12 μm in diameter, and some of these may prove suitable for use as primary reference materials for sizing red cells.[13]

Platelets

Glutaraldehyde-fixed platelets provide a useful reference preparation for platelet counting, as the shape of natural platelets is less affected in the diluent. Latex spheres of 2 μm diameter are useful as primary reference material for platelet sizing.[13]

Leucocytes

Three types of material are suitable as reference materials:

1. Leucocytes concentrated from human blood and fixed in a solution of glacial acetic acid 42 mg, sodium sulphate 7 g, sodium chloride 7 g, water to 1 l.[19]

2. Glutaraldehyde-fixed turkey or chicken erythrocytes resuspended in leucocyte-free mammalian whole blood.[12]

3. Latex particles 5–6 μm in diameter.[13]

Reference preparations are available for a number of other tests, and these will be referred to in the sections where these tests are described.

International reference preparations are, as a rule, biological materials with assigned values of activity which are available from the World Health Organization; in addition to Hb, they include erythropoietin, blood group sera, thromboplastin and several other coagulation factors.[23] These materials are not freely available for routine use but are intended to act as standards for assigning values to commercial (or laboratory produced) 'secondary standards' or calibrators.

In some countries national standards are available, while in Europe the Bureau of Reference (BCR)* of the EEC is establishing a number of reference materials.

QUALITY CONTROL MATERIAL

The best material for internal quality control procedures for blood counts is human, horse or donkey blood collected into ACD or CPD (see p. 432) and passed through a blood-infusion set to remove any clots. For different purposes it is necessary to use preserved blood, stabilized erythrocytes, or lysate. One unit of blood (500 ml) will be sufficient to provide about 75 ml of lysate or 200 ml of

* Bureau Communautaire de Référence

resuspended stabilized cells. For platelets a special collection procedure is required.

When human blood is used, it must first be checked to ensure that it is hepatitis-B (HBs)-antigen negative.

Preparation of preserved blood[22]

Collect a unit of blood into a blood transfusion donor bag containing ACD or CPD. Run the blood through a transfusion giving set into a sterile 2 l round-bottomed flask. The contents of the flask must be mixed continuously* throughout the subsequent steps and every effort must be made to minimize contamination by careful technique.

Adjust the RBC and WBC levels, as required:

1. To increase the red-cell count, sediment cells over exit vents of pack and run into the flask with a minimum of plasma.

2. To lower the red-cell count, add compatible plasma or a solution containing 1.5 volumes of ACD and 10 volumes of 9 g/l NaCl.

3. To raise the white-cell count, add fixed avian cells (p. 17).

4. To lower the white-cell count, pass blood through a leucocyte filter.†

Add one vial of penicillin-streptomycin (e.g. 'Crystamycin', Glaxo) per 500 ml total volume. Dispense into sterile containers and cap tightly. Store at 4°C. Assign values for Hb, RBC, WBC and PCV by 10 replicate measurements using the system on which the material will be used. The CV should not exceed 2%. Check dispensing by repeated counts on five randomly selected tubes. Before analysis, mix a sample on a roller mixer or continuously by hand for 5 min before opening. Unopened vials of human blood should keep in good condition for about 3 weeks at 4°C, equine blood for up to 3 months.[12]

Preparation of lysate

Collect blood as described above into a blood transfusion donor bag. Centrifuge at c 2000 g

for 20 min and remove the plasma aseptically. Add an equal volume of 9 g/l NaCl (saline), mix well, transfer to a sterile centrifuge bottle and re-centrifuge; discard the supernatant and the buffy coat. Repeat the saline wash three times to ensure complete removal of the plasma, white cells and platelets. Add to the washed cells half their volume of toluene, cap and then shake vigorously on a mechanical shaker or vibrator for 1 h: refrigerate overnight to allow the lipid/cell debris to form a semi-solid interface between the toluene and lysate. On the following day, centrifuge at c 2000 g for 20 min, remove the toluene and, using a gentle water-pump vacuum, syphon the lysate from under the lipid/cell debris into a clean sterile bottle or flask; re-centrifuge and syphon off more lysate. Then centrifuge the combined lysate, and by vacuum suction remove residual lipid/cell debris from the surface of the lysate. Using gentle water-pump suction, filter the centrifuged lysate through Whatman No. 42 filter paper in a Büchner funnel, changing the paper whenever the filtration slows down. It is important not to overload the funnel with lysate. To each 70 ml of lysate add 30 ml of glycerol. Mix well; if it is necessary to lower the haemoglobin concentration, add 30% glycerol in saline. To each 500 ml of glycerol-lysate add one vial of penicillin-streptomycin. Mix well and dispense aseptically into sterile containers* and cap tightly.

Assign a value for haemoglobin content by the spectrophotometric method (p. 32) by carrying out 10 replicate tests, taking samples at random from several tubes of the batch. The CV should be less than 2%. Stored at 4°C, the product should maintain its assigned value for at least 2 years.

Preparation of stabilized erythrocytes[22]

Sterility must be maintained throughout the procedure. Centrifuge blood at c 2000 g for

---

* A mixing unit which is particularly suitable is available.[5,20]
† e.g. Leuco-Pak, Fenwal.

* γ-irradiated containers are available from most laboratory suppliers. Autoclaving and dry heat sterilization distorts many containers and caps.

20 min and remove the plasma aseptically. Add an equal volume of 0.15 mol/l phosphate buffer, pH 7.4 (p. 436), mix and transfer to a sterile centrifuge bottle; re-centrifuge and discard the supernatant and buffy coat. Repeat the wash and centrifugation twice. To the washed cells, add 10 times their volume of glutaraldehyde fixative (0.25% in 0.15 mol/l phosphate buffer, pH 7.4). Leave overnight at 4°C. On the next day shake vigorously to ensure complete resuspension. Mix on a mechanical mixer for 1 h. To check that fixation has been complete, centrifuge 2–3 ml of the suspension, discard the supernatant and add water to the deposit. If lysis occurs, the stock glutaraldehyde requires replacement.

When fixation is complete, centrifuge the suspension at c 2000 g for 10 min and discard the supernatant. Add an equal volume of micropore-filtered water to the fixed cell deposit, resuspend and mix by stirring and shaking; again centrifuge at c 2000 g for 10 min and discard the supernatant; repeat twice. Resuspend the fixed cells in an appropriate volume of aqueous glycine (125 g/l) and mix well by vigorous shaking; place on a mechanical shaker for 24 h to break up microclumps. The addition of a few 8 mm diameter glass beads helps in this process. Add one vial of penicillin-streptomycin for every 500 ml of suspension. Mix well for at least 20 min and then, with continuous mixing by hand or in a mixing unit (p. 16) dispense into sterile containers, with two or three 3 mm glass beads. Cap tightly.

Establish the cell count by 10 replicate measurements by haemocytometry or electronic cell counting (p. 22). Fixed cells should only be used in low concentration in fully automated systems after predilution. Check dispensing by repeated counts on five randomly selected tubes. The CV should be less than 3%. For use, resuspend by vigorous shaking by hand or on a vortex mixer for 1 min and then mix on a mechanical mixer for at least 10 min before opening the tube. The unopened vials should be stable for several years.

Preparation of pseudo-leucocytes[22]

Stabilized chicken and turkey red blood cells are suitable for use as 'pseudo-leucocytes' in preserved blood. For this, 25 ml of blood collected into ACD (NIH-A)* is sufficient. The procedure for preparation is the same as for stabilized erythrocytes (p. 16). Before use, resuspend by vigorous shaking by hand followed by mechanical mixing until no clumps remain at the base of the container. Transfer the required volume of suspension to preserved blood or lysate (p. 16), mix well and dispense as described above. Although the 'pseudo-leucocyte' cell concentrate (c 2.5×10^{12}/l) is unsuitable for direct use in fully automated systems, no problems occur when it is diluted in preserved blood, or added to a haemolysate for the simultaneous control of Hb and WBC or after it has been diluted appropriately in 9 g/l NaCl. Establish the cell count by five replicate measurements by haemocytometry (p. 24) or 10 estimates by electronic cell counter (p. 22). Check the dispensing by repeated counts on 10 or more randomly selected tubes. The CV should be less than 5%.

Preparation of platelet control[15,22]

Reagents

0.15% glutaraldehyde in Isoton II (Coulter). Add 3 ml of 50% glutaraldehyde to 1 l of Isoton II and mix well. This reagent should be prepared and used immediately.

0.15% glutaraldehyde in glycerol/Isoton II. To each 600 ml of glycerol, add 400 ml of Isoton II and 3 ml of 50% glutaraldehyde and mix well.

Procedure

Sterility must be maintained throughout. Centrifuge well-mixed fresh blood at 200 g for 10 min; collect the platelet-rich plasma. Dispense 100-ml volumes of glutaraldehyde-Isoton II solution into a series of clean dry

---

* For formula, see p. 432.

150-ml screw-capped glass bottles and to each add 15 ml of the platelet-rich plasma. Cap and mix on a roller mixer for 20 min. (As the final platelet concentration in the plasma-glutaraldehyde-Isoton II mixture should not exceed about $250 \times 10^9/l$, less platelet-rich plasma must be used if it has a very high platelet content; larger volumes of fixative and plasma should not be mixed as this induces clumping.)

Pool the suspensions in a 2 l round-bottomed flask which has previously been cooled, and rotate at 4°C for 24 h. Pass the suspension through a 20 μm high capacity transfusion filter (Fenwal) to remove fibrin strands and any other debris. Dispense 50-ml volumes of glutaraldehyde-glycerol-Isoton II solution into another set of 150-ml screw-capped bottles; carefully layer on to this solution 50 ml of filtered fixed platelet suspension and cap. Stand at 4°C for 4 days to allow the fixed platelets to drift through the glycerol-based mixture so that the initially yellowish supernatant becomes clear and the lower layer milky. With gentle suction remove the supernatant and 2–3 ml of the lower layer. Adjustment to the platelet concentration may be made by removing more of the lower layer or by adding more of the glycerol-based mixture. Resuspend the platelets by shaking and roller mixing for 20 min before pooling in a 2 l flask or into a mixing unit. Add 1 vial of penicillin-streptomycin to every 500 ml of platelet suspension, and with continuous mixing, dispense 5–10 ml volumes into sterile glass containers and cap tightly.

Assign values by 10 replicate measurements by haemocytometer (p. 24) or by electronic counter (p. 22). To check dispensing, repeated counts should be done on five randomly selected samples. The CV should be less than 3%.

Standard deviation of control specimens

If a specimen is measured a number of times successively, the dispersion of results around the mean will define the error of reproducibility. This is expressed as the standard deviation (SD). When the distribution is normal (Gaussian) 68% of the results should be within ±1 SD of the mean, 95% within ±2 SD and 99.7% within ±3 SD*. Thus, by chance alone c 1 in 3 of the measurements might be expected to fall outside ±1 SD, 1 in 20 outside ±2 SD and only 1 in 333 outside ±3 SD. If the measurements are more widely dispersed this indicates an error in the test.

For replicate testing, 10–20 identical tests are carried out on samples of the specimen. The mean is calculated and the differences from the mean recorded for each measurement. The standard deviation is calculated from the formula:

$$SD = \pm \sqrt{\frac{\text{Sum of } d^2}{n-1}},$$

where d^2 = differences, squared, and n = number of tests.

Coefficient of variation (CV) is another way of expressing the dispersion of results. Its advantage is that it relates SD to the level of the measurements. It is calculated as follows:

$$CV\ (\%) = \frac{SD \times 100}{\text{Mean}}.$$

CONTROL CHART

Charts have been used in clinical chemistry for many years[7,11] but their usefulness has only recently become recognized for the control of haematological measurements. Samples of the control specimen are included with every batch of patients' specimens and the results checked on a control chart. To check precision it is not necessary to know the exact value of the control specimen. If, however, its value has been determined reliably, the same material can also be used to check accuracy or to calibrate an instrument. If possible, controls with high, low and normal values should be used. It is advisable to use one control sample per batch even if the batch is very small. As controls are intended to simulate random sampling, they must be treated exactly like the patient's specimen.

---

* More precisely, 68.27%, 95.45% and 99.73%, respectively.

The results obtained with the control samples are plotted on a chart as described below (Fig. 2.1).

The mean value of the control specimen is obtained as described above and the SD is calculated. Using arithmetical graph paper a horizontal line is drawn to represent the mean (as a base) and on an appropriate scale of quantity and unit, lines representing $+2$ SD and -2 SD are drawn above and below the mean (Fig. 2.1). The results of the control samples are plotted. The following indicate a fault in technique or in the instrument used:

A value outside the ± 2 SD limits.

Two or more results per 20 on the $+2$ SD or -2 SD lines.

Several consecutive values show a rising tendency.

Several consecutive values show a falling tendency.

Several consecutive values on one side of the mean.

CUMULATIVE SUM METHOD (CUSUM)[3,4]

This is another way to display the data obtained in the precision test; the CUSUM is the running total of the difference between each measurement and the established mean of the control tests, taking the plus and minus signs into account. At times, it is a more sensitive indicator of faulty technique or instrument, and it is especially useful for detecting a consistent change in performance due to drift.

The mean value and SD of the control specimen are established as for the control chart (p. 18). This mean value is subtracted from each subsequent observed value for the control specimen and the

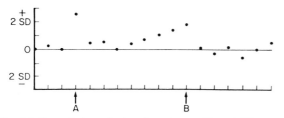

Fig. 2.1 Control chart. At time A a value outside $+2$ SD occurred as a result of a pipetting error. At time B several values had occurred consecutively on one side of the mean, due to deterioration of a reagent. When this was remedied the test was satisfactory.

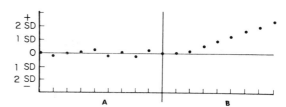

Fig. 2.2 Cusum chart. A illustrates satisfactory performance; B indicates a small consistent error.

difference is plotted on arithmetical graph paper (Fig. 2.2). Random changes tend to cancel each other out, so that, if the observed values are close to the established mean value, with only random differences, some of the differences will be positive and some negative: the CUSUM will then oscillate around zero, and the charted data will form an approximately horizontal line. Consistent differences in observed values will result in all values being either above or below the zero line and/or a change in the slope of the plotted line; the differences become significant if they reach 2 SD of the mean. The scale used for plotting the results should be such that each unit on the horizontal axis (e.g. 1 day) corresponds in scale to 2 SD on the vertical axis.

DUPLICATE TESTS ON PATIENTS' SPECIMENS

This provides another way of checking the precision of routine work.[2] Ten consecutive specimens are each tested in duplicate. The paired differences are calculated, and the standard deviation is calculated from the formula:

$$SD = \pm \sqrt{\frac{\text{sum of } d^2}{2 \times n}},$$

where d^2 = differences between duplicates, squared, and n = number of pairs. In all instances the duplicate tests should not differ from each other by more than 2 SD.

Check tests are similar to duplicate tests but they use specimens which have been measured originally in an earlier batch. The two tests should agree with each other within 2 SD. This procedure will detect deterioration of apparatus and reagents which may have developed between tests, if it is certain that the earlier specimen has not altered.

Clinical significance

±2 SD defines the range within which 95% of the duplicate or replicate tests will fall as the result of chance variation alone. If the result of a repeat test on a patient varies from a previous determination by more than 2 SD, there is less than one chance in 20 that the difference would have occurred as a result of chance. A change of less than 2 SD cannot be considered as having clinical significance.

STATISTICAL ANALYSIS OF OBSERVED VALUES

Normal data

When plotted as a frequency distribution, the haematological data obtained by carrying out tests on healthy subjects conform to a Gaussian Curve, and, in practice any abnormal values beyond ±2 SD should be ignored for the purpose of establishing reference values (see p. 6). In healthy individuals, however, the blood count data remain virtually constant day by day, subject only to the physiological changes already discussed (p. 7). When the measurements are made on a group of healthy subjects, deviation from the expected results indicates a constant error in the measurement or observation. Random errors, on the other hand, will produce an abnormally wide range of MCV, MCH and MCHC; the SD will be increased although the means may be unaffected. It is possible to use these observations for quality control in routine laboratory work by analysing the results of blood counts from 5–10 healthy subjects at intervals. The means for MCV, MCH and MCHC are determined each day. The SD for each is calculated from the formula:

$$SD = \pm \sqrt{\frac{\text{sum of } d^2}{n-1}},$$

where d^2 = difference of individual measurements from mean, squared, and n = number of measurements. The means should not vary by more than 2 SD and the SDs themselves should remain constant.

Patient data

In medium to large hospitals with a large number of patients being investigated each day, there should be no significant day-to-day or week-to-week variability in the means of their red-cell indices. Any significant change indicates a change in instrument calibration or a fault in its function. By using a computer interphased with an electronic counting system, it is possible to analyse the data continuously, using an algorithm and a desk-top programmable calculator to analyse the results on successive batches of 20 patients' specimens.[1,10]

A modification of this method uses modal values instead of mean values, as these are less likely to be affected by the presence of a few highly abnormal results on any one occasion.[17]

EXTERNAL QUALITY ASSESSMENT[6,9,16,21,22]

This is an important supplement to the internal control system used by an individual laboratory. Even when all possible precautions are taken to achieve accuracy and precision in the laboratory errors arise which are only detectable by external assessments. The principle is that the same material is sent from a national or regional centre to a large number of laboratories. All the laboratories send results back to the centre where they are analysed and the mean and SD are calculated. The laboratory can then compare its performance with that of other laboratories and with its own previous performance. A 'deviation index' can be calculated, i.e. the difference between the individual laboratory result and the mean (calculated from the results of all laboratories) related to the SD:

Deviation Index
$$= \frac{\text{Actual result} - \text{weighted mean for test}\star}{\text{Weighted SD}\star}.$$

When a laboratory uses more than one technique, the index obtained with the different methods will indicate their acceptability.

A deviation index (score) of less than 0.5 denotes excellent performance; a score between 0.5 and 1.0

★ 'Weighted' results are obtained by recalculation after excluding results outside ±2 SD.

is satisfactory and a score between 1.0 and 2.0 is still acceptable. A score above 2.0 indicates that there is a defect requiring attention.

ROUTINE QUALITY ASSURANCE PROGRAMME

The procedures which should be included in a comprehensive programme will vary with the tests undertaken, the instruments used (especially if these include a fully-automatic counting system), the size of the laboratory and the numbers of specimens handled, the computer facilities available and the amount of time which can be devoted to the programme. Some at least of the following must be carried out:

Instrument calibration (at intervals; some daily, others weekly): by means of reference preparations and standards; e.g. HiCN reference preparations, preserved blood (in ACD), stabilized (fixed) blood-cell standards.

Tests on control specimens (daily): control sample with each batch of specimens; control chart; CUSUM; duplicate measurements on patients' specimens (5 or more).

Statistical analysis (daily): mean of MCV, MCH, MCHC.

Interlaboratory tests (at intervals; usually monthly or 3-monthly).

Correlation assessment (at all times): by means of cumulative report forms (see p. 135); blood film appearances and numerical data; clinical state (see p. 132).

REFERENCES

[1] BULL, B. S. and KORPMAN, R. A. (1982). Intralaboratory quality control using patients' data. *Methods in Hematology*, **4**, 121.

[2] CARSTAIRS, K. C., PETERS, E. and KUZIN, E. J. (1977). Development and description of the 'random duplicates' method of quality control for a hematology laboratory. *American Journal of Clinical Pathology*, **67**, 379.

[3] CAVILL, I. (1971). Quality control in routine haemoglobinometry. *Journal of Clinical Pathology*, **24**, 701.

[4] CAVILL, I. and RICKETTS, C. (1974). Automated quality control for the haematology laboratory. *Journal of Clinical Pathology*, **27**, 757.

[5] CHAPPELL, D. A. and WARD, P. G. (1978). Safe and sterile mixer for biological fluids. *Laboratory Equipment Digest*, **16**, 75.

[6] GOGUEL, A. F. (1975). Inter-laboratory trial: surveys in France. In *Quality Control in Haematology*, Eds. S. M. Lewis and J. F. Coster, p. 69. Academic Press, London.

[7] HENRY, R. J. and SEGALORE, M. (1952). The running of standards in clinical chemistry and the use of the control chart. *Journal of Clinical Pathology*, **5**, 305.

[8] International committee for standardization in haematology (1978). Recommendations for reference method for haemoglobinometry in human blood (ICSH Standard EP 6/2: 1977) and specifications for international haemiglobincyanide reference preparation (ICSH Standard EP 6/3: 1977). *Journal of Clinical Pathology*, **31**, 139.

[9] KOEPKE, J. A. (1975). Inter-laboratory trials: the quality control survey programme of the College of American Pathologists. In *Quality Control in Haematology*, Eds. S. M. Lewis, J. F. Coster, p. 53. Academic Press, London.

[10] KORPMAN, R. A. and BULL, B. S. (1976). The implementation of a robust estimator of the mean for quality control on a programmable calculator or a laboratory computer. *American Journal of Clinical Pathology*, **65**, 252.

[11] LEVEY, S. and JENNINGS, E. R. (1950). The use of control charts in the clinical laboratory. *American Journal of Clinical Pathology*, **20**, 1059.

[12] LEWIS, S. M. (1975). Standards and reference preparations. In *Quality Control in Haematology*, Eds. S. M. Lewis and J. F. Coster, p. 79. Academic Press, London.

[13] LEWIS, S. M. (1981). The philosophy of value assignment. In *Advances in Hematological Methods: The Blood Count*. Eds. O. W. van Assendelft and J. M. England, p. 231. CRC Press, Florida.

[14] LEWIS, S. M. and BURGESS, B. J. (1966). A stable standard suspension for red-cell counts. *Laboratory Practice*, **15**, 305.

[15] LEWIS, S. M., WARDLE, J., COUSINS, S. and SKELLY, J. (1979). Platelet counting—development of a reference method and a reference preparation. *Clinical and Laboratory Haematology*, **1**, 227.

[16] POLLER, L., THOMSON, J. M. and YEE, K. F. (1979). Quality control trials of prothrombin time: an assessment of the performance in serial studies. *Journal of Clinical Pathology*, **32**, 251.

[17] PRANGNELL, D. R. and JOHNSON, P. H. (1977). A new method of quality control for the Coulter Model S counter. *Journal of Clinical Pathology*, **30**, 487.

[18] THOM, R. (1972). Hemocytometry: method and results by improved electronic blood-cell sizing. In *Modern Concepts in Hematology*, Eds. G. Izak, S. M. Lewis, p. 91. Academic Press, New York.

[19] TORLONTANO, G. and TATA, A. (1972). Stable standard suspensions of white blood cells suitable for calibration and control of electronic counters. In *Modern Concepts in Hematology*, Eds. G. Izak and S. M. Lewis, p. 230. Academic Press, New York.

[20] WARD, P. G., CHAPPELL, D. A., FOX, J. G. C. and ALLEN B. V. (1975). Mixing and bottling unit for preparing biological fluids used in quality control. *Laboratory Practice*, **24**, 577.

[21] WARD, P. G. and LEWIS, S. M. (1975). Interlaboratory trials—a national proficiency assessment scheme for Britain. In *Quality Control in Haematology*, Eds. S. M. Lewis and J. F. Coster, p. 37. Academic Press, London.

[22] WARD, P. G., WARDLE, J. and LEWIS, S. M. (1982). Standardization for routine blood counting—the role of interlaboratory trials. *Methods in Hematology*, **4**, 102.

[23] World Health Organization (1977). Biological substances: international standards, reference preparations, and reference reagents. WHO, Geneva.

3

Basic haematological techniques

THE TOTAL RED-CELL COUNT

The ease and speed with which a red-cell count can be obtained since the advent of electronic cells counters has increased enormously the practicability of such counts, whilst their high level of reproducibility has increased their diagnostic value. Some instruments are limited to particle counting; others have inter-related systems by means of which the size of cells can be measured, so as to provide PCV and MCV; Hb, as well, can be determined on the same sample.

Visual counting is, however, still a necessary procedure, not only for smaller laboratories which do not possess electronic counters but also because electronic counters have to be calibrated and visual counting is used as a reference method. Accordingly, all those working in a haematological laboratory should have training and experience in the method and have some knowledge of its difficulties and its limits of accuracy and precision.

COUNTING RED CELLS WITH ELECTRONIC COUNTERS

In recent years several different types of electronic equipment have been developed for the automatic counting of blood cells. The better known machines in current use are based on one of three principles.

Moldavan's capillary method[68]

A red-cell suspension flows through a cuvette in the form of an optical chamber which is aligned to a dark-field condenser. Each cell is illuminated briefly as it passes a focussed light. The light impulses produced are converted into electrical impulses in a photomultiplier tube and then counted and recorded. This is the basis of the Technicon system.

Laser light scatter[58]

A diluted red-cell suspension is injected into a stream of buffered saline in which the cells then flow in single file past a laser beam. The light which is diffracted and scattered by the cells is detected by a photovoltaic cell which generates pulses with a magnitude relative to the size. The pulses pass to an electronic system where they accumulate and are counted. This is the basis of the Ortho system.

Electrical impedance method[16]

This method, first described by Coulter in 1956,[16] depends on the fact that blood is a poor conductor of electricity, whereas certain diluents are good conductors. It is the basis of the Coulter Counters (Coulter Electronics Ltd.) and has also been used in the Toa Micro-cell Counter (Toa Electric Co. Ltd.)[42] and in several other counters which have been marketed in recent years.

For a cell count, blood is highly diluted in a buffered electrolyte solution. An external vacuum initiates movement of a mercury siphon which causes the sample to flow through an aperture tube of specific dimensions, usually about 100 μm in diameter and 70 μm in length. By means of a constant source of electricity a direct current is maintained between an electrode in the sample beaker and one inside the aperture tube. As a blood cell is carried through the orifice of the aperture tube, it displaces some of the conductive fluid and increases the electrical resistance. This produces a corresponding change in potential between the electrodes, which lasts as long as the passage of the cell through the aperture tube and assumes the shape of a pulse. The amplitude of the pulse is proportional to cell volume. The pulses are displayed on an oscilloscope screen, the volume of the cells being indicated by the height of the pulses. The pulses are led to a threshold circuit which has an amplitude discriminator for selecting the minimal pulse height which will be counted. The counting process stops when the mercury in the siphon reaches a second contact.

In choosing an instrument for a particular laboratory, account has to be taken of the daily workload, the rate at which specimens are received by the laboratory, and whether the laboratory is concerned primarily with health care screening or with providing a diagnostic service. For a small laboratory all its needs may be satisfied by a simple single-channel cell counting instrument, together with a haemoglobinometer. On the other hand, for large laboratories dealing with 300 or more blood samples daily, automated instruments such as Coulter Model S Plus are more suitable as they are designed specifically for a routine screening procedure, including platelet counting (see p. 46).

Detailed discussions of the physical and other aspects of electronic cell counting are beyond the scope of this book; they can be found in a number of other publications.[41,42,56,67,107] Nor will the actual use of the various instruments be described here, as detailed instructions for assembly and operation are supplied by the manufacturers when the instruments are delivered.

The necessary diluent requires some consideration. For counters based on the electrical impedance method it is necessary to avoid alterations in pH, temperature and rate of ionization, all of which influence the electrical field and may lead to artefactual alterations in the size, shape and stability of the blood cells in the diluent.[41,101]

For red-cell counting, several diluents have been described. For electrical impedance counters, a modified Eagle's solution, under the trade name Isoton, was originally recommended by Coulter Electronics. A suitable alternative solution can be prepared as follows[41]: NaCl 8.3 g, KCl 0.41 g,

$CaCl_2$ 0.011 g, Na_2HPO_4 1.0 g, NaN_3 1.0 g, glucose 1.0 g, water* to 1 l; sufficient 3 mol/l HCl is added to adjust the pH to 7.4. The (modified) solution now recommended by the manufacturers is known as Isoton II[2]: this is free of azide (a potentially explosive substance) and also ensures relatively constant red-cell size and shape.

Physiological saline (9 g/l NaCl), which has the advantages of simplicity and ready availability, can be used as a red-cell diluent, provided that the counts are performed immediately after dilution in order to avoid errors due to sphering. Another reason for counting immediately after dilution is to avoid loss of counts due to settling of the red cells.

The solution used for dilution must, as far as possible, be particle-free. Commercial solutions of saline (for intravenous use) are generally suitable; with other solutions it may be necessary to remove dust particles by filtration through a 0.22 or 0.45 μm micropore filter. The diluent should give a background count of less than 100 particles in the measured volume. For instruments in which several measurements are carried out consecutively on a single blood sample, it is necessary to add agents to lyse the red cells (for the leucocyte count) and to convert Hb to HiCN. Coulter Electronics Ltd recommends Isoton II with the addition of Lyse S for this purpose. Alternatively, a diluent containing potassium cyanide and potassium ferricyanide together with ethylhexadecyldimethyl ammonium bromide can be used.[1,84]

RELIABILITY OF ELECTRONIC COUNTERS

Electronic blood-cell counters vary considerably in ease of maintenance both from the mechanical and electronic standpoints. Because large numbers of cells can be enumerated, replicate counts correspond closely, and the coefficient of variation should only be a fraction of that of counts done visually on 500–1000 cells. Electronic counters thus have a very great potential advantage over visual methods of counting red cells. Not only can many thousands

---

* Throughout the book, 'water' refers to distilled or de-ionized water.

of cells be counted, but the actual time of counting (10–100 s according to the type of machine) is also far less than that necessary for a most perfunctory visual count. However, the actual count recorded may vary from instrument to instrument and even with different models of the same instrument.[7,57,88] This is likely to be due to incorrect setting of the threshold discrimination, variation in counting volume or flow rate, or the use of orifice tubes of different dimensions. Other factors include coincidence counts for which adequate correction may not be made, dead-time of the electrical circuit, air bubbles being counted as cells, recirculation of cells around the orifice, and adhesion of cells to the surface of the container in which the blood is diluted.

Errors of coincidence can be detected by carrying out a series of measurements at various dilutions of the specimen, and then extrapolating the results to zero concentration for the true value.[95] Loss of red cells by electrostatic adhesion to the container surface is more likely with polystyrene than glass.[60] It may be impossible to recognize the existence of erroneous results when measurements are carried out on a single machine, as the error may be constant in the particular instrument. The only adequate method of checking is to use a reference preparation to calibrate the instrument (p. 15) and, at frequent intervals, quality assurance procedures to check on precision and accuracy (see p. 21). Auto-agglutinated blood, due to the presence of high-thermal-amplitude cold agglutinins, may give erroneously low counts. However, the discrepancy should be obvious when the red-cell count is compared with PCV and Hb content and the cause of the error will be identified when a blood film is examined.

Counting red cells by visual means

Make a 1:200 dilution of blood in formal-citrate solution. This is most conveniently done by washing 20 μl of blood taken into a micropipette into 4 ml of diluting fluid contained in a glass or plastic 75 × 12 mm tube. After sealing the tube with a tightly fitting rubber or plastic bung, mix the diluted blood in a mechanical mixer or by hand for at least 2 min by tilting the tube through an angle of about 120° combined with rotation, thus allowing the air bubble to mix the suspension.

Fill a clean dry counting chamber, with its cover-glass already in position, without delay. This is simply accomplished with the aid of a Pasteur pipette or a length of stout capillary glass tubing which has been allowed to take up the suspension by capillarity. Care should be taken that the counting chamber is filled in one action and that no fluid flows into the surrounding moat. Leave the chamber undisturbed on a bench for at least 2 min for the cells to settle, but not much longer, for drying at the edges of the preparation may initiate currents which cause movement of the cells after they have settled. The bench must be free of vibrations and the chamber not exposed to draughts or to direct sunlight or other source of heat. It is important that the cover-glass should be of a special thick glass and perfectly flat, so that when laid on the counting chamber, diffraction rings are seen. The cover-glass should be of such a size that when placed correctly on the counting chamber the central ruled areas lie in the centre of the rectangle to be filled with the cell suspension. The preparation must be discarded and the filling procedure repeated using another clean dry chamber if any of the following filling defects occur:

1. Overflow into moat.
2. Chamber area incompletely filled.
3. Air bubbles anywhere in chamber area.
4. Any debris in chamber areas.

The type of counting chamber used and the arrangement of the rulings are matters of personal preference and availability. The Neubauer and improved Neubauer have become the commonest types in general use. The visiblity of the rulings is as important as the accuracy of calibration.

Count the cells using a 4 mm dry objective and ×6 or ×10 eyepieces. It is important to count as many cells as possible, for the accuracy of the count is increased thereby (see below); 500 cells should be considered the absolute minimum. With a Neubauer chamber (Figs. 3.1 and 3.2), count the

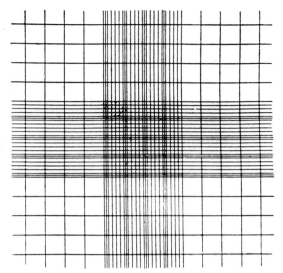

Fig. 3.1 Neubauer counting chamber. The total ruled area is 3 mm × 3 mm; the central ruled area is 1 mm × 1 mm. In the central area 16 groups of 16 small squares are separated by triple rulings.

cells in 4 or 8 horizontal rectangles of 1 mm × 0.05 mm (80 or 160 small squares) or in 5 or 10 groups of 16 small squares, including the cells which touch the bottom and left-hand margins of the small squares.

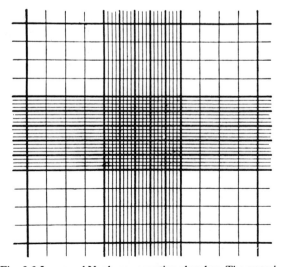

Fig. 3.2 Improved Neubauer counting chamber. The central area consists of 25 groups of 16 small squares separated by closely ruled triple lines (which appear as thick black lines in the photograph).

Calculation

Red-cell count (per l)

$$= \frac{\text{No. of cells counted}}{\text{volume counted } (\mu l)} \times \text{dilution} \times 10^6.$$

Thus, when 80 small squares of an improved Neubauer chamber are counted (total volume = 0.02 μl) and the blood is diluted 1 : 200, the red cell count will be:

$$\frac{N}{0.02} \times 200 \text{ per } \mu l \text{ or } \frac{N}{0.02} \times 200 \times 10^6 \text{ per l.}$$

Red-cell diluting fluid

A solution of 10 ml of 40% formalin, made up to 1 l with 32 g/l trisodium citrate is recommended. The solution is simple to prepare; it keeps well and does not need to be sterilized. The red cells maintain their normal disc-like form and are not agglutinated. The cells are well preserved and counts may be performed several hours after the blood has been diluted.

Occasionally, when the patient's blood is auto-agglutinated, as in some cases of auto-immune haemolytic anaemia, it is advantageous to use as a diluting fluid 32 g/l trisodium citrate solution without the addition of formalin. Auto-agglutination may disperse and enable a count to be carried out in the absence of formalin which appears to prevent, (?) by its fixing action, the clumps of agglutinated cells from breaking up.

Range of red-cell counts in health (see p. 8).

ERRORS OF VISUAL RED-CELL COUNTING

The errors associated with the count are of two main kinds: those due to inaccurate apparatus, indifferent technique or unrepresentative nature of the blood counted ('technical' errors) and that due to the distribution of the suspension of red cells in the counting chamber—the 'inherent' or 'field' error. The former errors can be minimized by careful technique, the latter error can be diminished by counting a large number of cells.

Technical errors

These include bad sampling of the blood due to an inadequate flow from a skin puncture; the prolonged use of a tourniquet; insufficient mixing of venous blood which has sedimented after collection; inaccurate pipetting and the use of badly calibrated pipettes or counting chambers; inadequate mixing of the red-cell suspension; faulty filling of the counting chamber, and careless counting of cells within the chamber.

It is essential that the accuracy of the apparatus be known so that, if necessary, appropriate correction factors can be applied. The British Standard for Haemocytometer Counting Chambers (BS 748: 1963) specifies a tolerance of dimensions which provides reasonable accuracy. But even so, the chance summation of all the tolerances for different parts of the apparatus in a single counting chamber would result in an error as large as ±7%.

The exact chamber depth depends also on the cover-glass, which should be free from bowing and sufficiently thick so as not to bend when pressed on the chamber. It must be free from scratches, and even the smallest particle of dust may cause unevenness in the lie of the cover-glass on the chamber.

Bulb diluting pipettes are not recommended; they are difficult to calibrate and easily broken. The volumes of blood used are unnecessarily small and the pipettes are difficult to label and handle. In particular, filling the counting chamber so that the exact amount of fluid is delivered from the pipette is an art difficult to master. 20 μl pipettes are relatively inexpensive and easy to calibrate. By the use of 4 ml of diluting fluid in a glass or plastic tube provided with a tightly fitting rubber or plastic bung, a suspension easy to label and handle is obtained, and with a little practice a perfect filling of the counting chamber can regularly be accomplished with the aid of a fine Pasteur pipette or stout glass capillary.

The accuracy of 20 μl pipettes may be checked, after careful cleaning by filling them to the mark with clean mercury, expelling the mercury and

weighing it.[87] 20 μl of mercury weigh 272 mg; 50 μl weigh 680 mg. It is convenient to draw up the mercury to the mark in the pipette by attaching to the pipette a small length of pressure tubing one end of which has been closed. The measured column of mercury is then expelled on to a previously weighed watch-glass and weighed in a balance sensitive to a difference of 1 mg.

Automatic diluter units are useful. These consist of a dual metering system which enables a volume of diluent and the appropriate volume of blood to be dispensed consecutively into a tube. A variety of automatic diluting systems are now available. Hand-held semi-automatic microsamplers with a detachable tip (e.g. Eppendorf, Oxford, Labora) are designed to operate as 'to deliver' pipettes. They are popular and they have good accuracy and precision.

Pipetting errors apply to all tests which involve dilution of the blood sample and they also occur with autodiluters which are liable to error with viscid fluids and when the delivery volume of the unit is not correctly adjusted. The inherent error, discussed below, is unique to visual cell counting.

Inherent error

The distribution of cells in a counting chamber is of an irregular (random) pattern, even in a perfectly mixed sample. However, the pattern of distribution conforms to a definite type. Theoretical considerations indicate that variation between the numbers of red cells which settle in areas similar in size should conform to a mathematical distribution (Poisson series) and that the standard deviation (SD) of the distribution of the number of cells in areas of equal size should be given by $\sqrt{m}$ where m is the mean number of cells in the areas. However, the movement of the cells in the chamber during the filling process causes them to collide and this influences their distribution which thus varies from the theoretical expectation of the SD.[63] This is given instead by $\sigma = 0.92 \sqrt{m}$. This means that if a counting chamber is filled with a red-cell suspension so that the mean number of cells in an area (say 80 small squares) is 100, σ would be 9.2. Then, if it were possible to count the number of cells in each of 100 similar areas, in 95 areas the number of cells encountered would range between 82 and 118, i.e.

$100 \pm 2\sigma$; in the remaining five areas the counts would be outside this range.

Clearly, this random distribution has a very important bearing on the accuracy of visual blood counts, for no amount of mixing will minimize the inherent variation in numbers between area and area.

The ratio σ/m is the coefficient of variation (CV) of the distribution and this calculated as a percentage gives a convenient way of expressing the inherent error of blood counts.

The inherent error in blood counting can be reduced in one of two ways: by counting more cells in one preparation or by making successive counts. The following calculations (Table 3.1) demonstrate that, in theory, the CV of the count varies in proportion to the square root of the number of cells counted, i.e. if four times the number of cells are counted, the coefficient of variation is halved. For example, if the imaginary (ideal) figures given in Table 3.1 are studied, it will be seen that 19 out of 20 counts based on the number of cells in 80 small squares will lie within the wide range of 5.16 to $6.04 \times 10^{12}/1$. If the cells in 320 small squares are counted, the range will be considerably narrower— 5.38 to $5.82 \times 10^{12}/1$. Causes of error of red-cell counts include personal bias from fore-knowledge of what the result should be, selection of counting areas and uneven distribution of cells within the counting chamber due to the momentum given to the cells as the chamber is filled.[82]

The method of making serial counts and taking the mean has been widely (perhaps unconsciously) used as a means of reducing the error of the red-cell count. If a sufficient number of counts are done, the truth is likely to reveal itself; not only will the inherent error be reduced by the counting of a large number of cells, but there is also a chance that errors in technique will cancel each other out.

Clearly, the errors of blood counting by visual means are very considerable. That due to the random distribution of the cells in the counting chamber can be reduced by counting the cells in a larger area, as already mentioned (see Table 3.1), but in ordinary laboratory practice there is rarely time to count carefully the cells in more than 160 small squares—about 1000 cells in a normal count. The practice of making counts in duplicate is a good one, but does not necessarily increase accuracy: it is always possible that the second count will be further from the truth than the first, due to the random distribution of cells. It is better to repeat a count using a second chamber and pipette than to count double the number of cells in a single filling of the counting chamber.

ESTIMATION OF HAEMOGLOBIN

The Hb content of a solution may be estimated by several methods: by measurement of its colour, its power of combining with oxygen or carbon monoxide and by its iron content. The clinical methods to be described are all colour or light-intensity matching techniques, which measure at the same time with different degrees of efficiency any proportion of inert pigments, i.e. methaemoglobin (Hi) or sulphaemoglobin (SHb), which may be present. The oxygen-combining capacity of blood is 1.34 ml O_2 per g Hb. Ideally, as a functional estimation of Hb, measurement of oxygen capacity should be carried out, but this is hardly practicable in clinical work. It gives results at least 2% lower than the

Table 3.1 Error of the red-cell count.

No. of small squares counted	No. of cells counted (m)	σ ($0.92 \times \sqrt{m}$)	Range (95%) $m \pm 2\sigma$	Calculated red-cell count ($x10^{12}/1$)	Coefficient of variation (CV) %
80	560	22	516–604	5.16–6.04	3.9
160	1120	31	1058–1182	5.29–5.91	2.8
320	2240	44	2152–2328	5.38–5.82	2.0
640	4480	62	4356–4604	5.44–5.75	1.4

Showing how the inherent error of red-cell counting may be reduced by counting large numbers of red cells.

other methods because a small proportion of inert pigment is probably always present. The iron content of Hb can be estimated accurately,[106] but again the method is impracticable for routine purposes. Estimations based on iron content are generally taken as authentic, but iron bound to inactive pigment is included. Iron content is converted into Hb content by assuming the following relationship: 0.347 g iron = 100 g Hb.[48]

MEASUREMENT OF HAEMOGLOBIN USING A PHOTOELECTRIC COLORIMETER

In the following section three procedures will be described and their merits and disadvantages discussed:

1. The cyanmethaemoglobin (haemiglobin-cyanide) (HiCN) method.
2. The oxyhaemoglobin (HbO$_2$) method.
3. The alkaline-haematin method.

There is little to choose in accuracy between the methods, although the alkaline-haematin procedure is probably less accurate than the others. A major advantage of the HiCN method is the availability of a stable and reliable reference preparation. Sahli's acid-haematin method is less accurate than any of the methods mentioned above as the colour which develops does not become stable but begins to fade almost immediately after it reaches its peak.

COLLECTION OF BLOOD SAMPLES FOR DETERMINATION OF HAEMOGLOBIN

Venous blood or free-flowing capillary blood added to any solid anticoagulant can be used. The concentration of anticoagulant is not critical. Measurements can be carried out on blood which has been stored at 4°C for several days, provided it has not become obviously infected, but the blood must be allowed to warm up to room temperature and be well mixed before it is sampled.

CYANMETHAEMOGLOBIN METHOD

The basis of the method is dilution of blood in a solution containing potassium cyanide and potassium ferricyanide.[19] Hb, Hi and HbCO (but not SHb) are all converted to HiCN. The absorbance of the solution is then measured in a photoelectric colorimeter at a wavelength of 540 nm or with a yellow-green filter (e.g. Ilford 625).

Diluent

This is based on Drabkin's cyanide-ferricyanide solution*.[19] The original Drabkin reagent had a pH of 8.6. The following modified solution, which has a pH of 9.6, is less likely to cause turbidity from precipitation of plasma proteins: it consists of potassium ferricyanide 200 mg, potassium cyanide 50 mg, water to 1 l.

The above solution reacts relatively slowly, and the diluted blood must stand for at least 10 min to ensure complete conversion of Hb. The following further modification, as recommended by the *International Committee for Standardization in Haematology*,[48] results in a shorter conversion time (<3 min), although it has the disadvantage that the presence of a detergent causes some degree of frothing. The pH should be 7.0–7.4: it consists of potassium ferricyanide 200 mg, potassium cyanide 50 mg, potassium dihydrogen phosphate 140 mg, Nonidet P40 (Shell Chemical Co.) 1 ml, water to 1 l. Other non-ionic detergents which can be used in place of Nonidet include Sterox SE (Harleco) 0.5 ml, Triton X-100 (Rohm and Haas) 1 ml and Saponic 218 (Alcoac Inc) 1 ml.

The reagent should be clear and pale yellow in colour. When measured against water as blank in a photoelectric colorimeter at a wavelength of 540 nm, the absorbance must read zero. If stored at room temperature in a brown borosilicate glass bottle, the solution keeps for several months. It must not be allowed to freeze, as this can result in its decomposition.[108] The reagent must be discarded if it becomes turbid, or if the pH is found to be outside the 7.0–7.4 range or if it has an absorb-

---

* Drabkin's solution may be conveniently prepared by means of Aculute Diluent Pellets (Ortho Pharmaceutical Ltd.).

ance other than zero at 540 nm against a water blank.

Cyanmethaemoglobin (HiCN) reference preparation

With the advent of HiCN as a stable solution other standards have become outmoded. *The International Committee for Standardization in Haematology* has defined specifications on the basis of a molecular weight of 64 458 and a millimolar coefficient extinction of 44.0*.[48] These specifications have been widely adopted; in Britain they have been incorporated into a British Standard (BS 3985: 1966) for a HiCN solution for photometric haemoglobinometry, and a WHO International Reference Preparation has been established.

Solutions of HiCN are stable for at least several years. Reference solutions which conform to the international specifications are available commercially. They contain 550–850 mg Hb per l and the exact concentration is indicated on the label. The solution is dispensed in 10 ml sealed ampoules, and, to ensure that contamination is avoided, any unused solution should be discarded at the end of the day on which the ampoule is opened. In use, the reference solution is regarded as a dilution of whole blood, and the original Hb concentration that it represents is obtained by multiplying the figure stated on the label by the dilution to be applied to the blood sample. Thus, if the standard solution contains 600 mg/l, it will have the same optical density as that of a blood sample containing 120 g Hb per l diluted 1 in 200, or as one containing 150 g Hb per l diluted 1 in 250*.

The HiCN reference preparation is intended primarily for direct comparison with blood which is also converted to HiCN. It can also be used for the standardization of a whole-blood standard in the HbO_2 method and for the calibration of Gibson and Harrison's standard used in the alkaline-haematin method (see p. 31).

---

* i.e. the absorbance of a solution containing 4×55.8 mg of Hb iron per l at 540 nm.

* Within the SI system many measurements are now expressed in terms of substance concentration, using the mole as unit. For clinical purposes, there are practical advantages in continuing to express Hb in mass concentration, i.e. as g/l; if substance concentration is used, the monomer should be the elementary entity used in calculation.[105]

Method

Add 20 μl of blood to 4 ml of diluent. Stopper the tube containing the solution and invert it several times. After being allowed to stand at room temperature for a sufficient period of time to ensure the completion of the reaction (3–10 min, see above), the solution of HiCN is ready to be compared with the standard and a reagent blank in a spectrophotometer at 540 nm or in a photoelectric colorimeter with a suitable filter.[†] Open an ampoule of HiCN standard (brought to room temperature if previously stored in a refrigerator) and measure the absorbance of the solution in the same spectrophotometer or photoelectric colorimeter against the blank. The standard should be discarded at the end of the day and during the day must be kept in the dark. The absorbance of the test sample must be measured within 6 h of its being diluted.

Calculation

$$\text{Hb g/l} = \frac{^{\ddagger}A^{540} \text{ of test sample}}{A^{540} \text{ of standard}} \times$$

$$\frac{\text{Conc std (mg/l)}}{1000} \times \text{dilution factor (e.g. 201)}.$$

Preparation of standard curve and standard table

When many blood samples are to be tested it is convenient to read the results from a standard curve or table relating absorbance readings to Hb concentration in g/l for the individual instrument. These can be prepared as follows.

Open an ampoule of HiCN reference solution (brought to room temperature) and measure the absorbance or transmittance of the solution against a blank of cyanide-ferricyanide reagent, in the same photometer as is to be used for the subsequent haemoglobinometry. Make readings with the same

---

† e.g. Ilford 625, Wratten 74 or Chance O Gr 1.

‡ i.e. absorbance; formerly called optical density. In some instruments, measurements are read as percentage transmittance.

standard solution diluted with the reagent 1 in 2, 1 in 3, 1 in 4, etc. Translate the Hb values of the solutions into terms of g/l, as described above. If the readings are in absorbance, plot them on linear graph paper using arithmetical scales, with absorbance as ordinates (vertical scale) and Hb (g/l) as abscissae (horizontal scale). If the readings are in percentage transmittance, use semilogarithmic paper with the transmittance recorded on the vertical (log) scale. As Lambert-Beer's law is valid for HiCN, the points should fit a straight line which passes through the origin. This provides a check that the calibration of the photometer is linear (assuming that the standard has been correctly diluted). From the standard curve it is possible to construct a table of readings and corresponding Hb values. The table may be more convenient than the graph when large numbers of measurements are made. Prepare a calibration curve whenever a new photometer is put into use.

It is important that the performance of the instrument should not vary and that its calibration remains constant in relation to Hb measurements. To ensure this, the reference preparations should be measured at frequent intervals, preferably with each batch of blood samples.

The main advantages of the HiCN method for Hb determination are that it allows direct comparison with the HiCN standard and that the readings need not be made immediately after dilution; it also has the advantage that all forms of Hb, except SHb, are readily converted to HiCN. The use of KCN in the preparation of Drabkin's solution is a potential hazard but the diluent itself, containing only 50 mg of KCN per l, is relatively inoccuous; 600–1000 ml would have to be swallowed to produce serious effects. As already referred to, a possible disadvantage is that the diluted blood has to stand for a period of time to ensure complete conversion of the Hb. Also, the rate of conversion is markedly slowed in blood containing carbon monoxide. This difficulty can be overcome by prolonging the reaction time to 3 h or by using a reagent with an increased concentration of potassium ferricyanide.[93]

Abnormal plasma proteins or a high leucocyte count may result in turbidity when the blood is diluted in the cyanide-ferricyanide reagent.[65,102] The turbidity can be avoided by centrifuging the diluted sample, by adding 5 g of NaCl per l to the reagent or by reducing the amount of potassium dihydrogen phosphate to 120 mg/l.[65]

OXYHAEMOGLOBIN METHOD

This is the simplest and quickest method for general use with a photoelectric colorimeter. Its disadvantage is that it is not possible to prepare a stable HbO_2 standard. The reliability of the method is not affected by a moderate rise in plasma bilirubin but it is not satisfactory in the presence of HbCO, Hi or SHb.

Method

Wash 20 μl of blood into 4 ml of 0.4 ml/l ammonia (sp gr 0.88) contained in a tube provided with a tightly fitting stopper. Mix by inverting the tube several times. The solution of HbO_2 is then ready for matching in the colorimeter. A yellow-green filter (e.g. Ilford 625) is employed. If the absorbance of the Hb solution exceeds 0.7, dilute the blood further with an equal volume of water.

Standard

At a dilution of 1 in 200, blood containing 146 g Hb/l, placed in a 1 cm cell, gives an extinction coefficient of 0.475, using a yellow-green filter (Ilford 625, Wratten 74 or Chance 0 Gr 1). A neutral grey filter of 0.475 density (Ilford or Chance) can, therefore, be used as a 146 g/l standard.

Colorimeters and light filters unfortunately differ sufficiently one from the other to make it essential to check the chosen standard at frequent intervals against a HiCN reference preparation in the colorimeter in which it is going to be used. It is probably preferable to use a new fresh whole-blood sample each day as a secondary standard after measuring its

Hb content by the HiCN method. Preserved blood (p. 16) or lysate (p. 16) can be used instead.

As originally used, a disadvantage of the HbO$_2$ method was the tendency for the solution of HbO$_2$ to fade.[91] This has been found to be due to the high dilution of the solution and the unnecessarily high pH, resulting from the use of 1 g/l sodium carbonate solution or relatively strong ammonia solution as diluent. However, using 0.4 ml/l ammonia, the solution appears to be stable for a day or more at room temperature.

ALKALINE-HAEMATIN METHOD

The alkaline-haematin method is a useful ancillary method under special circumstances as it gives a true estimate of total Hb even if HbCO, Hi or SHb is present. A true solution is obtained and the plasma proteins and lipids have little effect on the development of colour, although they cause turbidity unless the blood and alkali are quickly and thoroughly mixed.

A disadvantage of the method is that certain forms of Hb are resistant to alkali denaturation, in particular Hb-F and Hb-Barts (see p. 185), but this can be overcome by heating the solution in a boiling water-bath for 4 min. In normal circumstances the method is more cumbersome and less accurate than the HiCN or HbO$_2$ methods and is thus unsuitable for use as a routine method.

Two methods will be described:

1. The standard method,[15] using Gibson and Harrison's standard.[35]
2. The acid-alkali method.

Standard method

Add 50 μl of blood to 4.95 ml of 0.1 mol/l NaOH and heat in a boiling water-bath for exactly 4 min. Cool the sample rapidly in cold water and when cool match against the standard in a photoelectric colorimeter using a yellow-green filter (e.g. Ilford 625).

Standard. This is a mixture of chromium potassium sulphate, cobaltous sulphate and potassium dichromate in aqueous solution (for preparation, see p. 434). The solution is equal in colour to a 1 in 100 dilution of blood containing 160 g Hb per l.

It is essential to heat the standard along with the test sample. Only after heating, which alters the ionization of the salts it contains, does the ability of the standard to absorb green light approximate closely to that of alkaline haematin. A fresh sample of standard should be heated on each occasion and then discarded.

Acid-alkali method

A disadvantage of the alkaline-haematin method, as previously described, is that the solution of Hb in alkali has to be heated to ensure complete denaturation. This procedure can be omitted if the blood is collected first into acid and, after standing for 20–30 min, sufficient alkali is added to neutralize the acid and convert the acid haematin into alkaline haematin.

Wash 50 μl of blood into 4.0 ml of 0.1 mol/l HCl and mix immediately. After the tube has stood for 20–30 min, add 0.95 ml of 1 mol/l NaOH and invert the tube several times. After a further 2 min, measure the test sample in a photoelectric colorimeter. Use a yellow-green filter (e.g. Ilford 625), employing as a standard heated Gibson and Harrison's standard (see above) or a grey filter or solution[96] previously calibrated against blood of known Hb content treated by acid and then alkali as described above.

OTHER METHODS OF HAEMOGLOBINOMETRY

Direct-reading haemoglobinometers

These instruments have a built-in filter and a scale calibrated for direct reading of haemoglobin in g/dl or g/l. A recent development is the use of a light-emitting diode of appropriate wavelength.[73] The calibration of this type of instrument should be checked regularly, using HiCN reference solutions to ensure maintenance of accuracy and precision.

Spectrophotometry

The Hb content of blood can be determined accurately by spectrophotometry. The blood is diluted suitably (1 to 200 or 1 to 250) with cyanide-ferricyanide reagent (see p. 28) and the absorbance is measured at 540 nm. The Hb content is calculated as follows:

Concentration (g/l)

$$= \frac{A^{540}HiCN \times 64\,500 \times \text{dilution factor}}{44.0 \times d \times 1000},$$

where A^{540} HiCN = absorbance of the solution at 540 nm, 64 500 = molecular weight of Hb (derived from 64 458), dilution factor = 201 when 20 μl of blood are diluted in 4 ml of reagent, 44.0 = millimolar extinction coefficient, d = layer thickness in cm, and 1000 = conversion factor for mg to g.

The spectrophotometric method gives a direct measurement of the Hb content of the diluted blood. It does not require a HiCN standard, but both wavelength scale and absorbance scale must be calibrated. The wavelength scale of a spectrophotometer may be calibrated using the mercury emission line at 546.1 nm, the hydrogen emission lines at 656.3 and 486.1 nm or using a suitable filter with exactly known light absorption peaks. The absorbance scale is calibrated using a suitable filter with known absorption at a given wavelength, preferably near 540 nm (e.g. Shott glass NG-4) or with a solution of known content and known molar extinction, e.g. a haemiglobincyanide reference solution (see p. 29), or acidic potassium dicromate solution*.

DETERMINATION OF PACKED CELL VOLUME (PCV OR HAEMATOCRIT VALUE)

Haematocrit (literally 'blood separation') tubes are in daily use in many haematological laboratories where automated blood-count systems are not available, as the measurement of the PCV can be used as a simple screening test for anaemia. In addition, in conjunction with accurate estimations of Hb and red-cell count, knowledge of the PCV enables the calculation of 'absolute' values (see p. 34). The two methods of direct measurement of PCV which are in current use are:

1. A macro-method using Wintrobe tubes.
2. A micro-method using capillary tubes.

Although relatively less accurate, the latter is the more popular method as it has the advantages of a short time of centrifugation and better packing of the red cells.

Macro-method (Wintrobe's method)

Wintrobe tubes, 2.5–3 mm in internal diameter and about 110 mm in length calibrated at 1 mm intervals to 100 mm, are employed. They hold about 1 ml of blood.

Collect venous blood with minimal stasis and render it incoagulable by EDTA at a concentration of c 1.5 mg/ml or by heparin at a concentration of 15–20 iu/ml.

Centrifuge the sample with as little delay as possible and no longer than 6 h after collecting it, keeping the blood at 4°C until required.

Mix the blood carefully by repeated inversion and fill the haematocrit tube at once to the 100 mm mark by means of a glass capillary pipette. Centrifuge the tube at 2000–2300 **g** for 30 min*.

The height of the column of red cells is taken as the PCV (the volume occupied by the red cells expressed as a fraction of the total volume of the blood). Above the red cells and not included in the figure for the PCV will be seen a greyish-red layer of leucocytes and above this, just below the plasma, a thin creamy layer of platelets. These comprise the 'buffy coat'.

Range for packed cell volume in health (see p. 8).

---

* Obtainable on request from the National Bureau of Standards, Office of Standard Reference Materials, Washington DC 20234, USA.

* i.e. at a speed of 3000 rpm in a centrifuge of 22.5 cm radius or at a speed of 3800 rpm in a centrifuge of 15 cm radius (see p. 437).

Accuracy of macro-method

This is a potentially accurate method with reproducibility c 1%. However, a number of technical factors can lead to significant inaccuracies. These include

1. Specimen handling.
2. The tubes.
3. Centrifugation.

Specimen handling. Apart from inaccuracies due to delay in setting up the tests, failure to mix the samples of blood adequately or incomplete filling or faulty reading, EDTA anticoagulant in excess of 1.5 mg/ml of blood may lead to cell shrinkage. The degree of oxygenation of the blood also affects the result, as the PCV of venous blood is c 2% higher than that of fully aerated blood (which has lost CO_2 and taken up O_2). Storage of blood leads to changes in PCV. Although these changes take place relatively slowly and can be delayed by keeping the blood at 4°C, the measurement of PCV should be carried out with as little delay as possible, and preferably not longer than 6 h after collecting the blood.

Tubes. Variation in bore is the main cause of error. In tubes which conform to the British Standard for Apparatus for Measurement of Packed Red-Cell Volume (BS 4316: 1968) the bore is 2.55 mm and it does not vary by more than ±2% of the mean throughout.

Centrifugation. The aim is to achieve complete packing of the red cells. In addition to the centrifugal force applied, the speed of packing depends upon the density and the size of the cells, the viscosity of the suspending fluid and the relative densities of cells and fluid.

Centrifugation for 30 min at c 2000 g (within the capacity of most laboratory centrifuges) is sufficient to pack the red cells of an anaemic patient to a constant volume. With PCVs of about the normal range (0.36–0.54), an additional 30 min centrifuging will reduce the apparent red-cell volume by c 1%, whilst in polycythaemia, with a PCV exceeding 0.55, the further packing resulting from the prolonged centrifugation may amount to as much as 3% (e.g. from 0.60 to 0.58). The reason for these discrepancies is that the effective mean radius of the centrifuge (the distance from the spindle of the centrifuge to the mid-point of the packed cell mass) is greater with a low PCV than with a normal PCV. With an abnormally high PCV the effective mean radius of the centrifuge is less than with blood of a normal PCV. As the centrifugal force applied to the contents of the tube is a function of the speed of rotation and the effective radius of the centrifuge, the effective centrifugal force is greater with a low PCV than with a high PCV.

Under the usual conditions of the test procedure, trapped plasma may account for about 3% of the apparent red-cell column in normal blood and even more in certain abnormal conditions, notably iron deficiency, thalassaemia, spherocytosis and sickle-cell disease. While this is not a serious problem in routine clinical practice, it must be taken into account when a high degree of accuracy is required, for example, when estimating blood volume or for calibrating automated blood counters. A reference method has been described in which the amount of trapped plasma can be determined, using radioactive human serum albumin as an indicator.[50]

MICRO-METHOD

The use of haematocrit tubes of much smaller diameter and capacity than Wintrobe tubes is very convenient as a routine procedure in clinical work; furthermore, the tubes can be used with 'capillary' blood collected directly into them. Originally, Strumia et al.[90] employed a centrifuge with a maximum speed of 27 000 rpm; at this speed, using a microhaematocrit tube 32 mm in length, the centrifugal force was calculated to be c 28 000 g. Packing was completed in 1 min and no correction for trapped plasma was thought to be necessary. The machines now available provide a centrifugal force of c 12 000 g and 3–5 min centrifugation results in a constant PCV. When the PCV is greater than 0.5, it may be necessary to centrifuge for a further 5 min. When packing is as complete as possible the column of cells will appear translucent. The amount of trapped plasma is less than with the Wintrobe method. Garby and Vuille reported it as 1.1–1.5% (mean 1.3%).[33] Other authors have reported higher values, namely 2.5–3.5%,[92] 2.78% ± 0.117,[81] and 3%[30] with normal blood. There is a slightly increased amount of plasma trapping in macrocytic anaemias,[30] considerably more in the presence of spherocytes as in hereditary spherocytosis,[32] in thalassaemia,[21] in hypochromic anaemias[30] and in sickle-cell anaemia;[30] it may be as high as 20% in sickle-cell anaemia if all the cells are sickled.

Method

Capillary tubes which are 75 mm in length and have an internal diameter of about 1 mm are required. They can be obtained plain or coated inside with 2 iu of heparin. The latter type are suitable for the direct collection of capillary blood. Plain tubes are used for anti-coagulated venous blood.

Allow the blood to enter the tube by capillarity, leaving at least 15 mm unfilled. Then seal the tube by heating the dry end of the tube rapidly in a fine flame, e.g. the pilot light of a Bunsen burner, combined with rotation. After centrifugation for 5 min, measure the PCV using a reading device.

Accuracy of micro-method

The inaccuracies due to specimen handling described in the previous section apply equally to this method. Also variation in the bore of the tubes may cause serious errors. In one study various capillary tubes were found to have bore variations of up to 15.7%.[8]

Other errors unique to the micro-method are due to difficulty in heat-sealing the lower end of the tube so as to obtain a flat base and difficulties in reading. The former can be minimized by using capillaries made of low melting point soft glass. To avoid errors in reading with the special reading device a magnifying glass should be used. Alternatively, the ratio of red-cell column to whole column (i.e. red cells plus plasma) can be calculated from measurements obtained by placing the tube against arithmetic graph paper or against a ruler. In routine practice it is not customary to correct for trapped plasma, and it is perhaps best to establish a standard method and to recognize its limitations and possible errors. When accuracy is of especial importance, e.g. when the PCV is required for calculating blood volume, a correction factor of 2% should be applied when the PCV is less than 0.5. When it is more than 0.5, centrifugation should be continued for a further 5 min and a correction of 3% should be applied.[49] It is, however, preferable to use the reference method employing radioactive human serum albumin (p. 33), if possible.

MEASUREMENT OF PACKED CELL VOLUME FROM MEAN CELL VOLUME AND RED-CELL COUNT

With some electronic counters PCV can be derived indirectly from the red-cell count and MCV. The PCV obtained by this method is frequently 1.5–3% lower than the micro-haematocrit value; this is because errors due to trapped plasma and inadequate oxygenation are eliminated.[12] On the other hand, the accuracy of derived PCV measurement may be influenced by the shape of the red cells in the diluting medium and their orientation in the sensing zone, by other blood constituents and by the calibration settings of the instrument. Applying a calibration correction to the instrument settings in order to achieve comparability with PCV by centrifugation does not take into account the extent by which plasma trapping varies in different diseases.

MEASUREMENT AND CALCULATION OF SIZE OF RED CELLS

'ABSOLUTE' VALUES

The mean cell volume (MCV), mean cell Hb (MCH) and mean cell Hb concentration (MCHC) have been referred to as 'absolute' values. These values, calculated from the results of the red-cell count, Hb content and PCV have been widely used in the classification of anaemia.

With fully automated counting systems absolute values are measured simultaneously with the red-cell count. In the Coulter S series, MCV is calculated from the mean height of the pulses generated during the red-cell count; Hb is measured as HiCN in a standard procedure; PCV is deduced from the red-cell count and MCV; MCH is deduced from Hb and red-cell count; whilst MCHC is calculated from the measured Hb and the deduced PCV. All the measurements are stored by the machine as voltages which are compared automatically with the voltages generated by the calibration material. The results are expressed in proportion to the original calibration after conversion from analog to digital form. A similar process of measurement and calculation is used in the Ortho ELT system whilst in the Technicon H 6000 the sum of the generated pulses is totalled and the PCV is obtained from this measurement relative to the red-cell count. The MCV and other 'absolute' values are then calculated from this value.

In the Technicon Hemalog, PCV is measured directly by a micro-haematocrit technique.

Calculation of mean cell volume (MCV)

If the PCV and the number of red cells per l (or μl) are known, the MCV can be calculated:
e.g. if the PCV is 0.45, 1 l of blood contains 0.45 l of red cells.
Therefore, if there are 5×10^{12} red cells per l, they occupy a volume of 0.45 l.

$$\text{Therefore, volume of 1 cell} = \frac{0.45}{5 \times 10^{12}}$$

$$= 90 \text{ fl.}$$

In practice, the PCV (0.45) is divided by the red-cell count in millions per μl (5.0) and multiplied by 1000. The answer is expressed in femtolitres.

Calculation of mean cell haemoglobin (MCH)

This can be calculated if the Hb and red-cell count are known:
e.g. if there are 150 g of Hb per l of blood, and if there are 5×10^{12} red cells per l, the mean cell Hb is

$$\frac{150}{5 \times 10^{12}} = \frac{3}{10^{11}} = 30 \text{ picograms (pg).}$$

Calculation of mean cell haemoglobin concentration (MCHC)

This can be calculated if the Hb per l of blood and PCV are known:
e.g. if there are 150 g Hb per l of blood, of PCV 0.45, the MCHC is

$$150 \div 0.45 \text{ g/l} = 333 \text{ g/l.}$$

Range of 'absolute' values

The range of normal 'absolute' values varies slightly depending on whether they are based on automated measurements or on the PCV as determined by centrifuging blood at approximately 1500 **g** or at 2000–2300 **g** for 30 min, or by the micro-method at a much higher **g**, or whether the PCV has been 'corrected' for trapped plasma. In practice, the differences are small and without clinical significance except in iron-deficiency anaemia and thalassaemia in which the PCV is significantly lower by Coulter S Counter than by micro-haematocrit. This results in an automated MCHC which is less abnormally low than is the MCH. The normal range given below is based on micro-haematocrit data not corrected for trapped plasma. Measurements by electronic counters should be within this range but with a smaller SD.

Normal adults (mean ± 2 SD)

Mean cell volume (MCV) = 86 ± 10 fl.
Mean cell haemoglobin
(MCH) = 29.5 ± 2.5 pg.
Mean cell haemoglobin concentration
(MCHC) = 325 ± 25 g/l.

In disease

1. In macrocytic anaemias:
MCV increased up to about 150 fl (rarely higher).
MCH increased up to about 50 pg (rarely higher).
MCHC normal or diminished.

2. In microcytic hypochromic anaemias:
MCV diminished to 50 fl (rarely lower).
MCH diminished to 15 pg (rarely lower).
MCHC diminished to 220 g/l (rarely lower).

Accuracy of the calculation of 'absolute' values

A danger attached to the calculation of 'absolute' values from visual blood count measurements is that the observer may delude himself into a false sense of their accuracy, particularly when the results are expressed to one place of decimals, as has sometimes unjustifiably been done.

Until recently, the only measurement which could be relied upon was the MCHC calculated from the relatively accurate Hb and PCV measurements. MCVs and MCHs based on visual red-cell counts were too inaccurate to be of much clinical value. Now that electronic cell counters can give highly reproducible values for MCV and MCH, these have become much more reliable aids to the recognition of minor degrees of macrocytosis or in the diagnosis of the onset of iron deficiency at an early stage,[18,57,99] and for discriminating between iron deficiency and β-thalassaemia trait.[28,29,53] A formula for this discrimination is:

$$\text{MCV (fl)} - \text{RBC}(\times 10^{12}/1) - (0.5 \times \text{Hb(g/l)}) - k,$$

where k is a constant factor, dependent on the instrument calibration: a positive result indicates β-thalassaemia.[28,29] An analogous calculation has been shown to be useful in detecting α-thalassaemia trait.[40] The extent to which numerical data are a help in diagnosis is again considered in Chapter 8 (p. 132).

In health, when the Hb is normal, an individual's 'absolute' values are remarkably constant and they can be used for instrument calibration.[89]

RED-CELL SIZE DISTRIBUTION

RED-CELL DIAMETERS

Normally, even in health, a population of red cells can be seen to vary appreciably in size, and it was largely owing to the work of Price-Jones[75] that this normal variation was measured and recorded. He showed that if the diameters of a large number of red cells were measured and the cells grouped together in classes according to their diameters, the frequency-distribution curve of diameters was of the 'normal' type. Price-Jones applied statistical methods to his data and calculated limits of normal variation; and he also showed that characteristic deviations from normal were encountered in various types of anaemia. This work excited great interest and at one time the drawing of a Price-Jones curve was considered to be an almost essential step in the investigation of any obscure case of anaemia—although the labour expended contributed nothing to the understanding of the case and merely placed on paper what was to be seen by inspection of a stained film!

The measurement of red-cell diameters in dried films is a highly artificial method; not only do cells shrink on drying, their diameters being then 8–16% less than when the cells are suspended in plasma,[74] but their diameters also vary appreciably artefactually in different parts of a dried film. An area of film where the cells are neither distorted nor shrunken has therefore to be found before measurements can be made. Moreover, in anaemias such as severe pernicious anaemia it is extremely difficult, if not impossible, to measure accurately the diameters of the poikilocytes likely to be present. There is little doubt but that the laborious Price-Jones method of the individual measurement of red cells in dried films is less accurate than was at one time supposed.

For clinical purposes the measurement of 500 cells, as was recommended by Price-Jones, is superfluous, although this enables fairly smooth diameter-distribution curves to be drawn. The accuracy of estimation of the mean cell diameter is hardly increased by increasing the number of cells counted from 100 to 500; the standard deviation, on the other hand, will be less.

Various modifications of the Price-Jones technique have been introduced from time to time. Instead of actually measuring the images of projected red cells with a glass or plastic rule, diameters may be scored by finding the best fit with a series of black rings of different sizes. Alternatively, the images of the cells may be projected on to a ground glass screen. Another method available for the measurement of red-cell diameters is the use of an eye-piece micrometer.

Measurement of red-cell diameter with an eye-piece micrometer

The method has the advantages of directness and simplicity and can be quickly applied to stained blood films.

The scale of the eye-piece micrometer has to be calibrated in relation to the objective, eye-piece and tube-length employed, before it can be used. This is best done using a slide on which a scale, usually 1 mm in 0.01 mm (10 μm) intervals, has been engraved. Alternatively, the calibrations on a counting chamber can be utilized (the side of the smallest square is 0.05 mm in length).

It is convenient to have a conversion scale kept near the microscope, e.g. using a 2 mm objective and × 6 eye-pieces: 5.0 divisions = 6.6 μm, 5.5 divisions = 7.2 μm, 6.0 divisions = 7.9 μm, 6.5 divisions = 8.5 μm, etc.

The diameters of red cells can be measured to about 0.5 μm without difficulty with the aid of the eye-piece micrometer. The accuracy of measurement is dependent upon correct illumination, in accordance with Kohler's principle, and the objective used must have a minimum numerical aperture of 0.85. Inconstant optical conditions can result in considerable error. The method is useful although minor degrees of deviation from the normal will not be detected. Nevertheless, in practice, it is possible by measuring a few representative cells to confirm or refute a visual impression of abnormality. This does not mean that the observer should search for the largest or smallest cells to measure, for a few as large as 9 μm or as small as 6 μm may be seen in dried films of normal blood. It is much more significant to find an unusually high proportion of cells of 8.5 μm than a few outside these limits. Price-Jones gave normal limits for cells of the dimensions just referred to.[75]

Range of red-cell diameters in health (MCD)

Price Jones,
   dry films[75] 6.7–7.7 μm (mean 7.2 μm).
Houchin, Munn and Parnell[44]
   cells in rouleaux 8.1–8.7 μm (mean 8.3 μm).

Westerman, Pierce and Jensen[104]
   cells in rouleaux 8.3–9.1 μm (mean 8.7 μm).
   isolated cells 8.6 μm (mean).

CALCULATION OF MEAN RED-CELL THICKNESS (MCT)

Mean cell thickness can be calculated from the mean cell diameter and mean cell volume on the assumption that the red cell is a short cylinder rather than a biconcave disc. Thus the MCT, or more correctly MCAT (mean cell average thickness) is given by:

$$\frac{\text{MCV}}{\pi\left(\dfrac{\text{MCD}}{2}\right)^2} .$$

It is obvious that a figure for MCT, as derived above, is only an approximate measurement, and it is doubtful whether its calculation is of any practical value.

Red-cell surface area may be calculated from the diameter and thickness measurements.[44,104]

Normal range for red-cell thickness (MCT)

Dry films 1.7–2.5 μm.
Houchin, Munn and Parnell[44]
   cells in rouleaux 1.5–1.9 μm (mean 1.7 μm).
Westerman, Pierce and Jensen[104]
   cells in rouleaux 1.5–1.7 μm (mean 1.6 μm).

Normal range for red-cell surface area

Houchin, Munn and Parnell[44]
   128–144 μm^2 (mean 134 μm^2).
Westerman, Pierce and Jensen[104]
   132–160 μm^2 (mean 145 μm^2).

RED-CELL VOLUME

As the MCV is only a measure of the mean red cell volume, its measurement may miss a small but possibly significant degree of microcytosis or macrocytosis. It is now possible to obtain volume distribution curves using automated counters (see below). Curves obtained in this way are more sensitive than are the conventional red-cell indices for studying, for example, the early response to therapy in iron deficiency and megaloblastic anaemias, identifying multiple deficiency states or a dimorphic red-cell population and discounting the confusing presence of (normal) transfused cells in the blood of a patient whose own cells are abnormal.[5,26,31]

Cell size distribution curves can be obtained easily using a semi-automatic Coulter Counter (e.g. ZBI) to which is attached a Channelyzer C-1000 (Coulter Electronics); a similar unit is now incorporated in some of the newer automated counting systems. Results are presented as a frequency distribution histogram from which are calculated mean, median and modal cell volumes and their standard deviations. The normal curve appears to have a log-normal distribution[26]; its accuracy depends on the calibration of the instrument, but it may also be influenced by the non-axial flow of cells or their distortion as they pass through the orifice and by an effect of the diluent on the cells.[41,94]

The following data were derived from automated measurements of red-cell volume distribution curves in a series of healthy men and women:[26]

	Men	Women
Mean red-cell volume	87.7 fl.	87.6 fl.
Median red-cell volume	86.5 fl.	86.3 fl.
Modal red-cell volume	84.1 fl.	83.9 fl.
Size variation of 95% of cells	62–120 fl.	62–120 fl.

LEUCOCYTE COUNTS

Total counts by electronic methods

To get rid of the red cells before the leucocytes are counted, a lytic agent is required which destroys the red cells and eliminates red-cell stroma, but does not destroy the leucocytes, or at least only destroys them slowly. The following fluid appears to be satisfactory when used with the Coulter Counter:[22] Cetavlon 20 g, 10% formaldehyde (in 9 g/l NaCl (saline)) 2 ml, glacial acetic acid 16 ml, sodium citrate 14 g, NaCl 6 g and water to 1 l.

Dilute 20 μl of blood in 10 ml of saline, and add 2 drops of the above solution. Lysis is instantaneous. The count is stable for at least 40 min and the background count is low.

Saponin has also been extensively used as a lytic agent but it does not cause complete lysis of the red cells, the leucocytes swell and the background count is relatively high. Zaponin (Coulter), Zapoglobin (Coulter), Lysoton (Hyland) and similar commercial products appear to be more effective. With these, the cytoplasm is stripped, leaving leucocyte nuclei similar in size to the red cells. Thus, when calibrating the counter the same lytic agent and diluent should be used for routine counts.[56]

Total counts by visual method

Make a 1 in 20 dilution of blood by adding 20 μl of blood to 0.38 ml of diluting fluid in a 75 × 10 mm glass or plastic tube. Bulb pipettes are not recommended (see p. 26). After tightly corking the tube, mix the suspension by rotating in a cell-suspension mixer for at least 1 min. Fill the counting chamber by means of a Pasteur pipette or stout glass capillary, as for red-cell counts (p. 24).

The red cells are lysed by the diluting fluid (see below) but the leucocytes remain intact, their nuclei staining deep violet-black. View the preparation using a 4 mm objective and ×6 eye-pieces or a 16 mm objective and ×10 eyepieces. Count at least 100 cells in as many 1 mm² areas (0.1 μl in volume) as may be necessary—the ruled area in an improved Neubauer chamber consists of 9 of these areas.

Calculation

$$\text{count (/l)} = \frac{\text{No. of cells counted}}{\text{volume counted } (\mu l)} \times \text{dilution} \times 10^6.$$

Thus, if N cells are counted in 0.1μl, then the

leucocyte count per litre

$$= N \times 10 \times 20 \text{ (dilution)} \times 10^6$$

$$= N \times 200 \times 10^6$$

$$(= N \times 20 \text{ per } \mu l).$$

Diluting fluid

2% (20 ml/l) acetic acid coloured pale violet with gentian violet.
Range of the total leucocyte count in health (see p. 8).

Error of the total leucocyte count

The factors causing errors in counting leucocytes by the visual method are the same as in counting red cells. As many leucocytes as possible should be counted; 100 cells is a reasonable and practical figure for visual counts. The standard deviation (SD) of a 100-cell count is approximately $\sqrt{100} = 10$, and the coefficient of variation (CV) is thus 10%: 95% of counts of mean value 100 would thus lie within the range $100 \pm 2SD = 80$–120. Translated into actual results, this means that 95% of observed counts on a blood of true value 5.0×10^9 cells per l would lie within the range 4.0–6.0.

Fortunately, error in the leucocyte count is not nearly as important as error in red-cell counts; even an error as high as 20% does not matter much—the difference between 5.0 and 6.0×10^9 cells per l is of little practical significance. The error can be reduced by counting more cells, and with high counts this can be accomplished without the expenditure of much extra time. If 400 cells are counted, the CV is reduced to 5%

$$\left(\frac{\sqrt{400}}{400} \times 100 \right).$$

Other potential causes of error include mistaking dirt or clumped red-cell debris for leucocytes and the clumping of leucocytes. The latter—usually several leucocytes stuck to debris—seems to occur particularly in heparinized blood, especially when the concentration of heparin is high. The clumps are most frequently seen in blood which has been

allowed to stand for several hours before undertaking the count.

With electronic counters the major source of error is incorrect calibration. Other factors which may cause erroneous results include excessive debris from inadequately lysed red cells, adherence of leucocytes to the aperture of the sensing zone, air bubbles and carry over from the previous sample. This last is especially important as a potential source of error when the count is low; it can be prevented by washing the counter through three or four times with the diluent (e.g. Isoton II, Coulter), noting the blank reading on the cycle of the final wash and subtracting this from the subsequent leucocyte count.[45] Erroneously high leucocyte counts have been reported with cryoglobulinaemia.[38] In some counters results are unreliable when the leucocyte count is greater than $30 \times 10^9/l$.

DIFFERENTIAL LEUCOCYTE COUNT

Differential leucocyte counts are usually performed on blood films which are prepared on slides by the spread or 'wedge' technique. Unfortunately, even in well-spread films the distribution of the various cell types is not totally random (see below). To overcome this, a spin preparation method has been proposed by means of which the cells are evenly distributed on the slide as a monolayer.[46,71] The following description is concerned with differential leucocyte counts made on films spread on slides.

For an accurate differential leucocyte count, the film must not be too thin and the tail of the film should be smooth. To achieve this the film should be made with a rapid movement using a smooth glass spreader (see p. 50). This should result in a film in which there is some overlap of the red cells, diminishing to separation near the tail, and in which the leucocytes in the body of the film are not too badly shrunken. If the film is made too thinly, or if a rough-edged spreader is used, many of the leucocytes, perhaps even 50% of them, accumulate at the edges and in the tail (Fig. 3.3). Moreover, a gross qualitative irregularity in distribution is the rule: polymorphonuclear neutrophils and monocytes predominate at the margins and the tail, and

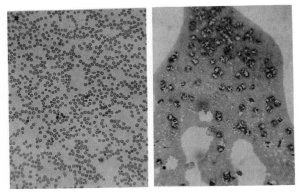

Fig. 3.3 Centre (left) and tail (right) of a badly made blood film. The centre of the film is almost devoid of leucocytes; in the tail neutrophils, particularly, are present in large numbers. ×100.

lymphocytes in the middle of the film (Fig. 3.4). This separation probably depends upon differences in stickiness, size and specific gravity among the different classes of cells.

Various systems of performing the differential count have been advocated. The problem is to overcome the differences in distribution of the various classes of cells, which are probably always present to a small extent even in well made films. No system of counting will compensate for the gross irregularities in distribution in a badly made film. It is a waste of time to attempt a differential count on such a film and, if this is attempted, futile to count only the cells in the centre of the film, where lymphocytes probably predominate, and to neglect altogether the tail, where most of the neutrophils lie. If the film has been well made, and many leucocytes are present in the body of the film and there is no great accumulation at the tail, the following technique of counting is recommended.

Method

Count the cells using a 4 mm dry or 3.7 mm oil-immersion lens, in a strip running the whole length of the film. Avoid the lateral edges of the film. Inspect the film from the head to the tail, and if less than 100 cells are encountered in a single narrow strip, examine one or more additional strips until at least 100 cells have been counted. Each longitudinal strip represents the blood drawn out from a small part of the original drop of blood when it has spread out between the slide and spreader (Fig. 3.5). If all the cells are counted in such a strip, the differential totals will approximate closely to the true differential count. This technique admittedly does not allow for any excess of neutrophils and monocytes at the edges of the film, but this preponderance is slight in a well made film and in practice makes little difference to the result.

The above technique is easy to carry out; with high counts (10.0–30.0 × 10⁹ cells per l) a short, 2–3 cm, film is desirable. In patients with very high counts (as in leukaemia) the method has to be abandoned and the cells should be counted in any well spread area where the cell types are easy to identify. Other systems of counting, such as the 'battlement' count,[62] seem to be more elaborate and have no advantage.

Most workers find it possible to remember accurately the differential counts of small groups of 20 to 25 cells, writing the results on

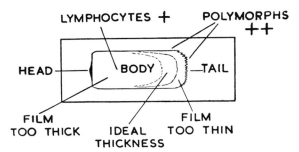

Fig. 3.4 Schematic drawing of a blood film made on a slide. The film has been spread from left to right. An indication is given of the way the leucocytes are distributed (see text).

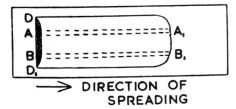

Fig. 3.5 Schematic drawing illustrating the longitudinal method of performing differential leucocyte counts. The original drop of blood spreads out between spreader and slide (D–D₁). The film is made in such a way that representative strips of films, such as A–A₁ and B–B₁, are formed from blood originally at A and B, respectively. In order to perform an accurate differential count, *all* the leucocytes in one or more strips, such as A–A₁ and B–B₁, should be inspected and classified.

paper when each small group has been surveyed. However, a multiple manual register is a help in recording the results of a count. With some sophisticated electronic registers, the differential count is entered directly into a computerized data processor alongside the results of the automated blood count.

The observed differential count depends not only on artefactual differences in distribution due to the process of spreading, but also on 'random' distribution; together they are by far the most important cause of unreliable differential counts.[24] Deviation of the counts of a major cell population is Gaussian*; that of a minor population is a Poisson distribution†.[109] In practical terms the random distribution means that, if a total of 100 cells are counted, with a true neutrophil proportion of 50%, the range ($\pm$2SD) within which 95% of the counts will fall, is of the order of about $\pm$14%, i.e. 36–64% neutrophils.

A 200-cell count can provide a more accurate estimate; in the above example, the $\pm$2SD range will be about 40–60%. In a 500-cell count the range would be reduced to 44–56% neutrophils. In the case of a minor population, if the true count is 3% in a 100-cell differential count, in 95 out of 100 counts, the count would range between 0% and 6%, whilst a true count of 10% is a likely to be counted as anything between 5% and 15%. Even 500-cell counts are little better for the counting of cells present in low percentages. An automated technique is the only practical way by which the large number of cells necessary may be scrutinized.

AUTOMATED DIFFERENTIAL LEUCOCYTE COUNTING[3,23,54]

Two methods have been developed—continuous flow cytochemistry and high resolution pattern recognition. Continuous flow cytochemistry is the principle of the Technicon Hemalog D and H 6000.[64,67,76] The blood, after dilution in an appropriate reagent, is directed into different channels where the leucocytes are differentiated by cytochemical reactions and size. In the H 6000, in one channel basophils are detected with alcian blue, in a second channel the remaining cells are classified by peroxidase activity and size. The major advantage of this system is that 10 000 cells are counted in 1 min, thus providing high precision. Some discrepancies have been noted when comparison is made with classification based on traditional morphology[14,54] but the discrepancies are not serious enough to prevent the system being useful as a screening procedure.

Pattern recognition

This is an adaptation of traditional differential leucocyte counting and, although it uses sophisticated computer technology for the pattern recognition, its basis is classification of cells by their morphological features in Romanowsky-stained films. These are scanned under a microscope by a high resolution photosensor which generates electronic signals corresponding to various features of the cells (e.g. size, shape, periphery, texture, granularity, nuclear-cytoplasmic ratio) and compares then with patterns of cells in the computer's memory. Thus, the reliability of the instrument in identifying cells will depend on how and to what extent it has been instructed; moreover, it is dependent on the staining of the test slides being similar to that of the original training set.

Several systems are available commercially (e.g. Abbott ADC 500; Perkin-Elmer Diff 3; Leitz Hematrak; Microx Omron Analyser). They differ in the range of cells which they have been programmed to identify and, thus, in the extent to which they are independent of technical supervision when a count is being carried out. This also effects their speed of performance; in the different systems a 500-cell count takes 2–6 mins.

A third method for distinguishing different types of cells is by leucocyte volume analysis using an electronic counter linked to a pulse height analyser.[25] At least two cell populations can be resolved—smaller cells which are mainly lymphocytes, and larger ones which are mainly neutrophils. This limited differential count can be used as a screening test. It has now been incorporated in

---

* 'Gaussian' distribution describes events (data) which occur symmetrically about a mean.
† 'Poisson' distribution describes rare events which are random in their occurrence.

the Coulter Model S Plus Phase II which gives the percentage and absolute numbers of lymphocytes (the smaller leucocytes) as part of the blood count.

Range of differential leucocyte counts in health (see p. 8).

EOSINOPHIL COUNTS BY COUNTING-CHAMBER METHOD

Although total eosinophil counts can be roughly calculated from the total and differential leucocyte counts, the staining properties of eosinophils make it possible to count them directly and more accurately in a counting chamber.

The principles underlying the counting-chamber or 'wet' eosinophil count were reviewed by Spiers.[86] Ideally, the diluent should stain the eosinophil granules brightly and distinctly and at the same time lyse the red cells and all other types of leucocytes.

Diluting fluids for eosinophil counts

The acetone group of diluents, introduced by Dunger,[20] contain:

1. An acid dye, such as eosin or phloxine.

2. Water to lyse the red cells and rupture the leucocyte membranes (the eosinophils seem more resistant than other leucocytes in this respect).

3. Acetone to inhibit the lytic action of water on the leucocytes according to the proportion used— about 5–10% seems to be the most useful concentration.

In later modifications of Dunger's diluent small amounts of a detergent[20] or alkali[86] were added to accelerate the staining of the eosinophil granules.

Method

Add 20 μl of EDTA blood to 0.38 ml of diluting fluid to give a 1 in 20 dilution. Mix the suspension for not longer than 30 s, and then fill the counting chamber using a stout glass capillary or Pasteur pipette. The eosinophils may be counted as soon as they have settled or the count may be postponed for 30 min or so if

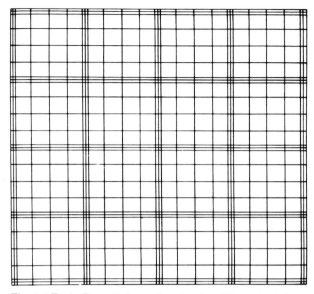

Fig. 3.6 Fuchs-Rosenthal counting chamber. The total ruled area is 4 mm × 4 mm, divided into 16 large squares, 1 mm × 1 mm, each containing 16 small squares.

the counting chamber is placed in a moist chamber (a Petri dish with cover containing a pledget of damp cotton wool).

Counting Chamber. A chamber with the Fuchs-Rosenthal ruling is suitable. The ruled area in a Fuchs-Rosenthal chamber is a 4 mm square (Fig. 3.6) and the chamber is 0.2 mm in depth (area 16 mm^2 and volume 3.2 μl).* With counts at the upper limit of the normal range (see below) the whole ruled area should be surveyed and the total number of eosinophils recorded. With lower counts several fillings of the counting chamber may be surveyed. It is convenient to use a 16 mm objective and ×10 eyepieces. In a good clean preparation the eosinophils should be easily identified; their granules stain deep red and the cells containing them should be intact.

As in ordinary leucocyte counts the accuracy of the count is largely determined by the number of cells counted. In a serious investigation 100 cells should be looked upon as the minimum, the counting chamber being

* A modified version is also available in which the ruled area is a 3-mm square, total area 9 mm^2.

filled several times, if necessary. The coefficient of variation due to the random distribution of the cells is c 10% in a 100-cell count.

Calculation

$$\text{Count (/l)} = \frac{\text{No of cells counted}}{\text{Volume counted (}\mu\text{l)}}$$
$$\times \text{ dilution} \times 10^6.$$

Thus, if N eosinophils are counted in 3.2 μl, then the total eosinophil count per litre

$$= \frac{N \times 20 \text{ (dilution)}}{3.2} \times 10^6$$

$$= N \times 6.25 \times 10^6$$

$$(= N \times 6.25 \text{ per } \mu\text{l}).$$

Diluting fluid

Eosin, aqueous, (200 g/l) 10 ml, acetone 10 ml, water 80 ml. The fluid will keep for 2–3 weeks at 4°C. It must be filtered before use.

Eosinophils slowly disintegrate in the diluting fluid and the count should not be delayed for more than 15–30 min. It is probably best to fill the counting chamber as soon as the blood is diluted and to avoid prolonged mixing, for in this way, clumping of the eosinophils may be prevented.[4]

Range of eosinophil count in health. 40–440 $\times 10^6$/1.[70,80]

There is normally considerable diurnal variation in the eosinophil count and differences amounting to as much as 100% have been recorded. The lowest counts are found in the morning (10 a.m. to noon) and the highest at night (midnight to 4 a.m.).[6,80,100] Muehrcke et al.[70] found that the counts of 42 healthy but fasting young males conformed to a log-normal distribution. Although the height of the count is controlled, to some extent at least, by the adrenal cortex[43] eosinophil counts are seldom now used as an index of adrenocortical activity.

PLATELET COUNTS

Many methods for counting platelets have been published and their number is doubtless due to real difficulties in counting small bodies which agglutinate and break up so easily, and which may be difficult to distinguish from extraneous matter. The reader is referred to the excellent earlier reviews of Tocantins[97,98] and more recent reviews[9,103] for technical and other details concerning mammalian platelets. The introduction of electronic counting systems has greatly improved counting precision. A visual direct method is described which is suitable for moderately low normal to high counts. A method is also described using plasma which is valuable when the count is low.

Visual method for whole blood[10]

The diluent consists of 1% ammonium oxalate in which the red cells are lysed. There is a possibility that red-cell debris may be mistaken for platelets but with some experience this should not cause any difficulties. The method described in the previous edition, using formal-citrate diluent is more likely to give incorrect results, incorrectly low counts being especially marked when the platelet count is low.[61]

Reagent

10 g/l ammonium oxalate. Not more than 500 ml should be made at a time, using scrupulously clean glassware and fresh glass-distilled or de-ionized water. The solution should be filtered through a micropore filter (0.22 μm) and kept at 4°C. For use, a small part of the stock is refiltered and dispensed in 1.9 ml volumes in 75 $\times$ 12 mm tubes.

Method

Collect blood into a dry plastic syringe using a short needle of 19 or 20 SWG. It is essential that the puncture is a clean one and that the blood flows into the syringe with the minimum of suction. Detach the needle from the syringe and deliver the requisite amount of blood without frothing into a vessel containing EDTA. Mix gently and without delay. If the collection of blood has been satisfactory, the dilution of the blood may be postponed for 3–4 h.

It is convenient to make a 1 in 20 dilution of the blood in the diluent by adding 0.1 ml of blood to 1.9 ml of the diluent. Mix the suspension on a mechanical mixer for 10–15 min.

Fill a Neubauer counting chamber with the suspension, using a stout glass capillary or Pasteur pipette. Place the counting chamber in a moist Petri dish and leave untouched for at least 20 min to give time for the platelets to settle.

Examine the preparation with the 4 mm objective and ×6 or ×10 eyepieces. The platelets appear under ordinary illumination as small (but not minute) highly refractile particles, if viewed with the condenser racked down; they are usually well separated and clumps are rare if the blood sample has been skilfully collected. They are more easily seen with the phase-contrast microscope. A special thin-bottomed (1 mm) counting chamber is best for optimal phase-contrast effect.

The number of platelets in one or more areas of 1 mm^2 should be counted. The total number of platelets counted should always exceed 200.

Calculation

$$\text{Count (/l)} = \frac{\text{No. of cells counted}}{\text{Volume counted } (\mu l)} \times \text{dilution} \times 10^6.$$

Thus, if N be the number of platelets counted in an area of 1 mm^2 (0.1μl in volume), the number of platelets per l blood

$= N \times 10 \times 20 \text{ (dilution)} \times 10^6$

$= N \times 200 \times 10^6$

$(= N \times 200 \text{ per } \mu l).$

Modified method using plasma in place of whole blood

This method is basically the same as that described in the preceding paragraphs.

However, instead of diluting whole blood, plasma is used; this enables low platelet counts (even as low as 10×10^9/l) to be carried out reliably. The blood is allowed to stand at room temperature (18–25°C) until a few mm of plasma are visible. Make a 1 in 10 dilution of the plasma by adding 0.1 ml of plasma to 0.9 ml of diluting fluid. Mix for 1 min, and then fill the counting chamber and leave the preparation to stand in a damp chamber for 20 min or even longer for all the platelets to settle before counting.

Calculation

$$\text{Count (/l)} = \frac{\text{No. of cells counted}}{\text{Volume counted } (\mu l)} \times \text{dilution} \times (1 - \text{PCV}) \times 10^6.$$

Thus, if N be the number of platelets counted in an area of 1 mm^2 (0.1 μl in volume), the number of platelets per l of blood

$= N \times 10 \times 10 \text{ (dilution)} \times (1 - \text{PCV}) \times 10^6$/l

$= N \times 100 \times (1 - \text{PCV}) \times 10^6$/l

$(= N \times 100 \times (1 - \text{PCV}) \text{ per } \mu l).$

The result is adjusted by multiplying by $(1 - \text{PCV})$ to allow for the fact that the count is carried out on plasma, not on whole blood. Alternatively, the correction factors given in Table 3.2 can be used.

Table 3.2 Platelet count correction factors.[13]

PCV : Factor	PCV : Factor	PCV : Factor
0.20 : 0.78	0.30 : 0.63	0.40 : 0.45
0.21 : 0.77	0.31 : 0.61	0.41 : 0.44
0.22 : 0.75	0.32 : 0.60	0.42 : 0.42
0.23 : 0.74	0.33 : 0.58	0.43 : 0.41
0.24 : 0.73	0.34 : 0.57	0.44 : 0.40
0.25 : 0.71	0.35 : 0.54	0.45 : 0.39
0.26 : 0.70	0.36 : 0.52	0.46 : 0.38
0.27 : 0.68	0.37 : 0.50	0.47 : 0.37
0.28 : 0.66	0.38 : 0.48	0.48 : 0.36
0.29 : 0.65	0.39 : 0.47	0.49 : 0.35
		0.50 : 0.34

To convert the plasma platelet count to a whole-blood platelet count, multiply the plasma count by the factor shown, according to the PCV of the original blood sample. The reliability of the correction factors has been questioned[37] but provided that the technique is used correctly, they appear to be valid.[59]

PLATELET COUNTS ON PERIPHERAL BLOOD

Platelet counts can be carried out on finger or ear-prick blood but the results are less satisfactory than those carried out on venous blood. Peripheral-blood counts are significantly lower than venous and less constant[11] and a variable number of platelets are probably lost at the site of the skin puncture.

PLATELET COUNTS BY ELECTRONIC METHODS

Electronic instruments with appropriate threshold calibration can be used for counting platelets. The method has been considered in a number of reviews.[36,39,59,66,77] Their reliability may be affected by errors connected with the instrument and its calibration and the tendency of platelets to aggregate, and by the presence in the diluent of particles which may be little smaller than platelets, and by overlap between large platelets and small red cells. Reference materials are now available to ensure correct instrument calibration (p. 17).[61] An additional and important source of difficulty is the separation of red cells from the platelet-containing plasma. A method which has been used extensively is based on the gravitational sedimentation of blood.[13] A modification of the method uses a special centrifuge to achieve accelerated sedimentation (Thrombofuge, Coulter). Both methods are satisfactory but they are liable to error due to variation in the level of supernatant plasma at which the sample is removed.[59] The differential centrifugation method described below overcomes this source of error, and is recommended. The sedimentation method is described later.

Differential centrifugation method[17]

Material

Pour 60 ml of 32.8% sodium metrizoate solution, sp gr 1.200 (±0.001) (Nyegaard, Olso) into a clean dry 150 ml glass bottle. Add 60 ml of Isoton II (Coulter Electronics) and mix well for 10 min on a roller mixer. Filter through a 0.22 μm micropore filter. Store at 4°C in the dark.

Method

Pour 10 ml of the fluid into a plastic 25 ml container. Add 0.1 ml of a well mixed sample of EDTA blood, using a clean dry pipette. Mix the blood with the fluid by rolling the tube in the palms of the hands for 30 s. Then centrifuge for 3 min at 2000 **g**. Remove approximately 8 ml of the red-cell-free supernatant into a clean plastic container. Remix for 30 s before removing 0.2 ml and diluting in 10 ml of Isoton II for electronic counting. By this procedure the original whole blood sample has been diluted 1:5151.

Sedimentation method

The advantage of this method over that described above is that it is particularly suitable for use with small volumes of blood.

Prepare sedimentation tubes from small-bore plastic (polyvinyl chloride, PVC) tubing, internal diameter 2 mm, as follows: seal the tubing every 8 cm (by means of a blood-bank tubing sealer) and then cut through at the seals and midway between them in order to form segments 4 cm in length, sealed at one end*. Dip the open end of a tube into a container of EDTA blood, and then gently squeeze the tube so that c 0.1 ml of the blood is sucked into the tube to a level above the open end. Then wipe the open end clean and place the tube with the sealed end up in a rack at an angle of 45°. Allow the sedimentation to proceed for sufficient time to provide an adequate amount of plasma. This usually takes 10–50 min. Then cut the tube through with scissors at or above the junction of red cells and plasma, and invert the upper part so that the residual red cells sediment rapidly through the plasma. Take a volume of the plasma layer into a

* Or available from Coulter Electronics Ltd.

capillary pipette and deliver into an appropriate volume of diluent for subsequent platelet counting. Correct the result of the count for PCV as described on p. 44. It is also necessary to take account of the fact that some plasma is trapped by the red cells as they sediment. The correction factors which convert the plasma platelet count to whole-blood platelet count are given in Table 3.2.[13]

For Coulter counting, take 3 μl of plasma in a micropipette and dilute it 1 in 3000 in particle-free 9 g/l NaCl or Isoton II.

Normal range of platelet count

In health there are approximately 150–400 $\times$ 10^9 platelets per l of blood. The counts in individual subjects have been reported as being relatively constant,[10,85] although there is some evidence of a diurnal variation. There may also be a sex difference (see p. 12); in women there is cycling with a slightly lower count at about the time of menstruation.[69]

The use of EDTA as anticoagulant has removed the one former major difficulty in platelet counting—namely, the clumping of platelets. In some cases, EDTA at a concentration of 1.5 mg/ml fails to prevent clumping. However, EDTA should not be used at a concentration greater than c 2 mg/ml, for the platelets then tend to swell and disrupt, and cause an erroneously high count. Accuracy in visual counting is only achieved by the most careful regard to detail, particularly with respect to the cleanliness of the preparation, and by experience, which alone can help in deciding what is and what is not a platelet. Under these circumstances the error should not exceed by much that of other chamber cell-counting methods. As already mentioned, the use of phase-contrast microscopy helps considerably in recognizing and counting platelets.

The 'normal' range for platelet counts in the literature is astonishingly large, being from 150 $\times$ 10^9 to 600 $\times$ 10^9/l or more.[85] Although there is clearly considerable individual variation, much of this wide range is probably due to differences in technique. There is certainly no reason to believe that high counts are necessarily correct; probably, fragments of platelets and other particles are included in the counts.

With the visual method the coefficient of variation (CV) is 8–10%. By electronic counting better reproducibility is obtained and a CV of 3–4% is possible. Electronic counting cannot, however, overcome error caused by platelet clumping and/or fragmentation.

MEASUREMENT OF PLATELET VOLUME

Some of the recently developed automated systems include measurement of platelet volume distribution.[79] Normally the platelet volume is distributed in a log-normal way;[72] in EDTA blood their mean volume is c 9 fl, median volume slightly less. The 'plateletcrit' is about 0.0015–0.003 (i.e. 0.15–0.3%).[78,79] Several studies have illustrated the potential value of these measurements. Thus, platelet volume appears to correlate fairly well with platelet aggregation and other tests of function;[51] in hypersplenism the mean platelet volume is less than in immune thrombocytopenia as large platelets appear to be preferentially sequestered in the spleen.[34,52,55] Platelet size can also be measured by the Channelyzer (Coulter Electronics).[51,78] Unfortunately the different systems give different results, and reference material with values determined by one method cannot be used to calibrate an instrument which uses a different system.[22,78] The results are also affected by the method of collection, type of anticoagulant used and storage time of the specimen.

AUTOMATED HAEMATOLOGY

The introduction of a comprehensive automated system usually means that the laboratory has to be organized to ensure efficient and effective use of the expensive equipment. In selecting a system, it is important to assess how it will fulfil the requirements of the laboratory. Account must be taken of the rate at which the equipment can operate (at present between 50 and 100 specimens can be handled per hour by different instruments): clearly the slower machines would be inadequate for a laboratory with a daily workload of 500 specimens or more. The cost of reagents and other materials must be ascertained, as reagents supplied specifically for an instrument are often more expensive, and are required in larger amounts, than those used in manual techniques. The availability of services (water, compressed air, drainage) has to be considered; whether a controlled environment is required, and the effect of the instrument on the environment in terms of vibration, noise and heat production. Also the training required and the extent to which this is provided by the manufacturer and the maintenance and repair service provided by the manufacturer or agent.

Guidelines have been published to help to choose an instrument suitable for the needs of an individual laboratory and also to assess its performance, as compared with the claims of the manufacturer, when it has been installed and is being used in routine practice.[47,83]

REFERENCES

[1] BALLARD, B. C. D. (1972). Lysing agent for the Coulter S. *Journal of Clinical Pathology*, **25**, 460.

[2] BARNARD, D. F., CARTER, A. B., CROSLAND TAYLOR, P. J. and STEWART, J. W. Comparison of Isoton and Isoton II. *Medical Laboratory Science*, **33**, 321.

[3] BENTLEY, S. A. and LEWIS, S. M. (1980). Aspects of automated differential leucocyte counting. *Topical Reviews in Haematology*, **1**, 50.

[4] BERGSTRAND, C. G., HELLSTRÖM. B. and JOHNSSON, B. (1950). Remarks on the technique of eosinophil counting. *Scandinavian Journal of Clinical and Laboratory Investigation*, **2**, 341.

[5] BESSMAN, J. D. and JOHNSON, R. K. (1975). Erythrocyte volume distribution in normal and abnormal subjects. *Blood*, **46**, 369.

[6] BEST, W. R. and SAMSTER, M. (1951). Variation and error in eosinophil counts of blood and bone marrow. *Blood*, **6**, 61.

[7] BOROVICZENY, C. G. (1966). On the standardization of the blood cell counts. *Bibliotheca haematologica (Basel)*, **24**, 2.

[8] BOROVICZENY, C. G. (1966). On the standardization of packed cell volume determination. *Bibliotheca haematologica (Basel)*, **24**, 83.

[9] BRECHER, G. (1971). Enumeration of blood platelets: methods and their validity. *International Academy of Pathology Monograph No. 11*, 358.

[10] BRECHER, G. and CRONKITE, E. P. (1950). Morphology and enumeration of human blood platelets. *Journal of Applied Physiology*, **3**, 365.

[11] BRECHER, G., SCHNEIDERMAN, M. and CRONKITE, E. P. (1953). The reproducibility and constancy of the platelet count. *American Journal of Clinical Pathology*, **23**, 15.

[12] BRITTIN, G. M., BRECHER, G. and JOHNSON, C. A. (1969). Evaluation of the Coulter counter model S. *American Journal of Clinical Pathology*, **52**, 679.

[13] BULL, B. S., SCHNEIDERMAN, M. A. and BRECHER, G. (1965). Platelet counts with the Coulter counter. *American Journal of Clinical Pathology*, **44**, 678.

[14] CAIRNS, J. W., HEALY, M. J. R., STAFFORD, D. M., VITEK, P. and WATERS, D. A. W. (1977). Evaluation of the Hemalog D differential leucocyte counter. *Journal of Clinical Pathology*, **30**, 997.

[15] CLEGG, J. W. and KING, E. J. (1942). Estimation of haemoglobin by the alkaline haematin method. *British Medical Journal*, **ii**, 329.

[16] COULTER, W. H. (1956). High speed automatic blood cell counter and cell size analyser. *Proceedings of National Electronics Conference*, **12**, 1034.

[17] COUSINS, S. and LEWIS, S. M. (1982). A rapid and accurate differential centrifugation method for platelet counts. *Journal of Clinical Pathology*, **35**, 114.

[18] DAVIDSON, R. J. L. and HAMILTON, P. J. (1978). High mean red cell volume: its incidence and significance in routine haematology. *Journal of Clinical Pathology*, **31**, 493.

[19] DRABKIN, D. L. and AUSTIN, J. H. (1932). Spectrophotometric studies: spectrometric constants for common haemoglobin derivatives in human, dog and rabbit blood. *Journal of Biological Chemistry*, **98**, 719.

[20] DUNGER, R. (1910). Eine einfache Methode der Zählung der eosinophilen Leukozyten und der praktische Wert dieser Untersuchung. *Münchener medizinische Wochenschrift*, **57**, 1942.

[21] ECONOMOU-MAVROU, C. and TSENGHI, C. (1965). Plasma trapping in the centrifuged red cells of children with severe thalassaemia. *Journal of Clinical Pathology*, **18**, 203.

[22] ELLIOT, W. G. and WOOD, J. A. (1969). A concentrated stromalytic solution for electronic leukocyte counts. *American Journal of Clinical Pathology*, **51**, 298.

[23] ENGLAND, J. M. (1979). Prospect for automated differential leucocyte counting in the routine laboratory. *Clinical and Laboratory Haematology*, **1**, 263.

[24] ENGLAND, J. M. and BAIN, B. J. (1976). Annotation: Total and differential leucocyte count. *British Journal of Haematology*, **33**, 1.

[25] ENGLAND, J. M., BASHFORD, C. C., HEWER, M. G., HUGHES-JONES, N. C. and DOWN, M. C. (1975), Simple method for automating the differential leucocyte count. *Lancet*, **i**, 492.

[26] ENGLAND, J. M. and DOWN, M. C. (1974). Red-cell-volume distribution curves and the measurement of anisocytosis. *Lancet*, **i**, 701.

[27] ENGLAND, J. M. and DOWN, M. C. (1979). À comparison of methods for analysing red cell and platelet volume distribution curves. *Clinical and Laboratory Haematology*, **1**, 47.

[28] ENGLAND, J. M. and FRASER, P. M. (1973). Differentiation of iron deficiency from thalassaemia trait by routine blood count. *Lancet*, **i**, 449.

[29] ENGLAND, J. M. and FRASER, P. M. (1973). Differentiation of iron deficiency from thalassaemia trait. *Lancet*, **i**, 1514.

[30] ENGLAND, J. M., WALFORD, D.M. and WATERS, D. A. W. (1972). Re-assessment of the reliability of the haematocrit. *British Journal of Haematology*, **23**, 247.

[31] ENGLAND, J. M., WARD, S. M. and DOWN, M. C. (1976). Microcytosis, anisocytosis and the red cell indices in iron deficiency. *British Journal of Haematology*, **34**, 589.

[32] FURTH, F. W. (1956). Effect of spherocytosis on volume of trapped plasma in red cell column of capillary and Wintrobe hematocrits. *Journal of Laboratory and Clinical Medicine*, **48**, 421.

[33] GARBY, L. and VUILLE, J.-C. (1961). The amount of trapped plasma in a high speed micro-capillary hematrocrit centrifuge. *Scandinavian Journal of Clinical and Laboratory Investigation*, **13**, 642.

[34] GARG, S. K., LACKNER, H. and KARPATKIN, S. (1972). The increased percentage of megathrombocytes in various clinical disorders. *Annals of Internal Medicine*, 77, 361.

[35] GIBSON, Q. H. and HARRISON, D. C. (1945). An artificial standard for use in the estimation of haemoglobin. *Biochemical Journal*, 39, 490.

[36] GLASS, U. H., WETHERLEY-MEIN, G., MILLS, R. T. and PRIEST, C. J. (1971). Automated platelet counting. *British Journal of Haematology*, 21, 529.

[37] GOTTFRIED, E. L., WEHMAN, J., and WALL, B. (1976). Electronic platelet counts with the Coulter Counter. Reassessment of a correction factor. *American Journal of Clinical Pathology*, 66, 506.

[38] HAENEY, M. R. (1976). Erroneous values for the total white cell count and ESR in patients with cryoglobulinaemia. *Journal of Clinical Pathology*, 29, 894.

[39] HANDIN, R. I., LAWLER, K. C. and VALERI, C. R. (1971). Automated platelet counting. *American Journal of Clinical Pathology*, 56, 661

[40] HEGDE, U. M., WHITE, J. M., HART, G. H. and MARSH, G. W. (1977). Diagnosis of α-thalassaemia trait from Coulter Counter's indices. *Journal of Clinical Pathology*, 30, 884.

[41] HELLEMAN, P. W. (1972). Chemical and physical aspects of electronic cell counting. In *Modern Concepts in Hematology*, Eds. G. Izak and S. M. Lewis. p. 164. Academic Press, New York and London.
HELLEMAN, P. W. (1972). *The Coulter Electronic Particle Counter: Aspects and Views in Counting and Sizing of Erythrocytes*. De Bilt, Holland.

[42] HELLEMAN, P. W. and BENJAMIN, C. J. (1969). The Toa Micro cell Counter. I. A study of the correlation between the volume of erythrocytes and their frequency distribution curve. *Scandinavian Journal of Haematology*, 6, 69.

[43] HILLS, A. G., FORSHAM, P. H. and FINCH, C. A. (1948). Changes in circulating leukocytes induced by the administration of pituitary adrenocorticotrophic hormone (ACTH) in man. *Blood*, 3, 755.

[44] HOUCHIN, D. N., MUNN, J. I. and PARNELL, B. L. (1958). A method for the measurement of red cell dimensions and calculation of mean corpuscular volume and surface area. *Blood*, 13, 1185.

[45] HURD, K. E., PALMER, M. K. and HULL, S. (1977). A comparative study for the enumeration of peripheral blood white cell counts below $2.0 \times 10^9/l$ using counting chambers and the Coulter Counter Model 'S'. *Journal of Clinical Pathology*, 30, 1005.

[46] INGRAM, M. and MINTER, F. M. (1969). Semiautomatic preparation of coverglass blood smears using a centrifugal device. *American Journal of Clinical Pathology*, 51, 214.

[47] International committee for standardization in haematology (1978). Protocol for type testing equipment and apparatus used for haematological analysis. *Journal of Clinical Pathology*, 31, 275.

[48] International committee for standardization in haematology (1978). Recommendations for reference method for haemoglobinometry in human blood and specifications for international haemiglobincyanide reference preparation. *Journal of Clinical Pathology*, 31, 139.

[49] International committee for standardization in haematology (1980). Recommended methods for measurement of red-cell and plasma volume. *Journal of Nuclear Medicine*, 21, 793.

[50] International committee for standardization in haematology (1980). Recommendation for reference method for determination by centrifugation of packed cell volume of blood. *Journal of Clinical Pathology*, 33, 1.

[51] KARPATKIN, S. (1978). Heterogeneity of human platelets. VI. Correlation of platelet function with platelet volume. *Blood*, 51, 307.

[52] KHAN, I., ZUCKER-FRANKLIN, D. and KARPATKIN, S. (1975). Microthombocytosis and platelet fragmentation associated with idiopathic/autoimmune thrombocytopenic purpura. *British Journal of Haematology*, 31, 449.

[53] KLEE, G. G., FAIRBANKS, V. F., PIERRE, R. V. and O'SULLIVAN, M. B. (1976). Routine erythrocyte measurements in diagnosis of iron-deficiency anemia and thalassemia minor. *American Journal of Clinical Pathology*, 66, 870.

[54] KOEPKE, J. A. (1978). Differential leukocyte counting: CAP Conference Aspen, 1977. *College of American Pathologists*, Skokie, Illinois.

[55] KRAYTMAN, M. (1973). Platelet size in thrombocytopenias and thrombocytosis of various origins. *Blood*, 41, 587.

[56] LEWIS, S. M. (1972). Cell counting—enumeration of blood cells and bacteria. In *Biomedical Technology in Hospital Diagnosis*. Eds. A. T. Elder and D. W. Neill, p. 211. Pergamon Press, Oxford.

[57] LEWIS, S. M. (1979). Clinical implications of automation in cell counting systems. *Clinical and Laboratory Haematology*, 1, 1.

[58] LEWIS, S. M. and BENTLEY, S. A. (1977). Haemocytometry by laser-beam optics: evaluation of the Hemac 630L. *Journal of Clinical Pathology*, 30, 54.

[59] LEWIS, S. M., SKELLY, J. V. and COUSINS, S. (1981). Automated platelet counting—a re-evaluation of the sedimentation method. *Clinical and Laboratory Haematology*, 3, 215.

[60] LEWIS, S. M. and STODDARD, C. T. H. (1971). Effects of anticoagulant and containers (glass and plastic) on the blood count. *Laboratory Practice*, 20, 787.

[61] LEWIS, S. M., WARDLE, J., COUSINS, S. and SKELLY, J. V. (1979). Platelet counting—development of a reference method and a reference preparation. *Clinical and Laboratory Haematology*, 1, 227.

[62] MACGREGOR, R. G., SCOTT RICHARDS, W. and LOH, G. L. (1940). The differential leucocyte count. *Journal of Pathology and Bacteriology*, 51, 337.

[63] MAGATH, T. B., BERKSON, J., and HURN, M. (1936). The error of determination of the erythrocyte count. *American Journal of Clinical Pathology*, 6, 568.

[64] MANSBERG, H. P., SAUNDERS, A. M. and GRONER, W. (1974). The Hemalog D white cell differential system. *Journal of Histochemistry and Cytochemistry*, 22, 711.

[65] MATSUBARA, T., OKUZONO, H. and TAMAGAWA, S. (1972). Proposal for an improved reagent in the hemiglobincyanide method. In *Modern Concepts in Hematology*. Eds. G. Izak and S. M. Lewis, p. 29. Academic Press. New York and London.

[66] MAYER, K., CHIN, B., MAGNES, J., THALER, T., LOTSPEICH, C. and BAISLEY, A. (1980). Automated platelet counters: a comparative evaluation of latest instrumentation. *American Journal of Clinical Pathology*, 74, 135.

[67] MELAMED, M. R., MULLANEY, P. F. and MENDELSOHN, M. L,. (1979). *Flow Cytometry and Sorting*, Wiley, New York.

[68] MOLDAVAN, A. (1934). Photo-electric technique for the counting of microscopical cells. *Science*, 80, 188.

[69] MORLEY, A. (1969). A platelet cycle in normal individuals. *Australasian Annals of Medicine*, 18, 127.

[70] MUEHRCKE, R. C. ECKERT, E. L. and KARK, R. M. (1952). A statistical study of absolute eosinophil cell counts in healthy young adults using logarithmic analysis. *Journal of Laboratory and Clinical Medicine*, 40, 161.

[71] NOURBAKHSH, M., ALWOOD, J. G., RACCIO, J. and

SELIGSON, D. (1978). An evaluation of blood smears made by a new method using a spinner and diluted blood. *American Journal of Clinical Pathology*, **70**, 885.

[72] PAULUS, J. M. (1975). Platelet size in man. *Blood*, **46**, 321.

[73] POCOCK, S. N. and RIDEOUT, J. M. (1979). Short technical description of the Mon A and Pot Lab colorimeters. *Journal of Automatic Chemistry*, **1**, 222.

[74] PONDER, E. (1948). *Hemolysis and Related Phenomena*, p. 18. Grune and Stratton, New York.

[75] PRICE-JONES, C. (1933). *Red Blood Cell Diameters*. Oxford University Press, London.

[76] ROSS, D. W. and BARDWELL, A. (1980). Automated cytochemistry and the white cell differential in leukaemia. *Blood Cells*, **6**, 455.

[77] ROWAN, R. M., ALLAN, W. and PRESCOTT, R. J. (1972). Evaluation of an automatic platelet counting system utilizing whole blood. *Journal of Clinical Pathology*, **25**, 218.

[78] ROWAN, R. M., FRASER, C. and GRAY, J. H. (1981). Comparison of Channelyzer and Model S Plus determined platelet size measurements. *Clinical and Laboratory Haematology*, **3**, 165.

[79] ROWAN, R. M., FRASER, C., GRAY, J. H. AND MCDONALD, G. A. (1979). The Coulter Counter Model S Plus—the shape of things to come. *Clinical and Laboratory Haematology*, **1**, 29.

[80] RUD, F. (1947). The eosinophil count in health and mental disease. *Acta Psychiatrica et Neurologica (København)*, Suppl **40**.

[81] RUSTAD, H. (1964). Correction for trapped plasma in micro-hematocrit determinations. *Scandinavian Journal of Clinical and Laboratory Investigation*, **16**, 677.

[82] SANDERS, C. and SKERRY, D. W. (1961). The distribution of blood cells on haemocytometer counting chambers with special reference to the amended British Standards Specification 748 (1958). *Journal of Clinical Pathology*, **48**, 298.

[83] SHINTON, N. K., ENGLAND, J. M. E. and KENNEDY, D. A. (1982). Guidelines for the evaluation of instruments used in haematological laboratories. Journal of Clinical Pathology, **35**, 1095.

[84] SKINNIDER, L. F. and MUSGLOW, E. (1972). A stromatolysing and cyanide reagent for use with the Coulter Counter Model S. *American Journal of Clinical Pathology*, **57**, 537.

[85] SLOAN, A. W. (1951). The normal platelet count in man. *Journal of Clinical Pathology*, **4**, 37.

[86] SPIERS, R. S. (1952). The principles of eosinophil diluents. *Blood*, **7**, 550.

[87] STEVENSON, C. F., SMETTERS, G. W. and COOPER, J. A. D. (1951). A gravimetric method for the calibration of hemoglobin micropipets. *American Journal of Clinical Pathology*, **21**, 489.

[88] STEWART, J. W. (1967). The use of electronic blood-cell counters in routine haematology. *British Journal of Haematology*, **13** (Suppl), 11.

[89] STEWART, J. W. CROSLAND-TAYLOR, P. J., CARTER, A. B. and BARNARD, D. F. (1972). Quality control of fully automatic blood counters. In *Modern Concepts in Hematology*. Eds. G. Izak and S. M. Lewis, p. 213. Academic Press, New York and London.

[90] STRUMIA, M. M., SAMPLE A. B. and HART, E. D. (1954). An improved microhematocrit method. *American Journal of Clinical Pathology*, **24**, 1016.

[91] SUNDERMAN, F. W., MACFATE, R. P., MACFADZEAN, D., STEVENSON, G. F. and COPELAND, B. E. (1953). Symposium on clinical hemoglobinometry. *American Journal of Clinical Pathology*, **23**, 519.

[92] SWAN, H. and NELSON, A. W. (1968). Canine trapped plasma factors at different microhematocrit levels. *Journal of Surgical Research*, **8**, 551.

[93] TAYLOR, J. D. and MILLER, J. D. M. (1965). A source of error in the cyanmethemoglobin method of determination of hemoglobin concentration in blood containing carbon monoxide. *American Journal of Clinical Pathology*, **43**, 265.

[94] THOM, R. (1972). Method and results by improved electronic blood-cell sizing. In *Modern Concepts in Hematology*. Eds. G. Izak and S. M. Lewis, p. 191. Academic Press, New York and London.

[95] THOM, R. (1981). Calibration in haematology. In *New Approaches to Laboratory Medicine*. Ed. S. B. Rosalki, p. 3. Ernst Giebeler, Darmstadt.

[96] THOMPSON, L. C. (1946). An inorganic grey solution. *Transactions of the Faraday Society*, **42**, 663.

[97] TOCANTINS, L. M. (1937). Technical methods for the study of the blood platelets. *Archives of Pathology*, **23**, 850.

[98] TOCANTINS, L. M. (1938). The mammalian blood platelet in health and disease. *Medicine (Baltimore)*, **17**, 155.

[99] UNGER, K. W. and JOHNSON, D. (1974). Red blood cell mean corpuscular volume: a potential indicator of alcohol usage in a working population. *American Journal of Medical Sciences*, **267**, 281.

[100] UHRBRAND, H. (1958). The number of circulating eosinophils: normal figures and spontaneous variations. *Acta Medica Scandinavica*, **160**, 99.

[101] UR, A. and LUSHBAUGH, C. C. (1968). Some effects of electrical fields on red blood cells with remarks on electronic red cell sizing. *British Journal of Haematology*, **15**, 527.

[102] VANZETTI, G. (1966). An azide-methemoglobin method for hemoglobin determination in blood. *Journal of Laboratory and Clinical Medicine*, **67**, 116.

[103] WERTZ, R. W. and KOEPKE, J. A. (1977). A critical analysis of platelet counting methods. *American Journal of Clinical Pathology*, **68**, 195.

[104] WESTERMAN, M. P., PIERCE, L. E. and JENSEN, W. N. (1961). A direct method for the quantitative measurement of red cell dimensions. *Journal of Laboratory and Clinical Medicine*, **57**, 819.

[105] World Health Organization (1977). The SI for the health professions. WHO, Geneva.

[106] ZIJLSTRA, W. G. and VAN KAMPEN, E. J. (1960). Standardization of hemoglobinometry. I. The extinction coefficient of hemoglobincyanide at $\lambda = 540\,\text{m}\mu$: ε_{HiCN}^{540}. *Clinica Chimica Acta*, **5**, 719.

[107] VAN ASSENDELFT, O. W. and ENGLAND, J. M. (eds.). (1981). *Advances in Hematological Methods: The Blood Count*. CRC Press, Florida.

[108] ZWEENS, J., FRANKENA, H. and ZIJLSTRA, W. G. (1979). Decomposition on freezing of reagents used in the ICSH recommended method for the determination of total haemoglobin in blood; its nature, cause and prevention. *Clinica Chimica Acta*, **91**, 339.

[109] BARNETT, R. N. (1979). *Clinical Laboratory Statistics*, 2nd edn., p. 30. Little, Brown and Company, Boston.

4

Preparation and staining methods for blood and bone-marrow films

THE PREPARATION OF BLOOD FILMS ON SLIDES

Blood films can be made on glass slides or cover-glasses. The latter have the single possible advantage of a more even distribution of the leucocytes, but in every other respect slides are to be preferred. Unlike cover glasses, slides are not easily broken; they are simple to label and when large numbers of films are to be dealt with, slides will be found much easier to handle.

Good films may be made in the following manner, using chemically cleaned slides wiped free from dust immediately before use.

Place a small drop of blood in the centre line of a slide about 1 or 2 cm from one end. Then, without delay, place a part of a slide to be used as a spreader at an angle of 45° to the slide and move it back to make contact with the drop. The drop should spread out quickly along the line of contact of the spreader with the slide. The moment this occurs, spread the film by a rapid, smooth, forward movement of the spreader.

The drop should be of such a size that the film is 3 or 4 cm in length (Fig. 4.1). It is essential that the slide used as a spreader should have a smooth edge and should be narrower in breadth than the slide on which the film is to be made, so that the edges of the film may be readily examined. If the edge of the spreader is rough, films with ragged tails, containing many leucocytes, result (Fig. 4.1; see also Fig. 3.3). It is worthwhile keeping selected smooth-edged slides for use as spreaders and to cut such slides transversely

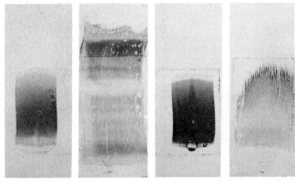

Fig. 4.1 Blood films made on slides. *Left*: a well made film. *Left centre*: a film which is too long, too wide, grossly irregular in thickness and which has been made on a greasy slide. *Right centre*: a film which is too thick. *Right*: a film which has been spread with an irregularly-edged spreader and which shows long tails (see also Fig. 3.3). (Slightly reduced.)

into sections approximately 2 cm in width. The spreader should be washed with running water and dried immediately after being used.

The faster a film is spread the more even and thicker it will be. A common mistake is to make a film too thin (Fig. 4.1). The ideal thickness is such that there is some overlap of red cells throughout much of the film's length, but separation and lack of distortion towards the tail of the film (see p. 40). The leucocytes should be easily recognizable throughout the length of the film. Their distribution in films is discussed on p. 41 . (The preparation of films of aspirated bone marrow is described on p. 122).

Spin method

This is an automated method by which 1 or 2 drops of blood, placed in the centre of a glass slide are briefly spun at high speed in a special centrifuge (e.g. Abbott, Perkin Elmer); the blood spreads on the slide in a monolayer.[18] By this method leucocytes and platelets are distributed uniformly and free of distortion.[33,42] The red cells show a tendency to become distorted, but this can be overcome by diluting 2 volumes of blood with 1 volume of 9 g/l NaCl immediately prior to putting the blood on the slide.[33]

Labelling blood films

A recommended method is to write the name of the patient and the date or a reference number in pencil (graphite) on the film itself. It will not be removed by staining. A paper label should be affixed to the slide later.

STAINING BLOOD AND BONE-MARROW FILMS

Romanowsky stains are universally employed for staining blood films as a routine, and very satisfactory results may be obtained. As far as possible films should be stained as soon as they have dried in the air; they certainly should not be left unfixed for more than a few hours. If the films are left unfixed for a day or more, it will be found that the background of dried plasma stains a pale blue and this is impossible to remove without spoiling the staining of the blood cells. Sometimes staining has to be postponed for up to several days, as when films are sent to the laboratory by post. It is advisable to fix such films before despatch if possible; even so, the results are likely to be less satisfactory than with freshly made films.

The remarkable property of the Romanowsky dyes of making subtle distinctions in shades of staining, and of staining granules differentially, depends on two components, namely, azure B (trimethylthionin) and eosin Y (tetrabromofluorescein).[23,43] The main cause of capricious staining is the presence of other dyes such as azure A, azure C, methyl violet etc. Some commercial stains contain as many as 10 different dyes identifiable by chromatography, and a variable amount of each in different batches of the same stain.[24] The

stains also contain a variable amount of metal salts which influences staining characteristics.[24] Other factors which affect the results are the staining time, dye concentration, ratio of azure B to eosin Y and the pH of the staining solution.

The original Romanowsky combination was polychrome methylene blue and eosin. Several of the stains used routinely which are based on azure B also include methylene blue, but the need for this is debatable. Its presence in the stain is thought by some to enhance the staining of nucleoli and polychromatic red cells; in its absence normal neutrophil granules tend to stain heavily and may resemble 'toxic granules' in conventionally stained films.[22,25]

As indicated above variation in staining is more likely to be due to contaminants in the commercial dyes, and a simple combination of pure azure B and eosin Y should be as suitable as more complex stains.[27,43] Amongst the Romanowsky stains now in use, Jenner's is the simplest and Giemsa's the most complex. Leishman's stain which occupies an intermediate position is still widely used in the routine staining of blood films, athough the results are inferior to those obtained by the combined Jenner-Giemsa method. Wright's stain, which is widely used in North America, gives results which are similar to those obtained with Leishman's stain.

A pH to the alkaline side of neutrality accentuates the azure component at the expense of the eosin and vice versa. A pH of 6.8 is recommended for general use, but to some extent this depends on personal preference. (When looking for malaria parasites a pH of 7.2 is recommended in order to see Schüffner's dots.) To achieve a uniform pH, 50 ml of 66 mmol/l Sörensen's phosphate buffer (see p. 436) may be added to each 1 l of the water used in diluting the stains and washing the films.

The mechanism by which certain components of a cell's structure stain with particular dyes and other components fail to do so, although staining with other dyes, depends on complex differences in binding of the dyes to chemical structures and interactions between the dye molecules. With Romanowsky dyes, the acidic groupings of the nucleic acids and proteins of the cell nuclei and primitive cytoplasm determine their uptake of the basic dye azure B, and, conversely, the presence of basic groupings on the Hb molecule results in its affinity for acidic dyes and its staining by eosin. The granules in the cytoplasm of neutrophil leucocytes are weakly stained by the azure complexes. Eosinophilic granules contain a spermine derivative with an alkaline grouping which stains strongly with the acidic components of the dye, whereas basophilic granules contain heparin which has an affinity for the basic component of the dye.

Staining methods

May-Grünwald-Giemsa's stain

Dry the films in the air, then fix by immersing in a jar of methanol for 10–20 min. Transfer to a staining jar containing May-Grünwald's stain freshly diluted with an equal volume of buffered water. After the films have been allowed to stain for *c* 15 min, transfer them without washing to a jar containing Giemsa's stain freshly diluted with 9 volumes of buffered water. After staining for 10–15 min, transfer the slides to a jar containing buffered water and rapidly wash in three or four changes of water and finally allow to stand undisturbed in water for a short time (usually 2–5 min) for differentiation to take place. This may be controlled by inspection of the wet slide under the low power of the microscope; with experience the naked-eye colour of the film is often a good guide. The slides should be transferred from one staining solution to the other without being allowed to dry. As the intensity of the staining is affected by any variation in the thickness of a film, it is not easy to obtain uniform staining throughout a film's length.

When differentiation is complete, stand the slides upright to dry. When thoroughly dry, cover the films by a rectangular No. 1 cover-glass, using for this purpose a mountant, which is miscible with xylol.* For a temporary mount, cedar-wood oil may be used.

The cover-glass should be sufficiently large to overlie the whole film, including both the edges and the tail. If a neutral mounting medium is used the staining should be preserved for at least 5–10 yr. Although it is probable that stained films keep best un-

* e.g. Diatex (R. A. Lamb).

mounted, there are objections to this course: it is almost impossible to keep the slides free from dust and from being scratched, and in the absence of a cover-glass the observer is tempted to examine the film solely with the oil-immersion objective, a practice which is to be deprecated (p. 62).

As an alternative to a neutral mountant and cover-glass, the slide may be covered with a layer of polystyrene or acrylic resin in solvent[†]. This has the advantage of speedy application and rapid drying. However, the resin tends to gather dust and finger marks which are less easily removed than from glass.

The May-Grünwald-Giemsa staining method described above is designed for staining a number of films at the same time. Single slides may be stained by flooding the slide with a combined fixative and staining solution (e.g. Leishman's stain).

A relatively prolonged fixation, at least 10 min, is required for good staining; particularly is this so in staining films of bone marrow. It is important to ensure that the methanol used as fixative is completely water-free. As little as 4% water may affect the appearance of the films, and a higher water content causes gross changes (Figs. 4.2, 4.3).

The diluted stains usually retain their staining powers sufficiently well for several batches of slides to be stained in them. They must be made up freshly each day, and it is probably best to stain the day's films all at the same time, or if this is not possible in consecutive batches. There is no need to filter the stains before use unless a deposit is present.

Jenner-Giemsa's stain

Jenner's stain may be substituted for May-Grünwald's stain in the above-described technique. The results are a little less satisfactory. The stain is used with 4 volumes of buffered water and the films, after being fixed in methanol, are immersed in it for approximately 4 min before being transferred to the Giemsa's stain. They should be allowed to stain in

† Acrylek (Fisons Ltd.); Trycolac (Aerosol Marketing & Chemical Co. Ltd.).

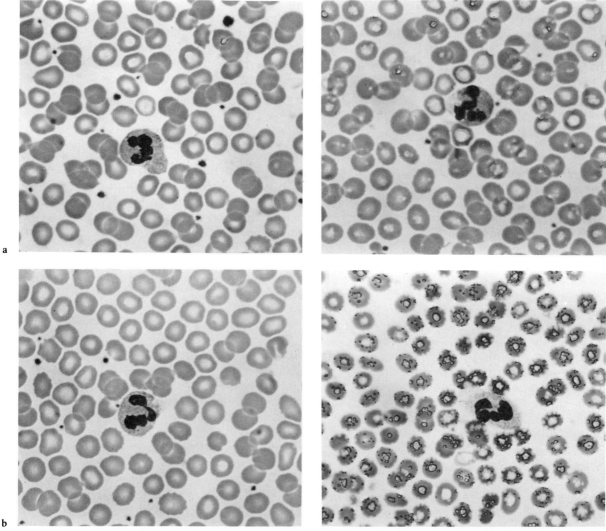

Fig. 4.2 Blood film appearances following methanol fixation. Photomicrographs of Romanowsky-stained blood films which have been fixed in methanol containing (a) 1% water and (b) 3% water. The erythrocytes and leucocytes are well fixed.

Fig. 4.3 Blood film appearances following methanol fixation. Photomicrographs of Romanowsky-stained blood films which have been fixed in methanol containing (a) 4% water and (b) 10% water. In (a) the erythrocytes are poorly fixed; in (b) they are very badly fixed.

the latter solution for 7–10 min. Differentiation is carried out as described above.

Leishman's stain

Dry the film in the air and flood the slide with the stain. After 2 min add double the volume of water and stain the film for 5–7 min. Then wash it in a stream of buffered water until it has acquired a pinkish tinge (up to 2 min).

After the back of the slide has been wiped clean, set it upright to dry.

Preparation of solutions of the Romanowsky dyes

May-Grünwald's stain. Weigh out 0.3 g of the powdered dye and transfer to a conical flask of 200–250 ml capacity. Add 100 ml of methanol and warm the mixture to 50°C. Allow the flask to cool to room temperature and shake several times during the day. After standing for 24 h, filter the solution. It is then ready for use, no ripening being required.

Jenner's stain. Prepare a 5 g/l solution in methanol in exactly the same way as described above for May-Grünwald's stain.

Giemsa's stain. Weigh 1 g of the powdered dye and transfer to a conical flask of 200–250 ml capacity. Add 100 ml of methanol and warm the mixture to 50°C; keep at this temperature for 15 min with occasional shaking, then filter the solution. It is then ready for use, but will improve on standing.

Buffered water. Make up 50 ml of 66 mmol/l Sörensen's phosphate buffer to 1 l with water (see p. 436). An alternative buffer may be prepared from Buffer Tablets which are available commercially. Solutions of the required pH are obtained by dissolving the tablets in water.

Automatic staining machines are available which enable large batches of slides to be handled. As a rule, staining is of a uniform high standard, but to achieve this reliable stains are required and the cycle time has to be carefully controlled.

Standardized Romanowsky stain[44]

The following stain which is based on the use of pure dyes has the advantage of being standardized; it thus ensures consistent results from batch to batch. The essential elements are azure B and eosin Y.

Reagents

Stock solution. Dissolve 300 mg of pure azure B perchlorate or thiocyanate* in 40 ml of dimethylsulfoxide (DMSO). Dissolve 100 mg of eosin Y[†] in 60 ml of methanol. When both dyes are completely dissolved, add the eosin Y solution to the azure B solution and

* R. Heyl, Goerzallee 253, W. Berlin; Aldrich Chemical Co., New Road, Gillingham, Dorset SP8 4JL.
[†] e.g. Koch Light Ltd.

stir well. This stock solution should remain stable for several months if kept at room temperature in the dark.

Staining solution. Immediately before use dilute 1 volume of the stock solution with 14 volumes of Hepes buffer, pH 6.5–6.6 (p. 435).

Method

Fix films for 5–10 min in methanol. Leave the slides in the diluted stain for 25 min. Rinse with water, air dry and mount.

The staining solution should be freshly made and should be renewed at intervals when several batches of films are being stained in succession. Loss of staining power is usually due to precipitation of the eosin Y and this will result in the nuclei staining blue instead of purple.

Rapid staining method

Field's method[12,13,14] was introduced to provide a quick method for staining thick films for malaria parasites (see below). With some modifications it can be used fairly satisfactorily for the rapid staining of thin films.

Stains

Stain A (polychromed methylene blue). Methylene blue 1.3 g, disodium hydrogen phosphate ($Na_2HPO_4.12H_2O$) 12.6 g, potassium dihydrogen phosphate (KH_2PO_4) 6.25 g, water 500 ml.

Dissolve the methylene blue and the disodium hydrogen phosphate in 50 ml of water. Then boil the solution in a water-bath almost to dryness in order to 'polychrome' the dye. Add the potassium dihydrogen phosphate and 500 ml of freshly boiled water. After stirring to dissolve the stain, set aside the solution for 24 h before filtering. Filter again before use. The pH is 6.6–6.8.

Azure I may be added to the methylene blue in the proportion of 0.5 g of azure I to 0.8 g of methylene blue. The dyes can then be dissolved directly in the phosphate buffer solution. No evaporation is necessary.

Stain B (eosin). Eosin 1.3 g, disodium hydrogen phosphate ($Na_2HPO_4.12H_2O$) 12.6 g, potassium dihydrogen phosphate (KH_2PO_4) 6.25 g, water 500 ml.

Dissolve the phosphates in warm freshly boiled water, and then add the dye. Filter the solution after standing for 24 h.

Method of staining

Fix the film for a few seconds in methanol. Pour off the methanol and drop on the slide 12 drops of diluted Stain B (1 volume of stain to 4 volumes of water). Immediately, add 12 drops of Stain A. Agitate the slide to mix the stains. After 1 min rinse the slide in water, then differentiate the film for 5 s in phosphate buffer at pH 6.6, wash the slide in water and then place it on end to drain and dry. Two-stage stains of this type are also available commercially (e.g. Diff-Quick, Harleco).

Making and staining thick blood films

Thick blood films are widely used in the diagnosis of malaria. A relatively large volume of blood may be scrutinized in a short time and parasites seen even if present in very small numbers. Methods of staining have been reviewed by Field and Sandosham.[14] Field's method of staining[12,13] is quick and usually satisfactory, but the method is not practical for staining large numbers of films; for this purpose the Giemsa method is more suitable. Both methods will be described.

Making thick films

Make a thick film by placing a small drop of blood in the centre of a slide and spread it out with a corner of another slide to cover an area about four times its original area. The correct thickness for a satisfactory film will have been achieved if, with the slide placed on a piece of newspaper, small print is just visible.

Allow the film to dry thoroughly for at least 30 min at 37°C before attempting to stain it. Alternatively, leave the slide on the top of a microscope lamp, where the temperature is 50°–60°C, for 7 min. Absolutely fresh films, although apparently dry, often wash off in the stain.

Field's method [12,13,14]

The preparation of the stains is described on p. 54. Dip the slide with the dried but otherwise unfixed film on it into Stain A for 1–2 s. Rinse it in buffered water (pH 6.8–7.0) until the stain ceases to flow from the film (5–10 s). Dip into Stain B for 1 s and then rinse rapidly in buffered water for 10 s. Shake off excess water and leave the slide upright to dry. Do not blot.

Giemsa's stain

Dry the films thoroughly as above, immerse the slides for 20–30 min in a staining jar containing Giemsa's stain freshly diluted with 15–20 volumes of buffered water. Gently wash the films with buffered water. Stand the slides upright to dry. Do not blot.

Sometimes the films are overlaid by a residue of stain or spoilt by the envelopes of the lysed cells being visible. These defects can be minimized either by soaking the stained and dried films for a few minutes in 9 g/l NaCl or by staining the films in the first instance in Giemsa's stain which has been diluted in buffered 9 g/l NaCl, pH 6.8, instead of water.[39]

Relative value of thick and thin films in the diagnosis of malaria

Thick films are extremely useful when parasites are scanty, but the identification of the parasites is less easy than in thin films. Mixed infections may be missed and there may be doubt as to the identification of any particular object. However, an experienced observer may be able to find and recognize with certainty parasites in badly stained thick films, whilst in a well stained film parasites should be easily recognized even by beginners. Five min spent in examining a thick film is equivalent to about 1 h spent in traversing a thin film. Rapid screening can also be carried out by fluorescent microscopy at low magnification, as malaria parasites fluoresce intensely with acridine orange.[40]

Study of thin films enables an exact diagnosis as to the species to be made. Seldom, if ever, should there be any doubt as to whether or not an object is a malarial parasite if the film has been well stained.

Thick films, if well stained, are also useful when there is severe leucopenia. It is possible to perform differential counts (or at least to estimate the proportion of polymorphonuclear to mononuclear cells) much more rapidly and more accurately than in thin films made from the same blood.

EXAMINATION OF BLOOD CELLS IN PLASMA

The examination of a drop of blood sealed between a slide and cover-glass is sometimes of considerable value.

The preparation may be examined in several ways; by ordinary illumination, by dark-ground or by Nomarski (interference) illumination. Chemically clean slides and cover-glasses must be used and the blood allowed to spread out thinly between them. If the glass surfaces are free from dust, the blood will spread out spontaneously, and pressure, which is undesirable, should not be necessary. The edges of the preparation may be sealed with a melted mixture of equal parts of petroleum jelly and paraffin wax.

Red cells

Rouleaux formation is usually seen in varying degrees in 'wet' preparations of whole blood and has to be distinguished from auto-agglutination.

Rouleaux formation versus auto-agglutination

The distinction between rouleaux formation and auto-agglutination is sometimes a matter of considerable difficulty, particularly when, as not infrequently happens, rouleaux formation is superimposed on agglutination. The rouleaux, too, may be notably irregular in haemolytic anemias characterised by spherocytosis, while the clumping due to massive rouleaux formation of normal type may closely simulate true agglutination.

'Pseudo-agglutination' due to massive rouleaux formation may be distinguished from true agglutination in two ways:

1. By noting that the red cells, although forming parts of larger clumps, are mostly arranged side by side as in typical rouleaux.

2. By adding 3–4 volumes of 9 g/l NaCl (saline) to the preparation. Pseudo-agglutination due to massive rouleaux formation should either disperse completely or transform itself into typical rouleaux. The addition of saline to blood which has undergone true agglutination may cause the agglutination to break up somewhat, but a major degree of it is likely to persist and typical rouleaux will not be seen.

Anisocytosis and poikilocytosis can be recognised in 'wet' preparations of blood, but the tendency to crenation and the formation of rouleaux tend to make observations on shape changes rather difficult. Such changes are best studied in well made air-dried films or in 'wet' blood which has been fixed immediately after collection by adding to it 10 volumes of 0.25% glutaraldehyde (10 ml of 25% glutaraldehyde in 1 l of iso-osmotic phosphate buffer, pH 7.4 (see p. 436). The sickling of red cells in 'wet' preparations of blood is described on p. 181.

Parasites

Wet preparations of blood are suitable for the detection of microfilariae and the spirochaetes of relapsing fever. The presence of small numbers of the latter is revealed by occasional slight agitation of groups of red cells.

Leucocytes

The motility of leucocytes can be readily studied if the microscope stage can be warmed to c 37°C. Usually only the granulocytes show significant progressive movements.

Leucocytes can also be examined under dark-ground illumination or phase-contrast microscopy, either unstained or after supravital staining with neutral red or Janus green dyes, or with fluorescent dyes such as acridine orange or auramine.

It seems doubtful whether supravital staining or the use of the phase-contrast, interference or fluorescent microscope helps in the day-to-day problems of diagnostic haematology, and no attempt will be made to describe the appearances of cells viewed by these methods. Excellent photographs of cells viewed with the phase-contrast microscope were given by Bessis.[3] Cell shape and surface structures are particularly well demonstrated by means of Nomarski interference microscopy.[3,4] Kosenow[20] and Jackson[19] illustrated the appearances of leucocytes which had taken up fluorescent dyes.

SEPARATION AND CONCENTRATION OF BLOOD CELLS

A number of methods are available for the concentration of leucocytes or abnormal cells when they are present in only small numbers in the peripheral blood. Concentrates are most simply prepared from the buffy coat of centrifuged blood.

Making a buffy-coat preparation

Defibrinate venous blood in a flask and then centrifuge a sample for 15 min in a Wintrobe haematocrit tube at 3000 rpm (1500 **g**). Remove the supernatant serum carefully with a fine pipette, and with the same pipette deposit the platelet and underlying leucocyte layers on to one or two slides. Emulsify the buffy coat in a drop of the patient's serum and then spread the films. Allow them to dry in the air and then fix and stain in the usual way.

When leucocytes are scanty or if many slides are to be made, it is worthwhile centrifuging the blood twice: first, c 5 ml are centrifuged and a haematocrit tube is then filled from the upper cell layers of this sample.

As an alternative to centrifugation, the blood may be allowed to sediment, with the help of sedimentation-enhancing agents such as fibrinogen, dextran, gum acacia, Ficoll or methyl cellulose.[5,8] Bøyum's reagent[6] (methyl cellulose and Isopaque) is particularly suitable for obtaining leucocyte preparations with minimal red-cell contamination and this is now a standard method is most haematology laboratories. Sodium metrizoate can be used to obtain platelet preparations (p. 45). Most methods of separation affect to some extent subsequent staining properties, chemical reactions and the viability of the separated cells.

The buffy coat

It is well known that atypical or primitive blood cells circulate in small numbers in the peripheral blood in health. Thus, atypical mononuclear cells, metamyelocytes and megakaryocytes may be found. Even promyelocytes, blasts and nucleated red cells may occasionally be seen, but only in very small numbers. Efrati and Rozenszajn[10] described a method for the quantitative assessment of the numbers of atypical cells in normal blood and gave figures for the incidence of megakaryocyte fragments (e.g. mean 21.8 per 1 ml of blood) and of atypical mononuclears and metamyelocytes and myelocytes. In cord blood the incidence of all types of primitive cells is considerably greater.[11]

In disease, leaving the leukaemias and allied disorders out of consideration, abnormal cells may be seen in buffy-coat preparations in much larger numbers than in films of whole blood. For instance, megakaryocytes and immature cells of the granulocyte series are found in relatively large numbers in disseminated carcinoma.[36] Megaloblasts so found may help in the diagnosis of a megaloblastic anaemia. Erythophagocytosis may be conspicuous in cases of auto-immune haemolytic anaemia, and in systemic lupus erythematosus a few LE cells may be found—this is, however, not the best way to demonstrate LE cells.

It is rash to attempt an accurate differential count on buffy-coat concentrates as the different leucocytes, having different densities, tend to sediment under the influence of gravity at different rates and form layer upon layer. In Bøyum's separation procedure lymphocytes especially are lost. However, in leucopenia there is a fairly satisfactory correlation between the buffy-coat differential count and the standard method.[35]

SEPARATION OF SPECIFIC CELL POPULATIONS

Differences in density of cells can be used to separate individual cell types, using gradient solutions of selected specific gravity. Thus, Ficoll has been used to separate various haemopoietic cells,[32] as has albumin.[45]

Another method is by density gradient using polyvinylpyrrolidone (PVP)-coated silica gel (Percoll, Pharmacia) which appears suitable for separating, progressively, myeloblasts at sp gr 1062, promyelocytes at 1073, myelocytes at 1077, metamyelocytes at 1080, neutrophils at 1086, eosinophils at 1090, monocytes at 1066 and lymphocytes at 1068.[34] An advantage of this procedure is that the coating renders the medium non-toxic to cells. Phthalate esters have been used to separate red cells of different ages.[9,21]

Isolation of tumour cells from blood

The methods used for demonstrating tumour cells in circulating blood involve elimination of the red cells and differential sedimentation or filtration of the leucocytes. Fleming and Stewart[15] assessed several methods critically and concluded that differential separation was to be preferred for routine use. They recommended a slight modification of the silicon flotation method of Seal.[37] Positive identifications are seldom made except in advanced cancer when the diagnosis is usually only too obvious.

THE RETICULOCYTE COUNT

Reticulocytes are juvenile red cells; they contain remnants of the ribosomes and the ribonucleic acid which were present in larger amounts in the cytoplasm of the nucleated precursors from which they were derived. Ribosomes have the property of reacting with certain dyes such as brilliant cresyl blue or New methylene blue to form a blue precipitate of granules or filaments. This reaction takes place only in vitally-stained unfixed preparations. The most immature reticulocytes are those with the largest amount of precipitable ribosome material; in the least immature only a few dots or short strands are seen.

If a blood film is allowed to dry and is afterwards fixed with methanol, reticulocytes appear as red cells staining diffusely basophilic if the film is stained with basophilic dyes. Complete loss of basophilic material probably occurs as a rule in the blood stream and, particularly, in the spleen[2] after the cells have left the bone marrow.[38] The ripening process is thought to take 2–3 days, of which about 24 h are spent in the circulation.

The number of reticulocytes in the peripheral blood is a fairly accurate reflection of erythropoietic activity, assuming that there is normal release of reticulocytes from the bone marrow, and that they remain in circulation for the normal period of time. These assumptions are not always valid as an increased erythropoietic stimulus leads to premature release into the circulation. The maturation time of these so-called 'stress' or stimulated reticulocytes will be prolonged for up to 3 days. In such cases, it is possible to deduce the reticulocyte maturation time and a corrected reticulocyte count by using plasma iron-turnover data.[16,17] Nevertheless, adequate information is usually obtained from a simple reticulocyte count, recorded as a percentage of the red cells or preferably, if the red-cell count is known, expressed as absolute numbers.

A technique for the reticulocyte count

Reliable results are obtained with the following technique using New methylene blue, which, in the authors' experience, is superior to brilliant cresyl blue. New methylene blue stains the reticulo-filamentous material in reticulocytes more deeply and more uniformly than does brilliant cresyl blue, which varies from sample to sample in it staining ability. Purified azure B seems to be a satisfactory substitute for New methylene blue; the dye does not precipitate.[26] It is used in the same concentration and the staining procedure is the same as with New methylene blue.

Staining solution

Dissolve 1.0 g of New methylene blue (CI 52030)* in 100 ml of citrate-saline solution (1 volume of 30 g/l sodium citrate to 4 volumes of 9.0 g/l NaCl). The mixture is filtered after the dye has dissolved and is then ready for use.

Method

Deliver 2 or 3 drops of the New methylene blue, by means of a Pasteur pipette, in to a 75 × 10 mm glass or plastic tube. Add 2–4 volumes of the patient's EDTA blood to the dye solution and mix. Keep the mixture at 37°C for 15–20 min. Resuspend the red cells by gentle mixing and make films on glass slides in the usual way. When dry, examine the films without fixing or counterstaining.

The exact volume of blood to be added to the dye solution for optimal staining depends upon the red-cell count. A larger proportion of anaemic blood, and a smaller proportion of polycythaemic blood, should be added than of normal blood. In a successful preparation the reticulo-filamentous material should be stained deep blue and the non-reticulated cells stained diffusely shades of pale greenish blue.

Films stained with New methylene blue should not be counterstained. The reticulo-filamentous material is not better defined after counter-staining and precipitated stain overlying cells may cause confusion. Moreover, Heinz bodies will not be visible in fixed and counterstained preparations. Satisfactory counts may be made on blood which has been allowed to stand (unstained) for as long as 24 h, although the count will tend to fall as some of the reticulocytes may ripen in vitro.[1]

Counting reticulocytes

An area of film should be chosen for the count where the cells are undistorted and where the staining is good. A common fault is to make the film too thin; however, the cells should not overlap. To count the cells use the 2-mm oil-immersion objective and if possible eyepieces provided with an adjustable diaphragm. If eyepieces with an adjustable diaphragm are not available, a paper or cardboard diaphragm, in the centre of which has been cut a small square with sides about 4 mm in length, can be inserted into an eyepiece and used as a less convenient substitute.

The counting procedure adopted should be appropriate to the number of reticulocytes present. Very large numbers of cells have to be surveyed for an accurate count when only small numbers of reticulocytes are present.[38]

For counts of less than 10%, a convenient method is to survey successive fields until, except in severe reticulocytopenia, at least 100 reticulocytes have been counted (recording the number on a simple hand counter) and to count the total cells in every tenth field. The total cells in at least ten fields should be counted. The calculation is then simple, e.g.:

Number of reticulocytes seen in 150 fields = 100;

total cells present in 15 fields = 300.

Therefore, approximate number of cells of all types in 150 fields = 3000;

$$\text{and reticulocyte percentage} = \frac{100}{3000} \times 100$$

$$= 3.3\%.$$

When the reticulocyte count exceeds 10%, a greater number of complete fields should be counted in proportion to the fields in which only reticulocytes are counted.

It is essential that the reticulocyte preparation be well spread and well stained. Other important factors which affect the accuracy of the count are the visual acuity and patience of the observer and the quality and resolving power of the microscope. The most accurate counts are carried out by a conscientious observer who has no knowledge of

---

* New methylene blue is chemically different from methylene blue which is a poor reticulocyte stain.

the supposed reticulocyte level, thus eliminating the effect of conscious or unconscious bias.

The decision as to what is and what is not a reticulocyte may be difficult, as the most mature reticulocytes contain only a few dots or threads of reticulo-filamentous material. Nizet,[31] who classified reticulocytes into groups according to the amount of basophilic material present, recommended the use of dark-ground illumination as a sensitive method of detecting the most mature reticulocytes. Unfortunately, this does not overcome the difficulty of differentiating reticulocytes from cells containing inclusions such as Pappenheimer bodies[29], found particularly in peripheral blood after splenectomy (see p. 107). Fortunately, in well-stained preparations, viewed under the light microscope, the Pappenheimer type of granular material—usually present as a single small dot, less commonly as multiple dots—stains a darker shade of blue than does the reticulo-filamentous material of the reticulocyte. If there is any doubt, Pappenheimer's bodies can be identified by post-staining the film for iron by Perls's reaction (see p. 108).

Hb-H undergoes denaturation in the presence of New methylene blue solution, resulting in round inclusion bodies which stain greenish-blue. These can be clearly differentiated from reticulo-filamentous material (see p. 111). Heinz bodies are also stained by New methylene blue, but a lighter shade of blue than the reticulo-filamentous material of reticulocytes.

Reticulocytes can be counted by fluorescent microscopy after adding 10 volumes of acridine orange solution (10 mg / 100 ml of 9 g/l NaCl) to 1 volume of blood.[41] RNA gives an orange-red fluorescence whilst nuclear material (DNA) fluoresces yellow. This is a useful method for distinguishing the particles which may cause confusion when stained with New methylene blue. All forms of RNA fluoresce with acridine orange. However, because special equipment is required and the preparation quickly fades, the method is not suitable for routine use in demonstrating reticulocytes.

Range of reticulocyte count in health

Adults and children	0.2–2.0%.
Infants (full-term, cord blood)	2–6%.

There are insufficient data as to the range of the absolute reticulocyte count in health. The upper limit was given by Myhre[30] as $84 \times 10^9/l$; however, according to Cline and Berlin[7] it is $40 \times 10^9/l$.

REFERENCES

[1] BALDINI, M. and PANNACCIULLI, I. (1960). The maturation rate of reticulocytes. *Blood*, **15**, 614.

[2] BERENDES, M. (1973). The proportion of reticulocytes in the erythrocytes of the spleen as compared with those of circulating blood, with special reference to hemolytic states. *Blood*, **14**, 558.

[3] BESSIS, M. (1973). *Living Blood Cells and their Ultrastructure.* Springer-Verlag, Berlin, Heidelberg and New York.

[4] BESSIS, M. and THIÉRY, J. P. (1957). Les cellules du sang vues au microscope à interférences (Système Nomarski). *Revue d'Hématologie*, **12**, 518.

[5] BLOEMENDAL, H. (Ed.) (1977). *Cell Separation Methods.* Elsevier-North Holland, Amsterdam.

[6] BØYUM, A. (1964). Separation of white blood cells. *Nature (London)*, **204**, 793.

[7] CLINE, M. J. and BERLIN, N. I. (1963). The reticulocyte count as an indicator of the rate of erythropoiesis. *American Journal of Clinical Pathology*, **39**, 121.

[8] CUTTS, J. H. (1970). *Cell Separation: Methods in Hematology.* Academic Press, New York and London.

[9] DANON, D. and MARIKOVSKY, Y. (1964). Determination of density distribution of red cell population. *Journal of Laboratory and Clinical Medicine*, **64**, 668.

[10] EFRATI, P. and ROZENSZAJN, L. (1960). The morphology of buffy coat in normal human adults. *Blood*, **16**, 1012.

[11] EFRATI, P., ROZENSZAJN, L. and SHAPIRA, E. (1961). The morphology of buffy coat from cord blood of normal human newborns. *Blood*, **17**, 497.

[12] FIELD, J. W. (1940–41). The morphology of malarial parasites in thick blood films. Part IV. The identification of species and phase. *Transactions of the Royal Society of Tropical Medicine and Hygiene*, **34**, 405.

[13] FIELD, J. W. (1941–42). Further notes on a method of staining malarial parasites in thick films. *Transactions of the Royal Society of Tropical Medicine and Hygiene*, **35**, 35.

[14] FIELD, J. W. and SANDOSHAM, A. A. (1964). The Romanowsky stains—aqueous or methanolic? *Transactions of the Royal Society of Tropical Medicine and Hygiene*, **58**, 164.

[15] FLEMING, J. A. and STEWART, J. W. (1967). A critical and comparative study of methods of isolating tumour cells from the blood. *Journal of Clinical Pathology*, **20**, 145.

[16] HILLMAN, R. S. (1969). Characteristics of marrow production and reticulocyte maturation in normal man in response to anemia. *Journal of Clinical Investigation*, **48**, 443.

[17] HILLMAN, R. S. and FINCH, C. A. (1969). The misused reticulocyte. *British Journal of Haematology*, **17**, 313.

[18] INGRAM, M. and MINTER, F. M. (1969). Semiautomatic preparation of coverglass blood smears using a centrifugal device. *American Journal of Clinical Pathology*, **51**, 214.

[19] JACKSON, J. F. (1961). Supravital blood studies, using acridine orange fluorescence. *Blood*, **17**, 643.

[20] KOSENOW, K. (1956). Lebende Blutzellen im Fluoreszenz- und Phasenkontrastmikroscop. *Bibliotheca Haematologica (Basel)*, Fasc 4.

[21] LEWIS, S. M. and VINCENT, P. C. (1968). Red-cell density in paroxysmal nocturnal haemoglobinuria. *British Journal of Haematology*, **14**, 513.

[22] MARSHALL, P. N. (1977). Methylene blue-azure B-eosin as a substitute for May-Grünwald-Giemsa and Jenner-Giemsa stains. *Microscopica Acta*, **79**, 153.

[23] MARSHALL, P. N. (1978). Romanowsky-type stains in haematology. *Histochemical Journal*, **10**, 1.

[24] MARSHALL, P. N., BENTLEY, S. A. and LEWIS, S. M. (1975). An evaluation of some commercial Romanowsky stains. *Journal of Clinical Pathology*, **28**, 680.

[25] MARSHALL, P. N., BENTLEY, S. A. and LEWIS, S. M. (1975). A standardized Romanowsky stain prepared from purified dyes. *Journal of Clinical Pathology*, **28**, 920.

[26] MARSHALL, P. N., BENTLEY, S. A. and LEWIS, S. M. (1976). Purified azure B as a reticulocyte stain. *Journal of Clinical Pathology*, **29**, 1060.

[27] MARSHALL, P. N., BENTLEY, S. A. and LEWIS, S. M. (1978). Standardization of Romanowsky stains: the relationship between stain composition and performance. *Scandinavian Journal of Haematology*, **20**, 206.

[28] MARSHALL, P. N., BENTLEY, S. A. and LEWIS, S. M. (1978). Staining properties and stability of a standardized Romanowsky stain. *Journal of Clinical Pathology*, **31**, 280.

[29] McFADZEAN, A. J. S. and DAVIS, L. J. (1947). Iron-staining erythrocytic inclusions with especial reference to acquired haemolytic anaemia. *Glasgow Medical Journal*, **28**, 237.

[30] MYHRE, E. (1961). Reticulocyte count. *Nordisk Medicin*, **65**, 37.

[31] NIZET, A. (1944). Recherches sur la physiopathologie des hématies. I. Nouvelles techniques pour l'étude et la distinction des hématies granuleuses. *Acta Medica Scandinavica*, **117**, 199.

[32] NOBLE, P. B., CUTTS, J. H. and CARROLL, K. K. (1968). Ficoll flotation for the separation of blood leukocyte types. *Blood*, **31**, 66.

[33] NOURBAKHSH, M., ATWOOD, J. G., RACCIO, J. and SELIGSON, D. (1978). An evaluation of blood smears made by a new method using a spinner and diluted blood. *American Journal of Clinical Pathology*, **70**, 885.

[34] OLOFSSON, T., GÄRTNER, I. and OLSSON, I (1980). Separation of human bone marrow cells in density gradients of polyvinyl pyrrolidone coated silica gel (Percoll). *Scandinavian Journal of Haematology*, **24**, 254.

[35] PFLIEGER, H., GAUS, W. and DIETRICH, M. (1979). Differential blood counts from cell concentrates. A comparison with routine differential blood counts. *Acta Haematologica*, **61**, 150.

[36] ROMSDAHL, M. M., McGREW, E. A., McGRATH, R. G. and VALAITIS, J. (1964). Hematopoietic nucleated cells in the peripheral venous blood of patients with carcinoma. *Cancer (Philadelphia)*, **17**, 1400.

[37] SEAL, S. H. (1959). Silicone flotation: a simple quantitative method for the isolation of free-floating cancer cells from the blood. *Cancer (Philadelphia)*, **12**, 590.

[38] SEIP, M. (1953). Reticulocyte studies: the liberation of red blood corpuscles from the bone marrow into the peripheral blood and the production of erythrocytes elucidated by reticulocyte investigations. *Acta Medica Scandinavica*, Suppl. 282.

[39] SHUTE, P. and MARYON, M. (1960). *Laboratory Technique for the Study of Malaria*, p. 9. Churchill, London.

[40] SODEMAN, T. M. (1970). The use of fluorochromes for the detection of malarial parasites. *American Journal of Tropical Medicine*, **19**, 40.

[41] VANDER, J. B., HARRIS, C. A. and ELLIS, S. R. (1963). Reticulocyte counts by means of fluorescence microscopy. *Journal of Laboratory and Clinical Medicine*, **62**, 132.

[42] WENK, R. E. (1976). Comparison of five methods for preparing blood smears. *American Journal of Medical Technology*, **42**, 71.

[43] WITTEKIND, D. (1979). On the nature of Romanowsky dyes and the Romanowsky Giemsa effect. *Clinical and Laboratory Haematology*, **1**, 247.

[44] WITTEKIND, D., KRETSCHMER, V. and SOHMER, I. (1982). Azure B eosin Y-stain as the standard Romanowsky-Giemsa stain. *British Journal of Haematology*, **51**, 391.

[45] ZUCKER, R. M. and CASSEN, B. (1969). The separation of normal human leukocytes by density and classification by size. *Blood*, **34**, 591.

5

Blood cell morphology in health and disease

Examination of a fixed and stained blood film is an essential part of a haematological investigation, and it cannot be emphasized too strongly that for the most to be made out of the examination the films must be well spread, well stained and examined systematically. Details of the recommended technique of examination are given below. It is clearly impossible to include in a book of this size and scope a comprehensive atlas of blood-cell morphology. However, the most important red-cell abnormalities, as seen in fixed and stained films, are described and illustrated in black and white, and some notes on their significance and importance in diagnosis are added. Leucocyte and platelet abnormalities are described more briefly; no illustrations are included because for these to be helpful many would be needed and reproduction in colour would be essential—a requirement which, if met, would too greatly increase the price of the book.

TECHNIQUE OF EXAMINATION OF BLOOD FILMS

The point has already been made that blood films must be well spread, well fixed and well stained and examined systematically. It is useless to place a drop of immersion oil anywhere on the film and then to examine it straightaway using the high-power 2 mm objective.

First, the film should be covered with a cover-glass using a neutral medium as mountant. Next, it should be inspected under a low magnification (with a 16 mm objective) in order to get an idea of the quality of the preparation and of the number, distribution and staining of the leucocytes, and to

find an area where the red cells are evenly distributed and are not distorted.

Having selected a suitable area, a 4 mm objective or 3.5 mm oil-immersion objective should then be used. A much better appreciation of variation in red-cell size, shape and staining can then be obtained with these objectives than with the 2 mm oil-immersion lens. The latter in combination with × 6 eyepieces should be reserved for the final examination of unusual cells and for looking at fine details such as cytoplasmic granules, punctate basophilia, etc.

As the diagnosis of the type of anaemia or abnormality present usually depends upon a comprehension of the whole picture which the film presents, the red cells, leucocytes and platelets should all be systematically examined.

MORPHOLOGY OF THE RED CELLS

In *health*, the red blood cells vary relatively little in size and shape (Fig. 5.1). In well spread dried films the great majority of cells have round smooth contours and have diameters within the comparatively narrow range (mean ±2 SD) of 6.0 to 8.5 μm. They stain quite deeply with the eosin component of Romanowsky dyes, particularly at the periphery of the cell in consequence of the cell's normal biconcavity. A small but variable proportion of cells in well made films (usually less than 10%) are definitely oval rather than round and a very small percentage may be contracted and have an irregular contour or appear to be cells which have lost part of their substance as the result of fragmentation. There may be a very occasional

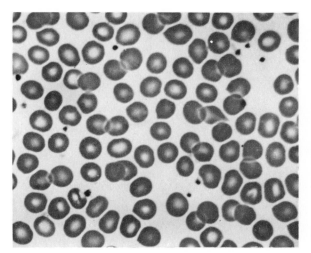

Fig. 5.1 Photomicrograph of a blood film. Film of a healthy adult. ×700.

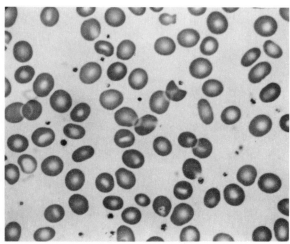

Fig. 5.2 Photomicrograph of a blood film. Ideal thickness for examination. ×700.

pyknocyte or schistocyte. According to Marsh the percentage of 'pyknocytes' and schistocytes in normal blood does not exceed 0.1% and the proportion is usually considerably less than this;[12] in normal full-term infants the proportion is higher, 0.3–1.9%,[12] and in premature infants still higher, up to 5.6%.[12]

Normal and pathological red cells are subject to considerable distortion in the spreading of a film and, as already referred to, it is imperative to scan films carefully to find an area where the red cells are least distorted before attempting to examine the cells in detail. Such an area can usually be found towards the tail of the film, although not actually at the tail. Rouleaux often form rapidly in blood after withdrawal from the body and may be conspicuous even in films made at a patient's bedside. They are particularly noticeable in the thicker parts of a film, which have dried more slowly. Ideally, red cells should be examined in an area in which little or no rouleaux have formed, but the film in the chosen area must not be so thin as to cause red-cell distortion. The very different appearances of different areas of the same blood film are illustrated in Figs. 5.2–5.4. The area illustrated in Fig. 5.2 would clearly be the best for looking at red cells critically.

In *disease*, abnormality in the red-cell picture stems from four main causes:

1. Abnormal erythropoiesis which may be effective or ineffective.

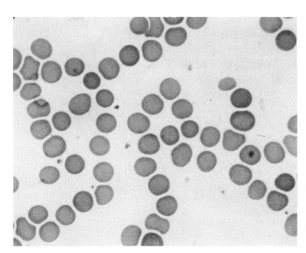

Fig. 5.3 Photomicrograph of a blood film. Film too thin. From same slide as Fig. 5.2 . ×700.

2. Inadequate haemoglobin formation.

3. Damage to, or changes affecting, the red cells after leaving the bone marrow.

4. Attempts by the bone marrow to compensate for anaemia by increased erythropoiesis.

These processes result, respectively, in the following abnormalities of the red cells:

1. Increased variation in size and shape (*anisocytosis* and *poikilocytocis*).

2. Reduced or unequal haemoglobin content (*hypochromasia* or *anisochromasia*).

3. *Spherocytosis, irregular contraction* or *fragmentation (schistocytosis).*

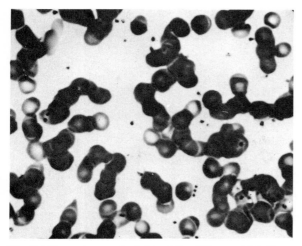

Fig. 5.4 Photomicrograph of a blood film. Film too thick. From same slide as Fig. 5.2. ×700.

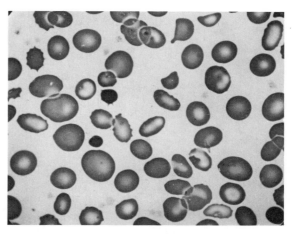

Fig. 5.6 Photomicrograph of a blood film. Shows a marked degree of anisocytosis, caused by the presence of both microcytes and macrocytes. ×700.

4. Signs of immaturity (*polychromasia*, *punctate basophilia* and *erythroblastaemia*).

INCREASED VARIATION IN SIZE AND SHAPE

Anisocytosis (ἄνισός, unequal) and **poikilocytosis** (πόικιλός, varied)

These are non-specific features of almost any blood disorder. The terms imply more variation in size than is normally present (Fig. 5.5). Anisocytosis may be due to the presence of cells larger than normal (*macrocytosis*) or cells smaller than normal

(*microcytosis*); frequently both macrocytes and microcytes are present together (Fig. 5.6).

Macrocytes

Classically found in megaloblastic anaemias (Figs. 5.7, 5.56), but they are also present in aplastic anaemia (and other dyserythropoietic anaemias). In one rare form of congenital dyserythropietic anaemia (Type III), the macrocytes are exceptionally large (Fig. 5.8). Another cause of macrocytosis is chronic liver disease. In this condition the red cells tend to be fairly uniform in size

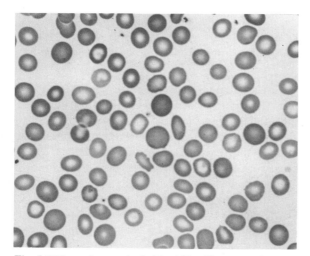

Fig. 5.5 Photomicrograph of a blood film. Shows a moderate degree of anisocytosis. ×700.

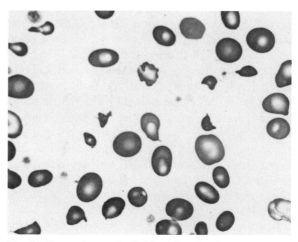

Fig. 5.7 Photomicrograph of a blood film. Pernicious anaemia. Shows macrocytes, poikilocytes and cell fragments (schistocytes), and extreme anisocytosis. ×700.

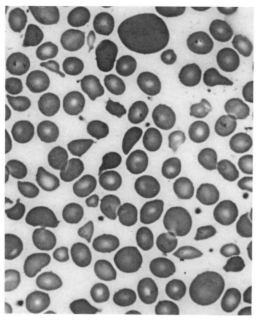

Fig. 5.8 Photomicrograph of a blood film. Congenital dyserythropoietic anaemia Type III. Shows unusually large macrocytes. ×700.

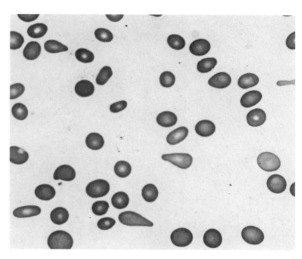

Fig. 5.9 Photomicrograph of a blood film. Myelosclerosis. Shows poikilocytosis and moderate anisocytosis. ×700.

and shape. Macrocytosis also occurs whenever there is increased erythropoiesis, because of the presence of reticulocytes. These are identified by them staining slightly basophilically, giving rise to polychromasia (p. 77) and their presence can be easily confirmed by a reticulocyte count.

Microcytes

Result from fragmentation of normally sized red cells (normocytes) or macrocytes, as occurs with many types of abnormal erythropoiesis, e.g. megaloblastic anaemia (Fig. 5.7). Microcytes are formed as such, or result from fragmentation, in iron-deficiency anaemia (Fig. 5.12) and thalassaemia (Fig. 5.13). In haemolytic anaemias, microcytes result from the process of spherocytosis or from fragmentation (Figs. 5.16–5.25).

Poikilocytes

Produced in many types of abnormal erythropoiesis, e.g. megaloblastic anaemia, iron-deficiency anaemia, thalassaemia, myelosclerosis; they also result from damage to circulating red cells, as in microangiopathic haemolytic anaemia. Poikilocyto-

sis (and anisocytosis) are illustrated in Figs. 5.7, 5.9 and 5.21–5.24.

Elliptocytosis

In disease a much higher proportion of oval or elliptical red cells may be found than in health. Elliptical or oval cells are thus frequent in megaloblastic anaemias and in hypochromic anaemias (Fig. 5.12); they may, too, be conspicuous in myelosclerosis (Fig. 5.10). The highest proportions are found in hereditary elliptocytosis and

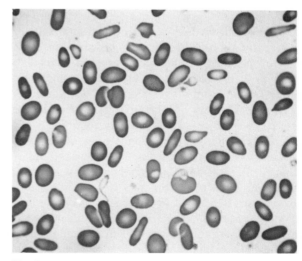

Fig. 5.10 Photomicrograph of a blood film. Myelosclerosis. Almost all the cells are elliptical or oval (cf Fig. 5.11). ×700.

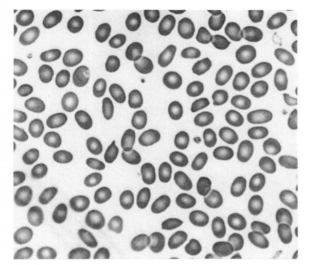

Fig. 5.11 Photomicrograph of a blood film. Hereditary elliptocytosis. Almost all the cells are elliptical. ×700.

hereditary ovalocytosis in which 90% or more of the adult red cells may be markedly elliptical or oval (Fig. 5.11). Remarkably, the reticulocytes in the above conditions are round in contour; that is to say, the cell assumes an abnormal shape only in the late stages of maturation.

INADEQUATE HAEMOGLOBIN FORMATION

Hypochromasia (υπόρ, under)

Present when red cells stain unusually palely. (In doubtful cases it is wise to compare the staining of the suspect film with that of a normal film stained at the same time.) There are two possible causes: a lowered haemoglobin concentration and abnormal thinness of the red cells. A lowered haemoglobin concentration results from impaired haemoglobin synthesis. This may stem from failure of haem synthesis—iron deficiency is a very common cause (Fig. 5.12), sideroblastic anaemia a rare cause—or failure of globin synthesis as in the thalassaemias (Fig. 5.13). Haemoglobin synthesis may also be interfered with by infections. It cannot be too strongly stressed that a hypochromic blood picture does *not* necessarily mean iron deficiency, although this is the most common cause. In iron deficiency the red cells are characteristically hypochromic and microcytic, but the extent of these abnormalities depends on the severity; hypochromasia may be

overlooked if the Hb exceeds 100 g/l. In homozygous β-thalassaemia, the abnormalities are greater than in iron deficiency at the same level of Hb, but it may not be possible to distinguish heterozygous β-thalassaemia from iron deficiency by the blood film.

Anisochromasia

A proportion only of the red cells stain palely. Can be seen in several circumstances: in a patient with

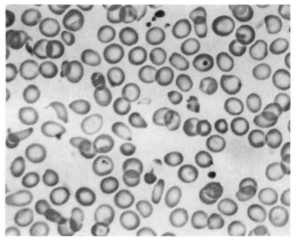

Fig. 5.12 Photomicrograph of a blood film. Iron-deficiency anaemia. Shows a marked degree of hypochromasia, microcytosis and anisocytosis, and a few poikilocytes and cell fragments. ×700.

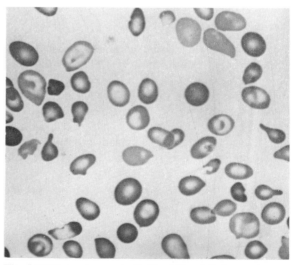

Fig. 5.13 Photomicrograph of a blood film. β-thalassaemia major. Shows hypochromasia and anisocytosis, and numerous poikilocytes and cell fragments. ×700.

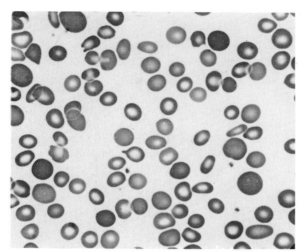

Fig. 5.14 Photomicrograph of a blood film. Iron-deficiency anaemia. Shows anisochromasia following treatment with iron. A macrocytic and orthochromic population contrasts with a microcytic and hypochromic one (dimorphic picture). ×700.

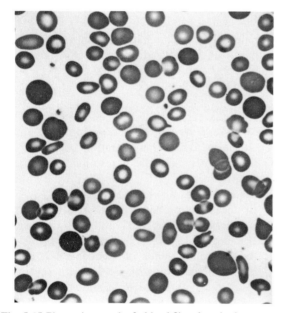

Fig. 5.15 Photomicrograph of a blood film. Acquired sideroblastic anaemia. Shows marked anisocytosis and anisochromasia (cf Fig. 5.14). ×700.

an iron-deficiency anaemia responding to iron therapy (Fig. 5.14), after the transfusion of normal blood to a patient with a hypochromic anaemia and in sideroblastic anaemia (Fig. 5.15). Such blood pictures have been referred to as 'dimorphic'.

Hyperchromasia ($\upsilon\pi\acute{\epsilon}\rho$, over).

Unusually deep staining of the red cells may be seen in macrocytosis when the red-cell thickness is increased and the haemoglobin concentration normal, as in neonatal blood and megaloblastic anaemias, and in spherocytosis in which the red-cell thickness is greater than normal and the MCHC slightly increased (Figs. 5.16–5.19).

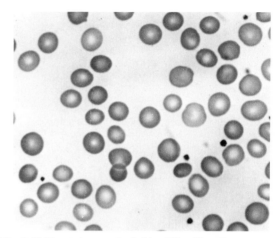

Fig. 5.16 Photomicrograph of a blood film. Hereditary spherocytosis. Shows a moderate degree of spherocytosis and anisocytosis. Note the round contour of the spherocytes. ×700.

DAMAGE TO RED CELLS AFTER FORMATION

Spherocytosis ($\sigma\phi\alpha\iota\rho\alpha$, a sphere).

Spherocytes are cells which are more spheroidal (i.e. less disc-like) than normal red cells. Their diameter is less and their thickness greater than normal. Only in extreme instances are they almost spherical in shape. Spherocytes may result from genetic defects of the red-cell membrane as in hereditary spherocytosis (Fig. 5.16), from the interaction between immunoglobulin- or complement-coated red cells and phagocytic cells, as in auto-immune haemolytic anaemia (Fig. 5.17) and from the action of bacterial toxins, e.g. *Cl. perfringens* lecithinase (Fig. 5.18).

Spherocytes typically appear perfectly round in contour in stained films; they have to be carefully distinguished from 'spherical forms' or 'crenated

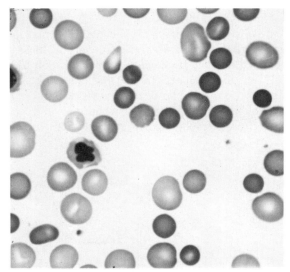

Fig. 5.17 Photomicrograph of a blood film. Auto-immune haemolytic anaemia. Shows a moderate degree of spherocytosis and anisocytosis. ×700.

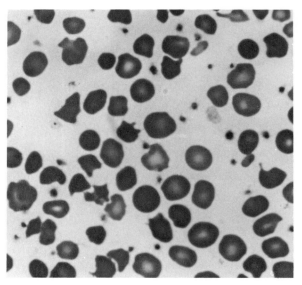

Fig. 5.19 Photomicrograph of a blood film. Congenital haemolytic anaemia, ? diagnosis. Shows many irregularly-contoured spherocytes; an unusual picture. ×700.

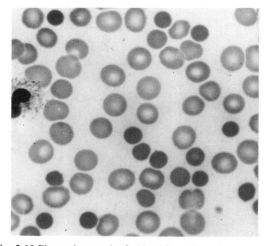

Fig. 5.18 Photomicrograph of a blood film. *Cl. perfringens* septicaemia. Shows an extreme degree of spherocytosis; note the round contour of the spherocytes. A markedly dimorphic picture. ×700.

spheres' (Fig. 5.43), the end-result of crenation or acanthocytosis (see p. 73); 'spherical forms' can develop as artifacts especially in blood which has been allowed to stand before films are spread. In rare and atypical hereditary haemolytic anaemias spherocytes may have an irregular contour (Fig. 5.19) and in haemolytic hereditary elliptocytosis any spherocytes present tend to be oval rather than round (Fig. 5.11). The blood film of a patient who has been transfused with stored blood may show a proportion of spherocytes.

Schistocytosis (fragmentation)($\sigma\chi\iota\sigma\tau\acute{o}\varsigma$, cleft).

Schistocytes, of varying shape, are found in many blood diseases. Thus fragmentation occurs:

1. In certain genetically determined disorders, e.g. thalassaemias (Fig. 5.13) and hereditary elliptocytosis and allied disorders (Fig. 5.20).

2. In acquired disorders of red-cell formation, e.g. megaloblastic (Fig. 5.7) and iron-deficiency anaemias (Fig. 5.12).

3. As the consequence of mechanical stresses, e.g. in the microangiopathic haemolytic anaemias (Figs. 5.21–5.23) and cardiac haemolytic anaemias (Fig. 5.24).

4. As the result of direct thermal injury as in severe burns (Fig. 5.25).

In all conditions in which fragmentation is occurring three types of cell can be distinguished:

1. Small fragments of cells of varying shape, sometimes with sharp angles or spines (spurs), sometimes round in contour, usually staining deeply but occasionally palely as the result of loss of haemoglobin at the time of fragmentation.

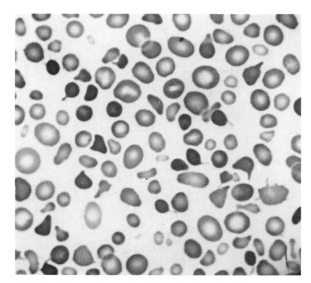

Fig. 5.20 Photomicrograph of a blood film. Hereditary haemolytic anaemia, a variant of hereditary ovalocytosis. Shows spherocytosis and numerous cell fragments, and a few elliptocytes. ×700.

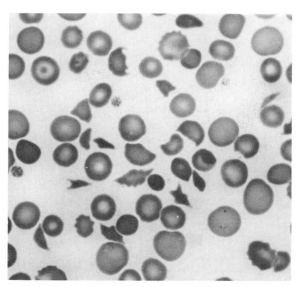

Fig. 5.22 Photomicrograph of a blood film. Microangiopathic haemolytic anaemia: haemolytic-uraemic syndrome. Shows spherocytosis and cell fragments, and marked crenation. ×700.

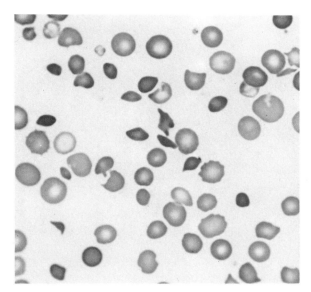

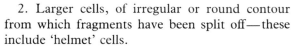

Fig. 5.21 Photomicrograph of a blood film. Microangiopathic haemolytic anaemia: renal cortical necrosis. Shows numerous small poikilocytes and cell fragments. ×700.

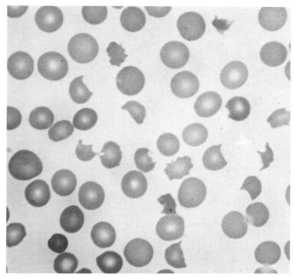

Fig. 5.23 Photomicrograph of a blood film. Microangiopathic haemolytic anaemia: disseminated carcinoma of breast. Shows many bizarre-shaped poikilocytes and cell fragments, and 'burr' cells. ×700.

2. Larger cells, of irregular or round contour from which fragments have been split off—these include 'helmet' cells.

3. Normal unfragmented adult red cells and reticulocytes.

Not infrequently, as for instance in the haemolytic-uraemic syndrome in children, the blood picture is made more bizarre by the superimposition of varying degrees of crenation (Fig. 5.22).

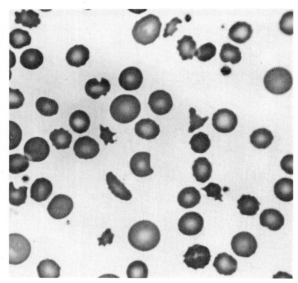

Fig. 5.24 Photomicrograph of a blood film. Post-cardiac surgery haemolytic anaemia. Shows numerous irregularly shaped cell fragments. Note presence of platelets. ×700.

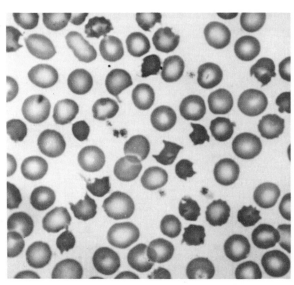

Fig. 5.26 Photomicrograph of a blood film. Haemolytic anaemia due to dapsone. Shows many irregularly-contracted cells. ×700.

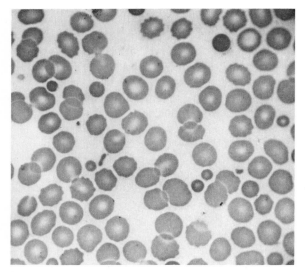

Fig 5.25 Photomicrograph of a blood film. Severe burns. Shows many very small rounded cell fragments, and a little crenation. ×700.

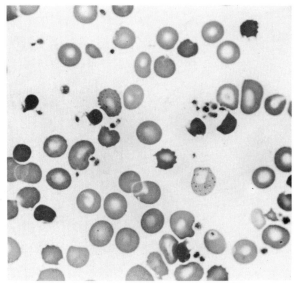

Fig. 5.27 Photomicrograph of a blood film. Phenacetin poisoning. Shows many markedly and irregularly contracted cells; also punctate basophilia. ×700.

Irregularly-contracted red cells

Several types of irregularly contracted cells can be distinguished. In drug- or chemical-induced haemolytic anaemias a proportion of the red cells are smaller than normal and unusually densely staining, i.e. they appear contracted, and their margins are slightly irregular and may be partly concave (Figs. 5.26, 5.27). These may be cells from which Heinz bodies have been extracted by the spleen. Similar cells may be seen in films of some unstable haemoglobinopathies, e.g. that due to the presence of Hb Köln (Fig. 5.28). An extreme

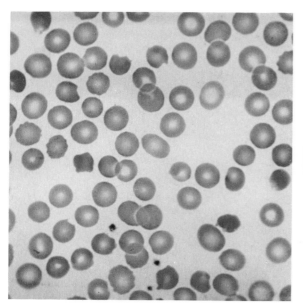

Fig. 5.28 Photomicrograph of a blood film. An unstable haemoglobinopathy (Hb Köln). Shows some moderately contracted cells with somewhat irregular contours. ×700.

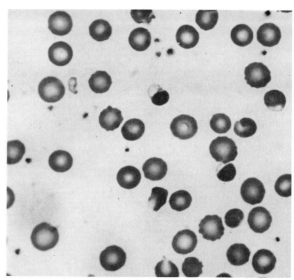

Fig. 5.30 Photomicrograph of a blood film. Favism. Shows numerous markedly contracted cells. Note condensation and contraction of Hb from the cell membrane. ×700.

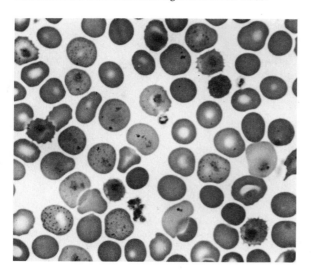

Fig. 5.29 Photomicrograph of a blood film. An unstable haemoglobinopathy (Hb Bristol). Shows contracted and crenated cells; also punctate basophilia and inclusions. ×700.

degree of irregular contraction is characteristic of severe favism, and it is typical to see that in some of the contracted cells the haemoglobin appears to have contracted away from the cell membrane (Fig. 5.30).

A type of irregular contraction of unknown origin has been described by the term pyknocytosis.[21] The pyknocytes closely resemble chemically damaged red cells. As already referred to (p. 63), a small number of pyknocytes may be found in the blood of infants in the first few weeks of life, especially in premature infants. The term 'infantile pyknocytosis' refers to an obscure transient haemolytic anaemia affecting infants in which many pyknocytes are present (Fig. 5.31).[10,21]

MISCELLANEOUS CHANGES

Leptocytosis (λεπτός, thin).

This term has been used to describe unusually thin red cells, as in severe iron deficiency or thalassaemia in which the cells may stain as rings of haemoglobin with large almost unstained central areas (Fig. 5.12). The term *target cell* refers to a leptocyte in which there is a central round stained area in addition to a rim of haemoglobin. Target cells are thought to result from cells having a surface which is disproportionately large compared with their volume. They are seen in films in chronic liver diseases in which the cell membrane may be loaded with chloesterol (Fig. 5.32), and in varying numbers in iron-deficiency anaemia and in thalasaemia. They are often conspicuous in certain haemoglobinopathies, e.g. Hb-CC disease

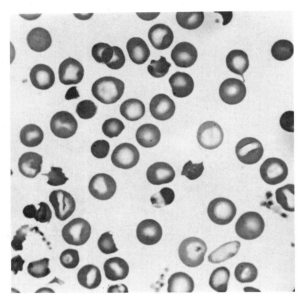

Fig. 5.31 Photomicrograph of a blood film. Infantile pyknocytosis. Shows irregularly-contracted cells similar to those seen in chemical or drug-induced haemolytic anaemias (cf Figs. 5.26 and 5.27). ×700.

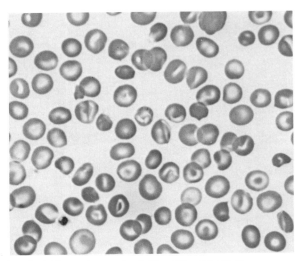

Fig. 5.33 Photomicrograph of a blood film. Hb CC disease. Shows many target cells. ×700.

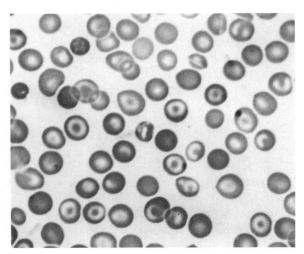

Fig. 5.32 Photomicrograph of a blood film. Chronic liver disease (obstructive jaundice). Shows many target cells. ×700.

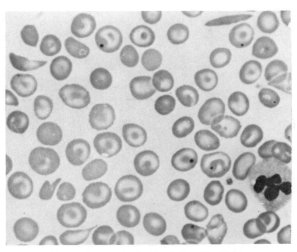

Fig. 5.34 Photomicrograph of a blood film. Hb SS disease. Shows a few sickled cells, target cells and Howell-Jolly bodies. ×700.

(Fig. 5.33), Hb-SS disease (Figs. 5.34–5.35), Hb-SC disease (Fig. 5.37), Hb-S/thalassaemia and Hb-EE disease. In Hb-CC disease crystals of haemoglobin may be seen (Fig. 5.38).

Target cells appear after splenectomy (Fig. 5.39), even in otherwise healthy subjects whose spleens have been removed for traumatic rupture. Splenectomy in thalassaemia may result in an extreme degree of leptocytosis and target cell formation (Fig. 5.40).

Sickle cells (drepanocytes)

The varied film appearances in sickle-cell disease are illustrated in Figs. 5.34–5.37. In homozygous sickle-cell (Hb-SS) disease sicked cells are probably

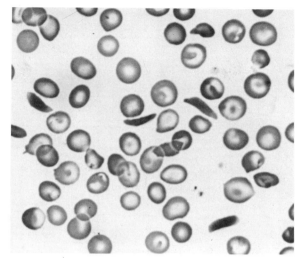

Fig. 5.35 Photomicrograph of a blood film. Hb SS disease. Shows sickled cells and target cells. ×700.

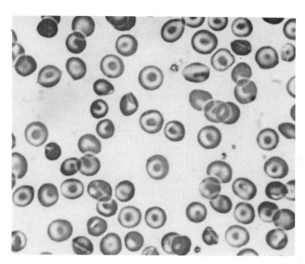

Fig. 5.37 Photomicrograph of a blood film. Hb SC disease. Shows numerous target cells. ×700.

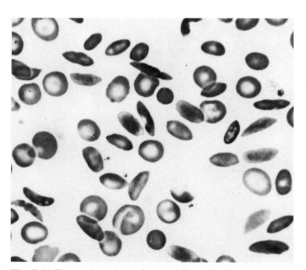

Fig. 5.36 Photomicrograph of a blood film. Hb SS disease. Shows numerous sickled cells. ×700.

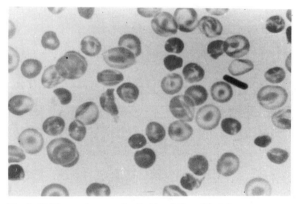

Fig. 5.38 Photomicrograph of a blood film. Hb CC disease. Shows an extracellular crystal. ×700.

Crenation

This term describes the process by which red cells develop many or numerous projections from their surface (Fig. 5.41). Described by Ponder[15] as disc–sphere transformations, crenation can result from many causes, e.g. by washing red cells free from plasma and suspending them in 9 g/l NaCl between glass surfaces particularly at a raised pH, from the presence of traces of fatty substances on the slides on which films are made and from the presence of traces of chemicals which at higher concentrations cause lysis. The end stages of crenation are the 'finely crenated sphere' and the

always present in films of freshly withdrawn blood. Sometimes many irreversibly sickled cells are present (Fig. 5.36) and in all cases massive sickling takes place when the blood is subjected to anoxia (see p. 181). In films of fresh blood the sickled cells vary in shape between elliptical forms, oat-shaped cells and genuine sickles. Target cells are also often a feature (Figs. 5.34, 5.35), and Howell-Jolly bodies are found when there is splenic atrophy.

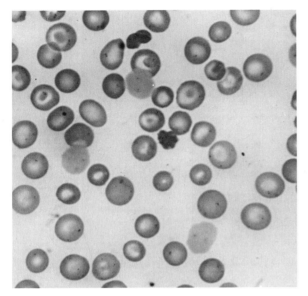

Fig. 5.39 Photomicrograph of a blood film. Pyruvate-kinase deficiency, post-splenectomy. Shows macrocytosis and target cells. ×700.

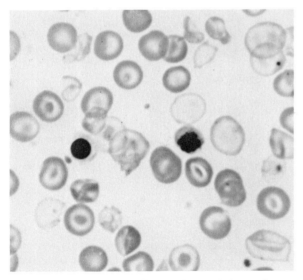

Fig. 5.40 Photomicrograph of a blood film. β-thalassaemia major, post-splenectomy. Shows many target cells and cells grossly deficient in Hb. Many of the target cells are normal cells which have been transfused. Two normoblasts are present. ×700.

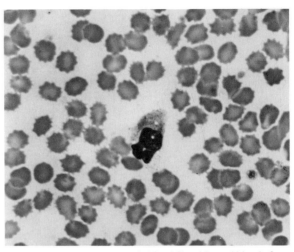

Fig. 5.41 Photomicrograph of a blood film. Normal blood after 18 h at c 20°C. Shows a marked degree of crenation. ×700.

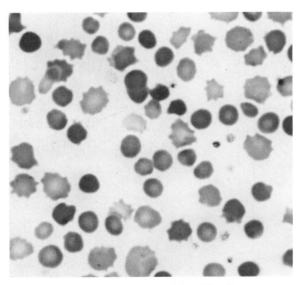

Fig. 5.42 Photomicrograph of a blood film. Hereditary spherocytosis. Shows marked spherocytosis and an unusual degree of crenation. ×700.

'spherical form' which closely resemble spherocytes (Figs. 5.42 and 5.43). The disc-sphere transformation may be reversible, e.g. that produced by washing cells free from plasma, and in this respect the contracted 'spherical form' (which has not lost surface) is quite distinct from the 'spherocyte' (which has lost surface), although they may closely resemble one another in stained films.

A varying degree of crenation may be seen in many blood films, even in those from healthy subjects. It regularly develops if blood is allowed to stand overnight at 20°C before films are made (Fig. 5.41). It may be a marked feature, for obscure and probably diverse reasons, in blood

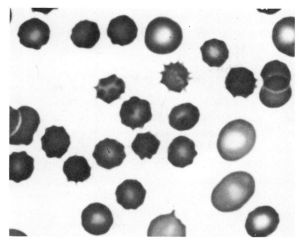

Fig. 5.43 Photomicrograph of a blood film. Acute renal failure following multiple bee stings. Shows crenation leading to finely-crenated spheres. × 1200.

films made from patients suffering from a variety of illnesses, e.g. uraemia. When crenation is superimposed on an underlying abnormality, the red cells may appear bizarre in the extreme (Fig. 5.22).

Acanthocytosis ($\dot{\alpha}\kappa\alpha\nu\theta\alpha$, spine)

The term acanthocytosis was introduced to describe an abnormality of the red cell associated with abnormal phospholipid metabolism (Fig. 5.44).[5,13,16] Characteristically, the majority of the red cells are coarsely crenated (acanthocytes),

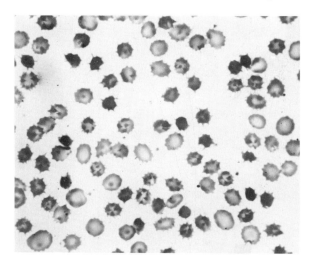

Fig. 5.44 Photomicrograph of a blood film. 'Acanthocytosis'. Many cells show marked crenation and contraction. ×700.

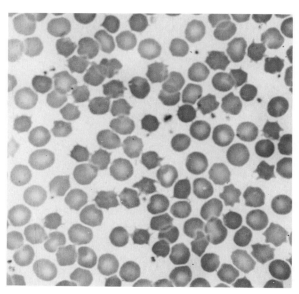

Fig. 5.45 Photomicrograph of a blood film. Hereditary spherocytosis, 11 yr after splenectomy. Shows spherocytosis and crenation (cf Fig. 5.53 for other features of splenic atrophy or post-splenectomy blood films). ×700.

the size and number of the projections varying. Some cells have moderate numbers of small regularly arranged projections from their surface, others have smaller numbers of less regularly arranged finer projections with sharper points. Morphologically, rather similar irregularly crenated cells (? acanthocytes) are to be seen, often in quite large numbers, in blood films made from splenectomized patients (Fig. 5.45); and somewhat similar cells may be seen in the films of some patients with anaemia and chronic liver disease ('spur cell' anaemia)[18] Yet another cause of acanthocytosis is the McLeod phenotype, caused by lack of the Kell antigen precursor (Kx) (Fig. 5.46).[24] The cause of these phenomena is obscure, but they may reflect an abnormality in the phospholipid content or phospholipid-cholesterol ratio of the red-cell membrane.

In another type of ? acanthocytosis, a proportion of the red cells bear small numbers of irregularly situated but often quite large projections with rounded tips (Fig. 5.47). Although usually less than 10% of the cells are affected, the appearances are unusual and distinctive. The cause of the abnormality is obscure; the phenomenon is not rare and its relationship, if any, to other types of acanthocytosis has not been determined. The

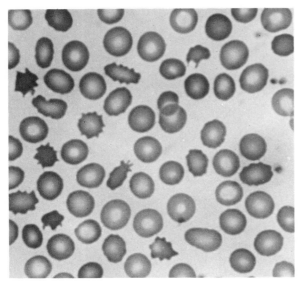

Fig. 5.46 Photomicrograph of a blood film. Spur cells. ×700.

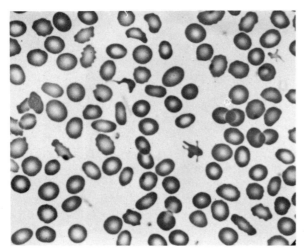

Fig. 5.47 Photomicrograph of a blood film. Acanthocytosis. Shows some bizarre shaped acanthocytes and cell fragments; also moderate anisocytosis and ovalocytosis. ×700.

change has not yet been found to correlate with any particular type of illness, and in some instances the patients have not been anaemic.

Burr Cells

The 'burr' abnormality was described by Schwartz and Motto[17] in the blood films of patients suffering from a variety of disorders, but particularly in uraemia. Burr cells are small cells or cell fragments

bearing one or a few spines. They are probably damaged or fragmented cells which have undergone a type of crenation (Figs. 5.22, 5.23).

Stomatocytosis (στόμα, mouth)

Stomatocytes are red cells in which the central biconcave area appears slit-like in dried films. The term was first used to describe the appearances of some of the cells in a rare type of hereditary haemolytic anaemia.[11] In 'wet' preparations, the stomatocyte is a cup-shaped red cell. Subsequently, stomatocytes have been recognized in small numbers in many films and occasionally many or even the majority of the cells present are stomatocytes (Fig. 5.48). They occur in alcoholism. Their presence in large numbers has been attributed to a genetic factor, stomatocytes having been described as being particularly frequent in films of Australians of Mediterranean origin.[4,14] There is a suspicion that in some films the occurrence of stomatocytosis may be an artifact and it is known that the change can be produced by decreased pH and as the result of exposure to cationic detergent-like compounds and non-penetrating anions.[22] However, it remains to be explained, if the stomatocytic change is usually an artifact, why the change is seen in some films and not in others and why some cells are affected and not others.

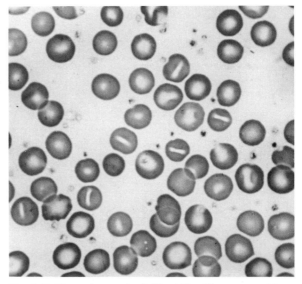

Fig. 5.48 Photomicrograph of a blood film. 'Stomatocytosis'. Many of the cells have slit-like central unstained areas. ×700.

The advent of the scanning electron microscope, which has a resolving power at least ten times that of the light microscope, has a great depth of focus and gives a three-dimensional view, has provided the stimulus and the means for a critical re-examination of red-cell morphology.

Bessis and his co-workers have published excellent photographs of pathological red cells and have introduced a new nomenclature to describe what they have seen.[1,2,22] They use the term *echinocyte* (ἐχῖνοζ, sea urchin) for the crenated cell and clearly differentiate the echinocyte from the acanthocyte. (The normal cell is referred to as a discocyte.) Echinocytes (e.g. crenated red cells as produced by adding oleic acid or lysolecithin to plasma) have 10–30 evenly distributed spicules, while acanthocytes (in congenital abetalipoproteinaemia) have 5–10 spicules of varying length which are irregularly distributed. Acanthocytes can undergo crenation, the product being termed an 'acanthoechinocyte'. Bessis and his co-workers stressed how the echinocytic and stomatocytic change can be superimposed on other pathological forms. Thus, they illustrated 'sickle-stomatocytes' and 'stomato-acanthocytes'. They also discussed the difficult question of the in vivo significance of crenation (echinocytic change) observed in vitro. It seems that neither echinocytosis nor acanthocytosis is necessarily associated with increased haemolysis. It cannot be concluded, too, that crenation is occurring in vivo, when the phenomenon is markedly evident in films made on glass slides. To ensure that cells are crenated in any blood sample as it is withdrawn, Brecher and Bessis recommended that the blood be examined immediately between plastic instead of glass cover-slips or slides, to avoid the known 'echinocytogenic' effect of glass surfaces, probably due to alkalinity.[2] Recently, marked echinocytosis has been reported in premature infants following exchange transfusion or transfusion of normal red cells.[6]

CHANGES ASSOCIATED WITH COMPENSATORY ERYTHROPOIESIS

Polychromasia (πολύς, many)
This term suggests that the red cells are being stained many colours. In practice, it denotes that some of the red cells stain shades of bluish grey—

these are the reticulocytes. Cells staining shades of blue, 'blue polychromasia', are unusually young reticulocytes. 'Blue polychromasia' is most often seen when there is extramedullary erythropoiesis, as, for instance, in myelosclerosis or carcinomatosis.

Punctate basophilia

'Classical' punctate basophilia is found, as a variant of diffuse basophilia, in many blood diseases, as well as in infections and intoxications such as lead poisoning. The granules of diffuse punctate basophilia are uniformly distributed in the cell (Figs. 5.49 and 5.50); they do not give a positive Perls's reaction for ionized iron in contrast to Pappenheimer bodies (see below) which do.

Erythroblastaemia

Erythroblasts may be found in the blood films of almost any patient with a severe anaemia; they are, however, very unusual in aplastic anaemia. They are more common in children than in adults and

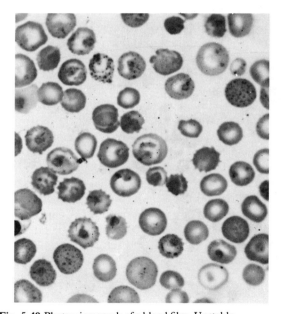

Fig. 5.49 Photomicrograph of a blood film. Unstable haemoglobinopathy (Hb Hammersmith); post-splenectomy. There is a remarkable degree of punctate basophilia. Also shows Pappenheimer bodies and circular bodies corresponding to Heinz bodies. ×700.

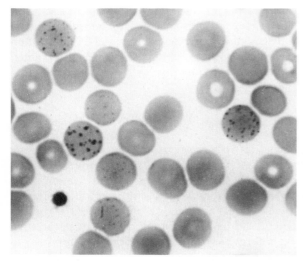

Fig. 5.50 Photomicrograph of a blood film. Punctate basophilia. Pyrimidine-5′-nucleotidase deficiency. ×1200.

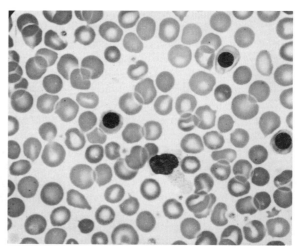

Fig. 5.51 Photomicrograph of a blood film. Myelosclerosis, post-splenectomy. Shows three normoblasts, and moderate anisocytosis and poikilocytosis; also a target cell and a cell fragment. ×700.

very characteristic of haemolytic disease of the newborn. Small numbers can be found in the cord blood of normal infants at birth and quite large numbers in that of premature infants.

When large numbers of erythroblasts are present, many of them are probably derived from extramedullary foci of erythropoiesis, e.g. in the liver and spleen. This seems likely to be true, for instance, in haemolytic disease of the newborn, leukaemia, myelosclerosis and carcinomatosis. In carcinomatosis the number of erythroblasts is often disproportionately high for the degree of anaemia, and a few immature granulocytes are usually present also (so-called leuco-erythroblastic anaemia).

Erythroblasts can usually be found in the peripheral blood after splenectomy and in the presence of extramedullary erythropoiesis the number may be very large (Fig. 5.51). Large numbers are frequently seen in the blood films of Hb-SS disease patients in painful crises. Small numbers of erythroblasts are not uncommon in blood from patients suffering from cyanotic heart failure or septicaemias.

Howell-Jolly bodies

These are nuclear remnants and (usually singly) may be seen in a small percentage of red cells in pernicious anaemia. Cells containing them are regularly present post-splenectomy and where there

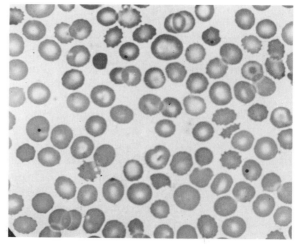

Fig. 5.52 Photomicrograph of a blood film. Steatorrhoea. Shows Howell-Jolly bodies, target cells and crenation, all consequences of splenic atrophy. ×700.

has been marked splenic atrophy. Usually only a few such cells are present, but they may be numerous in steatorrhoea in which there is splenic atrophy and some deficiency of folate (Fig. 5.52).

EFFECT OF SPLENECTOMY

Some of the changes have already been mentioned, namely, the occurrence of target cells, 'acantho-

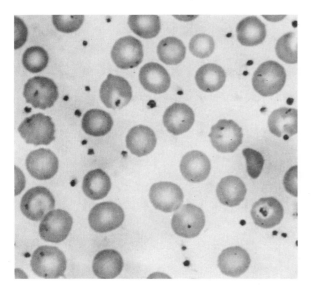

Fig. 5.53 Photomicrograph of a blood film. Pyruvate-kinase deficiency, post-splenectomy. Shows many macrocytes, the majority containing 'Pappenheimer bodies'. ×700.

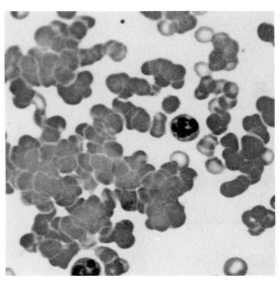

Fig. 5.55 Photomicrograph of a blood film. Shows massive auto-agglutination (cf Fig. 5.54). ×700.

cytes' (Figs. 5.29, 5.39 and 5.45) and Howell-Jolly bodies. Pappenheimer bodies are also regularly found. These are granules, usually minute and usually only present singly or in pairs. Not infrequently they may be found in the majority of circulating red cells (Fig. 5.53). They correspond to the siderotic granules of siderocytes and are never distributed uniformly throughout the cells as is classical punctate basophilia.

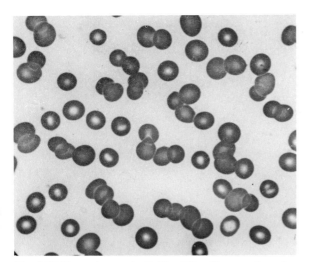

Fig. 5.54 Photomicrograph of a blood film. Shows rouleaux in a normal blood film (cf Fig. 5.55). ×700.

Rouleaux and auto-agglutination

The differences between rouleaux and agglutination are described on p. 56, and there is usually no difficulty in determining which is which in stained films (cf Figs. 5.54 and 5.55). However, in myelomatosis and in other conditions in which there is intense rouleaux formation the rouleaux may simulate auto-agglutination. Even so, if the film, apparently showing auto-agglutination, is carefully scanned an area in which rouleaux can be clearly seen will almost certainly be found. Rouleaux occur to some extent in all films, and their presence adds point, as has been mentioned, to the importance of careful selection of the area of film to be examined.

MORPHOLOGY OF LEUCOCYTES AND PLATELETS

It is difficult to describe shortly the normal morphology of the various types of leucocytes and still more difficult to describe even a selection of the abnormalities met with in disease. To do so adequately would require a lengthy text and many photomicrographs in colour. However, the recognition of leucocyte abnormalities and the appreciation of their significance are of such practical importance that the subjects cannot be omitted altogether. Relatively common abnormalities will be referred to; less common abnormalities, usually well illustrated in atlases, will not be described. The various types of leucocytes will be dealt with in order. (The descriptions refer to cells stained by Romanowsky dyes.)

NEUTROPHIL POLYMORPHONUCLEARS

The following are abnormalities to look for:

Granules

'Heavy', dark-staining, 'toxic' granules are characteristic of bacterial infections, although with some Romanowsky stains normal granules are also darkly stained. Large reddish-staining granules are frequently seen in aplastic anaemia and also sometimes in myelosclerosis. In myeloid leukaemias, on the other hand, the granules often stain poorly and the recognition of 'agranular' polymorphs may help in diagnosis; sometimes only a proportion of the neutrophils is affected, and the cells with easily visible granules can then act as a standard against which the cells with poorly visible granules can be compared.

Vacuoles

These are not normally visible in the neutrophils in stained films of fresh blood viewed with the optical microscope. In bacterial infections they are, however, not uncommon, and they develop, along with other changes, in normal blood allowed to stand in vitro after withdrawal (see p. 4).

Döhle bodies

These are small round or oval patches up to 2–3 μm in size, usually in the periphery of the cytoplasm of neutrophils, which stain blue-grey with Romanowsky dyes. They are mostly seen in bacterial infections, and are not characteristic of leukaemia. A similar structure occurs as a benign

inherited anomaly, known as May-Hegglin anomaly.

Nuclei

Segmentation of the nucleus of neutrophils is a normal phenomenon which, it has been suggested, enables the cells to pass through small spaces in the course of leaving blood vesels more easily than they would be able to if their nucleus was in one large piece. A shift to the 'left' or 'right', of the segmentation of the nuclei of neutrophils in the peripheral blood has been noticed and studied for years and has been recorded quantitatively by various, mostly obsolete, indices. There is no doubt, however, but that recognition of a right shift can help in the diagnosis of a megaloblastic anaemia (Fig. 5.56). Uraemia is another cause of a right shift, and atypical hypersegmented neutrophils may sometimes be seen in leukaemia.

A shift to the left, with band and stab forms and a few myelocytes, is a common consequence of severe sepsis and is usually accompanied by 'toxic' granulation etc. (Fig. 5.57). More pronounced left shifts, e.g. with promyelocytes and a few blasts present, are more likely to denote leucoerythroblastic anaemia or leukaemia but such a picture can be seen in severe infections.

Abnormalities in nuclear shape, e.g. unusually elongated or bizarre-shaped lobes, are not uncommon in some leukaemias, and at the opposite end of the scale, Pelger-like nuclei may be encountered,

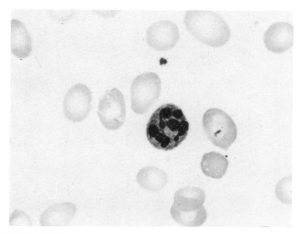

Fig. 5.56 Photomicrograph of a blood film. Pernicious anaemia. Shows a hypersegmented neutrophil. ×700.

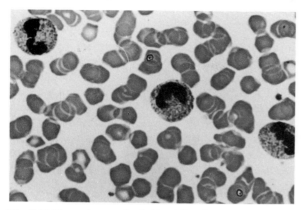

Fig. 5.57 Photomicrograph of a blood film. Severe infection. Shows neutrophil left shift and toxic granulation. ×700.

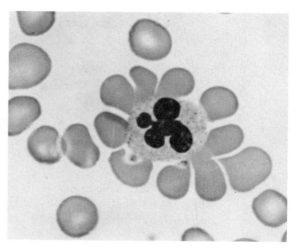

Fig. 5.58 Photomicrograph of a blood film. Adherence of red cells (and two platelets) to a neutrophil. Patient had acquired haemolytic anaemia, with negative direct antiglobulin test. ×1200.

too, in myeloid leukaemias. In such instances the nuclei are unusually densely staining and have rounded contours and there is a sharp distinction between acidophilic and basophilic chromatin. The majority of the cells will be unsegmented 'metamyelocytes', and at the most a polymorph consists of two regular almost equal lobes. In some cases Pelger 'myelocytes' with small round nuclei may be present. Pelger cells, as seen in leukaemia, are morphologically very similar to the neutrophils of the benign inherited Pelger-Hüet anomaly.

Occasionally, unusually large neutrophils may be seen in films. Such cells often appear to contain about twice the normal amount of nuclear material; they are in fact probably tetraploid. Such cells are most frequent in leukaemia but small numbers may be found in a variety of benign conditions.

Small numbers of dead or dying polymorphonuclears may be found in blood films; they are to be seen in their largest numbers in severe sepsis or in blood which has been allowed to stand 18 h or more in vitro. The nuclei of such cells are densely staining, small and rounded off.

An interesting phenomenon which has occasionally been observed is the adhesion of red cells to neutrophils (Fig. 5.58). At first sight an immune adherence phenomenon, the significance and mechanism of the occurrence is unknown.

LYMPHOCYTES

Normally, the majority of circulating lymphocytes are small cells with only a scanty rim of cytoplasm in which there are often a few scattered azurophil granules. About 10% of the lymphocytes in circulation are much larger cells with more abundant cytoplasm and a reduced nuclear : cytoplasmic ratio; the cytoplasm of these large lymphocytes frequently contains azurophil granules. In both small and large lymphocytes, the nucleus is relatively homogeneous but a few cells may have one to two discernible nucleoli. Lymphoblasts, with relatively small amounts of cytoplasm, larger nuclei, less dense nuclear pattern and well defined nucleoli probably do not circulate in health, except possibly in small numbers in the blood of infants. In acute lymphoblastic leukaemia they may be the predominant cell type. Sometimes, the cells, although clearly blasts, are quite small (microblasts) and do not exceed mature lymphocytes in size.

In certain lymphomas, lymphocytes with clefts in their nuclei, giving rise sometimes to overlapping lobes, are not uncommon; usually these are small cells with little cytoplasm. (Lymphocytes with well marked lobes are likely to be artifacts developing in blood allowed to stand in vitro [see p. 4]). Plasmacytoid lymphocytes, with deeply basophilic cytoplasm, are not uncommon in infections, particularly in virus infections, e.g. in rubella, measles, influenza, hepatitis and cytomegalovirus infection; but cells identical with, or very closely similar to, marrow plasma cells are rare in the peripheral blood and their presence (if more than very occasional) may indicate underlying myelomatosis.

The lymphocytosis of infectious mononucleosis is rather characteristic. More abnormal cells are likely to be present than in other virus infections and the cells themselves, 'reactive lymphocytes', although rather variable in size and appearance, tend to be large and to have abundant deeply basophilic cytoplasm.

Lymphocytes predominate in the blood films of infants and small children, and in such films large lymphocytes and reactive lymphocytes tend to be conspicuous.

A variety of lymphocyte types may be seen in chronic lymphocytic leukaemia (CLL). Usually the picture is relatively monotonous, the cells being superficially very similar and usually lacking the few azurophilic granules normally found in the cytoplasm of mature lymphocytes. On close scrutiny of CLL films a small proportion of larger younger cells with one or two visible nucleoli may be seen as well as a few lymphoblasts with multiple nucleoli. In lymphomas, pathological cells, if present, vary in type and if there is lymphocytosis the blood lymphocyte picture is usually far less uniform than in CLL.

MONOCYTES

Monocytes are normally easy to distinguish from lymphocytes and neutrophil polymorphonuclears. In disease, however, this distinction may be less easy. Thus, it is sometimes difficult to separate clearly monocytes from lymphocytes in infectious mononucleosis and monocytes from neutrophils in sepsis and in some types of myeloid leukaemia. Leukaemic monocytes or 'monocytoid cells' tend to differ in subtle ways from their normal counterparts, but the diagnosis of leukaemia, fortunately, does not depend on the recognition of individual cells as leukaemic or normal, respectively. Rarely, monocytes which have acted as macrophages are seen in peripheral blood films. The classic circumstance is bacterial endocarditis, particularly if films are made from ear-pick blood.

EOSINOPHILS AND BASOPHILS

Immature eosinophils, i.e. eosinophil myelocytes and promyelocytes, are seldom seen in peripheral blood films except in chronic granulocytic leukaemia. In non-leukaemic eosinophilias the vast majority of, if not all, the eosinophils are mature. In eosinophilic leukaemia, a varying number of the eosinophils may be partially or almost completely devoid of granules. The presence of such poorly granulated cells points toward leukaemia as the diagnosis but should not be taken as being absolute proof.

PLATELETS

It is possible, using EDTA as anticoagulant, to assess platelet numbers fairly closely by inspection of stained films. In films of native blood, platelets clump and this assessment cannot be done with any pretence of accuracy—except in rare conditions such as Glanzmann's disease in which the platelets fail to clump. Platelets normally vary considerably in size and a small proportion of large platelets, up to 3–5 μm in diameter, may be seen in health. More are present when platelets are being actively regenerated as after haemorrhage or in thrombocytopenic purpura. A higher proportion still of large platelets, and 'giant' platelets up to 7 μm in diameter, may be conspicuous features of thrombocythaemia or myelosclerosis (megakaryocytic myelosis) and in this group of disorders, megakaryocyte nuclei or fragments of nuclei may sometimes be found in peripheral blood films.

Although EDTA is a very convenient anticoagulant to use for routine platelet counts, occasionally the presence of EDTA causes the platelets to clump and the count to be falsely low.[8] The mechanism of this phenomenon and its incidence is unknown. EDTA also affects the staining of platelets, some of which swell and stain relatively palely if EDTA-containing blood is allowed to stand at c 20°C for 2 h or more. Exceptionally, failure to stain develops much more rapidly.[20]

An interesting phenomenon which is occasionally seen is the adhesion of platelets to neutrophils (Fig. 5.59).[3,7,19] Its significance is uncertain for it has been observed in blood withdrawn from

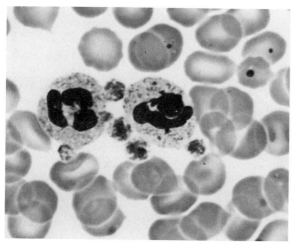

Fig. 5.59 Photomicrograph of a blood film. Idiopathic thrombocytopenic purpura post-splenectomy. Shows adhesion of platelets to neutrophils; also Howell-Jolly bodies. ×1200.

apparently healthy individuals. On the other hand, it has been seen in patients in whom platelet auto-antibodies have been demonstrated[23] and in other types of thrombocytopenia.[9] It is not seen in films made from uncoagulated blood.

REFERENCES

[1] BESSIS, M. (1972). Red cell shapes. An illustrated classification and its rationale. *Nouvelle Revue Française d'Hématologie*, **12**, 721.

[2] BRECHER, G. and BESSIS, M (1972). Present status of spiculated red cells and their relationship to the discocyte-echinocyte transformation: a critical review. *Blood*, **40**, 333.

[3] CROME, P. E. and BARKHAN, P. (1963), Platelet adherence to polymorphs. *British Medical Journal*, **ii**, 871.

[4] DUCROU, W. and KIMBER, R. J. (1969). Stomatocytes, haemolytic anaemia and abdominal pain in Mediterranean migrants: some examples of a new syndrome? *Medical Journal of Australia*, **ii**, 1087.

[5] ESTES, J. W., MORLEY, T. J., LEVINE, I. M. and EMMERSON, C. P. (1967). A new hereditary acanthocytosis syndrome. *American Journal of Medicine*, **42**, 868.

[6] FEO, C. J., TCHERNIA, G., SUBTIL, E. and LEBLOND, P. F. (1978). Observation of echinocytosis in eight patients: a phase contrast and SEM study. *British Journal of Haematology*, **40**, 519.

[7] FIELD, E.J. and MACLEOD, I. (1963). Platelet adherence to polymorphs. *British Medical Journal*, **ii**, 388.

[8] GOWLAND, E., KAY, H. E. M., SPILLMAN, J. C. and WILLIAMSON, J. R. (1969). Agglutination of platelets by a serum factor in the presence of EDTA. *Journal of Clinical Pathology*, **22**, 460.

[9] GREIPP, P. R. and GRALNICK, H. R. (1976). Platelet to leucocyte adherence phenomena associated with thrombocytopenia. *Blood*, **47**, 513.

[10] KEIMOWITZ, R., and DESFORGES, J. F. (1965). Infantile pyknocytosis. *New England Journal of Medicine*, **273**, 1152.

[11] LOCK, S. P., SEPHTON SMITH, R. and HARDISTY, R. M. (1961). Stomatocytosis: a hereditary red cell anomaly associated with haemolytic anaemia. *British Journal of Haematology*, **7**, 303.

[12] MARSH, G. W. (1966). Abnormal contraction, distortion and fragmentation in human red cells. London University MD Thesis.

[13] MIER, M., SCHWARTZ, S. O. and BOSHES, B. (1960). Acanthrocytosis [*sic*], pigmented degeneration of the retina and ataxic neuropathy: a genetically determined syndrome with associated metabolic disorder. *Blood*, **16**, 1586.

[14] NORMAN, J. G. (1969). Stomatocytosis in migrants of Mediterranean origin. *Medical Journal of Australia*, **i**, 315.

[15] PONDER, E. (1948). *Hemolysis and Related Phenomena*. Grune and Stratton, New York.

[16] SALT, H. B., WOLFF, O. H., LLOYD, J. K. FOSBROOKE, A. S., CAMERON, A. H. and HUBBLE, D. V. (1960). On having no beta-lipoprotein. A syndrome comprising a-beta-lipoprotinaemia, acanthocytosis, and steatorrhoea. *Lancet*, **ii**, 325.

[17] SCHWARTZ, S. O. and MOTTO, S. A. (1949). The diagnostic significance of 'Burr' red blood cells. *American Journal of Medical Sciences*, **218**, 563.

[18] SILBER, R., AMOROSI, E., LHOWE, J. and KAYDEN, H. J. (1966). Spur-shaped erythrocytes in Laennec's cirrhosis. *New England Journal of Medicine*, **275**, 639.

[19] SKINNIDER, L. F., MUSCLOW, C. E. and KAHN, W. (1978). Platelet satellitism—an ultrastructural study. *American Journal of Hematology*, **4**, 179.

[20] STAVEM, P. and BERG, K. (1973). A macromolecular serum component acting on platelets in the presence of EDTA—'Platelet stain preventing factor.' *Scandinavian Journal of Hematology*, **10**, 202.

[21] TUFFY, P., BROWN, A. K. and ZUELZER, W. W. (1959). Infantile pyknocytosis: a common erythrocyte abnormality of the first trimester. *American Journal of Diseases of Children*, **98**, 227.

[22] WEED, R. I. and BESSIS, M. (1973). The discocyte-stomatocyte equilibrium of normal and pathologic red cells. *Blood*, **41**, 471.

[23] WHITE, L. A., BRUBAKER, L. H., ASTER, R. H., HENRY, P. H. and ADELSTEIN, E. H. (1978). Platelet satellitism and phagocytosis by neutrophils: association with antiplatelet antibodies and lymphoma. *American Journal of Hematology*, **4**, 313

[24] WINNER, B. M., MARSH, W. L., TASWELL, H. F. and GALEY, W. R. (1977). Haematological changes associated with the McLeod phenotype of the Kell blood group system. *British Journal of Haematology*, **36**, 219.

6

Blood-cell cytochemistry and supplementary techniques
(*Written in collaboration with D. Catovsky*)

CYTOCHEMICAL TESTS

Cytochemical methods applied to haemopoietic cells allow the demonstration of specific enzymes or other substances in individual cells. They are particularly useful for the study of immature cells (e.g. blasts) and lymphocytes because conventional morphology, as seen in Romanowsky-stained films, is not sufficient to identify differentiation features. Most tests are applied to the diagnosis and classification of leukaemia:

1. In distinguishing the patterns of differentiation of early granulocytic and early monocytic cells in the acute leukaemias and in recognizing some types of acute lymphoblastic leukaemia (ALL).

2. In characterizing the cells in chronic lymphoid leukaemias, and, to some extent, in normal lymphocyte subsets.

3. In distinguishing leucocytoses and leukaemoid reactions from genuine myeloproliferative disorders.

4. In studying abnormalities and/or enzyme deficiencies of neutrophils, for example, in the myelodysplastic syndromes.[8]

In erythroid cells, free iron, Hb derivatives and red-cell enzymes can be demonstrated.

In special cases, methods of ultrastructural cytochemistry need to be applied, as the resolution of light microscopy may not suffice to demonstrate the localization of the reaction product. One such example is the platelet peroxidase reaction demonstrable in the endoplasmic reticulum and nuclear membrane of mature and immature cells of the megakaryocytic series.[2,16] A number of techniques for enzyme histochemistry can now also be applied to semi-thin sections of plastic-embedded bone-marrow trephine biopsies.[19]

THE MYELOPEROXIDASE REACTION

Myeloperoxidase is a lysosomal enzyme localized in the azurophil granules of neutrophils and monocytes.[3,83] Azurophil granules in granulocytic cells correspond to the relatively large electron-dense (primary) granules seen under the electron microscope.[3,85] The secondary (specific) granules are less electron dense and appear at the myelocyte stage.[3,16] In the monocytic series the azurophil granules are smaller[83] and are not the first to appear during maturation in these cells. Thus the designation primary for them is not appropriate. The lysosomal granules present in early monocytic cells (monoblasts) are very small and have acid phosphatase but lacks peroxidase activity.[85]

Myeloperoxidase can also be demonstrated in the specific granules of eosinophils and basophils. In eosinophils the specific granules are not newly formed but derive from primary granules which are also myeloperoxidase positive. The eosinophil peroxidase has been shown by chemical, cytochemical and immunological methods to be different from that of neutrophils and probably to be under separate genetic control.[1] The enzyme in eosinophils is cyanide-resistant and, in neutrophils, cyanide-sensitive.[122]

Most of the early methods for the demonstration of peroxidase use benzidine and hydrogen peroxide. The method of Kaplow[67] described in previous editions of this book uses benzidine dihydrochloride, a less carcinogenic compound. As there are difficulties, in some countries, in the use of methods which include benzidine, alternative and probably safer substrates should be considered. These are 3-amino-9-ethyl carbozole, o-tolidine, [50]

2,7-fluorenediamine(FDA)[10,57] and 3,3'-diamino-benzidine (DAB) tetrahydrochloride.[47] Some of them, like α-napthol, are less sensitive than benzidine-based methods and therefore are of little value in the study of leukaemic cells.[61]

DAB is the substrate of choice for ultrastructural studies because its oxidized product is electron-dense and can be intensified by post-fixation with osmium tetroxide.[16] DAB is also frequently used to visualize the immunoperoxidase reaction.[16] Hanker et al[47] described a method using DAB that we have found reliable in the diagnosis of acute myeloid leukaemia (AML).[34] This method, as well as one with the alternative substrate (FDA) described by Inagaki et al,[57] will be described here.

Method with DAB

Fixative. A mixture of 1.25% glutaraldehyde and 1% formaldehyde in 0.1 mol/l phosphate buffer (pH 7.3). Mix 50 ml of a 25% solution of glutaraldehyde, 27.8 ml of a 36% solution of formaldehyde and add the buffer up to 1000 ml.

Incubation mixture. DAB (Sigma Chemical Co.), 5 mg; tris-HCl buffer, 0.05 mol/l, pH 7.6, 10 ml; H_2O_2, 30% (w/v), 0.1 ml. Add the reagents in this order and mix well after each addition. This medium should be prepared just before use.

Enhancer. Dissolve $CuSO_4$, 0.5 g or $Cu(NO_3)_2 \cdot 3H_2O$, 0.5 g in 100 ml of tris-HCl buffer, 0.05 mol/l, pH 7.6.

Counterstain. Dissolve 10 g of Giemsa's stain in 100 ml of 0.066 mol/l phosphate buffer, pH 6.4.

Method

Fix peripheral-blood or bone-marrow films for 1 min and then rinse in 9 g/l NaCl (saline). Immerse the slides in the incubation mixture for 1 min in a Coplin jar at room temperature (20–25°C). Rinse briefly in tris-HCl buffer (three changes) and then immerse the slides in the reaction enhancer. Rinse in saline and keep in the saline until counterstained. Counterstain for 10 min, dry and mount in DPX.

Method with 2,7-FDA[10,57]

Fixative. 10% formal-ethanol solution: 9 volumes of 95% ethanol and 1 volume of 40% formaldehyde.

Incubation mixture. Dissolve 40 mg of 2,7-FDA(Koch-Light Laboratories Ltd.) in 40 ml of tris-HCl buffer (pH 8.6) in order to obtain a saturated solution. Stir vigorously for 5 min at room temperature and then filter to remove excess of precipitated substrate. The solution (without H_2O_2) is stable for at least 6 weeks at room temperature. Add just before use 2 drops of 30% H_2O_2 to the clear filtrate.

Giemsa counterstain. 10% Giemsa in 0.066 mol/l phosphate buffer (as above).

Method

Fix films for 1 min and rinse in water. Transfer the slides to a Coplin jar containing the incubation mixture. Incubate for 5 min at room temperature. Wash for a few seconds and counterstain with Giemsa for 15 min, dry and mount in DPX.

Technical considerations

Either reaction works well with films made from freshly withdrawn (uncoagulated) blood or bone marrow. Myeloperoxidase is not inhibited by heparin, oxalate or EDTA and films made from such blood may be stained adequately if the blood is not allowed to stand at *c* 20°C for more than 6 h. Once films are made they should be left to dry and then fixed; they may then be kept at 4°C for up to 1 week until the reaction is performed. The fixation procedure described above can be interchanged for both cytochemical reactions, and counterstaining may be modified according to individual needs. The methods described above were tested mainly on cells from cases of acute leukaemia.

Significance

Developing granulocytes always give positive reactions; the reaction is strong in promyelocytes and myelocytes but may be negative in very early myeloblasts. Almost all mature neutrophils give a positive reaction despite the fact that few azurophil granules are visible when the cells are stained with Romanowsky dyes. Eosinophils and basophils give positive reactions, as do promonocytes and monocytes. Monoblasts, lymphocytes and lymphoblasts fail to react.

The main value of the myeloperoxidase reaction is in the distinction between acute myeloid and acute lymphoblastic leukaemia (see below).[6,37,50,51] For practical purposes only immature cells that show myeloperoxidase activity can be confidently referred to as myeloblasts; if the reaction is negative they could be any other type of blast cell.

Auer rods nearly always react positively in leukaemic myeloblasts, and the reaction permits a better identification of these characteristic rods

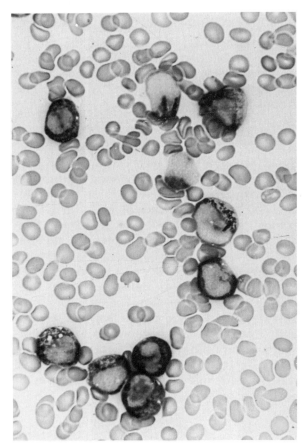

Fig. 6.1 Myeloperoxidase reaction (2,7-FDA method).
Bone-marrow cells from a case of acute myeloblastic leukaemia with maturation (M2). The cells are myeloperoxidase-positive. Note two blasts cells with positive Auer rods. ×800.

than the May-Grünwald-Giemsa stain. An interesting difference has been observed when using the above methods in AML cells. The method with DAB demonstrates a significantly higher percentage of positive rods than techniques with other substrates.[34,47] In particular, DBA allows the visualization of the so-called Phi bodies,[47] small fusiform-shaped rods, which appear to derive from catalase-containing granules, whilst Auer rods derive from primary granules. Thus the apparent greater sensitivity of the method with DBA in samples of AML may result from the known property of DBA to demonstrate catalase in microperoxisomes as well as myeloperoxidase activity.[34] Phi bodies are not seen using the reaction with 2,7-FDA but Auer rods are easily seen (Fig. 6.1). The latter give a clean brown reaction product without crystals or precipitates, which facilitates the morphological recognition of the cells reacting positively.

SUDAN BLACK B STAINING

Sudan Black B was used by Sheehan[105] and later by others to stain the granules of neutrophils, many of which appear to contain phospholipids. The close parallelism observed between sudanophilia and myeloperoxidase activity relates to the fact that both cytochemical reactions are positive in the azurophil granules of neutrophils and monocytes and in the specific eosinophil granules. The biochemical basis for the sudanophilia in these cells is poorly understood.[50] One possible view is that the Sudan Black B stains the lipid membrane of the granules whilst the enzyme myeloperoxidase is contained inside them. Another is that the dye stains through an enzymatic mechanism, perhaps linked to myeloperoxidase, and not just by physical solution in the lipids.[50] Both reactions are positive in mature and immature myeloid cells and thus are useful in the differential diagnosis and classification of the acute leukaemias.[37,50,51] The simplicity of the Sudan Black B reaction makes it mandatory in routine haematology laboratories. The method of Sheehan and Storey[106] which has been in use, almost unchanged, for the last 35 years, is given below.

Reagents

Fixative. 40% formaldehyde.

Staining solution. This is a mixture of two solutions, A and B.

(A) Sudan Black B. 0.3 g in 100 ml of absolute ethanol. Shake well to dissolve the stain and filter to remove particles.

(B) Buffer. 16 g of crystalline phenol in 30 ml of absolute ethanol. Add the phenol-ethanol mixture to 100 ml of water in which 0.3 g of disodium hydrogen phosphate ($Na_2HPO_4.12H_2O$) has been dissovled. Stir vigorously until all the phenol has dissolved and filter. Add 30 ml (or 60 ml) of solution A to 20 ml (or 40 ml) of solution B and filter. The mixture can be kept at 4°C for 2–3 months.

Counterstain. May-Grünwald-Giemsa, preferably, or safranin.

Method

Fix air-dried films of blood or bone marrow for 10 min in formalin vapour. This can be done by soaking filter paper in formalin and placing inside a 37°C incubator.* Wash gently in water for 5–10 min. Immerse in staining solution for at least 30 min; longer periods (e.g. 1 h) may result in stronger staining. Wash in 70% ethanol by waving the slides in the alcohol in a Coplin jar for 3–5 min. Wash with water for 2 min, dry, counterstain for 5 min and mount.

The reaction product in the cytoplasm is black; the nuclei stain blue (or red) depending on the counterstain used.

NEUTROPHIL ALKALINE PHOSPHATASE (NAP)

Alkaline-phosphatase activity can be demonstrated cytochemically in the cytoplasm of mature neutrophils, typically in segmented forms and only rarely in band forms. The enzyme is not demonstrable in other blood leucocytes but fibroblast-

---

* Alternatively, immerse the films for 5 min in a solution of 9 volumes of absolute ethanol and 1 volume of 40% formaldehyde.

like reticulum cells,[9] part of the bone marrow stroma, react strongly.

Recently, small amounts of NAP activity have been demonstrated in the membrane of some lymphoid cells[20] and shown histochemically in a type of B-cell lymphoma.[82]

NAP was thought initially to be localized in the specific (secondary) granules, by analogy with the findings in rabbit neutrophils,[3] or in late-appearing tertiary granules. Recent studies by Rustin et al[94] have shown that NAP is associated with a membranous component of the cytoplasm identified as an irregularly-shaped tubular structure distinct from primary or secondary granules or other cytoplasmic organelles.

Early cytochemical methods for the demonstration of NAP were based upon the hydrolysis of the substrate α-naphthyl phosphate at pH 9.0–10.0 and the coupling of the liberated naphthol to a diazotized amine to form an insoluble coloured precipitate. The intensity of the precipitate is a rough measure of the enzyme content of individual neutrophils. Later methods have used substituted naphthols as substrates,[68] e.g. naphthol AS,[100] AS-BI[66] or AS-MX phosphate; they all give highly chromogenic and insoluble reaction products which are superior to those developed in previously described methods. We describe here below the method of Rutenburg et al[100] which is simple and highly reproducible and gives an easily recognizable blue reaction product. This method can also be applied to tissue sections. For the technical aspects of the preparation and storage of films and the effects of fixation on NAP activity, refer to the detailed review by Kaplow.[68]

Reagents

Fixative. Absolute methanol, 9 volumes; neutral formalin (40% formaldehyde), 1 volume. The mixture should be kept at -20°C, or in the ice compartment of a refrigerator, and may be used for up to 2–3 weeks.

Stock substrate solution. Dissolve 30 mg of Naphthol AS phosphate in 0.5 ml of N,N-dimethylformamide and add 0.3 mol/l tris buffer (pH 9) (p. 436) to make the volume up to 100 ml. This solution is stable for several months at 2–4°C, but its pH should be checked before use.

Diazonium salt. Fast Blue BB or BBN.

Counterstain. 1 g/l aqueous neutral red.

Control. Each batch of slides to be stained should include two controls, a normal blood film and a blood film giving a strong reaction, e.g. from a patient with a polymorphonuclear leucocytosis due to infection.

Method

Make films, if possible from freshly withdrawn blood (no anticoagulant). Films from blood collected into EDTA are less satisfactory, and if anticoagulated blood has to be used, films should be made as soon as possible, and in any case within 30 min of collection.

When made, fix the films without delay for 30 s in the formal-methanol fixative at 0–5°C. Then wash the slides in running tap-water for 10–15 s, drain off excess water and allow to dry. If staining has to be delayed for more than 5–6 h, store the fixed films at −20°C.

Prepare the incubation mixture by dissolving 10 mg of the diazonium salt in 10 ml of the stock substrate solution. Then filter this on to the slides and allow the reaction to continue for 15 min at *c* 20°C. Then rinse the slides in four changes of tap water, allow them to dry and then counterstain the films with neutral red for 6 min. After drying, place a drop of neutral mountant on the slide, and cover the film with a cover-slip.

Scoring results

Alkaline phosphatase activity is indicated by a precipitate of bright blue granules; the cell nuclei are stained red. Based on the intensity of staining and the number of blue granules in the cytoplasm of the neutrophils, individual cells can be rated as follows:

  0: negative, no granules.
  1: positive but very few blue granules.
  2: positive with few to a moderate number of granules.
  3: strong positive with numerous granules.

  4: very strong positive with cytolasm crowded with granules.

The score in an individual film consists of the sum of the scores of 100 consecutive neutrophils. As this mode of assessment is subjective, each laboratory should establish its own normal range.

Significance

The normal range of NAP is wide, 35–100 in our laboratory. In a few normal individuals occasional neutrophils score 3, none 4. The score is higher in women and children than in men, and in newborn infants the range is 150–300.

High scores are found in the neutrophilia of infections, in leukaemoid reactions, liver cirrhosis, Down's syndrome and polycythaemia vera. The enzyme seems to be influenced by oestrogens and corticosteroids, which may explain the gradual rise in score in pregnancy.[89] High scores are found in active Hodgkin's disease but they are uncommon in other malignant lymphomas (lymphocytic or histiocytic); in Hodgkin's disease, however, the determination of NAP has no apparent advantage over simpler tests such as the ESR in the assessment of the activity of the disease.[86] Low scores are found in chronic granulocytic leukaemia in relapse and in myeloblastic leukaemias while the scores in lymphocytic leukaemias are normal or high. Intermediate scores, more often than not rather high, are found in monocytic and myelomonocytic leukaemias.

Low scores are found in paroxysmal nocturnal haemoglobinuria[75] and high scores in aplastic anaemia.[86] The development of PNH in a patient with aplastic anaemia is associated with a falling score.

The value of the NAP reaction in the differential diagnosis of the chronic myeloproliferative disorders and leukaemias will be discussed later (see p. 95).

PERIODIC ACID-SCHIFF (PAS) REACTION

The PAS reaction depends on the liberation of carbohydrate radicals from combination with pro-

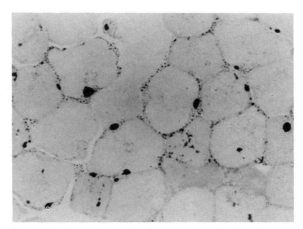

Fig. 6.3 PAS reaction in cells from cerebrospinal fluid. Cytocentrifuge preparation; acute lymphoblastic leukaemia. Most of the cells are PAS-positive with medium-size granules and single blocks. ×1200.

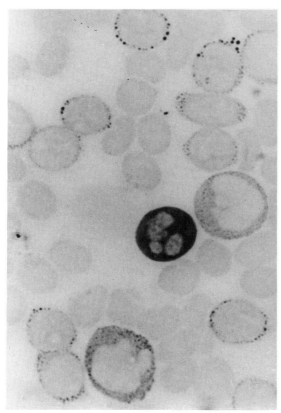

Fig. 6.2 PAS reaction in cells from a peripheral-blood film. Chronic lymphocytic leukaemia. Most of the lymphoid cells are PAS-positive with medium-size granules; two large cells with fine granules are monocytes and in the centre there is a neutrophil showing a diffuse positive reaction. ×1200.

tein and their oxidation to aldehydes by the Schiff reagent. A positive reaction usually denotes the presence of glycogen. This can be confirmed by demonstrating that the positive reaction disappears when the film is treated with saliva or diastase before it is stained. Other PAS-positive material is unchanged by diastase digestion.

Developing granulocytes react positively at all stages of development. Mature polymorphonuclear neutrophils react most strongly (Fig. 6.2) and their cytoplasm contains large amounts of positively-staining material in the form of small granules. Myeloblasts and myelocytes contain fewer positively-staining granules but the cytoplasm stains diffusely pale pink. In eosinophils the background cytoplasm is PAS-positive but the large specific granules are PAS-negative.

Lymphocytes normally contain much less staining material than granulocytes but a few fine or even coarse granules may often be demonstrated. Monocytes contain a small amount of fine, scattered, positively-staining material. The cytoplasm of normoblasts does not normally stain at any stage of development.

The PAS reaction of blood cells differs from the normal in disease and the findings have some diagnostic value.

Lymphocytes in the B-lymphoproliferative disorders (e.g. chronic lymphocytic leukaemia and prolymphocytic leukaemia) often contain an increased number of positively-staining granules (Fig. 6.2); in lymphoblasts, 'blocks' of staining material may be present.[37,50,51] This is the typical reaction in the common type of childhood lymphoblastic leukaemia (Fig. 6.3); in the less common T-cell variant the PAS reaction is, however, often weakly positive.[22]

Erythroblasts may react positively in disease. Deep diffuse staining has been observed in erythroleukaemia[90] and in thalassaemia; and lesser degrees of staining may be seen in iron-deficiency anaemia, cord-blood erythroblasts, sideroblastic anaemia, myelosclerosis, various types of leukaemia and in various types of haemolytic anaemia. Positive reactions have also been recorded in pernicious anaemia, aplastic anaemia, lead poisoning and polycythaemia vera.

The reaction is best carried out on fresh blood or bone-marrow films but old methanol-fixed films or films stained by Romanowsky dyes months or years before can be quite satisfactorily stained.[52]

Reagents

Periodic acid ($HIO_4 . 2H_2O$), 10 g/l.

*Schiff's reagent (leucobasic fuchsin).** Basic fuchsin, 1.0 g; boiling water to 400 ml.

Cool the solution to 50°C and then filter. To the filtrate add 1 ml of thionyl chloride ($SOCl_2$) and allow the solution to stand in the dark for 12 h. Then add 2.0 g of activated charcoal and after shaking for 1 min filter the preparation. Store in the dark at 0–4°C.*

Rinsing solution. Sodium metabisulphite, 100 g/l, 6 ml; 1 mol/l HCl, 5 ml; water to 100 ml.

Counterstain. Mayer's haemalum or Harris's aqueous haematoxylin, 2.0 g; water to 100 ml.

Method

Fix the films in methanol for 5–15 min. Then wash in running tap-water for 15 min. Expose the films for diastase digestion to diastase solution (1 g in 1 l of 9 g/l NaCl) for 1 h at room temperature. Thereafter, allow both treated and untreated slides to stand in the periodic acid solution for 10 min, then wash and immerse them in Schiff's reagent for 30 min at room temperature in the dark. Rinse the slides three times in the rinsing solution, then wash in distilled water for 5 min, counterstain with haematoxylin for 10 min and then blue in tap water for 5 min. Finally, dry in the air and mount in a neutral mountant.

ACID PHOSPHATASE REACTION

There are several techniques for the demonstration of acid phosphatase in leucocytes in films and tissue sections. Some utilize the same reagents used

---

for the demonstration of NAP but at pH 5.0. For example, the method of Li et al uses naphthol AS-BI phosphate and Fast Garnet GBC and gives a highly chromogenic reaction product;[77] it is easily reproducible and suitable for demonstrating the enzyme in the granulocytic series. For lymphocytes and monocytes, a method using naphthol AS-BI phosphate coupled with freshly hexazotized para-rosanilin buffered to pH 5.0[41] may be better, although its final reaction product is less distinctly granular than when Fast Garnet GBC is used.[50] Another good coupling agent is Fast red ITR salt.

Acid phosphatase activity is present in the lyso-somes of many types of haemopoietic cell, i.e. myelocytes, polymorphonuclear neutrophils, lymphocytes, plasma cells, megakaryocytes, platelets, and all the cells of the mononuclear phagocyte system (monoblasts, promonocytes, monocytes and macrophages). It is one of the few acid hydrolases that can be demonstrated in lymphoid cells, and is of diagnostic value in the differential diagnosis of lymphoproliferative conditions (see below). Studies in tissue sections have demonstrated a greater enzyme content in T-cell-dependent areas than in B-cell-dependent areas (e.g. germinal centres) of lymphoid tissues from man and rodents.[112] The activity of acid phosphatase increases after lymphocyte transformation with phytohaemagglutinin and very markedly during the transition from monocyte to tissue macrophage. The technique of Goldberg and Barka[41] has been shown, in our hands, to be reliable in the study of lymphocytic and monocytic proliferations.[18,20,21,22]

Reagents

Fixative. Methanol, 10 ml; acetone, 60 ml; water, 30 ml; citric acid, 0.63 g. This solution should be adjusted to pH 5.4 with 1 mol/l NaOH and controlled weekly.

Stock solutions.

A. Buffer, pH 5.0. Sodium acetate, trihydrate, 19.5 g; sodium barbiturate, 29.5 g; water to 1 l.

B. Substrate. Naphthol AS-BI phosphate (R. A. Lamb or Sigma) dissolved in N-N dimethylformamide, 10 mg/ml (i.e. 25 mg in 2.5 ml).

C. Sodium nitrite ($NaNO_2$). 4% aqueous solution.

D. Pararosanilin hydrochloride (Sigma). 2 g in 50 ml of 2 mol/l HCl. Heat gently, without boiling; cool down to room temperature and filter.

Solutions A, B and D can be stored at 4°C; solution C should be freshly made each time or can only be stored for up to 1 week at 4°C.

Working solution. Mix together 92.5 ml of solution A, 2.5 ml of solution B, 32.5 ml of water and 4 ml of hexazotized pararosanilin solution. Make the latter by mixing well 2 ml of solution C and 2 ml of solution D; allow to stand for 2 min before adding to the other constituents. Mix well and adjust the pH of the working solution to pH 5.0 with 1 mol/l NaOH.

Counterstain. 1% methyl green in veronal acetate buffer, pH 4.0.

Mounting medium. Glycerol/gelatin (Sigma). Add 15 g of gelatin to 100 ml of glycerol and 100 ml of water.

Method

Dry the films well before starting the reaction (it is desirable to leave them for this purpose for at least 24 h at room temperature). Fix the films for 10 min, then rinse the slides well in water. They can now be kept for 1–2 weeks at −20°C if required.

Incubate the slides for 1 h at 37°C in the working solution; rinse in tap water, counterstain the films for 1 min, rinse in tap water and mount whilst still wet. For this, the glycerol/gelatin mixture has to be in liquid phase; i.e. warmed to 37°C or higher.

The cytoplasmic reaction product is bright red; the nuclei stain pale green.

Test of tartrate resistance

This is often carried out in parallel with the above reaction, particularly for the study of hairy cells. Add 375 mg of crystalline L(+)-tartaric acid (Sigma) to 50 ml of the working solution; the final concentration is then 0.05 mol/l. Then carry out the reaction as described above. Most positively-reacting leucocytes are tartrate-sensitive and fail to react in the presence of tartrate. The majority

of hairy cells react equally positively in both solutions.[123]

Significance

The most important application of the acid phosphatase reaction is in the classification of lymphoproliferative disorders. Almost all acute and chronic T-cell lymphoproliferations are characterized by a strong acid phosphatase reaction. In T-ALL (Fig. 6.4)[18,22] the reaction is localized to an area of the cytoplasm which at ultrastructural level corresponds to the Golgi zone.[20] In the chronic T-cell leukaemias the reaction is also positive but with variable consistency. For example, most cases of T-cell chronic lymphocytic leukaemia (CLL) but only two-thirds of those with T-cell prolymphocytic leukaemia (PLL) have cells which react strongly positively. The enzyme activity in these cases is almost always tartrate-sensitive.

In normal T-cells, acid phosphatase activity is an early differentiation feature, e.g. the reaction is positive in fetal thymocytes and it persists in some mature T-lymphocytes.[5] In the B-cell disorders the reaction is often weak or negative with the exception of hairy cell leukaemia (HCL), the cells of which show a strong acid phosphatase activity[77] resistant to inhibition by tartrate in the majority of cases.[123] This enzyme corresponds to a unique isoenzyme 5 found predominantly in hairy cells.[123] Tartrate-resistant cells have not been found in the peripheral blood of normal individuals but a few

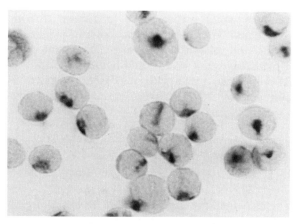

Fig. 6.4 Positive acid phosphatase reaction in a peripheral-blood film. Acute lymphoblastic leukaemia of T-cell type. ×1200.

such cells can be found in normal bone marrow.[80] In B-cell PLL *c* one-third of the cells show a positive acid phosphatase reaction if tested by the method of Goldberg and Barka[41] and these cells, too, have been shown to be tartrate-resistant, as in HCL.[22]

In AML, blasts of the monocytic lineage react more strongly than those of the granulocytic lineage. The reaction in monoblasts is diffuse over the whole cytoplasm and can be seen at ultra-structural level to be localized in the first generation of lysosomal granules.[85] The reaction may be of value in the distinction of the various types of AML (see below).

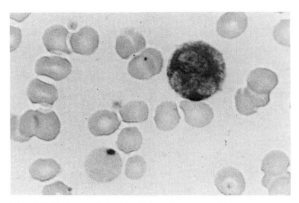

Fig. 6.5 Alpha-naphthyl acetate esterase reaction. ANAE-positive reaction in normal cells. A lymphocyte (presumably T) has a characteristic single 'dot-like' reaction; a monocyte shows a strong diffuse reaction over the whole cytoplasm. ×1200.

ESTERASES

These are a group of hydrolases with a wide range of pH activity which vary in their localization in cells of different bone-marrow lineages. It is best to consider separately the results obtained with the various substrates used for their cytochemical demonstration. Those currently in use are: α-naphthol acetate, α-naphthol butyrate, naphthol AS[118] (or AS-D[37]) acetate and naphthol AS-D chloracetate.

Li et al described nine esterase isoenzymes in leucocytes:[76] 1, 2, 7, 8 and 9 represent the 'specific' esterases of granulocytes which can be demonstrated by means of naphthol AS-D chloractetate; 3, 4, 5 and 6 represent the so-called 'non-specific' esterases which are sensitive to sodium fluoride (NaF) and are found in monocytes, megakaryocytes and platelets, and are demonstrated by α-naphthol esters (acetate and butyrate). Naphthol AS (or AS-D) reacts with most isoenzymes but is inhibited by NaF in its reaction with the non-specific esterases.

α-NAPHTHOL ACETATE ESTERASE (ANAE)

The cytochemical reaction for ANAE is of practical value because it gives distinct patterns in lymphocytes (a dot-like reaction)[20,72,81,91] and in monocytes (a diffuse positive reaction)[15,21] as illustrated in Fig. 6.5. The localized reaction in lymphocytes is resistant to NaF[20,91] whilst that in monocytes is NaF-sensitive.[102] In normal blood there is a good correlation between the proportion of E-rosettes (a T-cell marker) and the percentage of ANAE-positive lymphocytes. The reaction in immature T-cells (thymocytes) is also localized but it is weak and seen in only one-third of those cells. The dot-like reaction in peripheral-blood T-lymphocytes is seen mainly in the subset with Fc receptors for IgM, Tμ cells.[30] Results with the substrate α-naphthyl butyrate are, in general, very similar to those obtained with ANAE. Some authors have made a distinction between the ANAE reaction carried out at different pHs, acid or alkaline, the latter favouring the reaction in monocytes and the former being more specific for T-lymphocytes. The method of Yam et al[122] at pH 6.1 permits the adequate demonstration of the distinct reaction in both cell types.[20,21]

Reagents

Fixative. Phosphate buffered acetone-formaldehyde. Acetone, 40 ml; 35% formaldehyde, 25 ml; Na_2HPO_4, 20 mg, and KH_2PO_4, 100 mg, in 30 ml of water. Filter the solution before use; it must be clear. It will keep at room temperature for 1 month.

Stock solutions.

A. α-Naphthyl acetate. 50 mg dissolved in 2.5 ml of 2-methoxyethanol.

B. Phosphate buffer. 0.1 mol/l, pH 7.6, 44.5 ml.

C. Hexazotized pararosanilin. 3 ml. This is prepared by mixing equal volumes of pararosanilin solution (solution D of the acid phosphatase reaction, see p. 91) and fresh 4% aqueous NaNO₂ for 1 min just before use.

Incubation mixture. Mix solutions A and B and add to them the freshly prepared solution C. Adjust the pH to 6.1 with 1 mol/l NaOH. Filter before use; the solution must be clear.

Counterstain and mounting medium. As for acid phosphatase (methyl-green and glycerol/gelatin).

Method

Fix the films for 30 sec, rinse the slides well in water and allow to dry. Incubate the slides for 45 min in the incubation mixture. After the incubation, wash the slides in tap water and counterstain for 1 min and mount whilst still wet.

The reaction is seen as dark red granules; the nuclei stain pale green.

Inhibition with sodium fluoride (NaF)

Add 75 mg of NaF to 50 ml of the incubation mixture (concentration 1.5 mg/ml = 37.5 mmol/l). Carry the test out simultaneously with the ANAE reaction to investigate the NaF sensitivity of a cell population. This may be necessary for the identification of monocytes within a mixture of mononuclear cells or to characterize a particular leukaemic cell type.

Significance[4,20,30,56,72,122]

The ANAE cytochemical reaction is often applied to the study of normal and leukaemic cell populations. In normal samples it helps to distinguish between T-lymphocytes and monocytes because of the different pattern of reaction and the different sensitivity to NaF (see above). In leukaemias and lymphoproliferative disorders it has three main applications:

1. In AML it facilitates the diagnosis of monocytic leukaemia, the cells of which give a strong diffuse reaction sensitive to NaF.

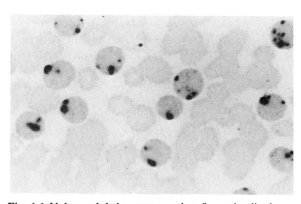

Fig. 6.6 Alpha-naphthyl acetate reaction. Strong localized ANAE reaction in peripheral blood cells of a T-cell prolymphocytic leukaemia. ×1200.
(Photograph by courtesy of Dr. A. D. Crockard).

2. In ALL, together with the acid phosphatase reaction, it helps to identify T-ALL.[4,56]

3. In the chronic B and T lymphoid leukaemias it helps to distinguish T-PLL (positive reaction) (Fig. 6.6) from B-PLL (negative reaction). The typical dot-like pattern of normal T-lymphocytes is not observed, however, in T-CLL. This probably relates to a similar finding in the cell subset that is the normal counterpart of T-CLL (Tγ lymphocytes[30]).

Erythroblasts are normally ANAE-negative. However, they can react positively in megaloblastic anaemia and erythroleukaemia;[98] weak reactions have also been described in thalassaemia and sideroblastic anaemia.

NAPHTHOL AS (OR AS-D) ACETATE ESTERASE

Both substrates are commonly used: naphthol AS acetate (NASA) or naphthol AS-D acetate (NASDA) can demonstrate non-specific esterase activity in monocytic cells. They do not show, as does ANAE, a consistent localized reaction in T-lymphocytes. The reaction with both substrates is carried out at pH 6.9.[122] At this pH, however, prolonged incubation can result in hydrolysis of the substrate by the chloracetate esterase of granulocytes,[76] thus making the reaction less specific for monocytes. Therefore, the simultaneous incubation with NaF is needed to improve the recognition of promonocytes and monocytes and to distinguish them from promyelocytes and myelocytes. NaF is less necessary with ANAE (or α-naphthol butyrate) because the reaction is strong in monocytic cells and is weak or negative in granulocytes. The reaction product with NASDA is often stronger than with NASA and diffuses less; it is thus the substrate of choice.[37] The main value of the reaction is in differentiating between the myeloblastic types (M1 and M2) and the monocytic types (M5a and M5b) of AML.[6] In myelomonocytic leukaemia (M4), it helps in assessing the relative size of the monocytic component.

CHLORACETATE ESTERASE

The specific esterase present in granulocytes and mast cells is distinct from that in monocytes and megakaryocytes; it can be demonstrated by using naphthol AS-D chloracetate as substrate and Fast Garnet GBC,[79] Fast Red Violet or Fast Blue BB[50] as coupling agents. The enzyme is optimally active at pH 7.0–7.6 and is not inhibited by NaF. The reaction is found in mature and immature granulocytes and, in general, the reactions parallel those of myeloperoxidase and Sudan Black B in the granulocytic lineage; Auer rods are often positive. Little or no enzyme activity is demonstrated in lymphocytes and monocytes.

One advantage of the chloracetate method is the possibility of demonstrating enzyme activity in paraffin-embedded histological sections of formalin-fixed material. It can be applied as well to material from other tissues, being particularly useful for the diagnosis of granulocytic sarcoma (chloroma).

The chloracetate esterase reaction has been widely used on haematological material in combination with ANAE or α-naphthol butyrate esterase in a single method: the so-called combined or dual esterase reaction.[50,122] The end-result is the demonstration, in the same preparation, of both types of esterase; they can be distinguished by the colour of the reaction products by using different coupling agents, e.g. blue when using Fast Blue BB for the chloracetate esterase and dark red using hexazotized pararosanilin for ANAE. This procedure simplifies the cytochemical characterization of leukaemic cells. In acute myelomonocytic leukaemia (M4) it helps to identify both the granulocytic and monocytic components.

OTHER ACID HYDROLASES

Two enzymes, β-glucuronidase[37] and β-glucosaminidase,[39] have been shown in histochemical methods to be present in high concentrations in T-cell-dependent areas of lymphoid tissues and to be either absent or present in small amounts in the B-cell-dependent areas.[112] Both enzymes have now been shown to be useful markers of leukaemic T-lymphocytes. The reaction product in cells of chronic B-cell leukaemias is usually weak or negative.[30]

LYSOZYME ACTIVITY

A simple cyto-bacterial method for the demonstration of lysozyme (muramidase) activity based on the technique of Briggs et al,[17] as modified by Syren and Raeste,[111] is described below.

Reagents

Fixative. 10% neutral formalin (1 volume) and 96% ethanol (2 volumes).
Substrate. A fresh suspension of dried *Micrococcus lysodeikticus* (Difco) (60 mg in 1 ml of 9 g/l NaCl) is prepared in a small tissue grinder and homogenized gently.
Buffer. 0.01 mol/l phosphate buffer, pH 7.0.

Method

The test has to be performed within 1 h of collecting the sample. Allow blood or bone marrow collected in EDTA to sediment, or centrifuge it, if the WBC is less than 10×10^9/l, in order to separate the buffy-coat layer. Mix equal volumes of the leucocyte suspension (in the supernatant or buffy coat) and of the substrate (0.25–0.5 ml of each) in a tube and shake gently for 5–10 s. Make films from the mixture and allow them to dry in the air. Once dried, fix them for 1 min and rinse in buffer. Then incubate at 37°C in the phosphate

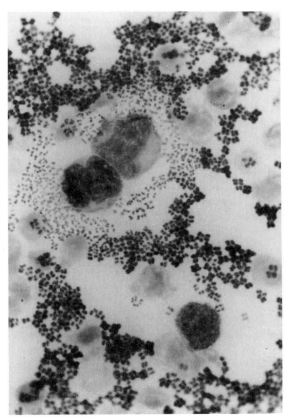

Fig. 6.7 Cyto-bacterial test for lysozyme. Acute monocytic leukaemia. An area of lysis is seen around two leukaemic cells. ×1200.

buffer in a Coplin jar for 10 min. After drying, counterstain the films with May-Grünwald-Giemsa. The myeloperoxidase reaction can also be carried out on slides prepared by this method, thus combining two cytochemical reactions in one film.

Positive lysozyme activity is seen as an area of bacterial lysis of variable size in the immediate vicinity of cells (Fig. 6.7).

Normal blood monocytes and neutrophils always give positive lysis but lymphocytes do not. In normal bone marrow, lysozyme activity can be demonstrated in granulocytes as far back as the myelocyte stage. In acute leukaemia, myeloblasts and lymphoblasts are lysozyme-negative but promonocytes and monocytes and sometimes monoblasts, give positive reactions.

Because lysozyme appears relatively late during monocyte maturation, at the promonocyte stage, this reaction is consistently positive in differentiated forms of monocyte leukaemia, i.e. in M4, M5D and CMML of the FAB classification,[23] but may be negative in the poorly differentiated type, i.e. M5PD. In the former case, a high proportion of leukaemic monocytes (50–90%) are lysozyme-positive. In general, the number of lysozyme-positive cells in the circulation and the serum lysozyme concentration are closely correlated.[23]

PRACTICAL VALUE OF CYTOCHEMICAL REACTIONS

There are three major groups of malignancies of haemopoietic cells in which the cytochemical methods described above have been found to be useful for a correct diagnosis and classification:

1. The acute leukaemias, proliferations of immature haemopoietic precursors (blast cells).

2. The chronic myeloproliferative disorders, proliferations of differentiated cells of the myeloid lineage.

3. The chronic lymphoproliferative disorders, malignancies of mature-looking lymphoid cells.

The so-called myelodysplastic syndromes,[8] a group of conditions distinct from, but possibly related to, the acute leukaemias should also be considered in the differential diagnosis.

Well-prepared peripheral-blood and bone-marrow films stained with May-Grünwald-Giemsa are the basis for any classification. The cytochemical tests provide clues regarding the type and direction of cellular differentiation and should be regarded as complementing and not substituting for the morphological analysis.

DIFFERENTIAL DIAGNOSIS OF THE ACUTE LEUKAEMIAS—THE FAB CLASSIFICATION[6]

Two main forms of acute leukaemia are recognized: myeloid (AML), more frequent in adults (>20 years), and lymphoblastic (ALL), predominantly in children (<15 years).

AML

Six types of AML can be identified by morphology with the help of cytochemistry. The main features of each type (M1–M6) are summarized in Table 6.1. Certain cytochemical reactions are essential in distinguishing AML from undifferentiated forms of ALL (e.g. L2). This is particularly so in cases where the cells are immature, e.g. in M1 (myeloblastic leukaemia without maturation) and M5PD (monoblastic leukaemia, poorly differentiated). The peroxidase, Sudan Black B and chloracetate esterase reaction reveal granulocytic differentiation in the M1, M2, M3 and M4 types of AML whilst the non-specific esterases (NASDA and ANAE ± NaF), and the acid phosphatase and lysozyme reactions, demonstrate monocytic differentiation. In addition to the cyto-bacterial test described on p. 94, lysozyme can be investigated in samples of serum and urine by turbimetric methods.

Although most cases of hypergranular promyelocytic leukaemia (M3) can be diagnosed in May-Grünwald-Giemsa stained films, an M3-variant characterized by having fewer azurophil granules may require for its identification a positive reaction with the cytochemical methods for granulocytic cells (Table 6.1). Because of their (typical) bilobed nuclei, cells of the M3-variant can sometimes be confused with atypical monocytes (as in M4 or M5 leukaemias). However, the non-specific esterase reactions are usually weak or negative in M3.

In erythroleukaemia (M6) the PAS reaction may be strongly positive, with a diffuse or granular pattern being found in erythroblasts and sometimes in erythrocytes, too; the ANAE reaction may also be positive in red-cell precursors.[98]

A rare form of AML, as yet not specifically designated in the FAB classification, is acute megakaryoblastic leukaemia. The blast cells appear undifferentiated, and may resemble lymphoblasts.[2] The cytochemical profile of these cells is similar to that of megakaryocytes: i.e. positive reactions with PAS, acid phosphatase and ANAE (NaF-sensitive

Table 6.1 Classification and cytochemistry of AML

Reaction	Myeloblastic M1	M2	Promyelocytic M3	Myelomonocytic M4	Monocytic M5	Erythroleukaemia M6
May-Grünwald-Giemsa stain	Blasts with few or no granules (90%); Auer rods	Blasts (>30%). Maturation beyond promyelocytes. Abnormal neutrophils	Hyper-granular promyelo-cytes; faggots. Bilobed nuclei. Hypogranular variant	Blasts (>30%). Evidence of granulocytic and monocytic differentiation	(a) Monoblasts; (b) Monoblasts, promonocytes & monocytes. (a) & (b) >80% monocytic cells.	Over 50% of eryth-roid cells, often bizarre. Myeloblasts with Auer rods
Peroxidase / Sudan Black B	+ or ++ (>5% blasts)	++	+++	+ or ++ (2 populations)	− or +	+ (blasts)
Esterases						
1. Chloroacetate	+	++	+++	+ or ++	− or ±	+
2. NASDA	+	+	++	+ or ++*	+++*	+
3. ANAE	−	±	±	+ or ++*	+++*	− or + (erythro-blasts)
Acid phosphatase	− or +	+	+ or ++	+ or ++	+++	±
Lysozyme	−	−	±	+ or ++	± or +++	−
PAS	+ diffuse	+ diffuse	++ diffuse	+ or ++ variable	+/++ granules	+ (erythroblasts)

* NaF sensitive.
Degree of reaction: − negative; ± weak (few positive cells); + moderate, ++ moderate to strong; +++ most of the cells strongly positive. Cytochemical reactions that are useful for differential diagnosis are printed in bold type.

as in monocytes). A specific test for megakaryo-blasts, the so-called 'platelet peroxidase' reaction, can be demonstrated by electron microscopy in the nuclear membrane and endoplasmic reticulum of these cells although not in the Golgi apparatus.[2,16]

The enzyme content of mature neutrophils in AML, particularly in M2 and M6, can often be shown by negative cytochemical reactions to be deficient. The NAP score is often low in M2 (myeloblastic leukaemia with maturation),[63] especially in M2 cases with the chromosome transloca-tion t 8; 21. An interesting difference between the low NAP values seen in CGL and in M2 has been reported by Kamada et al[63]—namely, that if the leukaemic cells are suspended in liquid culture for 1 week the NAP score increases in CGL whilst it remains unchanged in M2. The peroxidase, Sudan Black B and chloracetate reactions may also be negative in variable proportions of neutrophils in AML, more frequently in M2 and M6.[24,52] In contrast, the neutrophils in AML and in M5 react positively in these reactions to about the same degree as do normal neutrophils. The NAP scores are usually normal and high in ALL and M5.

ALL

Three morphological types have been described by the FAB group: L1, L2 and L3.[6,7] The differ-ences in age incidence (L1 is more common in children and L2 more frequent in adults), the strong correlation of L3 with B-ALL (with mono-clonal membrane immunoglobulins) and the differ-ence in prognosis between L1 and L2 (worse in L2) within similar age groups together suggest that the three morphological types may reflect true biologi-cal differences.

L1 lymphoblasts tend to be small and to have scanty cytoplasm; the nucleo-cytoplasmic (N:C) ratio is high in the majority and they have a small and not easily visible nucleolus; the nuclear mem-brane is often regular. L2 lymphoblasts, in contrast to L1, are larger, have more abundant cytoplasm (low N:C ratio) and have one or more prominent nucleoli; the nuclear outline is irregular in over 25% of cells. The differences between L1 and L2 can be more easily resolved in borderline cases by the simple scoring system proposed by the FAB group.[7] L3 (or Burkitt type) cells, because of their resemblance to cells of the endemic African lym-phoma are uniformly large, have finely stippled nuclear chromatin and, characteristically, a deep basophilic cytoplasm often associated with promin-ent vacuolation.[6]

Three cytochemical tests are useful in the study of ALL; the PAS, acid phosphatase and ANAE reactions. They do not correlate with the L1, L2 or L3 morphological types but they do show a relationship to the immunological subtypes of ALL (Table 6.2). In cases in which the cells are undif-ferentiated (usually L2 blast cells in adult patients), it is important to exclude AML (usually M1 and M5a). For this, the peroxidase, Sudan Black B and NASDA reactions should be shown to be negative. ANAE can show in ALL a granular reaction, but this is not the strong diffuse pattern (NaF-sensitive) seen in M5. The PAS reaction is often positive in ALL—at least, in a proportion of blasts, as shown by coarse granules or blocks of positively-reacting material (usually glycogen). This pattern of reaction, particularly with a nega-tive background, is rarely seen in AML; it is more typical of the common form of childhood ALL which can be defined by immunological tests for

Table 6.2 Cytochemistry and the immunological classification of ALL*

Method	Common-ALL	Null-ALL	T-ALL	B-ALL
Morphology	L1-L2	L1-L2	L1-L2	L3
PAS	+ or ++ coarse granules	− or ++	− or +	−
Acid phosphatase	− or +	− or ++	++ or +++	−
ANAE	−	− or +	+ or ++	−
Peroxidase	−	−	−	−
Sudan black B				
Lysozyme	−	−	−	−

* For details of the membrane and enzyme markers in ALL, see Table 6.4.
  Degree of reaction as in Table 6.1

the ALL antigen described by Greaves et al[43] as non-B, non-T ALL (negative B and T markers) or common-ALL.

In T-ALL (positive T-cell markers), the PAS reaction is negative in two-thirds of cases; in B-ALL it is negative in the majority. The differences shown by the PAS reaction probably reflect the different proliferation kinetics of the immunologically-defined subtypes of ALL. For example, in B-ALL (PAS-negative) a greater number of cells are in cycle; this is also reflected in the numerous mitotic figures seen in bone marrow with L3 morphology. The acid phosphatase test gives a consistently localized positive reaction in T-ALL and pre-T-ALL blast cells.[4,18,56]

Chronic myeloproliferative disorders

Low NAP scores are typical of untreated chronic granulocytic leukaemia (CGL) and high NAP scores are characteristic of polycythaemia vera, leucocytoses and leukaemoid reactions secondary to infection or neoplasia and of most cases of myelosclerosis. Normal scores are often found in secondary polycythaemia due to hypoxia, 'stress' or renal disorders. In CGL the low initial scores may change to normal or high in about one-third of patients during remission; scores become high during severe infections, after splenectomy and in up to 50% of cases undergoing blast-cell transformation.

The possibility of characterizing more precisely the type of blast cells seen during the transformation of CGL has improved significantly in the last 5 years. The cytochemical methods applied to the study of AML may provide useful information. Often, however, CGL blasts are very undifferentiated by cytological and cytochemical criteria. Ultrastructural studies, e.g. the platelet-peroxidase reaction may help in the diagnosis of megakaryoblastic transformation (15% of cases).[16] A 'lymphoid' transformation occurs in 20% of cases of CGL; most cytochemical tests are negative in this form, but the PAS reaction may show granular positivity. Lymphoblastic transformation can now be diagnosed by positive criteria by demonstrating the common ALL-antigen[59] and the enzyme terminal deoxynucleotidyl transferase (TdT).[13] A mixed population of blast cells is not rare during transformation of CGL; thus mixed lymphoid and myeloid blast crises have been documented.[21]

Myelodysplastic syndromes (MDS)

Precise diagnostic criteria for the MDS were recently proposed by the FAB group.[8] All of them are characterized by hypercellular bone marrows. Five conditions are included under the broad term MDS:

1. Refractory anaemia (RA), with erythroid hyperplasia and/or dyserythropoiesis.

2. RA with ring sideroblasts, also designated as acquired idiopathic sideroblastic anaemia (AISA), the main feature being the presence of ring sideroblasts in at least 15% of erythroblasts (see p. 108 for staining techniques).

3. RA with excess of blasts (RAEB) which shows dyspoiesis in the three bone-marrow cell lineages, dysgranulopoiesis being always conspicuous. The percentage of bone-marrow blasts is between 5 and 20%; these cells may have a few or no azurophil granules.

4. Chronic myelomonocytic leukaemia (CMML), with many features of RAEB plus a significant peripheral blood monocytosis (usually over $1 \times 10^9/l$).

5. RAEB in transformation, a group close to AML and defined by the presence of blasts in the peripheral blood (over 5%) and between 20 and 30% in the bone marrow.

In addition to staining for iron, the other cytochemical methods used in AML may be useful for the study of the MDS. They may help to define the monocytic component in CMML or the type of blasts in RAEB and they are particularly useful in demonstrating dysgranulopoiesis, e.g. by the presence of neutrophils negative for peroxidase and/or Sudan Black B reactions or giving extremely low NAP scores.

CHARACTERIZATION OF CHRONIC LYMPHOPROLIFERATIVE DISORDERS[20,30]

Analysis using immunological membrane markers shows that the majority of lymphoproliferative disorders are of the B-cell type (Table 6.3). In the most common of these, chronic lymphocytic leukaemia (CLL), and in prolymphocytic leukae-

Table 6.3 Cytochemistry of chronic lymphoproliferative disorders and relation to membrane phenotype

Disease	Immunological subtype*	Relative incidence[†]	ANAE	Acid phosphatase	β-glucuronidase β-glucosaminidase
CLL[‖]	B	98.5%	−	−	−
	T	1.5%	− or ±	+ +	+ + +
PLL[¶]	B	82%	−	− or +	−
	T	18%	+ + +	± or + +	+ + +
Lymphomas	B	88%	−	− or +	−
	T[‡]	12%	+ +	+ or + + +	+ +
HCL**	B	99%	−/+	+ +[§]	−

* *B-cell markers*: membrane bound and/or cytoplasmic monoclonal immunoglobulins; mouse RBC rosettes, etc. *T-cell markers*: sheep RBC rosettes, heteroantisera and monoclonal antibodies to T-cell antigents, etc.
[†] Based on 934 cases studied in the MRC Leukaemia Unit Laboratories by D.C.
[‡] Includes Sézary syndrome and adult T-cell lymphoma-leukaemia.
[§] Resistant to tartaric acid.
[‖] Chronic lymphocytic leukaemia.
[¶] Prolymphocytic leukaemia.
** Hairy cell leukaemia.

mia (PLL), the PAS reaction is often positive in a granular form.[22] This reaction is variable, often negative, in the chronic T-cell disorders.

The reactions for acid hydrolases (acid phosphatase, ANAE, β-glucoronidase and β-glucosaminidase) are positive in most T-cell disorders and negative in the B-cell types (Table 6.3). The non-specific esterase reaction can also help to diagnose the rare 'true' histiocytic lymphomas within the group of large-cell lymphomas, which are usually of B-cell type. True histiocytic lymphomas are tumours of monocytic lineage and show strong diffuse positivity with NASA, NASDA or ANAE, the reactions being NaF-sensitive. These cytochemical reactions are negative in the majority of B-cell lymphomas.

DEMONSTRATION OF DNA AND RNA

DNA

The Feulgen reaction is generally held to be a cytochemical test for desoxyribonucleic acid, an important component of nuclear chromatin. The reaction depends on the liberation of free pentose aldehyde groups from DNA after hydrolysis with HCl and the subsequent combination of these groups with leucobasic fuchsin to give a magenta colour. When applied to films of bone marrow or peripheral blood, the nuclei of the adult cell types stain most intensely and the nuclei of primitive cells least intensely. Nucleoli do not stain; Howell-Jolly bodies, however, do stain, i.e. they are Feulgen-positive, and chromosomes stain particularly well. The stain is thus well suited to the study of mitoses and to the (negative) demonstration of nucleoli.

The best staining results are obtained after wet-fixation with Susa fluid, but dry-fixed films can be stained. The method of staining was described in the 2nd edition of this book. In a well stained preparation the nuclear chromatin is sharply stained shades of purple. The results of Feulgen staining were illustrated by Gardikas and Israëls.[39] Greig described an acid-hydrolysis technique which is a simple substitute for the Feulgen reaction and gives results which appear to parallel it: nucleoli do not stain but appear as holes, whereas chromatin and chromosomes stain shades of blue-black.[45]

RNA

The Unna-Pappenheim stain is a combination of pyronin with methyl green. The pyronin stains the cell components containing ribonucleic acid bright red, e.g. nucleoli and the cytoplasm of primitive cells and of mature cells such as plasma cells in which synthesizing capacities persist. The methyl green part of the stain complex demonstrates the nuclear chromatin, which stains greenish-black. A satisfactory method was described by White[119] whose paper included illustrations.

Other methods have been used for staining RNA, e.g. Chromotrope-Giemsa[40] and Azure C.[96] These are not specific RNA stains but nevertheless they do stain RNA-containing material selectively and are useful for demonstrating nucleoli.

CELL MARKERS

Cells can now be identified, not only by their morphology and cytochemistry, but also by the presence of characteristic receptors and antigens on the cell membrane, immunoglobulin molecules on the membrane (SmIg) and/or in the cytoplasm (CyIg) and by enzymes such as terminal deoxynucleotidyl transferase (TdT) in the nucleus.[13] By this means it is possible to distinguish B and T lymphocytes and also subsets within the major types of lymphocytes. Marker studies help in identifying the lineage of immature cells; they have also contributed to the study of early and late stages of lymphoid differentiation,[59,73] and to the diagnosis and classification of the acute and chronic lymphoid leukaemias.[13,14,19,43,44,60,94,97]

Separation of mononuclear (MN) cells

For most cell marker studies it is necessary to separate the MN cell fraction containing lymphocytes, monocytes, blasts and other mononuclear cells (according to the sample) and to exclude neutrophils, eosinophils, basophils and erythrocytes. Methods include density gradient centrifugation with Ficoll-Triosil, Hypaque or Lymphoprep (Nyegaard, Oslo). The method with Lymphoprep is described below. When necessary, platelets can also be excluded by defibrinating the blood before separation.

Method

Dilute 10 ml of the anticoagulated (e.g. heparin) blood with an equal volume of 9 g/l NaCl (saline). Add the diluted blood drop by drop to 7.5 ml of Lymphoprep and then centrifuge at *400 g* for 30 min. The MN layer separates from the upper plasma layer and from the RBC and neutrophils (which settle to the bottom of the tube). After separation take up the MN cell layer into another tube and wash three times with TC 199.

ROSETTE TESTS

These are based on the affinity of red cells (RBC) to bind specifically to membrane receptors. This binding can be demonstrated with the RBC of various species (sheep, mouse, ox, etc.) which form rosettes (Fig. 6.8) with various types of lympho-

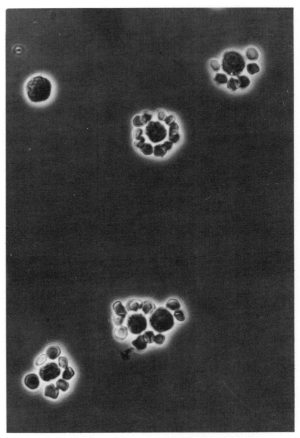

Fig. 6.8 E-rosette formation. Leukaemic T-cells from a case of T-PPL are seen forming rosettes with sheep RBC. Viewed under phase-contrast microscopy. ×400.

Table 6.4 Cell markers in the classification of acute lymphoblastic leukaemia (ALL)

ALL-type	E-rosettes OKT11	Other anti-T sera*	SmIg	Anti-ALL serum; J-5 [43,59,97]	Anti-HLA-Dr (Ia-like)	TdT[†]	Incidence Children (<15 years)	Incidence Adults (>15 years)
Common-ALL	−	−	−	**+**	+	+	75%	42%
Null-ALL	−	−	−	−	+	**+**	10%	38%
Pre B-ALL[‡]	−	−	−	+	+	+	15%	8%
B-ALL	−	−	**+**	−/+	+	−	1%	5%
T-ALL	**+**	+	−	−	−	+	14%	15%
Pre T-ALL[§]	−	**+**	−	−or±	−	+	4%	5%

* Heteroantisera (HUTLA)[59]; for details of anti-T monoclonal antibodies, see references 44, 73, 94, 117.
[†] Indirect immunofluorescence assay with rabbit anti-TdT[13] or biochemical assay[29]. The former is simpler and possibly more sensitive.
[‡] Pre B-ALL is considered a variant of Common-ALL.
[§] Pre T-ALL is considered an immature variant of T-ALL.
Tests that are essential for the diagnosis of a particular type of ALL are printed in bold type.

cytes. There are two types of rosette, immune and spontaneous, depending on whether the RBC are coated or not by Ig molecules.

Immune rosettes are used to demonstrate receptors for the Fc part of IgG (Fc gamma) or IgM (Fcμ) in B and T lymphocytes. For the latter, isolated T cells are incubated with ox RBC coated with IgG or IgM antibodies to identify the Tμ and Tγ subsets.[59] Human RBC (Rh positive) coated with anti-D can also be used to detect high affinity Fc receptors in monocytes.

Spontaneous binding of sheep or mouse RBC has been used, respectively, as markers for T-lymphocytes[14,59,65,78,121] and for a subset of B lymphocytes, chiefly those proliferating in B-CLL.[19,26,109]

SHEEP RED BLOOD CELLS (SRBC) ROSETTES (E-ROSETTES)[65,120]

This test is used as a marker of T-lymphocytes. Almost all peripheral-blood T-lymphocytes and most mature T-lymphocytes in other organs form E-rosettes. The receptor for SRBC appears early during T-cell maturation, and thus it is present also on immature T-cells, including most thymocytes. Because of this, it is usually considered a good marker for T-cell leukaemias, both acute (T-ALL) and chronic (T-CLL, T-PLL, etc.). The only exceptions are cases of pre-T-ALL, an immature variant constituting 25–30% of T-ALL cases

(Table 6.4) in which some T-antigens are present but few or no E-rosettes form. In the chronic T-cell lymphoproliferative disorders (Table 6.5) E-rosettes are, as a rule, demonstrable.

As the formation of E-rosettes requires active cell metabolism, viable cells are necessary. The sensitivity of the test can be increased by treating the SRBC with papain, neuraminidase[59] or the sulphydryl compound AET.[65,78] AET treatment results in the highest values for E-rosettes and it gives consistent reactions with strong rosettes which are resistant to disruption. In T-ALL, results are obtained which are comparable with those with anti-thymocyte sera. A positive reaction is sometimes obtained in cases which are negative with anti-T reagents;[78] however, in pre-T-ALL the reverse may be the case.[56] An interesting property of E-rosettes is their temperature dependence. Mature T-lymphocytes form a maximum number of rosettes at 4°C and these dissociate at 37°C. Thymocytes, on the other hand, form rosettes at 4°C and 37°C. This property has been used in the diagnosis of T-ALL where the proliferating cells have characteristics of thymic cells.[14]

Reagents

Sheep red cells. Wash SRBC three times in 9 g/l NaCl (saline); then treat with AET (see below). It is convenient to use formalized SRBC, obtainable from Tissue Culture Services Ltd (UK).

Table 6.5 Membrane markers in the classification of chronic lymphoid leukaemias/lymphomas

Disease		E-rosettes, (sheep RBC)	OKT mon. antibodies					Fluorescence intensity		Mouse RBC-rosettes†	Anti-HLA-Dr (Ia)
			T3	T4	T6	T8	T11	SmIg	CyIg		
CLL	B	−	−	−	−	−	−	± or +	−	+++	−
	T	+	+	−	−	+	+	−	−	−	− or +
PLL	B	−	−	−	−	−	−	+++	− or ++	− or +	+
	T	+	+	+	−	−	+	−	−	−	−
Lymphomas	B	−	−	−	−	−	−	++	− or +	± or ++	−
	T	+	−	+	−★	+	+	−	−	−	− or +
HCL Sézary syndrome		−	−	−	−	−	−	++	− or ++	± or +	+
		+	+	+	−	−	+	−	−	−	−

★ OKT6 and TdT are positive in T-lymphoblastic (thymic) lymphomas but not in mature (lymph node based) lymphomas.[25,44,73,94]
† The proportion of rosettes varies in the various B-cell disorders. Values for peripheral blood samples and neuraminidase treated lymphocytes are: +++ = >50%, ++ = 30–49%, + = 15–29%, ± = 5–14%, − = <5%.

Lymphocytes. Fresh normal blood human lymphocytes (10×10^6/ml) in saline suspension.

Fetal calf serum (FCS). Absorb 4 volumes of FCS with 2 volumes of SRBC for 2 h at 37°C. Then centrifuge, transfer the supernatant serum to another tube and inactivate it for 30 min at 56°C. Store in 5–10 ml volumes at −20°C.

Method

Add to 0.1 ml of AET-treated SRBC (1% suspension in TC 199) 0.05 ml of absorbed, inactivated FCS and 0.05 ml of lymphocyte suspension.

Centrifuge at 150 *g* for 5 min and then allow the mixture to stand (without resuspension) at 4°C for 1 h—the mixture can stand overnight, if convenient.

Resuspend the cells gently and add 2 drops of 0.05% methylene blue. Fill a counting chamber and inspect 200 lymphocytes.

The E-rosette test is considered to be positive when three or more SRBC are bound to a lymphocyte. With normal T-lymphocytes, six or more SRBC are usually bound. It is important to visualize a lymphocyte in the centre of a rosette and to distinguish between rosetting and agglutination of SRBC.

AET treatment of SRBC

AET. 2-aminoethyl*iso*thiouronium bromide [Sigma]. Dissolve 400 mg of AET in 10 ml of water and adjust the pH to 9.0 with 4 mol/l NaOH. The AET solution should be prepared immediately before use.

AET-treated SRBC. Add 1 volume of packed washed SRBC to 4 volumes of AET and incubate the mixture for 15 min at 37°C. Then wash the cells 3 times in saline and prepare finally a 1% suspension of the cells in TC 199 (e.g. 0.1 ml of washed packed SRBC in 10 ml of TC 199).

The AET-treated SRBC can be kept at 4°C for 5–7 days before use.

Mouse RBC (M) rosettes[19,26,109]

The principles of this test are similar to the E-rosette test. Mouse RBC are freshly drawn by cardiac puncture from a laboratory mouse, e.g. CBA strain. One ml of blood is added to 1 ml of 32 g/l trisodium citrate and 9 ml of saline. These cells have to be used within 3 days. The best results in B-CLL (Table 6.5) are obtained when lymphocytes are pre-treated with neuraminidase type VI (Sigma).[19] At least half the B-lymphocytes of normal peripheral blood (5–10%) form M-rosettes. A high percentage of B-CLL cells (usually over 50%, up to 90%) react similarly. This finding is useful for distinguishing B-CLL from other B-cell lymphoproliferative disorders (Table 6.5), where the percentages of M-rosettes are low or zero. These observations apply only to tests on peripheral-blood samples. For unknown reasons, even in B-CLL, the percentages of cells giving M-rosettes are lower in bone marrow samples;[26] and the differences shown in Table 6.5 are only seen in blood samples.

Immunofluorescence tests

In general, to detect surface antigens, SmIg, CyIg, and TdT, antibodies conjugated with fluorescein*iso*thiocyanate (FITC) or tetraethyl-rhodamine*iso*thiocyanate (TRITC) are used. For details of the methods to demonstrate antigens in immature haemopoietic cells and some blast cells, e.g. the common-ALL antigen, see Greaves et al,[44] and Janossy.[59] The method for SMIg will be described below. Most mature and immature B-cells fluoresce with anti-SmIg sera (Tables 6.4 and 6.5). In the B-lymphoproliferative disorders, the degree of positivity (intensity of immunofluorescence) can help to distinguish the various conditions (Table 6.5).

Whilst the presence of SmIg is looked for with viable cells in suspension, CyIg is sought in cells fixed on a slide, usually prepared by means of a cytocentrifuge (Cytospin). A good fluorescent microscope equipped with incident illumination and an appropriate filter system is essential.

Demonstration of surface membrane immunoglobulins (SMIg) by fluorescent antibody staining

Reagents

Acetate buffered saline, pH 5.5[59]. Add 8.8 ml of 0.2 mol/l (12 ml/l) glacial acetic acid to 41.2 ml of 0.2 mol/l (16.4 g/l) anhydrous sodium acetate and make the volume up to 200 ml with water. To each 200 ml add 1.8 g of NaCl and 0.2 g of anhydrous $CaCl_2$. Store in 10-ml volumes at $-20°C$.

Phosphate buffered saline (PBS), pH 7.4. See p. 436.

Azide. 0.02% sodium azide in PBS. This solution will keep for up to 1 month at 4°C without loss of potency.

Fluorescent antibodies. Preferably, use $F(ab)_2$ reagents, i.e. antibodies which have been treated with papain to destroy the Fc region. Such treatment leaves the $F(ab)_2$ antigen-binding fragment intact. This is essential when using rabbit antisera, although it may not be necessary with goat or sheep immunoglobulins.[59]

Pipettes. Use Eppendorf-type pipettes (e.g. Oxford sampler system) and tips and plastic tubes throughout the test.

Method

Wash the separated lymphocytes in 9 g/l NaCl (saline), and resuspend in acetate buffered saline, e.g. 0.2 ml of cell suspension $(1-2 \times 10^6$ cells) in 2 ml of buffer. Incubate the mixture at 37°C for 15 min.

Wash the cells twice in PBS and then incubate the deposited cells in 5 ml of TC 199 at 37°C for 1 h to remove cytophilic antibodies.

Centrifuge the cells, remove the supernatant and resuspend the cells in 0.2 ml of the azide solution. (The cell concentration should be $10-15 \times 10^6$/ml.)

Add 2 ml of diluted (usually 1 in 20) anti-Ig fluorescent conjugated antiserum. Mix the cell suspension well and allow to stand at 4°C or (preferably) in crushed ice for 30 min. Then top up the tube containing the cell suspension with TC 199 and centrifuge for 5 min at 400 ***g*** (to remove unbound conjugates). Discard the supernatant and wash the deposited cells twice in PBS.

Remove the supernatant and add to the deposited cells 1 drop of a mixture of equal volumes of PBS and glycerol.* Resuspend the cells and place 1 drop on a slide; cover with a cover-slip and seal with nail varnish.

Examine under the fluorescent microscope.

Monoclonal antibodies

A significant development in the last few years has been the possibility of producing antibodies of great purity by means of hybridoma technology. The principles of their preparation have been reviewed by Janossy.[59] A great number of reagents reactive with membrane antigens present on haemopoietic cells are now available. So far the major applications have been in discriminating between the stages of T-lymphocyte differentiation from early thymic cells to mature (peripheral blood) T-cells; this in turn has resulted in a more precise classification of the T-cell malignancies.[44,94] Monoclonal antibodies to early haemopoietic cells are also now available. For example, the common ALL antigen[43,59], a membrane glycoprotein of 100 000 mol wt, can now be demonstrated by means of the monoclonal antibody J-5 (Table 6.4).[97] The most widely used antibodies are those of the OKT series (Orthoclone)[73] which help to identify all the peripheral blood T-cells (T3), the T-helper (T4) and the T-cytotoxic/suppressor cells (T8). These antibodies are now available commercially. OKT 11 reacts with the receptors of SRBC, and thus the results with both tests are very similar (Table 6.5). OKT 6 reacts only with cortical thymocytes and gives a positive reaction in T-lymphoblastic lymphoma.[44,94] Findings in the T-cell leukaemias and lymphomas with these reagents are summarized in Table 6.5.

Instructions for using these antibodies are usually provided by the manufacturer. Their use involves indirect immunofluorescence. The first layer is the monoclonal antibody which is a mouse antibody of IgG or IgM class; the second layer is an FITC anti-mouse Ig, prepared in goats or rabbits. Careful controls omitting the first layer and/or using normal mouse serum should be used.

---

* To reduce fading during examination the following alternative mixture has been recommended[62]. Add 10 ml of PBS containing 10 mg of *p*-phenylenediamine (Hopkins and Williams) to 90 ml of glycerol. Adjust the pH to 8.0 with 0.5 mol/l carbonate-bicarbonate buffer, pH 9.0.

TERMINAL TRANSFERASE (TdT)[13,27,29,59,60]

This remarkable DNA polymerase can be demonstrated by a biochemical assay[29] or an immunofluorescence test.[13,59] Both methods give similar results[13,27,29] but the demonstration of TdT in cell nuclei by immunofluorescence is to be preferred because of its speed, simplicity and sensitivity to low numbers of cells. As shown in Table 6.4, tests for TdT are positive in all types of ALL with the exception of the rare B-ALL. Thus, it is the method of choice to distinguish ALL from AML. However, it should be noted that 5–10% of cases of AML, particularly immature forms, may show TdT activity.[60] On the other hand, the common-ALL antigen is almost never demonstrable in AML. By combining both methods the majority of cases of ALL can now be diagnosed confidently. If the tests for the common ALL antigens and TdT are positive the likelihood of a case being AML is remote. In our experience two sorts of AML cases may show TdT activity: in rare mixed ALL/AML cases the test for TdT is positive in lymphoblasts and in some true AML cases with myeloperoxidase-positive blast cells TdT activity persists or is aberrant. Three other situations in which the TdT assay gives useful information are:

1. In blast crisis of CGL, in which the TdT test is almost always positive in the lymphoblastic type of transformations (20% of cases).

2. In T-lymphoblastic lymphoma, which is the only non-Hodgkin's lymphoma with positive TdT activity.[13,44]

3. In the chronic (mature) T-cell proliferations, in which TdT activity is always absent, contrasting with the positive findings in acute (immature) T-cell proliferations (T-ALL, pre-T-ALL and T-lymphoblastic lymphoma).[25,44]

Slide assay for terminal deoxynucleotidyl transferase (TdT)

Reagents

Anti-TdT. This can be purchased from Bethesda Research Laboratories Inc (USA). For use dilute 1 in 10 in phosphate buffered saline (PBS), pH 7.4 (p. 436).

Fluorescent-conjugated (FITC) goat anti-rabbit Ig serum. For use dilute 1 in 10 in phosphate buffered saline. (Rhodamine-conjugated antibodies and porcine anti-rabbit Ig may be used instead of the goat antiserum.)

Mounting medium. Glycerol 48 ml, PBS 48 ml, formalin 4 ml.

Method

Make cytocentrifuge (Cytospin) preparations, using 250 μl of a I $\times$ 10^6/ml cell suspension per slide. Centrifuge for 1 min at 300 rpm (*c* 7 *g*) and allow the film to dry in the air. Ring the deposited cells with a wax pencil.

Such slides may be stored at room temperature for up to a week but it is preferable to carry out the test as soon as possible.

Fix the film in methanol for 15 min at 4°C. Then wash in PBS for 10 min in a jar provided with a magnetic stirrer. Wipe off the excess PBS around the ring of cells and cover the ring with 10 μl of the diluted anti-TdT serum. Leave for 10 min at room temperature in a moist chamber.

Wash the slides in PBS for a further 15 min using a magnetic stirrer as before.

Wipe off the excess PBS around the ring of cells and cover the cells with 10 μl of the diluted fluorescent-conjugated anti-rabbit Ig serum. Allow to stand for 30 min at room temperature in a moist chamber.

Wash the slide in PBS for 15 min at room temperature, as before; then cover the ring of cells with a cover-glass, using as mountant the glycerol/PBS/formalin mixture.

Examine under the fluorescent microscope. A positive reaction is denoted by nuclear fluorescence. Using the appropriate filters, this will be bright yellow with fluorescein conjugation and bright red with rhodamine conjugation.

Controls

Negative. Carry out the test leaving out the anti-TdT and also on cells known not to react (e.g. B-CLL cells).

Positive. Use a common ALL cell line (e.g. NALM-1) or cells from a patient with a known common ALL who is not in remission.

DEMONSTRATION OF CHROMOSOMES

The demonstration of human chromosome abnormalities has become a subject of increasing importance in clinical haematology. Description of how to obtain adequate mitosis and of the various methods of chromosomes banding (Q: quinacrine mustard; G: Giemsa stain; R: reverse banding pattern) are beyond the scope of this book. Details can be found in the references at the end of this chapter.[101,113,124]

For analysis, chromosomes are usually studied in mitoses arrested at metaphase by the addition of colchicine, demecolcine or vinblastine. Bone-marrow aspirates provide the best material for study in cases of leukaemia; peripheral blood may be adequate when the leucocyte count is very high, particularly in CGL. Blood lymphocytes should be studied simultaneously to define the normal constitutional karyotype. This is done by short-term culture with the mitogen phytohaemagglutinin (PHA).

Since the discovery of the Philadelphia (Ph^1) chromosome, due to the translocation of material from the long arm (q) of chromosome 22 (22q$-$) to the long arm of chromosome 9 (9q$+$), numerous haemopoietic malignancies have been found to be associated with specific abnormalities.[101,104,113,114,124,125] These are summarized in Table 6.6.

The abnormalities in a karyotype may be numerical, e.g. trisomy (an extra chromosome) or monosomy (only one chromosome of the pair) or structural. The modal number of chromosomes, 46 in man, may be less than 46 (hypodiploid) or more than 46 (hyperdipolid). For example, a hyperdiploid karyotype (47 chromosomes or more) is seen in 23% of children with ALL (114). A modal chromosome number greater than 50 is associated with the best prognosis in childhood ALL.[114]

Table 6.6 Non-random*, acquired[†] chromosome abnormalities in haemopoietic malignancies

* t(9q+; 22q−)	CGL and adult-ALL (17%)
* t(8q−; 21q+)	AML (M2)
* t(15q+; 17q−)	APL (M3) and M3-variant
* t(4q−; 11q+)	ALL (5%)
* 6q−	ALL (4%)
* t(8q−; 14q+)	Burkitt's lymphoma; B-ALL (L3)
* 14q+	Non-Hodgkin's lymphoma; B-PLL
* Trisomy 12	B-CLL (50%)
* Trisomy 8	AML and CGL in blast crisis
* Iso 17	CGL in blast crisis
* 5q−	RAEB[‡]
* Monosomy 7	MDS[§]

* Present in the majority of the abnormal metaphases.
[†] Present in the leukaemic cell population but not in normal cells (e.g. T-lymphocytes, fibroblasts, etc.).
[‡] Refractory anaemia with excess of blasts.
[§] Myelodysplastic syndrome.

Marker chromosomes are structurally abnormal chromosomes in banded or unbanded karyotypes. When the banding pattern can be recognized it should be described by the standard nomenclature.[95] Non-random abnormalities refer to consistent changes seen in a particular cell population which are unlikely to have occurred by chance. A clone refers to a population of cells, presumably derived from a single progenitor cell, which is characterized by the same marker chromosome(s).

The karyotype of the bone-marrow cells of a particular leukaemia (e.g. AML) may show that all the metaphases are abnormal (AA), or that some are normal and others abnormal (AN), or that all the metaphases are normal (NN). AA suggests that no normal cells are present and has usually a bad prognosis.[101,104] AN represents a mixture of normal and leukaemic cells; recent studies suggest that examination of mitotic figures after 24–48 h culture may yield more abnormal metaphases compared with direct preparations of the same material.[125] NN indicates either that there are no gross abnormalities, this depending also on the sensitivity of the method, or that only the karyotype of normal cells is being analysed rather than that of the leukaemic population.

The more sensitive techniques for the study of human chromosomes (long chromosomes, prometaphase banding) now becoming available may be expected to provide more information. For example, finely banded chromosome preparations can be obtained by high-resolution techniques, in particular those using culture techniques, and cell synchronization with amethopterin.

NUCLEAR SEXING OF LEUCOCYTES

Sex chromosome anomalies are not uncommon and they can usually be identified readily by nuclear sexing. Buccal mucosa is the material usually examined but in experienced hands valuable information can also be gained by inspection of the neutrophil leucocytes. The feature to be identified is a nuclear appendage, the drumstick, which is present in a proportion of the neutrophils in normal females but not in normal males. The drumstick represents one X chromosome and is equivalent to the single Barr body seen in normal (XX) females.

Method

Make blood films, stain them and cover with a cover-glass in the usual way. Then scan them systematically with an oil-immersion lens for drumsticks of the correct size and staining quality. The use of a micrometer ocular may be necessary to measure the drumsticks.

The drumsticks are pedunculated nuclear appendages, with a spherical or oval head of between 1.4 and 1.6 μm in diameter, formed of densely staining chromatin attached by a thread-like neck to the rest of the nucleus (Fig. 6.9). Very often a small space or chink can be seen in the chromatin of the head of the drumstick. These sex drumsticks have to be distinguished from non-specific nodules which may be of smaller or larger size, irregular in shape, and sometimes deficient in chromatin. Sessile chromatin sex nodules of the same size as drumsticks may also be seen; they stain densely and project by more than half their diameter beyond the nuclear membrane (Fig. 6.9). They also occur only in females, but they are less easily distinguished from other non-specific nodules and appendages which have no diagnostic significance.

As a screening test, scrutinize at least 50 neutrophils for drumsticks (and sessile

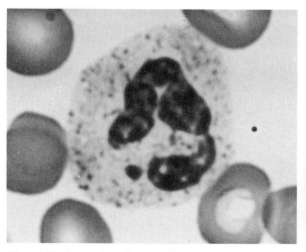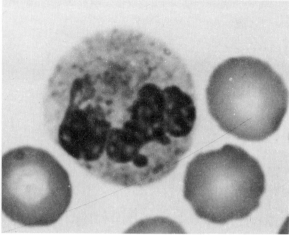

Fig. 6.9 Nuclear sexing of neutrophils. Photomicrographs of neutrophils showing female sex appendages. The left-hand cell has a 'drumstick'; the right-hand cell has a sessile nodule. ×3000.

nodules). In females, three or more definite sessile nodules and one or more drumsticks are usually seen in the first 50 cells. On the other hand, in males no drumsticks and no definite sessile nodules should be seen. If there is any doubt, examine further cells, and if at least two definite drumsticks and accompanying sessile nodules are identified in the first 500 cells, it can reliably be assumed that the cells are chromatin-positive and the subject female (XX). Usually at least six definite drumsticks are found in less than 200 neutrophils. If neither drumsticks nor sessile nodules are seen in the first 200 neutrophils, the cells can be regarded as chromatin-negative and the subject male (XY) or XO. When there is a shift to the left in the segmentation of the neutrophil nuclei it is more difficult to arrive at a clear-cut answer, and it may be necessary to examine many more cells.

SIDEROCYTES

Siderocytes, or red cells containing granules of non-haem iron, were originally described by Grüneberg[46] in small numbers in the blood of normal rat, mouse and human embryos, and in large numbers in mice with a congenital anaemia. The granules are formed of a water-insoluble complex of iron, lipid, protein and carbohydrate. This siderotic material (or haemosiderin) gives a positive Prussian blue (Perls's) reaction. It also stains by Romanowsky dyes and then appears as basophilic granules which have been referred to as 'Pappenheimer bodies' (Fig. 6.10).[88] By contrast, ferritin, which is a water-soluble compound of iron with the protein apoferritin is not detectable by Perls's reaction. Ferritin is normally present in all cells in the body whereas haemosiderin is mainly concentrated in recticulo-endothelial cells, except when the body is overloaded with iron as in haemochromatosis or transfusional haemosiderosis.

Iron is transported in plasma attached to a β-globulin, transferrin, and passes selectively to the bone marrow where, at the surface of the erythroblast, the iron is released and enters the cell. Most of the iron is rapidly converted to haem in the mitchondria. The non-haem residue is in the form of ferritin. Degradation of the ferritin turns some of it into haemosiderin which can be stained by Perls's reaction and visualized under the light microscope.

In health, siderotic granules are normally found in the cytoplasm of many of the normoblasts of human bone marrow and in marrow reticulocytes.[35,64] However, they are not normally found in human peripheral-blood red cells. After splenectomy, on the other hand, siderocytes can always be found in the peripheral blood, often in large numbers. The reason for this is probably

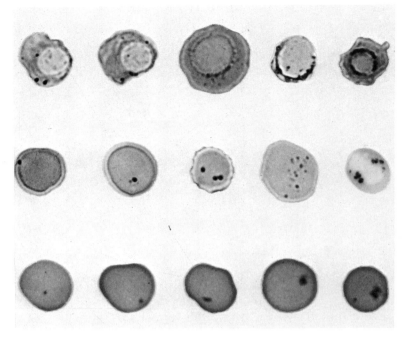

Fig. 6.10 Siderotic granules and 'Pappenheimer bodies'. Photomicrographs of normoblasts and red cells stained by the acid-ferrocyanide method to show siderotic granules (top two rows) and stained by Jenner-Giemsa's stain to demonstrate 'Pappenheimer bodies' (bottom row). ×1000.

because reticulocytes, after delivery from the marrow, are normally sequestered for a time in the spleen and there complete haem synthesis and utilize, for this purpose, the iron stored in their cytoplasm within the siderotic granules. After splenectomy, this stage of reticulocyte ripening has to take place in the blood stream, with the result that a small percentage of siderocytes can then be demonstrated in the peripheral blood.[33] The spleen is also probably able to remove large siderotic granules—as may be found in disease—from red cells by a process of pitting,[31] and in its absence such granules persist in the red cells of the peripheral blood throughout their life-span.

Method of staining siderocytes

Air-dry films of peripheral blood or bone marrow and fix with methanol for 10–20 min. When dry, place the slides in a solution of 10 g/l potassium ferrocyanide in 0.1 mol/l HCl made by mixing equal volumes of 47 mmol/l (20 g/l) potassium ferrocyanide and 0.2 mol/l HCl immediately before use.

Leave the slides in the solution for about 10 min at c 20°C. Wash well in running tap-water for 20 min, rinse thoroughly in distilled water and then counterstain with 1 g/l aqueous safranin or eosin for 10–15 s. Care must be taken to avoid contamination by iron which may have been present on the slides or in staining dishes. Prepare the glassware by soaking in 2 mol/l HCl before washing (see p. 329).

Prussian-blue staining can be applied to films which have previously been stained by Romanowsky dyes, even after years of storage. It is advisable to let the films stand in methanol overnight to remove most of the Romanowsky stain. Sundberg and Bromann described a technique whereby films were stained first by a Romanowsky dye (Wright's stain) and then overstained by the acid-ferrocyanide method.[110] This can give beautiful pictures but the small blue-stained iron-containing granules tend to be masked in young erythroblasts by the general basophilia of the cell cytoplasm. Hayhoe and Quaglino described a method for combined PAS and iron staining.[49] A rapid method has been described for demonstrating siderotic granules by staining with 1% bromochlorphenol blue for 1 min.[69] Iron-containing granules stain dark purple.

Significance of siderocytes

Siderocytes contain one or more (rarely many) small iron-containing unevenly distributed granules which stain a Prussian-blue colour. Sideroblasts normally only contain a few very small scattered iron-containing granules[64] and these may be difficult to see by light microscopy. The percentage of erythroblasts recognizable as sideroblasts is increased in haemolytic anaemias and megaloblastic anaemias and in haemochromatosis and haemosiderosis, in proportion to the degree of saturation of transferrin. A disproportionate increase in sideroblasts occurs when there is disturbed synthesis of Hb, in which case the granules in sideroblasts are both more numerous and larger than normal. When there is a defect in haem synthesis, the granules are frequently arranged in a collar aound the nucleus (Fig. 6.11) giving the 'ring sideroblasts' characteristic of sideroblastic anaemias. In contrast, the distribution of the granules within the cell is normal in conditions in which globin synthesis alone is affected, e.g. in thalassaemia, or when there is iron overload.

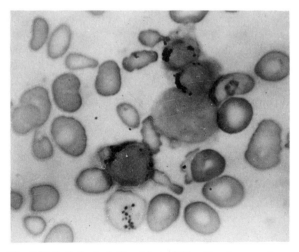

Fig. 6.11 Pathological sideroblasts. Sideroblastic anaemia (hereditary type). Three normoblasts are shown, in the cytoplasm of which is a massive accumulation of iron-containing granules. Perls's acid-ferrocyanide reaction. ×1100.

Several types of sideroblastic anaemia have been recognized.[55] These include the primary acquired and congenital (hereditary) types. Pyridoxine (vitamin-B_6) deficiency also results in a sideroblastic anaemia, and B_6-antagonists, e.g. drugs used in anti-tuberculosis therapy, produce the same effect. Secondary sideroblastic anaemia can also complicate alcoholism, lead poisoning and occasionally rheumatoid arthritis and other 'medical' diseases; and ring sideroblasts are not uncommonly seen in primary haematological disorders, notably myelosclerosis, myeloblastic leukaemia and erythroleukaemia.

In the primary acquired type, erythroblasts at all stages of maturity may be loaded with siderotic granules; whereas in some of the secondary sideroblastic anaemias and in the hereditary types the more mature cells seem most affected.

In addition to the siderotic granules within erythroblasts, haemosiderin can normally be seen in marrow films as accumulations of small granules, lying free or in phagocytes in marrow fragments.[92] The granules will be markedly increased in number in patients with large iron stores, and reduced or absent in iron-deficiency anaemias. In infections the iron stores may be increased, with much siderotic material in phagocytes but little or none visible in erythroblasts. Markedly excessive iron in phagocytes is also a feature of dyserythropoietic anaemias. In practice, staining to demonstrate iron stores in marrow fragments and siderotic granules in erythroblasts is a simple and valuable diagnostic procedure and should be applied to marrow films as a routine.

There is no cytochemical method of demonstrating ferritin. Methods of assay are described in Chapter 20.

CYTOCHEMICAL DEMONSTRATION OF HAEMOGLOBIN DERIVATIVES

HEINZ BODIES IN RED CELLS

Heinz, in 1890, was the first to describe in detail inclusions in red cells developing as the result of the action of acetylphenylhydrazine on the blood.[54] Now it is known that 'Heinz' bodies may be produced by the action on red cells of a wide range of aromatic nitro- and amino-compounds, as well as by inorganic oxidizing agents such as potassium chlorate. In man, the finding of Heinz bodies in the blood is either a sign of chemical poisoning or drug intoxication or G6PD deficiency, or the presence of an unstable haemoglobin, e.g. Hb Köln. When of chemical or drug origin, Heinz bodies are likely to be visible in the red cells only if the patient has been splenectomized previously or when massive doses of the chemical or drug have been taken. When due to an unstable Hb, they seem never to be visible in freshly withdrawn red cells except after splenectomy. They, nevertheless, develop in vitro when pre-splenectomy blood is incubated for 24–48 h.[32]

Heinz bodies represent an end-product of the degradation of Hb. Reviews dealing with Heinz bodies include those by Jacob[58] and by White.[120]

Demonstration of Heinz bodies

Unstained preparations

Heinz bodies may be seen as refractile objects in dry unstained films, if the illumination is cut down by lowering the microscope condenser, and they can be seen by dark-ground illumination or phase-contrast microscopy. However, it is preferable to look for them in stained preparations (see below). The size of the particles varies from 1 to 3 μm. One or more may be present in a single cell. They are usually close to the cell membrane, and in wet preparations may move around within the cells in a slow Brownian movement.

Stained preparations

Methyl violet stains the bodies excellently.

Dissolve c 0.5 g of methyl violet in 100 ml of 9 g/l NaCl and filter. Add 1 volume of blood (in any anticoagulant) to 4 volumes of the methyl violet solution and allow the suspension to stand for c 10 min at c 20°C. Then prepare films and allow them to dry or view the suspension of cells between slide and cover-glass. The Heinz bodies stain an intense purple (Fig. 6.12).

Heinz bodies also stain with other basic dyes. Brilliant green stains them well and none of the

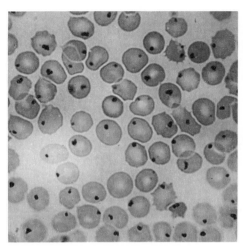

Fig. 6.12 Unstable haemoglobin disease. Hb-Köln (after splenectomy). Many of the cells contain large Heinz bodies. Stained supravitally by methyl violet. ×700.

stain is taken up by the remainder of the red cell.[103] Rhodanile blue (5 g/l solution in 10 g/l NaCl) stains them rapidly[108], i.e. within 2 min, at which time reticulocytes are only weakly stained. Compared with methyl violet, Heinz bodies stain less intensely with brilliant cresyl blue or New methylene blue. Nevertheless, they may be readily seen as pale blue bodies in a well-stained reticulocyte preparation, if the preparation is not counterstained.

If permanent preparations are required, fix the vitally stained films by exposure to formalin vapour for 5–10 min. Then counterstain the fixed films with 1 g/l eosin or safranin, after thoroughly washing in water. If films are fixed in methanol, the bodies are decolourized.

In β-thalassaemia major, methyl violet staining of the bone marrow will demonstrate precipitated α-chains. These appear as large irregular inclusions in late normoblasts, usually single and closely adhering to the nucleus. If such patients are splenectomized, inclusions are also found in reticulocytes and red blood cells.

DEMONSTRATION OF HAEMOGLOBIN H

Patients with α-thalassaemia, who form Hb H (β-4), have red cells which on exposure to brilliant cresyl blue, as in reticulocyte preparations, form multiple blue-green spherical inclusions (Fig. 6.13).[42]

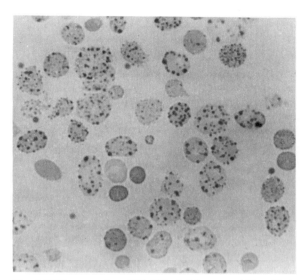

Fig. 6.13 Denaturation of Hb-H by brilliant cresyl blue. The round bodies of varying size consist of precipitated Hb-H. ×900.

Method

Mix together c equal volumes of fresh blood and 10 g/l cresyl blue in citrate-saline in a small tube as for staining reticulocytes. Leave the preparation at 37°C for 1–3 h before making films. Allow the films to dry and examine without counterstaining. Hb-H precipitates as multiple pale-staining greenish-blue almost spherical bodies of varying size which can be clearly differentiated from the darker staining reticulo-filamentous material of reticulocytes.

The number of cells containing inclusions varies according to the type of α-thalassaemia. In α-thalassaemia-1 trait only 0.01–1% of the red cells contain inclusions, but this finding provides a significant clue to diagnosis. In Hb-H disease (α-thalassaemia-1/α-thalassaemia-2), as a rule at least 10% of cells contain inclusions and, in some cases, the percentage is considerably greater.

CYTOCHEMICAL TESTS FOR DEMONSTRATING DEFECTS OF RED-CELL METABOLISM

Chemical tests for the recognition of defects of red-cell metabolism are described in Chapter 10.

Cytochemical methods have been developed by means of which some of these defects can be demonstrated in individual cells. Thus tests have been described for demonstrating red cells deficient in glucose-6-phosphate dehydrogenase (G6PD).[36,38,116] The principle on which the methods are based is that red cells are treated with sodium nitrite to convert their oxyhaemoglobin (HbO_2) to methaemoglobin (Hi). In the presence of G6PD, Hi reconverts to HbO_2, but in G6PD deficiency Hi persists. The blood is then incubated with a soluble tetrazolium compound (MTT) which will be reduced by HbO_2 (but not by Hi) to an insoluble formazan form.[70] Alternatively, the presence of Hi can be demonstrated by converting it to HiCN with potassium cyanide and then adding hydrogen peroxide which elutes HiCN but not HbO_2.[38] The cells are then stained, e.g. with eosin, and the HbO_2-containing cells can be readily distinguished from unstained ghosts, which had contained the Hi and which do not stain.

When G6PD activity is normal, all the red cells are stained. In G6PD hemizygotes the majority of the red cells are unstained. In heterozygotes mosaicism is usually easily seen, a proportion of cells behaving as normal and the remainder being devoid or almost devoid of stainable material. These cytochemical procedures are, however, not more sensitive in the demonstration of G6PD deficiency than are the screening tests described on p. 159.

DEMONSTRATION OF FETAL HAEMOGLOBIN, CARBOXYHAEMOGLOBIN AND METHAEMOGLOBIN IN RED CELLS BY CYTOCHEMICAL MEANS

FETAL HAEMOGLOBIN

An acid-elution cytochemical method was introduced by Kleihauer et al in 1957.[71] It is a sensitive procedure which identifies individual cells containing Hb-F even when few are present, and their detection in the maternal circulation provided valuable information on the pathogenesis of haemolytic disease of the newborn.

The identification of cells containing Hb-F depends upon the fact that they resist acid-elution to a greater extent than do normal cells; thus, in the technique described below, they appear as isolated darkly-stained cells amongst a background of palely-staining ghost-cells. The occasional cells which stain to an intermediate degree are less easy to evaluate; some may be reticulocytes as these also resist acid-elution to some extent. The following method in which elution is carried out at pH 1.5 is recommended.[84]

Reagents

Fixative. 80% ethanol.

Elution solution.

Solution A: 7.5 g/l haematoxylin in 90% ethanol.

Solution B: $FeCl_3$, 24 g; 2.5 mol/lHCl, 20 ml; doubly-distilled water to 1 l.

For use, mix well 5 volumes of A and 1 volume of B. The pH is approximately 1.5. The solution can be used for *c* 4 weeks: if a precipitate forms, the solution should be filtered.

Counterstain. 1 g/l aqueous erythrosin or 2.5 g/l aqueous eosin.

Method

Prepare fresh air-dried films. Immediately after drying, fix the films for 5 min in 80% ethanol in a Coplin jar. Then rinse the slides rapidly in water and stand vertically on blotting paper for about 10 min to dry. Next, place the slides for 20 s in a Coplin jar containing the elution solution. Rinse in tap-water and allow them to dry in the air. Fetal cells stain red and adult ghost-cells stain pale pink (Fig. 6.14).

A number of modifications of the Kleihauer method have been proposed. In one, New methylene blue is incorporated in the buffer solution, the reaction time is prolonged and buffer is used for washing the films.[28] The advantage of this technique is that reticulocytes stain blue, whilst cells containing Hb F stain pink.

An immunofluorescent staining method has been developed based on the use of a specific antibody against Hb F which does not react with Hb A.[115] A similar method employing an anti-Hb S antibody has been use for the identification of Hb S in red cells.[53,87]

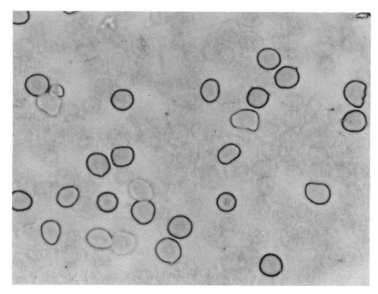

Fig. 6.14 Cytochemical demonstration of fetal haemoglobin. Acid elution method. The preparation consists of a mixture of cord blood and normal adult blood. ×700.

CARBOXYHAEMOGLOBIN

HbCO can be demonstrated in intact red cells in a blood film by a modification of the methaemoglobin elution technique.[11,12] This is based on the fact that HbO_2 is oxidized by nitrite to Hi whereas HbCO is not. The method has, however, only limited practical value.

METHAEMOGLOBIN

The peroxidatic capacity of Hi, but not of HbO_2, is reduced by cyanide. The peroxidatic activity prevents elution of Hb by citric acid in the presence of hydrogen peroxide. Thus normal red cells containing HbO_2 will remain intact and take up a counterstain whereas cells containing Hi will appear as ghosts when subjected to elution. Based on this principle, Kleihauer and Betke devised a simple method for demonstrating Hi in red cells in blood films.[70]

REFERENCES

[1] ARCHER, G. T., AIR, G., JACKAS, M. and MORELL, D. B. (1965). Studies on rat eosinophil peroxidase. *Biochimica et Biophysica Acta*, **99**, 96.

[2] BAIN, B. J., CATOVSKY, D., O'BRIEN, M., PRENTICE, H. G., LAWLOR, E., KUMARAN, T. O., McCANN, S. R. MATUTES, E. and GALTON, D. A. G. (1981). Megakaryoblastic leukemia presenting as acute myelofibrosis. A study of four cases with the platelet-peroxidase reaction. *Blood*, **58**, 206.

[3] BAINTON, D. F., ULLYOT, J. L. and FARQUHAR, M. G. (1971). The development of neutrophilic polymorphonuclear leukocytes in human bone marrow. *Journal of Experimental Medicine*, **134**, 907.

[4] BASSO, G., COCITO, M. G., POLETTI, A., MESSINA, C., COLLESELLI, P. and ZANESCO, L. (1980). Study of cytochemical markers ACP and ANAE in childhood lymphoma and leukaemia. *British Journal of Cancer*, **41**, 835.

[5] BASSO, G., COCITO, M. G., SEMENZATO, G., PEZZUTTO, A. and ZANESCO, L. (1980). Cytochemical study of thymocytes and T lymphocytes. *British Journal of Haematology*, **44**, 577.

[6] BENNETT, J. M., CATOVSKY, D., DANIEL, M. T., FLANDRIN, G., GALTON, D. A. G., GRALNICK, H. R. and SULTAN, C. (1976). Proposals for the classification of the acute leukaemias. *British Journal of Haematology*, **33**, 451.

[7] BENNETT, J. M., CATOVSKY, D., DANIEL, M. T., FLANDRIN, G., GALTON, D. A. G., GRALNICK, H. R. and SULTAN, C. (1981). The morphological classification of acute lymphoblastic leukaemia—concordance among observers and clinical correlations. *British Journal of Haematology*, **47**, 553.

[8] BENNETT, J. M., CATOVSKY, D. DANIEL, M. T. FLANDRIN, G., GALTON, D. A. G., GRALNICK, H. R. and SULTAN, C. (1982). Proposals for the classification of the myelodysplastic syndromes. *British Journal of Haematology*, **51**, 189.

[9] BECKSTEAD, J. H., Halverson, P. S., RIES, C. A. and BAINTON, D. F. (1981). Enzyme histochemistry and immuno histochemistry on biopsy specimens of pathologic human bone marrow. *Blood*, **57**, 1088.

[10] BENAVIDES, I. and CATOVSKY, D. (1978). Myeloperoxidase cytochemistry using 2,7-fluorenediamine. *Journal of Clinical Pathology*, **31**, 1114.

[11] BETHLENFALVAY, N. C. (1971). Cytologic demonstration of carboxyhemoglobin: clinical and in vitro studies in man. *Journal of Laboratory and Clinical Medicine*, **77**, 453.

[12] BETKE, K. and KLEIHAUER, E. (1967). Cytological demonstration of carboxyhaemoglobin in human erythrocytes. *Nature (London)*, **214**, 188.

[13] BOLLUM, F. J. (1979). Terminal deoxynucleotidyl transferase as a hematopoietic cell marker. *Blood*, **54**, 1203.

[14] BORELLA, L. and SEN, L. (1975). E-receptors on blasts from untreated acute lymphocytic leukaemia; comparison of temperature dependence of E-rosettes formed by normal and lymphoid cells. *Journal of Immunology*, **114**, 187.

[15] BOZDECH, M. J. AND BAINTON, D. F. (1981). Identification of α-napthylbutyrate esterase as a plasma membrane ectoenzyme of monocytes and as a discrete intracellular membrane-bounded organelle in lymphocytes. *Journal of Experimental Medicine*, **153**, 182.

[16] BRETON-GORIUS, J., GOURDIN, M. F. and REYES, F. (1981). Ultrastructure of the leukemic cell. In *The Leukemic Cell*, Ed. D. Catovsky, Chapter 4. Churchill Livingstone, Edinburgh.

[17] BRIGGS, R. S., PERILLIE, P. E. and FINCH, S. C. (1966). Lysozyme in bone marrow and peripheral blood cells. *Journal of Histochemistry and Cytochemistry*, **14**, 167.

[18] CATOVSKY, D., CHERCHI, M., GREAVES, M. F., PAIN, C., JANOSSY, G. and KAY, H. E. M. (1978). The acid phosphatase reaction in acute lymphoblastic leukaemia. *Lancet* **i**, 749.

[19] CATOVSKY, D., CHERCHI, M., OKOS, A., HEGDE, U. and GALTON, D. A. G. (1976). Mouse red cell rosettes in B-lymphoproliferative disorders. *British Journal of Haematology*, **33**, 173.

[20] CATOVSKY, D. and COSTELLO, C. (1979). Cytochemistry of normal and leukaemic lymphocytes: a review. *Basic and Applied Histochemistry*, **23**, 255.

[21] CATOVSKY, D., CROCKARD, A. D., MATUTES, E. and O'BRIEN, M. (1981). Cytochemistry of leukaemic cells. In *Histochemistry: the widening horizons*. Eds. P. J. Stoward and J. M. Polak, Chapter 6. John Wiley & Sons, Chichester.

[22] CATOVSKY, D., GALETTO, J., OKOS, A., MILIANI, E. and GALTON, D. A. G. (1974). Cytochemical profile of B and T leukaemic lymphocytes with special reference to acute lymphoblastic leukaemia. *Journal of Clinical Pathology*, **27**, 767.

[23] CATOVSKY, D. and GALTON, D. A. G. (1973). Lysozyme activity and nitroblue-tetrazolium reduction in leukaemic cells. *Journal of Clinical Pathology*, **26**, 60.

[24] CATOVSKY, D., GALTON, D. A. G. and ROBINSON, J. (1972). Myeloperoxidase-deficient neutrophils in acute myeloid leukaemia. *Scandinavian Journal of Haematology*, **9**, 142.

[25] CATOVSKY, D., LINCH, D. C. and BEVERLEY, P. C. L. (1982). T-cell disorders in haematological diseases. *Clinics in Haematology*, **11**, 661.

[26] CHERCHI, M. and CATOVSKY, D. (1980). Mouse RBC rosettes in chronic lymphocytic leukaemia—different expression in blood and tissues. *Clinical and Experimental Immunology*, **39**, 411.

[27] CIBULL, M. L., COLEMAN, M. S., NELSON, O., HUTTON, J. J., GORDON, D. and BOLLUM, F. J. (1982). Evaluation of

methods of detecting terminal deoxynucleotidyl transferase in human hematologic malignancies. *American Journal of Clinical Pathology*, **77**, 420.

28 CLAYTON, E. M., FELHAUS, W. D. and PHYTHYON, J. M. (1963). The demonstration of fetal erythrocytes in the presence of adult red blood cells. *American Journal of Clinical Pathology*, **40**, 487.

29 COLEMAN, M. S. and HUTTON, J. J. (1981). Terminal transferase. In *The Leukemic Cell*, Ed. D. Catovsky, p. 203. Churchill Livingstone, Edinburgh.

30 CROCKARD, A. D., CHALMERS, D., MATUTES, E. and CATOVSKY, D. (1982). Cytochemistry of acid hydrolases in chronic B and T cell leukemias. *American Journal of Clinical Pathology*, **78**, 437.

31 CROSBY, W. H. (1957). Siderocytes and the spleen. *Blood*, **12**, 165.

32 DACIE, J. V., GRIMES, A. J., MEISLER, A., STEINGOLD, L., HEMSTED, E. H., BEAVEN, G. H. and WHITE, J. C. (1964). Hereditary Heinz-body anaemia. A report of studies on five patients with mild anaemia. *British Journal of Haematology*, **10**, 388.

33 DACIE, J. V. and MOLLIN, D. L. (1966). Siderocytes, sideroblasts and sideroblastic anaemia. *Acta Medica Scandinavica*, **179**, Suppl. 445, p. 237.

34 DE SALVO CARDULLO, L., MORILLA, R. and CATOVSKY, D. (1981). Significance of Phi bodies in acute leukaemia. *Journal of Clinical Pathology*, **34**, 153.

35 DOUGLAS, A. S. and DACIE, J. V. (1953). The incidence and significance of iron-containing granules in human erythrocytes and their precursors. *Journal of Clinical Pathology*, **6**, 307.

36 FAIRBANKS, V. F. and LAMPE, L. T. (1968). A tetrazolium-linked cytochemical method for estimation of glucose-6-phosphate dehydrogenase activity in individual erythrocytes: applications in the study of heterozygotes for glucose-6-phosphate dehydrogenase deficiency. *Blood*, **31**, 589.

37 FLANDRIN, G. and DANIEL, M. T. (1981). Cytochemistry in the classification of leukemias. In *The Leukemic Cell*. Ed. D. Catovsky, Chapter 2. Churchill Livingstone, Edinburgh.

38 GALL, J. C., BREWER, G. J. and DERN, R. J. (1965). Studies of glucose-6-phosphate dehydrogenase activity of individual erythrocytes: the methaemoglobin-elution test for identification of females heterozygous for G6PD deficiency. *American Journal of Human Genetics*, **17**, 359.

39 GARDIKAS, C. and ISRAËLS, M. C. G. (1948). The Feulgen reaction applied to clinical haematology. *Journal of Clinical Pathology*, **1**, 226.

40 GILLIS, E. M. and BAIKIE, A. G. (1964). Method for the demonstration of nucleoli in lymphocytes and other blood and bone marrow cells. *Journal of Clinical Pathology*, **17**, 573.

41 GOLDBERG, A. F. and BARKA, T. (1962). Acid phosphatase activity in human blood cells. *Nature (London)*, **195**, 297.

42 GOUTTAS, A., FESSAS, Ph., TSEVRENIS, H. and XEFTERI, E. (1955). Description d'une nouvelle variété d'anémie hémolytique congénitale. *Sang*, **26**, 911.

43 GREAVES, M. F., JANOSSY, G., PETO, J. and KAY, H. (1981). Immunologically defined subclasses of acute lymphoblastic leukaemia in children: their relationship to presentation features and prognosis. *British Journal of Haematology*, **48**, 179.

44 GREAVES, M. F., RAO, J., HARIRI, G., VERBI, W., CATOVSKY, D., KUNG, P. and GOLDSTEIN, G. (1981). Phenotypic heterogeneity and cellular origins of T cell malignancies. *Leukemia Research*, **5**, 281.

45 GREIG, H. B. W. (1959). A substitute for the Feulgen staining technique. *Journal of Clinical Pathology*, **12**, 93.

46 GRÜNEBERG, H. (1941a). Siderocytes: a new kind of erythrocytes. *Nature (London)* **148**, 114. (1941b). Siderocytes in man. *Nature (London)*, **148**, 469.

47 HANKER, J. S., AMBROSE, W. W., JAMES, C. J., MANDELKORN, J., YATES, P. E., GALL, S. A., BOSSEN, E. H., FAY, J. W., LAZLO, J. and MOORE, J. O. (1979). Facilitated light microscopic cytochemical diagnosis of acute myelogenous leukemia. *Cancer Research*, **39**, 1635.

49 HAYHOE, F. G. J. and QUAGLINO, D. (1960). Refractory sideroblastic anaemia and erythraemic myelosis: possible relationship and cytochemical observations. *British Journal of Haematology*, **6**, 381.

50 HAYHOE, F. G. J. and QUAGLINO, D. (1980). *Haematological Cytochemistry*. Churchill Livingstone, Edinburgh.

51 HAYHOE, F. G. J., QUAGLINO, D. and DOLL, R. (1964). *The Cytology and Cytochemistry of Acute Leukaemias: A study of 140 Cases*. Her Majesty's Stationery Office, London.

52 HAYHOE, F. G. J., QUAGLINO, D. and FLEMANS, R. J. (1960). Consecutive use of Romanowsky and periodic-acid-Schiff techniques in the study of blood and bone-marrow cells. *British Journal of Haematology*, **6**, 23.

53 HEADINGS, V., BHATTACHARYA, S., SHUKLA, S., ANYAIBE, S., EASTON, L., CALVERT, A. and SCOTT, R. (1975). Identification of specific hemoglobins within individual erythrocytes. *Blood*, **45**, 263.

54 HEINZ, R. (1890). Morphologische Veränderungen der rother Blutkörperchen durche Gifte. *Virchows Archiv*, **122**, 112.

55 HOFFBRAND, A. V. (1981). Iron. In *Postgraduate Haematology*, 2nd edn., p. 57. Heinemann, London.

56 HUHN, D., THIEL, E., RODT, H. and ANDREEWA, P. (1981). Cytochemistry and membrane markers in acute lymphatic leukaemia (ALL). *Scandinavian Journal of Haematology*, **26**, 311.

57 INAGAKI, A., UNO, S., YONEDA, M. and OHKAWA, K. (1976). 2,7-fluorenediamine and 2,5-fluorenediamine as peroxidase reagents for blood smears. *Journal of Laboratory and Clinical Medicine*, **88**, 334.

58 JACOB, H. S. (1970). Mechanisms of Heinz body formation and attachment to red cell membrane. *Seminars in Hematology*, **7**, 341.

59 JANOSSY, G. (1981). Membrane markers in leukemia. In *The Leukaemic Cell*. Ed. D. Catovsky, Chapter 5. Churchill Livingstone, Edinburgh.

60 JANOSSY, G., HOFFBRAND, A. V., GREAVES, M. F., GANESHAGURU, K., PAIN, C., BRADSTOCK, K. F., PRENTICE, H. G., KAY, H. E. M. and LISTER, T. A. (1980). Terminal transferase enzyme assay and immunological membrane markers in the diagnosis of leukaemia—a multiparameter analysis of 300 cases. *British Journal of Haematology*, **44**, 221.

61 JOHAIS, T., DANIEL, M. T. and FLANDRIN, G. (1981). Valeur comparée des réactions à la benzidine et à l'α-naphthol pour la mise en évidence de l'activité peroxydase dans les cellules leucémiques. *Pathologie Biologie*, **29**, 189.

62 JOHNSON, G. D. and NOQUEIRA ARAUJO, G. M. de C. (1981). A simple method of reducing the fading of immunofluorescence during microscopy. *Journal of Immunological Methods*, **43**, 349.

63 KAMADA, N., DOHY, H., OKADA, K., OGUMA, N., KURAMOTO, A., TANAKA, K. and UCHINO, H. (1981). In vivo and in vitro activity of neutrophil alkaline phosphatase in acute myelocytic leukemia with 8; 21 translocation. *Blood*, **58**, 1213.

[64] KAPLAN, E., ZUELZER, W. W. and MOURIQUAND, C. (1954). Sideroblasts. A study of stainable nonhemoglobin iron in marrow normoblasts. *Blood*, **9**, 203.

[65] KAPLAN, M. E. and CLARK, C. J. (1974). An improved rosetting assay for detection of human T-lymphocytes. *Journal of Immunological Methods*, **5**, 131.

[66] KAPLOW, L. S. (1963). Cytochemistry of leukocyte alkaline phosphatase. Use of complex naphthol AS phosphates in azo dye-coupling technics. *American Journal of Clinical Pathology*, **39**, 439.

[67] KAPLOW, L. S. (1965). Simplified myeloperoxidase stain using benzidine dihydrochloride. *Blood*, **26**, 215.

[68] KAPLOW, L. S. (1968). Leukocyte alkaline phosphatase cytochemistry: applications and methods. *Annals of New York Academy of Sciences*, **155**, 911.

[69] KASS, L. and EICKHOLT, M. M. (1978). Rapid detection of ringed sideroblasts with bromchlorphenol blue. *American Journal of Clinical Pathology*, **70**, 738.

[70] KLEIHAUER, E. and BETKE, K. (1963). Elution procedure for the demonstration of methaemoglobin in red cells of human blood smears. *Nature (London)*, **199**, 1196.

[71] KLEIHAUER, E., BRAUN, H. and BETKE, K. (1957). Demonstration von fetalem Hämoglobin in den Erythrocyten eines Blutausstrichs. *Klinische Wochenschrift*, **35**, 637.

[72] KULENKAMPFF, J., JANOSSY, G. and GREAVES, M. F. (1977). Acid esterase in human lymphoid cells and leukaemic blasts: marker for T lymphocytes. *British Journal of Haematology*, **36**, 235.

[73] KUNG, P. C., GOLDSTEIN, G., REINHERZ, E. L. and SCHLOSSMAN, S. F. (1979). Monoclonal antibodies defining distinctive human T cell surface antigens. *Science*, **206**, 347.

[74] LENNOX, B. and DAVIDSON, W. M. (1964). Nuclear sexing. *Association of Clinical Pathologists Broadsheet* No. 47.

[75] LEWIS, S. M. and DACIE, J. V. (1965). Neutrophil (leucocyte) alkaline phosphatase in paroxysmal nocturnal haemoglobinuria. *British Journal of Haematology*, **11**, 549.

[76] LI, C. Y., LAM, K. W. and YAM, L. T. (1973). Esterases in human leukocytes. *Journal of Histochemistry and Cytochemistry*, **21**, 1.

[77] LI, C. Y., YAM, L. T. and LAM, K. W. (1970). Acid phosphatase isoenzyme in human leukocytes in normal and pathologic conditions. *Journal of Histochemistry and Cytochemistry*, **18**, 473.

[78] MELVIN, S. L. (1979). Comparison of techniques for detecting T-cell acute lymphocytic leukemia. *Blood*, **54**, 210.

[79] MOLONEY, W. C., McPHERSON, K. and FLIEGELMAN, L. (1960). Esterase activity in leukocytes demonstrated by the use of naphthol AS-D chloracetate substrate. *Journal of Histochemistry and Cytochemistry*, **8**, 200.

[80] MOVER, S., LI, C. Y. and YAM, L. T. (1972). Semiquantitative evaluation of tartrate-resistant acid phosphatase activity in human blood cells. *Journal of Laboratory and Clinical Medicine*, **80**, 711.

[81] MUELLER, J., BRUN DEL RE, G., BUERKI, H., KELLER, H.-U., HESS, M. W. and COTTIER, H. (1975). Nonspecific esterase activity: a criterion for differentiation of T and B lymphocytes in mouse lymph nodes. *European Journal of Immunology*, **5**, 270.

[82] NANBA, K., JAFFE, E. S., BRAYLAN, R. C., SOBAN, E. J. and BERARD, C. W. (1977). Alkaline phosphatase-positive malignant lymphoma—a subtype of B-cell lymphoma. *American Journal of Pathology*, **68**, 535.

[83] NICHOLS, B. A., BAINTON, D. F. and FARQUHAR, M. G. (1971). Differentiation of monocytes—origin, nature and fate of their azurophil granules. *Journal of Cell Biology*, **50**, 498.

[84] NIERHAUS, K. and BETKE, K. (1968). Eine vereinfachte Modifikation der sauren Elution für die cytologische Darstellung von fetalem Hämoglobin. *Klinische Wochenschrift*, **46**, 47.

[85] O'BRIEN, M., CATOVSKY, D. and COSTELLO, C. (1980). Ultrastructural cytochemistry of leukaemic cells: characterization of the early small granules of monoblasts. *British Journal of Haematology*, **45**, 201.

[86] OKUN, D. B. and TANAKA, K. R. (1978). Leukocyte alkaline phosphatase. *American Journal of Hematology*, **4**, 293.

[87] PAPAYANNOPOULOU, Th., McGUIRE, T. C., LIM, G., GARZEL, E., NUTE, P. E. and STAMATOYANNOPOULOS, G. (1976). Identification of haemoglobin S in red cells and normoblasts, using fluorescent anti-Hb antibodies. *British Journal of Haematology*, **34**, 25.

[88] PAPPENHEIMER, A. M., THOMPSON, K. P., PARKER, D. D. and SMITH, K. E. (1945). Anaemia associated with unidentified erythrocytic inclusions, after splenectomy. *Quarterly Journal of Medicine*, **14**, 75.

[89] PRITCHARD, J. A. (1957). Leukocyte phosphatase activity in pregnancy. *Journal of Laboratory and Clinical Medicine*, **50**, 432.

[90] QUAGLINO, D., and HAYHOE, F. G. J. (1960). Periodic-acid-Schiff positivity in erythroblasts with special reference to Di Guglielmo's disease. *British Journal of Haematology*, **6**, 26.

[91] RANKI, A. and HÄYRY, P. (1979). Histochemical distinction between lymphocytic and monocytic acid α-naphthyl acetate (ANAE) esterases. *Journal of Clinical and Laboratory Immunology*, **1**, 333.

[92] RATH, C. E. and FINCH, C. A. (1948). Sternal marrow hemosiderin: a method for the determination of available iron stores in man. *Journal of Laboratory and Clinical Medicine*, **33**, 81.

[93] REED, C. E. and BENNETT, J. M. (1975). N-Acetyl-β-glucosaminidase activity in normal and malignant leukocytes. *Journal of Histochemistry and Cytochemistry*, **23**, 752.

[94] REINHERZ, E. L., KUNG, P. C., GOLDSTEIN, G., LEVEY, R. H. and SCHLOSSMAN, S. F. (1980). Discrete stages of human intrathymic differentiation: analysis of normal thymocytes and leukemia lymphocytes of T cell lineage. *Proceedings of the National Academy of Sciences, USA*, **77**, 1588.

[95] Report of the Standing Committee on Human Cytogenetic Nomenclature (1978). An international system for human cytogenetic nomenclature: ISCN, 1978. *Cytogenetics and Cell Genetics*, **21**, 309.

[96] RIDWAY, J. C. and GARRETT, J. V. (1974). Demonstration of lymphocyte nucleoli. *Journal of Clinical Pathology*, **27**, 337.

[97] RITZ, J., PESANDO, J. M., NOTIS-McCONARTY, J., LAZARUS, H. and SCHLOSSMAN, S. F. (1980). A monoclonal antibody to human acute lymphocyte leukaemia. *Nature (London)*, **283**, 583.

[98] ROZENSZAJN, L., LEIBOVICH, M., SHOHAM, D. and EPSTEIN, J. (1968). The esterase activity in megaloblasts, leukaemic and normal haemopoietic cells. *British Journal of Haematology*, **14**, 605.

[99] RUSTIN, G. J. S., WILSON, P. D. and PETERS, T. J. (1979). Studies on the subcellular localisation of human neutrophil alkaline phosphatase. *Journal of Cell Science*, **36**, 401.

[100] RUTENBURG, A. M., ROSALES, C. L. and BENNETT, J. M. (1965). An improved histochemical method for the

demonstration of leukocyte alkaline phosphatase activity: clinical application. *Journal of Laboratory and Clinical Medicine*, **65**, 698.

[101] SANDBERG, A. A. (1980). *Chromosomes in human cancer and leukemia*. Elsevier, New York.

[102] SCHMALZL, F., and BRAUNSTEINER, H. (1970). The cytochemistry of monocytes and macrophages. *Series Haematologica*, **iii**, 2, 93.

[103] SCHWAB, M. L. L. and LEWIS, A. E. (1969). An improved stain for Heinz bodies. *American Journal of Clinical Pathology*, **51**, 673.

[104] Second International Workshop on Chromosomes in Leukemia—1979 (1980). Cytogenetic, morphologic and clinical correlations in acute non-lymphocytic leukemia with t(8q−;21q+), *Cancer Genetics and Cytogenetics*, **2**, 99.

[105] SHEEHAN, H. L. (1939). The staining of leucocyte granules by sudan black B. *Journal of Pathology and Bacteriology*, **49**, 580.

[106] SHEEHAN, H. L. and STOREY, G. W. (1947). An improved method of staining leucocyte granules with Sudan Black B. *Journal of Pathology and Bacteriology*, **59**, 336.

[107] SIMMONS, A. V., SPIERS, A. S. D. and FAYERS, P. M. (1973). Haematological and clinical parameters in assessing activity in Hodgkin's disease and other malignant lymphomas. *Quarterly Journal of Medicine*, **42**, 111.

[108] SIMPSON, C. F., CARLISLE, J. W. and MALLARD, L. (1970). Rhodanile blue: a rapid and selective stain for Heinz bodies. *Stain Technology*, **45**, 221.

[109] STATHOPOULOS, G. and ELLIOTT, E. V. (1974). Formation of mouse or sheep red-blood-cell rosettes by lymphocytes from normal and leukaemic individuals. *Lancet*, **i**, 600.

[110] SUNDBERG, R. D. and BROMANN, H. (1955). The application of the Prussian blue stain to previously stained films of blood and bone marrow. *Blood*, **10**, 160.

[111] SYRÉN, E. and RAESTE, A.-M. (1971). Identification of blood monocytes by demonstration of lysozyme and peroxidase activity. *Acta Haematologica (Basel)*, **45**, 29.

[112] TAMAOKI, N. and ESSNER, E. (1969). Distribution of acid phosphatase, β-glucuronidase and N-acetyl-β-glucosaminidase activities in lymphocytes of lymphatic tissues

of man and rodents. *Journal of Histochemistry and Cytochemistry*, **17**, 238.

[113] TESTA, J. R. and ROWLEY, J. D. (1981). Chromosomes in leukaemia and lymphoma with special emphasis on methodology. In *The Leukaemic Cell*. Ed. D. Catovsky, Chapter 6. Churchill Livingstone, Edinburgh.

[114] Third International Workshop on Chromosomes in Leukemia—1980 (1981). *Cancer Genetics and Cytogenetics*, **4**, 95.

[115] TOMODA, Y. (1964). Demonstration of foetal erythrocyte by immunofluorescent staining. *Nature (London)*, **202**, 910.

[116] TÖNZ, O. and ROSSI, E. (1964). Morphological demonstration of two red cell populations in human females heterozygous for glucose-6-phosphate dehydrogenase deficiency. *Nature (London)*, **202**, 606.

[117] UNGERLEIDER, R. S. (Ed.) (1981). Conference on Cell Markers in Acute Leukemia. *Cancer Research*, **41**, 4749.

[118] WACHSTEIN, M. and WOLF, G. (1958). The histochemical demonstration of esterase activity in human blood and bone marrow smears. *Journal of Histochemistry and Cytochemistry*, **6**, 457.

[119] WHITE, J. C. (1947). The cytoplasmic basophilia of bone-marrow cells. *Journal of Pathology and Bacteriology*, **59**, 223.

[120] WHITE, J. M. (1976). The unstable haemoglobins. *British Medical Bulletin*, **32**, 219.

[121] WYBRAN, J., CHANTLER, S. and FUDENBERG, H. H. (1973). Isolation of normal T-cells in chronic lymphatic leukaemia. *Lancet*, **i**, 126.

[122] YAM, L. T., LI, C. Y. and CROSBY, W. H. (1971). Cytochemical identification of monocytes and granulocytes. *American Journal of Clinical Pathology*, **55**, 283.

[123] YAM, L. T., LI, C. Y. and LAM, K. W. (1971). Tartrate-resistant acid phosphatase isoenzyme in the reticulum cells of leukemic reticuloendotheliosis. *New England Journal of Medicine*, **284**, 357.

[124] YUNIS, J. J. (1981) Chromosomes and cancer: new nomenclature and future directions. *Human Pathology*, **12**, 494.

[125] YUNIS, J. J. (1981). New chromosome techniques in the study of human neoplasia. *Human Pathology*, **12**, 540.

7

Bone-marrow biopsy

Biopsy of bone marrow is an indispensible adjunct to the study of diseases of the blood and may be the only way in which a correct diagnosis can be made. There are three ways in which marrow can be obtained—needle aspiration, microtrephine biopsy and surgical biopsy.[6] *Needle biopsy* is the simplest method and has many advantages over the surgical method: it is simple, safe and relatively painless, and it can be repeated many times and even performed on out-patients. It seems to be safe in almost all circumstances even in thrombocytopenic purpura. However, it should never be attempted when there is a major disorder of coagulation as in haemophilia. *Microtrephine biopsy* is a little less simple, but it is now widely used and has almost replaced surgical biopsy. It, too, is relatively painless and can be performed on out-patients.

The disadvantage of aspiration biopsy is that the arrangement of the cells in the marrow and the relationship of one cell to the other are more or less destroyed by the process of aspiration and in fibrotic marrows little but blood may be aspirated. On the other hand, when marrow is aspirated, individual cells in well made films are perfectly preserved and, after staining, subtle differences from one cell to another can be recognized to a far greater degree than is possible with sectioned material. If present, particles of aspirated marrow can, too, be concentrated and subsequently sectioned and this allows the structure of small pieces of marrow to be studied. The great value of microtrephine or surgical biopsy is that they can provide, if expertly carried out, a perfect view of the structure of relatively large pieces of marrow—that is, if the material obtained by the biopsy has been skilfully processed.

Microtrephines of 2 mm bore or less can be inserted into the sternum, vertebral spines or iliac crest; the larger trephines should only be inserted into the iliac crest. Studies on large numbers of cases have demonstrated that, whereas trephine-biopsy specimens are superior to films of aspirated material in some circumstances, e.g. for diagnosing marrow involvement by lymphoma or non-haematological neoplastic diseases, the simple procedure of aspiration marrow biopsy seldom fails to provide important information in patients who have a blood disease.[14,23] We regard both techniques as having an important and complementary role in their investigation.

Surgical biopsy has several disadvantages over microtrephine biopsy (see p. 121), including the fact that it can seldom be repeated. Its sole advantage is that it allows a larger piece of marrow to be sectioned.

TECHNIQUE OF NEEDLE (ASPIRATION) BIOPSY OF THE BONE MARROW

Satisfactory samples of bone marrow can be aspirated from the sternum, iliac crest or anterior or posterior iliac spines and from the spinous processes of the lumbar vertebrae, and in children aged <2 yr from the upper end of the tibia. Puncture of the sternum is perhaps most generally undertaken, but the other sites, particularly the posterior iliac spine, have their advocates and advantages.

Puncture of the sternum

The usual site for puncture is the manubrium or the first or second pieces of the body of the sternum. The manubrium contains rather denser bone than does the body of the sternum, and, in elderly subjects at least, it tends to contain more fatty marrow than is found elsewhere in the sternum.[15] It is also sometimes less easy to be certain that the needle point has reached the cavity of the bone. However, completely satisfactory samples are obtained more often than not from the manubrium. If serial punctures are being performed, a different site should be selected for each, in order to avoid marrow possibly disorganized by haemorrhage resulting from previous punctures.

Only needles designed for the purpose should be used. They should be stout and made of hard stainless steel, about 7–8 cm in length, with a well-fitting stilette, and must be provided with an adjustable guard. The point of the needle and the edge of the bevel must be kept well sharpened. The most commonly used ones are the Salah and the Klima needles (Fig. 7.1). The patient lies on his back in a semi-recumbent position and the skin covering the upper part of the sternum is cleansed with 70% ethanol or 0.5% chlorhexidine (5% diluted 1 in 10 in ethanol). If hairy, the site must be shaved. The skin, subcutaneous tissue and periosteum overlying the site selected for the puncture are carefully infiltrated with a local anaesthetic such as 2% lignocaine.

If the manubrium is selected, the site of the puncture should be about 1 cm above the sterno-manubrial angle and slightly to one side of the mid-line; if the body of the bone is to be punctured, this should be done opposite the second or third intercostal spaces slightly to one side of the mid-line.

Puncture the skin and pierce the subcutaneous tissues. When the needle-point reaches the periosteum, adjust the guard on the needle to allow it to penetrate for about 5 mm further, and fix the guard tightly in position. Then push the needle with a boring motion into the cavity of the bone. The amount of force required varies, but may need to be considerable. It is usually easy to appreciate when the cavity of the bone has been entered. Then remove the stilette and with a well fitting 2 or 5 ml syringe suck up not more than 0.3 ml of marrow contents—bone marrow diluted with a variable amount of blood. As a rule, material can be sucked into the syringe without difficulty; occasionally it may be necessary to re-insert the stilette and to push the needle in a little further and to suck again.

Make films from some of the aspirated material without delay (see p. 122). The remainder of the material may then be delivered into a suitable fixative for the preparation of histological sections (see p. 123). Fix some of the films in absolute methanol as soon as they are dry for subsequent staining by a Romanowsky method or by PAS or for iron. Further films should be fixed in formal-ethanol if other cytochemical staining is to be carried out (p. 84). If there has been a 'dry tap', insert the stilette into the needle and push any material in the lumen of the needle on to a slide; in lymphomas and carcinomas, especially, sufficient material may be obtained to make a diagnosis.[19]

Puncture of the ilium

The iliac crest is another site from which active marrow may be withdrawn. Pass the

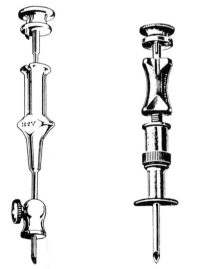

Fig. 7.1 Salah (left) and Klima (right) marrow-puncture needles (reduced ×3/4).

needle perpendicularly into the cavity of the ilium at a point just posterior to the anterior superior iliac spine or 2 cm posterior and 2 cm inferior to the anterior superior iliac spine. As with spinous-process puncture the bone is often appreciably harder to pierce than is the sternum. The anterior superior iliac spine can also be punctured and the bone overlying it is said to be thinner than that of the iliac crest.[33]

The posterior iliac spine overlies a large marrow-containing area and relatively large volumes of marrow can be aspirated from this site.[8] An advantage of puncturing the ilium is that the patient can lie on his side and cannot see what is happening, and several attempts at puncture and aspiration can be made, if necessary, in the same anaesthetized area. Posterior iliac puncture can be carried out with the patient lying prone or on his side.

Puncture of spinous processes

Good samples of marrow may be obtained from adults by puncturing the spines of lumbar vertebrae.[36] Puncture is not difficult since the bones lie superficially, but rather more pressure is required than for sternal puncture.

Pass the needle into the spine of a lumbar vertebra slightly lateral to the mid-line in a direction at right angles to the skin surface, with the patient either sitting up or lying on his side as for a lumbar puncture. With this technique, too, the patient cannot see what is happening.

Comparison of the different sites for needle puncture

There is considerable variation in the composition of cellular marrow withdrawn from adjacent or different sites. Aspiration from only one site may give misleading information;[27] especially is this true in aplastic anaemia as the marrow may be affected patchily.[21,35] In general, however, the overall cellularity and type of maturity of haemopoiesis and the balance between erythropoiesis and leucopoiesis are similar.[2,20] In practice, it is a distinct advantage to have a choice of several sites for puncture, particularly when puncture at one

site results in a 'dry tap' or when blood alone is withdrawn. Aspiration at a different site may yield cellular marrow or strengthen suspicion of a widespread change affecting the bone marrow, such as fibrosis or hypoplasia. In aplastic anaemia several punctures may be necessary in order to arrive at the diagnosis.

Which site is used is a matter of personal preference. The sternum is probably the easiest bone to puncture and on the whole seems to yield the most cellular marrow samples.[2] Sternal puncture, however, has the disadvantage that the patient is aware of what is happening and is often not unreasonably apprehensive.

The actual risks of sternal puncture, in particular of perforating the sternum, are extremely small in adults. Care and the use of a guarded needle should reduce the incidence to zero. In children aged <12 yr the risks are greater and a site for puncture other than the sternum should be chosen (see below).

NEEDLE BIOPSY OF THE BONE MARROW IN CHILDREN

In very young children, from birth to 2 yr, the medial aspect of the upper end of the tibia just below the level of the tibial tubercle may be punctured and active marrow withdrawn. In older children the tibial cortical bone is usually too dense and the marrow within is normally less active. Iliac puncture, particularly in the region of the posterior crest,[18] is then the method of choice. Sternal puncture, although possible, is not free from danger, for the bone is thin and the marrow cavities are small. The dimensions of the marrow cavities in the sternum of children were given by Diwany.[16]

ASPIRATION OF BONE MARROW FOR TRANSFUSION

Bone-marrow grafting has led to the introduction of techniques suitable for obtaining large volumes (1–1.5 l) of bone marrow from a donor. The method in general use is the multiple puncture technique which was described by Thomas and Storb.[46] They devised a special needle with a 45°

bevel to avoid plugging of the lumen during aspiration, but ordinary marrow puncture needles (p. 118) can be used satisfactorily.

PERCUTANEOUS TREPHINE BIOPSY OF THE BONE MARROW

Türkel and Bethell described a microtrephine of about 2 mm bore which could be passed through a hollow introducing needle only slightly larger than a marrow aspirating needle.[48] No skin incision is necessary and the instrument can be safely used on the sternum. However, the cylinders of bone and underlying marrow obtained are small, and they are apt to break up while being prepared for sectioning.

Needles of the Vim-Silverman type[12] are suitable for use in posterior iliac-crest punctures; but they yield smaller specimens of marrow than most other needles. However, the specimens are as a rule free from bone dust and the procedure can be carried out in the ward. A disadvantage of the use of marrow trephines is that not infrequently the specimen is crushed and its architecture altered. The Jamshidi needle*[30] which has a tapering end appears to overcome this problem. The trephine should be inserted by to and fro rotation through approximately 90°. It should not be continuously rotated as this tends to distort and twist the core of marrow. Sometimes, however, the sample fractures while being extracted from the needle and in other cases the biopsy specimen does not detach readily from its base and efforts to detach it by movement of the needle result in it being crushed.

These disadvantages have been overcome by having a core-securing device, as in the Islam trephine†.[29] This makes it possible to obtain a long uniform core of marrow containing bone without the marrow architecture being distorted (Figs. 7.2 and 7.3).

A larger trephine is sometimes of value as it may provide, without recourse to surgery, sufficient material for an accurate diagnosis when the result of a smaller and perhaps less representative biopsy is inconclusive. The Williams and Nicholson modification of the Sacker-Nordin

* A. R. Horwell Ltd., London NW6 2BP.
† Downs Surgical Ltd., Mitcham, Surrey.

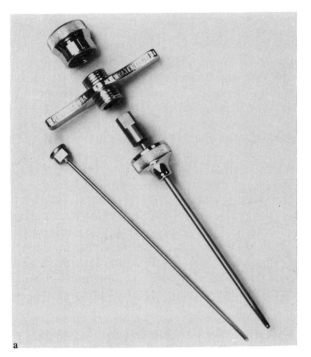

a

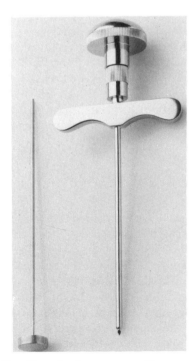

b

Fig. 7.2 Trephines for bone-marrow biopsy. a. Jamshidi, b. Islam.

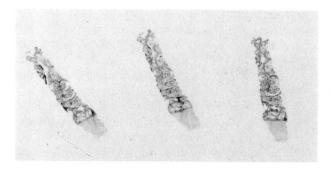

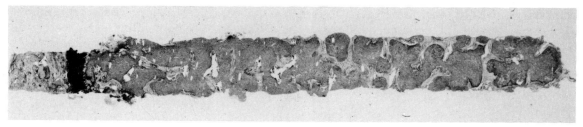

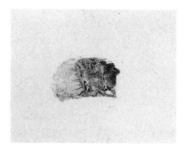

Fig. 7.3 Biopsy specimens of human bone marrow from iliac crest. Obtained using a. Jamshidi trephine (× 3), b. Islam trephine (×5) and c. Sacker-Nordin trephine (× 3).

trephine has a bore of 5 mm;[51] it can safely be used on the iliac crest. The instrument can be inserted under local anaesthesia, but as a small skin incision is necessary the biopsy should be performed in the operating theatre where full aseptic precautions can be taken. It was illustrated in the 5th edition of this book; it is no longer in general use.

SURGICAL BIOPSY OF THE BONE MARROW

As already mentioned, surgical biopsy of the bone marrow has several disadvantages: the biopsy has to be carried out in an operating theatre using a full aseptic technique and it can seldom be repeated; it may be dangerous if the patient has a bleeding diathesis or granulocytopenia, and in leukaemia particularly, the incision may fail to heal. On the other hand, the method has the advantage of providing a relatively large amount of bone and marrow. All in all, however, with the trephines which are now available surgical biopsy should rarely be required.

Biopsy may be carried out on the sternum, iliac crest or rib. However, as biopsy of the sternum may leave an ugly scar which the patient can see, the two latter sites are preferable.

Aspiration of bone marrow in laboratory animals

Several procedures have been suggested for obtaining marrow from small animals without having to kill them. In one method a dental drill is used and bone marrow is aspirated through the hole thus made, by means of a pipette[50] or a fine needle attached to a syringe.[39] Archer et al have designed a needle which, attached to an ordinary 5-ml syringe, can be used to puncture the femur: marrow can be aspirated readily and repeatedly.[1]

Examination of aspirated bone marrow

Quite large volumes of marrow (plus blood) can be aspirated, but the more material aspirated the greater is the proportion of contaminating blood. There is, as already stated, little if any advantage in aspirating more than 0.3 ml of marrow fluid. The material aspirated can be dealt with in at least four ways: films can be made of the material as aspirated; films can be made after it has been concentrated; 'particle smears' can be made, and histological sections can be cut.

Bone-marrow films

Careful preparation is essential and it is desirable, if possible, to concentrate the marrow cells at the expense of the blood in which they are diluted.

The following simple manoeuvre is generally satisfactory. Deliver single drops of aspirate on to slides about 1 cm from one end and then quickly suck off most of the blood with a fine Pasteur pipette applied to the edge of each drop. The irregularly shaped marrow fragments tend to adhere to the slide and most of them will be left behind. Then make films, 3–5 cm in length, of the marrow fragments and the remaining blood using a smooth-edged glass spreader of not more than 2 cm in width (Fig. 7.4). The marrow fragments are dragged behind the spreader and leave a trail of cells behind them. (It is in these cellular trials that differential counts should be made, commencing from the marrow fragment and working back towards the head of the film; in this way smaller numbers of cells from the peripheral blood become incorporated in a differential count.)

The preparation can be considered satisfactory only when marrow particles as well as free marrow cells can be seen in stained films, as is usual with the above technique. No attempt should be made to squash the marrow particles. Their structure—whether hypocellular or hypercellular—can readily be appreciated without recourse to squashing.

Fix the films of bone marrow and stain them with Romanowsky dyes as for peripheral-blood films (p. 51). However, a longer fixation time (at least 20 min in methanol) is essential for high quality staining. Films should be stained by Perls's method as a routine to demonstrate iron (see p. 108).

Some workers add the aspirated marrow routinely to an anticoagulant, e.g. dried EDTA, in a tube and prepare films on return to the laboratory. While this is convenient, the technique requires care. In particular, it is all too easy to use an excess of anticoagulant. When films are spread of marrow containing a gross excess of anticoagulant (as when a few drops of marrow are added to a tube containing sufficient EDTA to prevent the clotting of 5 ml of blood) masses of pink-staining amorphous material may be seen and some of the erythroblasts and reticulocytes may clump together.

Concentration of bone marrow by centrifugation

Centrifugation can be used to concentrate the marrow cells and to assess the relative proportions of marrow cells, peripheral blood and fat in aspirated material. While concentration of poorly cellular samples is useful, it is unnecessary when the aspirated material is of average or increased cellularity. Volumetric data, too, are of little value in individual patients because of the wide range of values encountered even in health.

Methods for separation of marrow cells are described on p. 58.

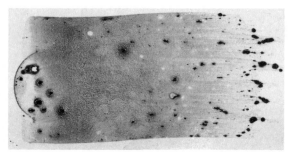

Fig. 7.4 Film of aspirated bone marrow. The marrow particles are easily visible, mostly at the tail of the film (×1.5).

'Particle smears'

Some workers deliberately isolate aspirated marrow particles and make 'smears' of them on slides or between two cover-slips using slight pressure.[42] While this technique undoubtedly gives preparations of authentic marrow cells, squashing and smearing out of the particle causes disruption and distortion of cells, and the resultant thick preparations are difficult to stain really well. The authors feel that this technique has no advantages over the method described on p. 122.

Preparation of films of post-mortem bone marrow

Films made of bone marrow obtained post mortem are seldom satisfactory. When the marrow is spread in the ordinary way the majority of the cells tend to break up and appear as smears. Berenbaum described how the blood cells are much better preserved if the marrow is suspended in albumin before the films are made.[4] He recommended that a small piece of marrow be suspended in 1–2 ml of 5% bovine albumin (one volume 30% albumin, five volumes 9 g/l NaCl). The suspension is then centrifuged and the deposited marrow cells are resuspended in a volume of supernatant approximately equal to, or slightly less than, that of the deposit. Films are made of this suspension in the usual way. Berenbaum also pointed out that the addition of albumin to blood so as to give a 5% concentration improves the preservation of lymphocytes in cases of lymphocytic leukaemia in which many 'smear cells' are often seen in films of peripheral blood prepared in the ordinary way.

The rate and pattern of cellular autolysis during the first 15 h after death has been studied and the differences between the changes of post-mortem autolysis and those which occur in life as a result of blood diseases have been defined.[28]

PREPARATION OF HISTOLOGICAL SECTIONS OF ASPIRATED BONE MARROW

Sections give a better picture of the marrow architecture than can be deduced from films. In a good preparation the relationship between cellular marrow and fat spaces is preserved, hypoplasia or hyperplasia can be recognized, and tumour cells and granulomata can be seen. However, as already emphasized, for cytological detail sectioned material is much less satisfactory. The subtle differences between cells such as normoblasts and megaloblasts, which are usually easy to appreciate in well stained films, are difficult to recognize in sections and it may sometimes be difficult even to differentiate erythroblasts from leucocytes with complete certainty—particularly is this true of trephine material which has had to be decalcified and is paraffin-embedded.

The fragments of bone marrow aspirated by the puncture technique are small, rarely greater than 1 mm in size, and a careful technique in handling them is required. They are usually free from bone and the marrow architecture is well preserved, but their usefulness is limited because their small size makes it uncertain how representative of the bone marrow they are. A more serious disadvantage of a puncture technique is that fragments are often not obtained by suction in just those patients—with perphaps marrow hypoplasia, myelosclerosis or invasion by tumour—in whom histological evidence of any marrow abnormality is particularly required. In these patients trephine biopsy may be necessary.

A number of methods of dealing with aspirated fragments have been published which differ in the details of handling and concentrating the fragments, fixation and embedding.[14,32,43] The following method gives adequate concentration of the marrow particles and is simple to carry out (Fig. 7.5). Fixation is good and sections may be successfully stained by Romanowsky dyes as well as by other methods.

Method of preparing histological sections of aspirated bone-marrow particles[43]

Fixative

Absolute ethanol is diluted with an equal volume of 15% formalin (150 ml/l 40% formaldehyde). The sp gr of the mixture is 0.93, almost exactly the same as that of human fat. When a marrow aspirate is added to this fixative, the blood remains in suspension

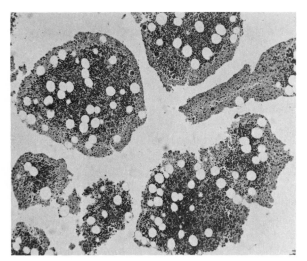

Fig. 7.5 Section of aspirated bone-marrow particles. Method of Raman.[38] × 60.

while the marrow particles rapidly sediment. Even fatty marrow settles down in a few seconds.

Method

Add 0.25 ml of bone-marrow aspirate to 20 ml of the fixative in a stoppered container and mix thoroughly. Allow it to fix overnight at room temperature.

The following morning resuspend the sediment by inversion. With a Pasteur pipette provided with a teat, pick out the coarser marrow fragments after they have re-settled to the bottom of the bottle, which usually takes only a few seconds. Then transfer them to a round-bottomed test-tube, provided with a rubber bung, containing 70% (v/v) ethanol. Leave for at least 15 min, then dehydrate with two changes of absolute ethanol, leaving the particles for 1 h in each. Then drain off the ethanol and replace with toluene. After 1 h decant off the toluene and replace it by a toluene-paraffin wax mixture and then by two changes of paraffin wax. Free the block by breaking the tube when the wax has cooled and hardened. The marrow fragments will have settled as a small mass at the bottom of the block and little or no trimming will be required.

Preparation of histological sections

Fix the specimen in 10% formal saline, buffered to pH 7.0, or preferably in Helly's fluid (potassium dichromate 2.5 g, mercuric chloride 5 g, formalin [40% formaldehyde] 5 ml, water 100 ml) for 12–48 h. Then wash in running water overnight before decalcifying, dehydrating and embedding in paraffin wax by the usual histological procedure. Then cut and stain 4–5 μm thick sections. The relatively thick sections prepared in this way, together with cell shrinkage and the distortion produced by decalcification make it difficult to interpret cellular detail. Almost all these disadvantages can be overcome by 'plastic embedding'. In this process the undecalcified biopsy specimen is embedded in glycol or methyl methacrylate. Sections 1–2 μm thick can then be obtained using a tungsten carbide knife and a purpose-built microtome, e.g. Reichert-Jung Autocut.[9,25] Not only does this provide clearer detail of cell morphology but cell and tissue relationships are maintained and the embedding procedure is less damaging to the tissue than paraffin embedding.

Sections of marrow should be stained by haematoxylin and eosin (H & E) and by a reticulin impregnation method as a routine. It is worthwhile also to stain sections by Giemsa's stain, and for iron by Perls's reaction. H & E staining is excellent for demonstrating the cellularity and pattern of the marrow and for revealing pathological changes such as fibrosis or the presence of granulomata or carcinoma. Haemopoietic cells, on the other hand, may be more easily identified in a Romanowsky-stained preparation (Figs. 7.6 and 7.7). In Fig. 7.8 is shown the extent to which the cellularity of the marrow varies in health.

Silver impregnation stains the glycoprotein matrix which is associated with connective tissue.[47] The bone marrow always contains a small amount of this material which is referred to as 'reticulin' and which is actually a type of collagen.[3] The reticulin content of normal iliac bone marrow is shown in Fig. 7.9 and for comparison the gross increase in reticulin that may be seen in myelosclerosis.

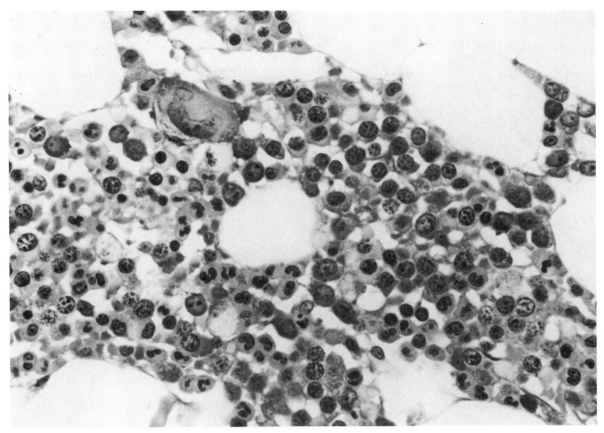

Fig. 7.6 Photomicrograph of section of normal bone marrow. Iliac crest biopsy. Methacrylate embedding. Stained by May-Grünwald-Giemsa. ×300.

Increased reticulin is also found to various degrees in acute and chronic leukaemias, polycythaemia vera and other myeloproliferative conditions.[10,34,44] Morphologically, two forms of argyrophilic fibres may be seen— thin branched fibrils and coarse wavy fibres. The latter type predominate in myelosclerosis.

Method of staining sections of bone marrow by May-Grünwald-Giemsa's stain

The many techniques which have been recommended for staining sectioned bone marrow by Romanowsky dyes are evidence of the real difficulty in obtaining good results. The following method is fairly satisfactory. It may be applied to aspirated marrow fragments, trephine or post-mortem material.

Place the sections which have been processed, as described on p. 124, when cut, in Lugol's iodine for 2 min. Then wash in several changes of water and finally rinse in water buffered to pH 6.8. Stain the sections for 1 h in May-Grünwald's stain diluted with an equal volume of buffered water. Then stain for a further 2 h in a fresh solution of the diluted stain. The sections become grossly overstained and deep blue in colour. Rinse in buffered water (pH 6.8) before differentiation.

Differentiate the sections by covering with a small volume of glycerin-ether, freshly diluted with four volumes of absolute ethanol. Differentiation takes place quickly and is usually adequate in a few seconds. Next dehydrate

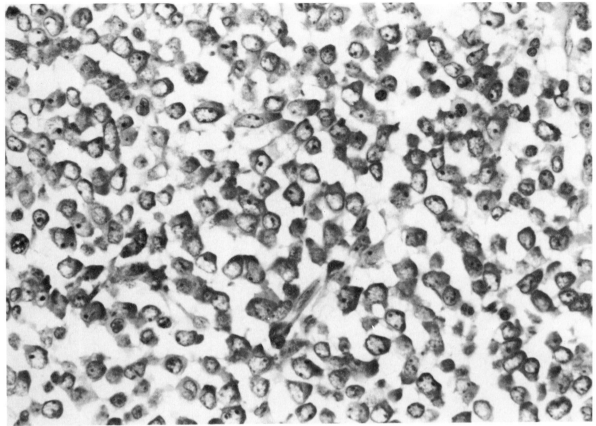

Fig. 7.7 Photomicrograph of section of bone marrow. Iliac crest biopsy. Methacrylate embedding. Myeloblastic leukaemia. Stained by May-Grünwald-Giemsa. ×300.

the sections by a rapid dip in absolute etha- nol, clear them in xylol and finally mount them in a xylol-miscible mounting medium (e.g. Diatex, R. A. Lamb). The use of glycerin- ether helps to prevent 'blueing' of the section during dehydration.

In a successfully stained section the cyto- plasm of primitive cells should be blue, that of myelocytes and segmented neutrophils pale pink, the eosinophil granules should be bright red and the cytoplasm of the red cells orange. Neutrophil granules are not as a rule easily seen.

QUANTITATIVE CELL COUNTS ON ASPIRATED BONE MARROW

A number of figures for the cell content of aspirated normal bone marrow have been given in the literature.[40,49] That the variation is extremely wide is hardly surprising, in view of the tendency of the marrow to be aspirated in the form of particles of varying size as well as free cells and the uncontroll- able factor of dilution with peripheral blood, which according to some authors may amount to 40– 100% in 0.25–0.5 ml bone-marrow samples.[5]

For the above reasons quantitative cell counts seem hardly worth carrying out; instead, the degree of cellularity can be assessed within broad limits as increased, normal or reduced by inspection of a stained film containing marrow particles, and for practical purposes this is all that is usually neces- sary. The proportion of fatty to cellular marrow in the sternum of healthy adults was given by Berman and Axelrod as 21–52%.[7] As a rough guide it may be taken that if less than one-quarter of the particle is occupied by haemopoietic cells it is probably hypocellular, and if more than 75–80% it is hyper- plastic.

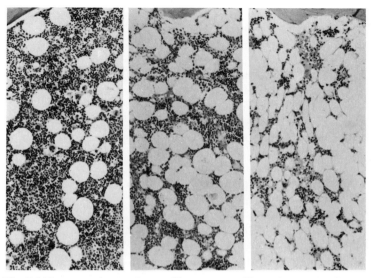

Fig. 7.8 Biopsy specimens of normal bone marrow. Photomicrographs of sections of iliac-crest bone marrow illustrating range of cellularity in health. ×100.

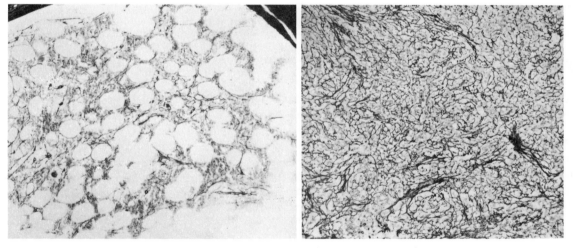

a
b

Fig. 7.9 Photomicrographs of sections of bone marrow. Iliac crest biopsy. Stained for reticulin by silver impregnation method. a. Normal; b. myelofibrosis. ×100.

Physiological variation in the cellular content has to be taken into account. The cellularity of the marrow is affected by age. In adults, as is well known, a smaller proportion of the marrow cavity is occupied by haemopoietic marrow than in children[13] and the proportion of fat cells to active cellular marrow is increased. In elderly subjects aged 70 or over the marrow tends to become still more fatty;[26] this is particularly true of that in the manubrium sterni. The marrow undergoes slight to moderate hyperplasia in pregnancy.[37]

DIFFERENTIAL CELL COUNTS ON ASPIRATED BONE MARROW; THE 'MYELOGRAM'

Many workers perform differential counts on marrow films and by presenting the data in the form of a myelogram express the incidence of the various cell types as percentages. Such figures are not as accurate as they might appear. Films made from aspirated material inevitably include cells from the peripheral blood as well as from the bone marrow, and the variable dilution with blood involves an error for which no compensation is possible. In addition, the more fixed and primitive cells may resist aspiration or, if aspirated, tend to remain embedded in marrow fragments. Megakaryocytes in particular are most irregularly distributed and tend to be carried to the tail of the film.

Ideally, differential counts should be performed on sectioned material. However, difficulties in identification make this impractical, although methacrylate embedding offers a better opportunity for correctly identifying cells. Fadem and Yalow recommended that differential counts be done on preparations made by the particle-smear technique.[20] As mentioned on p. 122, a fairly reliable method is to count the cells in the trails of cells left behind the marrow particles as they are carried to the tail during spreading.

Because of the naturally variegated pattern of the bone marrow and the irregular distribution of the marrow cells when spread in films, differential cell counts on marrow aspirated from normal subjects vary widely in health—so widely that minor degrees of deviation from the normal occurring in disease are difficult to establish. Lymph follicles occur in the bone marrow as a normal constituent, and chance aspiration at the site of such a follicle would result in a film with an unusually high proportion of lymphocytes. Follicles have been reported to occur especially in infants, although in one large study they were reported to be quite rare in children and more common in middle-aged and elderly people.[38]

The normal values given in Table 7.1 can only be taken as an approximate guide. Glaser et al gave figures for the cellular composition of the bone marrow in normal infants, children and young adults, based on 151 samples.[24] Variation is marked in the first year, particularly so in the first month. The proportion of erythroblasts falls from birth, and at 2–3 weeks they comprise only c 10% of the nucleated cells. Myeloid cells (granulocyte precursors) increase during the first two weeks of life, following which a sharp fall occurs at about the third week, but by the end of the first month c 60% of the cells are myeloid. Lymphocytes comprise up to 40% of the nucleated cells in the marrow of small infants; the mean value at 2 yr is c 20%, falling to c 15% during the rest of childhood. The proportion

Table 7.1 Normal ranges for differential counts on aspirated bone marrow

Reticulum cells	0.1– 2%
Myeloblasts	0.1– 3.5%
Promyelocytes	0.5– 5%
Myelocytes	
neutrophil	5 –20%
eosinophil	0.1– 3%
basophil	0 – 0.5%
Metamyelocytes	
young forms	
stab forms	10 –30%
Polymorphonuclears	
neutrophil	7 –25%
eosinophil	0.2– 3%
basophil	0 – 0.5%
Lymphocytes	5 –20%
Monocytes	0 – 0.2%
Megakaryocytes	0.1– 0.5%
Plasma cells	0.1– 3.5%
Proerythroblasts	0.5– 5%
Normoblasts*	
polychromatic	2 –20%
pyknotic†	2 –10%

* or erythroblasts.
† The term 'pyknotic' is preferred to 'orthochromatic' as a description of the most mature normoblasts. Cells with fully ripened cytoplasm (orthochromatic in the strict sense) are rarely met with in normal bone marrow.

of plasma cells is especially low from infancy up to the age of 5 yr.[45]

The hyperplasia which occurs in pregnancy affects both erythropoiesis and granulopoiesis, the latter proportionately less, though with some increase in the relative proportion of immature cells.[37] The hyperplasia is maximal in the third trimester; a return to normal begins in the puerperium but is not completed until at least 6 weeks post partum.

Ratios

Ratios based on a count of 200–500 cells provide useful qualitative information without recourse to more time-consuming differential counts.

The *myeloid: erythroid ratio* has been widely used. Leucocytes of all types and stages of maturation are lumped together. The very wide normal range, 2.5–15:1, reflects the variegated pattern of normal marrow.

As an alternative, the *leuco-erythrogenetic ratio* can be calculated; for this mature leucocytes are excluded. The normal ratio has been reported as 0.56–2.67:1.[41]

ROYAL POSTGRADUATE MEDICAL SCHOOL
HAMMERSMITH HOSPITAL

CASE No

DATE OF BIRTH

HAEMATOLOGY
BONE MARROW REPORT

SURNAME

SEX

FIRST NAMES

WARD

CONSULTANT

DATE TAKEN

LAB. No. | BM

Site(s)

Aspiration

Consistency of Bone

Cellularity

Erythropoiesis

Leucopoiesis

Megakaryocytes

Plasma Cells

Reticulum Cells

Abnormal Cells

Iron

Mitoses

Myeloid-Erythroid Ratio
(Normal Range   2.5-15 : 1)

CONCLUSION

Signature   Date

BM

LAB. No.

DISEASE CLASSIFICATION

NAME

Fig. 7.10 Report form for bone-marrow films in use at the Royal Postgraduate Medical School.

The myeloid:lymphoid ratio varies widely, 1:1–17:1, and the lymphoid:erythroid ratio is similarly a wide one 0.2–4.0:1.[22] These ratios seem to have little value.

REPORTING ON BONE-MARROW FILMS

The first thing to do is to look with the naked eye at a selection of slides and to choose from them several of the best spread films containing easily visible marrow particles. The particles should then be examined with a low-power (16 mm) objective with particular reference to their cellularity, and an estimate of whether the marrow is hypoplastic, normoplastic or hyperplastic can usually be made without much difficulty, if sufficient particles are available for study. The next step is to select for detailed examination—still using the 16 mm objective— a highly cellular area of the film where the nucleated cells are well stained and well spread. Areas such as these can usually be found towards the tails of films in the vicinity of marrow particles. The cells in these cellular areas should be examined first with the 4 mm objective and ×6 eyepieces, and subsequently, if necessary, with the 2 mm oil-immersion objective. Megakaryocytes should be looked for at this stage of the examination; they are most often found towards the tail of the film.

Systematic examination, backed by a knowledge of the patient's peripheral blood count and his history, will usually enable a diagnosis to be made without recourse to a differential count. A detailed 'myelogram' is, in fact, not often required in clinical practice. A description of the general cellularity of the marrow and the type of erythropoiesis (e.g. whether normoblastic, megaloblastic or dyserythropoietic) and of the general maturity of the erythropoietic and leucopoietic cells, and perhaps an estimate of the myeloid: erythroid ratio, are all that are usually needed when reporting on bone-marrow films for diagnostic purposes.

This is not to say that detailed differential counts are never useful and need never be done. Thus, changes in the proportion of primitive to maturing myeloid cells reflect response to treatment in leukaemia or recovery from agranulocytosis, and the actual percentage of blast cells may be of significance in the differentiation of obscure chronic refractory anaemias.[17] On the other hand, time is often much better spent in examining a series of slides than in performing a detailed differential count as a routine on the first few hundred cells looked at in the marrow film of each patient. A wide search may, for instance, in a case of obscure anaemia, settle the diagnosis by revealing isolated groups of metastatic carcinoma cells. In addition, a film should always be stained and examined for iron.

Other features of possible diagnostic value, include the presence of erythrophagocytosis, abnormal numbers of phagocytic reticulum cells, excess plasma cells, non-haemopoietic cells and degenerate or necrotic cells. Bone marrow necrosis is a not uncommon complication of sickle-cell disease; it also occurs occasionally in lymphomas, myeloproliferative diseases and metastatic carcinoma as well as in septicaemia and tuberculosis.[11,31]

It is helpful in reporting on bone-marrow films to have a printed form on which the report and conclusion can be set out in an ordered fashion (Fig. 7.10).

REFERENCES

[1] ARCHER, R. K., RILEY, J. and GWILLIAM, R. V. E. (1981). Aspiration of bone marrow from laboratory rats. *British Journal of Haematology*, **48**, 165.

[2] BENNIKE, T., GORMSEN, H. and MØLLER, B. (1956). Comparative studies of bone marrow punctures of the sternum, the iliac crest and the spinous process. *Acta Medica Scandinavica*, **155**, 377.

[3] BENTLEY, S. A., ALABASTER, O. and FOIDART, J. M. (1981). Collagen heterogeneity in normal human bone marrow. *British Journal of Haematology*, **48**, 287.

[4] BERENBAUM, M. C. (1956). The use of bovine albumin in the preparation of marrow and blood films. *Journal of Clinical Pathology*, **9**, 381.

[5] BERLIN, N. I., HENNESSY, T. G. and GARTLAND, J. (1950). Sternal marrow puncture: the dilution with peripheral blood as determined by P^{32} labelled red cells. *Journal of Laboratory and Clinical Medicine*, **36**, 23.

[6] BERMAN, L. (1953). A review of methods for aspiration and biopsy of bone marrow. *American Journal of Clinical Pathology*, **23**, 385.

[7] BERMAN, L. and AXELROD, A. R. (1950). Fat, total cell and megakaryocyte content of sections of aspirated marrow of normal persons. *American Journal of Clinical Pathology*, **20**, 686.

[8] BIERMAN, H. R. and KELLY, K. H. (1956). Multiple marrow aspiration in man from the posterior ilium. *Blood*, **11**, 370.

[9] BURKHARDT, R. (1970). *Colour Atlas of Clinical Histopathology of Bone Marrow and Bone*. Springer, Berlin, New York.

[10] BURSTON, J., and PINNIGER, J. L. (1963). The reticulin content of bone marrow in haematological disorders. *British Journal of Haematology*, **9**, 172.

[11] CONRAD, M. E. and CARPENTER, J. T. (1979). Bone marrow necrosis. *American Journal of Haematology*, **7**, 181.

[12] CONRAD, M. E. and CROSBY, W. H. (1961). Bone marrow biopsy: modification of the Vim-Silverman needle. *Journal of Laboratory and Clinical Medicine*, **57**, 642.

[13] CUSTER, R. P. and AHLFELDT, F. E (1932). Studies on the structure and function of the bone marrow: II. Variations in cellularity in various bones with advancing years of life and their relative response to stimuli. *Journal of Laboratory and Clinical Medicine*, **17**, 960.

[14] DEE, J. W., VALDIVIESO, M. and DREWINKO, B. (1976). Comparison of the efficacies of closed trephine needle biopsy, aspirated paraffin-embedded clot section and smear preparation in the diagnosis of bone-marrow involvement by lymphoma. *American Journal of Clinical Pathology*, **65**, 183.

[15] DENST, J. and MULLIGAN, R. M. (1950). The distribution of bone marrow in the human sternum. *American Journal of Clinical Pathology*, **20**, 610.

[16] DIWANY, M. (1940). Sternal marrow puncture in children. *Archives of Disease in Childhood*, **15**, 159.

[17] DREYFUS, B., SULTAN, C., ROCHANT, H., SALMON, C., MANNONI, P., CARTRON, J. P., BOIVIN, P. and GALAND, C. (1969). Anomalies of blood group antigens and erythrocyte enzymes in two types of chronic refractory anaemia. *British Journal of Haematology*, **16**, 303.

[18] EMERY, J. L. (1957). The technique of bone marrow aspiration in children. *Journal of Clinical Pathology*, **10**, 339.

[19] ENGESET, A., NESHEIM, A. and SOKOLOWSKI, J. (1979). Incidence of 'dry tap' on bone marrow aspirations in lymphomas and carcinomas. Diagnostic value of the small material in the needle. *Scandinavian Journal of Haematology*, **22**, 417.

[20] FADEM, R. S. and YALOW, R. (1951). Uniformity of cell counts in smears of bone marrow particles. *American Journal of Clinical Pathology*, **27**, 541.

[21] FERRANT, A. (1980). Selective hypoplasia of pelvic bone marrow. *Scandinavian Journal of Haematology*, **25**, 12.

[22] FRISCH, B. and LEWIS, S. M. (1974). The bone marrow in aplastic anaemia: diagnostic and prognostic features. *Journal of Clinical Pathology*, **27**, 231.

[23] GARRETT, T. J., GEE, T. S., LIEBERMAN, P. H. and MCKENZIE, S. (1976). The role of bone marrow aspiration and biopsy in detecting marrow involvement by nonhematogenic malignancies. *Cancer*, **38**, 2401.

[24] GLASER, K., LIMARZI, L. R. and PONCHER, H. G. (1950). Cellular composition of the bone marrow in normal infants and children. *Pediatrics*, **6**, 789.

[25] GREEN, G. H. and KURREIN, F. (1981). Glycol methacrylate embedding in general histopathology. ACP Broadsheet No. 97, Association of Clinical Pathologists, London.

[26] HARTSOCK, R. J., SMITH, E. B. and PETTY, C. S. (1965). Normal variations with aging of the amount of hematopoietic tissue in bone marrow from the anterior iliac crest. *American Journal of Clinical Pathology*, **43**, 326.

[27] HASHIMOTO, M. (1960). The distribution of active marrow in the bones of normal adults. *Kyushu Journal of Medical Science*, **11**, 103.

[28] HOFFMAN, S. B., MORROW, G. W. Jnr, PEASE, G. L. and STROEBEL, C. F. (1964). Rate of cellular autolysis in postmortem bone marrow. *American Journal of Clinical Pathology*, **41**, 281.

[29] ISLAM, A. (1981). A new bone marrow biopsy needle with core securing device. *Journal of Clinical Pathology*, **35**, 359.

[30] JAMSHIDI, K. and SWAIM, W. R. (1971). Bone marrow biopsy with unaltered architecture: a new biopsy device. *Journal of Laboratory and Clinical Medicine*, **77**, 335.

[31] KIRALY, J. F. and WHEBY, M. S. (1976). Bone marrow necrosis. *American Journal of Medicine*, **60**, 361.

[32] KUPER, S. W. A. (1965). Preparation of sections from bone marrow aspirates and cellular exudates using soluble plastic centrifuge tubes. *Journal of Clinical Pathology*, **18**, 255.

[33] LEFFLER, R. J. (1957). Aspiration of bone marrow from the anterior superior iliac spine. *Journal of Laboratory and Clinical Medicine*, **50**, 482.

[34] LENNERT, K., NAGAI, K. and SCHWARZE, E.-W. (1975). Patho-anatomic features of the bone marrow. *Clinics in Haematology*, **4**, 331.

[35] LEWIS, S. M. (1965). Course and prognosis in aplastic anaemia. *British Medical Journal*, **i**, 1027.

[36] LOGE, J. P. (1948). Spinous process puncture. A simple clinical approach for obtaining bone marrow. *Blood*, **3**, 198.

[37] LOWENSTEIN, L. and BRAMLAGE, C. A. (1957). The bone marrow in pregnancy and the puerperium. *Blood*, **12**, 261.

[38] MAEDA, K., HYUN, B. H. and REBUCK, J. W. (1977). Lymphoid follicles in bone marrow aspirates. *American Journal of Clinical Pathology*, **67**, 41.

[39] MCFADZEAN, A. J. S. (1948). Marrow biopsy in laboratory animals. *Journal of Pathology and Bacteriology*, **60**, 332.

[40] OSGOOD, E. E. and SEAMAN, A. J. (1944). The cellular composition of normal bone marrow as obtained by sternal puncture. *Physiological Reviews*, **24**, 46.

[41] PONTONI, L. (1936). Su alcuni rapporti citologici ricavati dal mielogramma; metodica e valutazione fisopatognostica generale. *Haematologica*, **17**, 833.

[42] PROPP, S. (1951). An improved technic of bone marrow aspiration. *Blood*, **6**, 585.

[43] RAMAN, K. (1955). A method of sectioning aspirated bone-marrow. *Journal of Clinical Pathology*, **8**, 265.

[44] ROBERTS, B. E., MILES, D. W. and WOODS, C. G. (1969). Polycythaemia vera and myelosclerosis: a bone marrow study. *British Journal of Haematology*, **16**, 75.

[45] STEINER, M. L. and PEARSON, H. A. (1966). Bone marrow plasmacyte values in childhood. *Journal of Pediatrics*, **68**, 562.

[46] THOMAS, E. D. and STORB, R. (1970). Technique for human marrow grafting. *Blood*, **36**, 507.

[47] TOMLIN, S. G. (1953). Reticulin and collagen. *Nature (London)*, **171**, 302.

[48] TÜRKEL, H. and BETHELL, F. H. (1943). Biopsy of bone marrow performed by a new and simple instrument. *Journal of Laboratory and Clinical Medicine*, **28**, 1246.

[49] VAUGHAN, S. L. and BROCKMYRE, F. (1947). Normal bone marrow as obtained by sternal puncture. *Blood*, *Special Issue*, No. 1, p. 54.

[50] VIGRAM, M. (1947). A method of bone marrow biopsy from the rat. *Journal of Laboratory and Clinical Medicine*, **32**, 102.

[51] WILLIAMS, J. A. and NICHOLSON, G. I. (1963). A modified bone-biopsy drill for outpatient use. *Lancet*, **i**, 1408.

8

Use of haematological techniques in clinical work

There are three ways in which the techniques described in this book may be useful:

1. Screening a blood sample for an abnormality.
2. Making a tentative diagnosis of a blood disorder.
3. Investigating in detail a patient in whom a tentative diagnosis of a particular blood disorder has been made.

Radiological and other non-haematological investigations are frequently helpful in arriving at a diagnosis. However, a description of their value and scope, and also of the clinical examination of the patient, is beyond the scope of this book.

SCREENING FOR ANAEMIA

The approach to screening tests depends on what facilities are available, especially whether an automatic counting system is used. Although electronic counters are in daily use in many laboratories, there are still a large number where they are not yet available. In these, measurement of PCV, Hb estimation and inspection of a stained film may be all that is practicable as a minimum 'screening' procedure. The measurement of PCV and Hb estimation provide a check of one measurement against the other and the MCHC, if subnormal, gives a presumptive indication of iron deficiency. If a leucocyte or platelet abnormality is suspected, total counts of these should be undertaken.

The availability of an electronic counter allows blood-count data to be obtained quickly and with considerable accuracy. In particular, the figures obtainable for red-cell count, MCV and MCH are far more reliable and consequently more valuable than those obtained by visual counting. However,

in relation to screening for anaemia the main value of automated equipment lies in the speed with which blood-count data can be obtained.

Irrespective of the degree to which automatic procedures can be used in blood counting, it is still necessary to make and examine blood films. It is ideal, although not always practical, to make films from every sample of blood submitted to the laboratory even if the PCV or Hb is normal. Inspection of a film may reveal signs of an unsuspected blood disease, for example, compensated haemolytic anaemia or chronic lymphocytic leukaemia, which might not be revealed by quantitative counts, as well as interesting abnormalities such as hereditary elliptocytosis or the Pelger-Hüet leucocyte abnormality, and the presence in the film of excessive rouleaux may draw attention to a protein abnormality.

Ideally, all blood films—and not necessarily only those showing a definite abnormality—should be filed away and kept for as long as possible. From time to time it will be important to have available a film made many years previously. Re-examination may show, for instance, the early stages of an abnormality which had been missed, but had become more obvious later, or that the earlier film was normal. Each type of information may be important in a particular case.

DIAGNOSIS OF THE TYPE OF BLOOD DISORDER

When a patient's blood has been shown to be abnormal as the result of a screening procedure, it is necessary to make an accurate diagnosis. Sometimes this can be arrived at simply by examination of a well stained and well spread blood film, supplemented by a reticulocyte count and the quantitative cell count data already available. In other cases, no certain diagnosis is possible without bone-marrow aspiration or trephine biopsy. The great majority of anaemias and leucocyte disorders can be diagnosed in this simple manner, namely, from knowledge of the blood-cell counts, by examination of the stained blood film and in some instances by examination of the bone marrow. Other simple tests which may be helpful in appropriate cases are the ESR, glycerol lysis time (p. 156), and the direct antiglobulin test. Only occasionally when, for example, a patient has a haemolytic anaemia, haemoglobinopathy or haemorrhagic disorder, have more complicated laboratory tests to be undertaken before even a tentative diagnosis can be made.

FURTHER HAEMATOLOGICAL INVESTIGATION OF A PATIENT AFTER A TENTATIVE DIAGNOSIS HAS BEEN MADE

The patient is investigated further usually for one of two reasons:

1. The diagnosis is not in doubt but further studies are required to elucidate the cause and mechanism of the patient's blood disorder or to classify it more precisely.

2. The diagnosis is not yet clear and further investigations are required in order to arrive (if possible) at the correct diagnosis.

The choice of tests and procedures to be undertaken depends upon the results of the preliminary tests already carried out and the facilities and time available. Recommended procedures for the further investigation of the more important types of blood disorder are given below. The more valuable and informative procedures are given first; the less important or more complicated tests, only applicable in certain circumstances, follow.

Hypochromic anaemias

Chemical tests for occult gastro-intestinal bleeding; bone-marrow aspiration (including staining for iron), if not already undertaken; measurement of serum iron and total iron-binding capacity; tests for malabsorption syndrome; tests for absorption of iron; measurement of blood loss using ^{51}Cr. If thalassaemia or a haemoglobinopathy is suspected: haemoglobin electrophoresis; Hb-F and Hb-A$_2$ estimation; tests for an unstable haemoglobin; family studies; globin chain synthesis; globin chain analysis.

Megaloblastic anaemias. See Chapter 20.

'Secondary anaemias'

These include too wide a range of blood disorders and mechanisms of anaemia to be summarized here. The haematologist should direct his efforts towards explaining the patient's anaemia, which may be dyshaemopoietic, haemolytic and/or due to blood loss, and excluding a 'primary' blood disease or replacement of normal haemopoietic marrow by tumour. When an anaemia remains unexplained, blood volume measurements may show that it is a 'pseudoanaemia'.

Aplastic anaemia

Bone-marrow aspiration or trephine biopsy, possibly in more than one site, if not already undertaken; acidified-serum test for PNH; test for haemosiderin in urine deposit; neutrophil alkaline phosphatase; ^{59}Fe (and ^{52}Fe scan if available) to study red-cell production; red-cell survival study using ^{51}Cr, including measurement of blood loss in the faeces.

Haemolytic anaemias. See Chapters 9–12 and 23.

Haemorrhagic disorders. See Chapters 13–15.

Leucopenia

Bone-marrow aspiration, if not already undertaken; serial observations on peripheral leucocyte count to test for cyclical neutropenia; tests for leucocyte agglutinins (see p. 410).

Acute leukaemia

Bone-marrow aspiration, if not already undertaken, including PAS staining and staining for iron; alkaline-phosphatase reaction of neutrophils;

myeloperoxidase reaction of neutrophils and precursor cells; other cytochemical and enzyme tests and immunological studies on cells from blood and marrow to identify cell type (see Chapter 6); serum-protein estimation; serum-B_{12} estimation; tests for abnormal haemoglobins, e.g. Hb H; chromosome studies.

Chronic granulocytic leukaemia

Bone-marrow aspiration; alkaline-phosphatase reaction of neutrophils; chromosome studies.

Chronic lymphocytic leukaemia

Bone-marrow aspiration, cytochemical and enzyme tests and immunological studies (see Chapter 6); serum-protein estimation; lymph-node biopsy (aspiration and/or surgical).

Myelomatosis

Bone-marrow aspiration; serum-protein estimation; tests for Bence-Jones and other urine proteins; tests of renal function; serum Ca; X-ray examination of skeleton.

Polycythaemia

Blood-volume estimation; bone-marrow aspiration or trephine biopsy; alkaline-phosphatase reaction of neutrophils; serum uric acid; renal function tests and pyelogram; oxygen saturation; oxygen dissociation; spleen scan and measurement of red-cell pool; identification of abnormal haemoglobin; erythropoietin assay.

Myelosclerosis

Bone-marrow trephine; serum folic acid; alkaline-phosphatase reaction of neutrophils; serum uric acid; use of ^{59}Fe (or ^{52}Fe) to demonstrate extramedullary erythropoiesis and ^{51}Cr to demonstrate rate and site of red-cell destruction; spleen scan and measurement of red-cell pool.

Pancytopenia and splenomegaly

Bone-marrow aspiration; lymph-node biopsy (if lymph nodes enlarged); liver biopsy; ^{51}Cr to study red-cell survival and sites of haemolysis; ^{59}Fe (or ^{52}Fe) to demonstrate extramedullary haemopoiesis; spleen scan; measurement of splenic red-cell pool.

DOCUMENTATION OF BLOOD-COUNT DATA

It is essential that adequate records be kept in the haematology department. By using a filing card on which the results of tests are recorded serially it is possible to see at a glance whether there has been any change in a patient's blood values (Fig. 8.1). The trend of a blood count is even better appreciated when the figures are plotted as a time-related graph, and this is of special value in assessing the effects of therapy on the blood picture (Fig. 8.2). An arithmetical scale should be used for haemoglobin, reticulocytes and red-cell counts, while leucocyte and platelet counts are best recorded on a logarithmic scale. On the horizontal scale of the chart illustrated in Fig. 8.2 each small square represents 1 day; and there are prominent vertical lines every 7 days.

USE OF COMPUTERS

The processing, storage and retrieval of laboratory data can be facilitated by using a computer system. Two systems are available—on-line and off-line.

In the on-line system the results of laboratory tests are entered into the computer store as they become available and reports are printed out automatically; they are updated continuously and cumulative reports can be produced, together with the results of all other tests performed on the same patient. With appropriate ancillary equipment reports can be displayed on a video-screen or cathode-ray tube or typed by teletype printer in wards or other sites away from the laboratory.

When only off-line facilities are available the data are processed at intervals throughout the day, depending on the availability of the computer, which will, as a rule, be shared by other users. Obviously, if information on work in pro-

ROYAL POSTGRADUATE MEDICAL SCHOOL HAMMERSMITH HOSPITAL		CASE No.		DATE OF BIRTH
HAEMATOLOGY **BLOOD COUNT**		SURNAME		SEX
CONSULTANT		FIRST NAMES		WARD

CARD No

RACF

DISEASE CLASSIFICATION

NAME

DATE					
%					
WBC x 10³/µl					
RBC x 10⁶/µl					
Hb g/100ml					
PCV %					
MCV fl					
MCH pg					
MCHC %					
Retics %					
Platelets x 10³/µl					
	% /µl	% /µl	/µl		/µl
Blasts					
Promyelocytes					
Myelocytes					
Metamyel					
Neutrophils					
Eosinophils					
Basophils					
Lymphocytes					
Monocytes					
Film morphology					
Signature					

For Lab. use only

Fig. 8.1 Example of blood-count record card. As used at Royal Postgraduate Medical School before introduction of a computer method for data presentation.

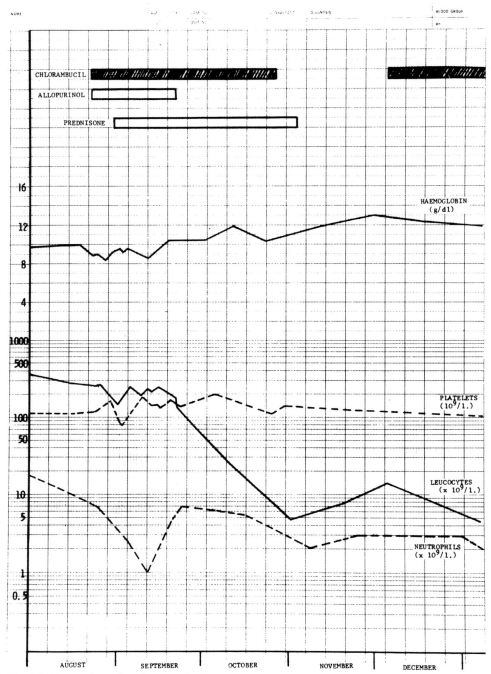

Fig. 8.2 Haematology chart for recording blood-count data as a time-related graph. The course in a patient with chronic lymphocytic leukaemia is illustrated.

gress is to be immediately available and for urgent reports an on-line facility is necessary. By interphasing the computer with a cell counter, it can be used for continuous quality control (see p. 20). It can also provide data for research and administrative records. A further refinement of programming enables the computer to include information on the use of blood and blood products both for the patients' records and for blood bank stock control.

The scope of a computer's performance depends, essentially, on its storage capacity. For a laboratory with a workload of up to 1000 tests a day, a core store of at least 16 K (K = 1024 locations) is necessary. A complete system to include all tests in a busy laboratory might require a capacity of 56–120 K. Even so, in most cases, only 2–3 months of cumulative reports can be stored for ready access. A number of reviews on the use of computers in haematological work have been published in recent years.[1-6]

REFERENCES

[1] CAVILL, I., RICKETTS, C. and JACOBS, A. (1975). *Computers in Haematology*. Computers in Medicine Series, Butterworth, London.

[2] CHALMERS, D. G. (1979). Minicomputer systems in clinical laboratories. *Clinical and Laboratory Haematology*, **1**, 153.

[3] CLARKE, A. A., COLEMAN, S. J., PRALL, A. and WOOTTON, I. D. P. (1980). Data processing in pathology laboratories: the extension of the Phoenix system into haematology. *Clinical and Laboratory Haematology*, **2**, 63.

[4] NELSON, M. G., FARRINGTON, C. L., ROGERS, J. D. and PURDY, G. W. (1980). Processing haematological data on a dedicated computer. *Journal of Clinical Pathology*, **33**, 926.

[5] PAGE, C. F. (1979). Minicomputer systems in clinical laboratories. *Clinical and Laboratory Haematology*, **1**, 153.

[6] PAGE, C. F. and ENGLAND, J. M. (1979). A minicomputer laboratory data-management system: the St. Mary's system and its haematology applications. *Clinical and Laboratory Haematology*, **1**, 165.

9

Laboratory methods used in the investigation of the haemolytic anaemias

The investigation of patients suspected of suffering from haemolytic anaemia comprises several distinct stages: recognizing increased haemolysis; determining the type of haemolytic mechanism; making the precise diagnosis; and, if facilities are available, carrying out tests of scientific rather than of strictly diagnostic or prognostic value. In practice, the procedures are often telescoped, for the diagnosis in some instances may be obvious to the experienced observer from a glance down the microscope at the patient's blood film.

The following practical scheme of investigation is recommended. The tests are arranged 1, 2, 3 and 4 in order of importance and practicability.

Is there evidence of increased haemolysis?

1. Hb estimation; reticulocyte count; inspection of a stained blood film for presence of spherocytes, elliptocytes, irregularly-contracted cells, schistocytes or auto-agglutination (see Chapter 5).
2. Glycerol lysis test; osmotic-fragility test; serum bilirubin estimation; demonstration of haptoglobins; test for increased excretion of faecal and urinary urobilinogen.
3. Bone-marrow examination.
4. Measurement of life-span of patient's red cells (^{51}Cr method).

What is the type of haemolytic mechanism?

1. Direct antiglobulin test.
2. Test for haemosiderin and Hb in urine; estimation of plasma Hb.
3. Measurement of life-span of normal red cells transfused to patient; determination of sites of haemolysis by surface counting.

What is the precise diagnosis?

Which test should be done depends upon the results of the tests which have already been carried out. Not all are appropriate in every case.

1. If a hereditary haemolytic anaemia is suspected:

Osmotic-fragility determination after 24 h incubation at 37°C; autohaemolysis test ± the addition of glucose; screening test for red-cell G6PD deficiency; red-cell pyruvate kinase assay; assay of other red-cell enzymes involved in glycolysis; estimation of red-cell glutathione.

Electrophoresis for abnormal haemoglobins; estimation of Hb-A$_2$; estimation of Hb-F; tests for sickling; tests for heat-labile Hb (Hb-Köln, etc.).

2. If an auto-immune acquired haemolytic anaemia is suspected:

Direct antiglobulin test using anti-Ig and anti-complement (C) sera; tests for auto-antibodies in the patient's serum; titration of cold agglutinins; Donath-Landsteiner test; electrophoresis of serum proteins.

3. If the haemolytic anaemia is suspected of being drug-induced:

Screening test for red-cell G6PD; glutathione stability test; staining for Heinz bodies; identification of methaemoglobin (Hi) and sulphaemoglobin (SHb); tests for drug-dependent antibodies.

4. In all instances of haemolytic anaemia of obscure type (and in all cases of aplastic anaemia):

Acidified serum test (Ham's test) for paroxysmal nocturnal haemoglobinuria (PNH); sucrose lysis test etc.

Tests primarily of scientific interest

1. Red-cell glucose consumption; red-cell lactate production.
2. Elution of auto-antibodies and determination of antibody specificity (of practical but not diagnostic importance); tests for agglutination and/or lysis of enzyme-treated cells by auto-antibodies; tests for lysis of normal cells by auto-antibodies; demonstration of thermal range of auto-antibodies.

In this and subsequent chapters, descriptions will be given of most of the tests which have been referred to. This chapter will include tests of general importance in providing evidence of increased haemolysis. The investigation of hereditary haemolytic anaemias is described in Chapter 10, haemoglobinopathies in Chapter 11, PNH in Chapter 12 and auto-immune acquired haemolytic anaemias in Chapter 23. Some relevant tests, which are normally carried out in clinical chemistry laboratories will not be described in detail. Instead, recommended methods are mentioned. In general, readers are referred to *Micro-analysis in Medical Biochemistry*, by I. D. P. Wootton,[38] *Methods of Enzymatic Analysis*, edited by H. V. Bergmeyer[2] and *Biochemical Methods in Red-Cell Genetics*, edited by J. J. Yunis.[40]

ESTIMATION OF PLASMA HAEMOGLOBIN

The technique described in the previous edition was Crosby and Furth's[8] modification of Wu's original peroxidase method.[39] The benzidine base used in the reaction is now thought to be potentially carcinogenic; its manufacture is limited and in some countries it is no longer readily available. Less toxic derivatives such as tetramethyl benzidine have been recommended as a substitute[19,32]

although they are possibly less reliable, as the end-point of the reactions is less well defined and the colour produced is less stable. When the plasma Hb concentration is >50 mg/l it can be measured by means of a spectrophotometer at 540 nm by a modification of the whole-blood haemoglobin-cyanide method.[23]

Sample preparation

Every effort must be made to prevent haemolysis during the collection and manipulation of the blood. A clean venepuncture is essential; a relatively wide-bore needle should be used and the syringe, first rinsed with sterile 9 g/l NaCl (saline), should fill spontaneously with blood. When the required amount of blood has been withdrawn, the needle should be detached and 9 volumes of blood added to 1 volume of 32 g/l sodium citrate. All glassware must be scrupulously clean.

In order to reduce haemolysis to a minimum, Hanks and his colleagues recommended that blood should be collected through a wide-bore needle direct into a siliconized centrifuge containing heparin.[13] The blood is then lightly centrifuged and the supernatant recentrifuged after being transferred to a clean tube. With this technqiue, the upper limit for plasma Hb in health was found to be as low as 6 mg/l.

Peroxidase method[8]

Principle. The catalytic action of haem-containing proteins brings about the oxidation of benzidine by hydrogen peroxide to give a green colour which changes to blue and finally to reddish violet. The intensity of the colour may be compared in a photoelectric colorimeter with that produced by solutions of known Hb content. Methaemalbumin and Hb are measured together.

Reagents

Benzidine reagent. Dissolve 1 g of pure benzidine base (or 3,3′,5,5′ tetramethyl benzidine) in 90 ml of glacial acetic acid and make up to 100 ml with water. The solution will keep for several weeks in a dark bottle at 4°C.

Hydrogen peroxide. Dilute 1 volume of 3% ('10 vols') H_2O_2 with 2 volumes of water before use.

Acetic acid. 100 g/l glacial acetic acid.

Standard. A blood sample of known Hb content is diluted with water to a final concentration of 200 mg/l. It is convenient to use a HiCN standard solution (p. 29) as the source of Hb.

Method

Add 20 μl of plasma to 1 ml of the benzidine reagent in a large glass tube. At the same time set up a control tube, in which 20 μl of water are substituted for the plasma, and a standard tube, containing 20 μl of the Hb standard. Add 1 ml of the H_2O_2 solution to each tube and mix the contents well.

Allow the mixture to stand at *c* 20° for 20 min and then add 10 volumes of the acetic acid solution to each tube and, after mixing, allow the tubes to stand for a further 10 min. Compare the coloured solutions at 515 nm or in a photoelectric colorimeter provided with a green (e.g. Ilford 624) filter, using the colour developed by the control tube as a blank. When tetramethyl benzidine is used as the reagent, read the absorbance at 600 nm. If the Hb content of the plasma to be tested is abnormally high, the plasma should be diluted with saline until it is just visibly tinged red.

Normal range. 10–40 mg/l;[7] up to 6 mg/l.[13]

Significance of raised plasma-haemoglobin concentrations

Hb liberated from the intracellular or extracellular breakdown of red cells interacts with the plasma haptoglobins to form a Hb-haptoglobin complex which is subsequently removed from the circulation by, and degraded in, reticulo-endothelial cells. Hb in excess of the capacity of the haptoglobins is partly cleared in the urine in an uncomplexed form, resulting in haemoglobinuria, and partly degraded in the plasma into haem and globin. The haem complexes with albumin forming methaemalbumin and with haemopexin (see p. 142); the globin competes with Hb to form a complex with haptoglobin. In effect, the plasma-Hb level is significantly raised in haemolytic anaemias when haemolysis is sufficiently severe for the available haptoglobin to be fully bound. The highest levels are found when heamolysis takes place predominantly in the blood stream (intravascular haemolysis). Thus marked haemoglobinaemia, with or without haemoglobinuria, may be found in paroxysmal nocturnal haemoglobinuria, paroxysmal cold haemoglobinuria, the cold-haemagglutinin syndrome, blackwater fever, and in march haemoglobinuria and in other mechanical haemolytic anemias, e.g. that after cardiac surgery. In warm-type auto-immune haemolytic anaemias, sickle-cell anaemia and severe Mediterranean anaemia, the plasma-Hb level may be slightly or moderately raised, but in hereditary spherocytosis, in which haemolysis occurs predominantly in the spleen, the levels are normal or only very slightly raised.

It cannot be over-emphasized that the presence of excess Hb in the plasma is a reliable sign of intravascular haemolysis *only* if the observer can be sure that the lysis has not been caused during or after the withdrawal of the blood. Chaplin et al reported 5–30-fold rises above their upper normal level of 6 mg/l as the result of violent exercise,[5] and similar rises have been recorded by Vanzetti and Valente.[37]

ESTIMATION OF SERUM HAPTOGLOBINS

Hb binds with haptoglobins in plasma or serum to form a complex which can be differentiated from free Hb by column chromatographic separation on Sephadex[27] or by its altered rate of migration on electrophoresis. For electrophoretic separation, paper,[18] cellulose acetate,[3,34] starch gel[31] and acrylamide gel[14] have been used. The method described below uses cellulose-acetate electrophoresis.

Another method for the estimation of haptoglobins is by means of radial immunodiffusion on a plate of agarose gel containing a monospecific equine or goat antiserum to human haptoglobin (see p. 441). In this method the test sample and a series of reference samples of known haptoglobin concentration are dispensed into wells in the plate and left for 18 h. Precipitation rings form by the reaction of haptoglobin with the antibody; the diameter of each ring is proportional to the concentration of haptoglobin in the sample. A calibration graph is prepared from the reference samples. The reagents for this procedure are available in a test kit (Endoplate Haptoglobin Test Kit, Kallestad Laboratories). Technical instructions are provided with the kit.

Electrophoretic method

Principle. A known amount of haemoglobin is added to serum. The Hb–haptoglobin complex is separated by electrophoresis on cellulose acetate, and the relative amounts of bound and free Hb are estimated by scanning the electrophoretic strips after staining. The concentration of haptoglobin can then be expressed as mg Hb-binding capacity per l serum.

Reagents

Buffer (pH 7.0, ionic strength 0.05): Na_2HPO_4 7.1 g/l, 2 volumes; $NaH_2PO_4.H_2O$ 6.9 g/l, 1 volume. Store at 4°C.

Haemolysate. Prepare as described on p. 179. Adjust the Hb concentration to 35–40 g/l with water. This solution is stable at 4°C for c 1 week.

Stain. Dissolve 0.5 g of *o*-dianisidine (3,3′-dimethoxybenzidine)* in 70 ml of 95% ethanol); prior to use add 10 ml of acetate buffer, pH 4.7 (sodium acetate 2.92 g, glacial acetic acid 1 ml, water to 1 l), 2.5 ml of 3% (10 vol) H_2O_2 and water to 100 ml.

Clearing solution. Glacial acetic acid 25 ml, 95% ethanol 75 ml.

Acetic acid rinse. Glacial acetic acid, 50 ml/l.

* This compound is considered to be safer than benzidine but should also be handled with care.

Method

Serum is obtained from blood allowed to clot undisturbed at 37°C. As soon as the clot starts to retract, remove the serum by pipette and centrifuge it to rid it of suspended red cells. The serum may be stored at −20°C until used.

Mix well 1 volume of haemolysate with 9 volumes of serum. Allow to stand for 10 min at room temperature.

Impregnate cellulose acetate membrane filter-strips (12 × 2.5 cm) in buffer solution and blot to remove all obvious surface fluid. Apply 0.75 μl samples of the serum-haemolysate mixture across the strips as a thin transverse line, and electrophorese at 150 V. Good separation patterns about 5–7 cm in length should be obtained in 30 min (Fig. 9.1).

After electrophoresis is completed, immerse the membranes in freshly prepared

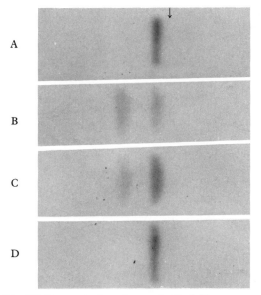

Fig. 9.1 Demonstration of serum haptoglobins.
A. Aqueous solution of haemoglobin (0.4 g/l) run as a reference. The band appears in the β globulin position.
B. Normal serum with added haemoglobin; bands appear in both the β globulin position (Hb) and in the α_2 globulin position (Hb-haptoglobin complex).
C. Slightly reduced haptoglobins; the β globulin band is denser than that of the α_2 globulin band (cf B).
D. Serum from a case of haemolytic anaemia; haptoglobins are absent and the haemoglobin appears only in the β globulin position. The line of origin is indicated by the arrow.

o-dianisidine stain for 10 min. Then rinse with water and immerse in 50 ml/l acetic acid for 5 min. Remove the membranes and place in 95% ethanol for exactly 1 min.

Transfer the membranes to a tray containing freshly prepared clearing solution and immerse for exactly 30 s. While still in the solution, position the membranes over a glass plate placed in the tray. Remove the glass plate with the membranes on it, drain the excess solution from the membranes, transfer the glass plate to a ventilated oven preheated to 100°C, and allow the membranes to dry for 10 min.

After the plate has cooled, scan the membranes by a densitometer at 450 nm with a 0.3 mm slit width.

Calculation

Calculate the density of the haptoglobin band as a fraction of the total Hb in the electrophoretic strip:

$$\text{Haptoglobin (g/l)} = \text{Haptoglobin fraction} \times \text{Hb conc (g/l)}.$$

Significance of haptoglobin levels

In normal sera, haptoglobins are present in sufficient amounts to bind 0.3–2.0 g of Hb/l. A mean value has been given as 1.1 g.[26] It has been thought that normal haptoglobin values differ to some extent according to haptoglobin group, and that the values are higher in men than in women.[26]

Haptoglobins begin to be depleted when the daily Hb turnover exceeds about twice the normal.[3] This occurs irrespective of whether the haemolysis is predominantly extravascular or intravascular; but rapid depletion, often with the formation of methaemalbumin, occurs as a result of small degrees of intravascular haemolysis, even when the daily Hb turnover is not increased appreciably above normal. Low concentrations of haptoglobins, in the absence of haemolysis, may be found in hepatocellular disease, and are characteristic of congenital ahaptoglobinaemia. Low concentrations may also be found in megaloblastic anaemias, probably, because of increased haemolysis, and following haemorrhage into tissues.

An increase in haptoglobin concentration may be found in pregnancy, chronic infections, malignancy, tissue damage, Hodgkin's disease, rheumatoid arthritis, systemic lupus erythematosus, biliary obstruction and as a consequence of steroid therapy or the use of oral contraceptives. Under these circumstances a normal haptoglobin concentration does not exclude increased haemolysis.

DEMONSTRATION OF SERUM HAEMOPEXIN

Haem derived from Hb, which fails to bind to haptoglobins, complexes with either albumin or haemopexin. The latter has a much higher affinity, and when complexed the haem is eliminated from the circulation, e.g. by the liver Kupffer cells.

Haemopexin is a haem-binding serum globulin.[24] In normal adults of both sexes its concentration is 0.5–1 g/l;[25] in newborn infants there is much less, c 0.3 g/l, but adult levels are reached by the end of the first year of life. In severe intravascular haemolysis haemopexin levels are low or zero when haptoglobins are depleted. With less severe haemolysis, although haptoglobins are likely to be reduced or absent, haemopexin may be normal or only slightly lowered, and it has been suggested that the haemopexin level gives a more reliable measure of haemolysis than does the haptoglobin level. Haemopexin seems to be disproportionately low in thalassaemia major,[25] and low levels may be found in certain pathological conditions other than haemolytic disease, namely, renal and liver diseases. The concentration is raised in diabetes mellitus, infections and carcinoma.[25]

Haemopexin can be measured by starch-gel electrophoresis[15] or immunochemically by radial immunodiffusion.[14]

Examination of plasma (or serum) for methaemalbumin

A simple but not very sensitive method is to examine the plasma using a hand spectroscope.

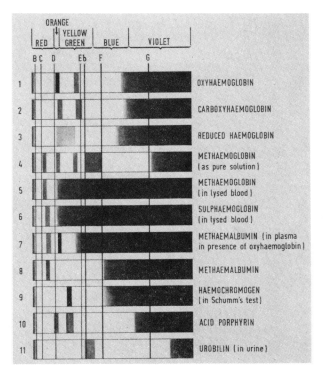

Fig. 9.2 Absorption spectra of derivatives of human haemoglobin. The absorption bands are shown in relation to the Fraunhofer lines, the positions of which are as follows: B at 686.7 nm, C at 656.3 nm, D at 589 nm, E at 527 nm, b at 518.4 nm, F at 486.1 nm and G at 430.8 nm.

Free the plasma from suspended cells and platelets by centrifuging at 1200–1500 **g** for 15–30 min. Then view it in bright daylight with a hand spectroscope using the greatest possible depth of plasma consistent with visibility. Methaemalbumin gives a rather weak band in the red (at 624 nm) (Fig. 9.2). As HbO_2 is usually present as well, its characteristic bands in the yellow-green may also be visible. The position of the methaemalbumin absorption band in the red can be readily differentiated from that of Hi by means of a reversion spectroscope.

Presumptive evidence of the presence of small quantities of methaemalbumin, giving an absorption band too weak to recognize, can be obtained by extracting the pigment by ether and then converting it to an ammonium haemochromogen which gives a more intense band in the green (Schumm's test).

Schumm's test

Method

Cover the plasma (or serum) with a layer of ether. Add a one-tenth volume of saturated yellow ammonium sulphide and mix it with the plasma. Then view it with a hand spectroscope. If methaemalbumin is present, a relatively intense narrow absorption band will be seen in the green (at 558 nm) (Fig. 9.2).

Significance of methaemalbuminaemia

Methaemalbumin is found in the plasma when haptoglobins are absent in haemolytic anemias in which lysis is predominantly intravascular. It was first observed by Fairley and Bromfield in black-water fever.[11] It is a haem-albumin compound formed subsequent to the degradation of Hb liberated into plasma. In contrast to haptoglobin-bound Hb and haemopexin-bound haem, the haem-albumin complex is thought to remain in circulation until the haem is transferred from albumin to the more highly avid haemopexin.[25]

Quantitative estimation of methaemalbumin by a spectrophotometric method[6]

To 2 ml of plasma (or serum) add 1 ml of iso-osmotic phosphate buffer, pH 7.4. Centrifuge the mixture for 30 min at 1200–1500 **g** and measure its absorbance in a spectrophotometer at 569 nm. Add c 5 mg of solid sodium dithionite to the supernatant diluted plasma. Shake the tube gently to dissolve the dithionite and leave for 5 min to allow complete reduction of the methaemalbumin. Remeasure the absorbance. The difference between the two readings represents the absorbance due to methaemalbumin; its concentration can be read off from a calibration graph.

The calibration graph is constructed as follows: solutions containing 10–100 mg/l methaemalbumin are obtained by dissolving appropriate amounts of haemin (e.g. BDH Ltd.; Sigma) in a minimum volume of 40 g/l human serum albumin. The absorbance of each solution is measured in a spectrophotometer at 569 nm, and a graph drawn from the figures obtained.

Demonstration of haemosiderin in urine

Method

Centrifuge 10 ml of urine at 1200**g** for 10–15 min. Transfer the deposit to a slide, spread out to occupy an area of 1–2 cm and allow to dry in the air. Fix by placing the slide in methanol for 10–20 min and then stain by the method used to stain blood films for siderocytes (p. 108). Haemosiderin, if present, appears in the form of isolated or grouped blue-staining granules, usually from 1 to 3 μm in size (Fig. 9.3). If haemosiderin is present in

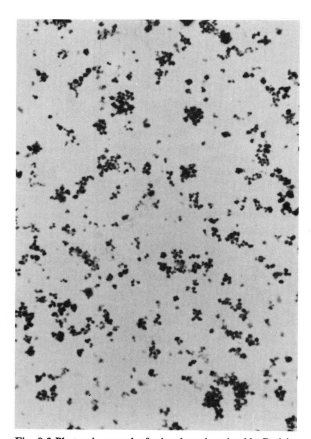

Fig. 9.3 Photomicrograph of urine deposit stained by Perls's reaction. Numerous granules of haemosiderin are present. ×1200.

small amounts, and especially if distributed irregularly on the slide, or if the findings are difficult to interpret, the test should be repeated on a fresh sample of urine collected into an iron-free container and centrifuged in an iron-free tube. (For the preparation of iron-free glassware, see p. 329.)

Significance of haemosiderinuria[9]

Haemosiderinuria is a sequel to the presence of Hb in the glomerular filtrate. It is a valuable sign of chronic intravascular haemolysis, for the urine will be found to contain iron-containing granules even if there is no haemoglobinuria at the time. However, haemosiderinuria is not found in the urine at the onset of a haemolytic attack even if this is accompanied by haemoglobinaemia and haemoglobinuria, as the haemoglobin has first to be absorbed by the cells of the renal tubules. The intracellular breakdown of Hb liberates iron which is then re-excreted. Haemosiderinuria may persist for several weeks after a haemolytic episode.

CHEMICAL TESTS OF HAEMOGLOBIN CATABOLISM

Measurement of serum bilirubin, urinary urobilin and faecal urobilogen can provide important information in the investigation of haemolytic anaemias. As these tests come within the province of the clinical chemist, they are, nowadays, seldom performed in a haematological laboratory. Accordingly, the principles of the tests and their interpretation will be described but details of the techniques will not be given.

SERUM BILIRUBIN

Bilirubin is present in serum in two forms: as unconjugated prehepatic bilirubin and bilirubin conjugated to glucuronic acid. Normally, the serum-bilirubin concentration is <17 μmol/l (10 mg/l) and is mostly unconjugated.

In haemolytic anaemias the serum bilirubin usually lies between 17–50 μmol/l (10–30 mg/l) and most is unconjugated. Sometimes the level may be normal, despite a considerable increase in haemolysis. Levels >85 μmol/1 (50 mg/1) and/or a large proportion of conjugated bilirubin suggest liver disease. Tisdale et al, who reported on the concentration of direct-reacting (conjugated) pigment in haemolytic jaundice, concluded that some of this type of bilirubin may often be regurgitated into the blood stream from the bile when the excretion of pigment is high, even in the absence of overt liver disease.[33]

In haemolytic disease of the newborn (HDN) the bilirubin level is an important factor in determining whether an exchange transfusion should be carried out, as high values of unconjugated bilirubin are toxic to the brain and can lead to kernicterus. In normal newborn infants the level may often reach 85 μmol/l, whilst in HDN infants levels of 350 μmol are not uncommon and need to be urgently lowered by exchange transfusion.

Moderately raised serum-bilirubin levels are frequently found in dyshaemopoietic anaemias, e.g. pernicious anaemia, where there is ineffective haemopoiesis. Although part of the bilirubin comes from red cells which have circulated, a major proportion is derived from red-cell precursors in the bone marrow which have failed to complete maturation.

Estimation of bilirubin is based on its reaction with aqueous diazotised sulphanilic acid. A red colour is produced which is compared in a photo-electric colorimeter with that of a freshly prepared standard. Only conjugated bilirubin reacts directly with this aqueous reagent; unconjugated bilirubin, which is bound to albumin, requires the addition of ethanol to free it from albumin to enable it to react or the action of an accelerator such as methanol or caffeine. Wootton[38] recommended the method of Michaelsson et al[21] who used caffeine benzoate as the accelerator.

Bilirubin is destroyed by exposure to direct sunlight or any other source of ultraviolet light, including fluorescent lighting. Solutions are stable for 1–2 days if kept at 4°C in the dark.

UROBILIN AND UROBILINOGEN

Urobilin and its reduced form urobilinogen are formed by bacterial action on bile pigments in the intestine. The excretion of faecal urobilinogen is increased in patients with haemolytic anaemias. Estimations are best expressed as mg of urobilinogen per 100 g of circulating Hb. In health this amounts to 18–35 μmol (11–21 mg) per day.[23]

The estimation of faecal urobilinogen is, however, a crude and often unsatisfactory method of assessing rates of haemolysis, and minor degrees are more reliably demonstrated by red-cell life-span studies. Urobilinogen excretion is also increased in dyshaemopoietic anaemias such as pernicious anaemia because of ineffective erythropoiesis.

The amount of urobilinogen in the urine is a still less reliable index of haemolysis, for excessive urobilinuria can be a consequence of liver dysfunction as well as of increased red-cell destruction.

For estimation in the faeces the bile-derived pigments (stercobilin) are reduced to urobilinogen which is extracted with water. The solution is then treated with Ehrlich's dimethylaminobenzaldehyde reagent to produce a pink colour which can be compared with either a natural or an artificial standard in a quantitative assay.[38]

Qualitative test for urobilinogen and urobilin in urine[38]

Zinc test

To 5 ml of urine, add 2 drops of N-iodine to convert urobilinogen to urobilin. After mixing and standing for 1–2 min, add 5 ml of a 100 g/l suspension of zinc acetate in ethanol and centrifuge the mixture. A green fluorescence becomes apparent in the clear supernatant if urobilin or urobilogen is present.

If a spectroscope is available the fluid may be examined for the broad absorption band (due to urobilin) at the green-blue junction (Fig. 9.2).

PORPHYRINS

The three porphyrins of clinical importance in man are: protoporphyrin, uroporphyrin and coproporphyrin. Protoporphyrin is widely distributed in the body, and, in addition to its main role as a precursor of haem in Hb and myoglobin, it is a precursor of cytochromes and catalase. Uroporphyrin and coproporphyrin, which are precursors of protoporphyrin, are normally excreted in small amounts in urine and faeces, and red cells, too, normally contain a small amount of free protoporphyrin and coproporphyrin.

Estimation of red-cell porphyrins

Principle. Porphyrins are extracted from washed red cells by a mixture of ethyl acetate and acetic acid. The preparation is treated with ether. Coproporphyrin is extracted from the ethereal solution by 0.1 mol/l HCl and protoporphyrin by 1.6 mol/l HCl. The porphyrin concentration in each extract is determined by a spectrophotometric method. Details of the procedure are given by Rimington.[28]

Demonstration of porphobilinogen in urine

Principle. Ehrlich's dimethylaminobenzaldehyde reagent reacts with porphobilinogen to produce a pink aldehyde compound which can be differentiated from that produced by urobilinogen by the fact that the porphobilinogen compound is insoluble in chloroform or *n*-butanol. The latter solvent is to be preferred.

Ehrlich's reagent. Dissolve 0.7 g of *p*-dimethylaminobenzaldehyde in a mixture of 150 ml of conc HCl and 100 ml of water.

Method

The test is best carried out on a freshly passed specimen of urine. Mix a few ml of urine and an equal volume of Ehrlich's reagent in a large test-tube. Add 2 volumes of a saturated solution of sodium acetate. The urine should then have a pH of about 5.0, giving a red reaction with Congo red indicator paper.

If a pink colour develops in the solution, add a few ml of *n*-butanol and shake the mixture thoroughly to extract the pigment. The colour due to urobilinogen or indole will be extracted by the butanol, whereas that due to porphobilinogen will not, and remains in the supernatant aqueous fraction. When present, the concentration of porphobilinogen in the urine may be estimated quantitatively by a spectrophotometric method.[28,30]

Demonstration of porphyrins in urine

Principle. Porphyrins exhibit pink-red fluorescence when viewed by UV light (at 405 nm). Uroporphyrin can be distinguished from coproporphyrin by the different solubilities of the two substances in acid solution.

Method

Mix 25 ml of urine with 10 ml of glacial acetic acid in a separating funnel and extract twice with 50 ml volumes of ether. Set the aqueous fraction (Fraction 1) aside. Wash the ether extracts in a separating funnel with 10 ml of 1.6 mol/l HCl and collect the HCl fraction (Fraction 2). View both fractions in UV light (at 405 nm) for pink-red fluorescence. Its presence in Fraction 1 indicates uroporphyrin; in Fraction 2, coproporphyrin. The presence of the porphyrins should be confirmed spectroscopically (see below).

If uroporphyrin has been demonstrated, the reaction can be intensified by the following procedure. Adjust the pH of Fraction 1 to 3.0–3.2 with 0.1 mol/l HCl and extract the fraction twice with 50 ml volumes of ethyl acetate. Combine the extracts and extract three times with 2 ml volumes of 3 mol/l HCl. View the acid extracts for pink-red fluorescence in UV light and spectroscopically for acid porphyrin bands.

Spectroscopic examination of urine for porphyrins

This is carried out on extracts, made as described above, or on urine which is acidified with a few drops of conc HCl. If porphyrins are present, a narrow band will appear in the orange at 596 nm and a broader band in the green at 552 nm (Fig. 9.2).

Qualitative tests are adequate for screening purposes. Accurate determinations require the use of fluorimetric analysis[29] or spectrophotometry.[28] It is possible to adapt the qualitative test for quantitative analysis by repeating the procedure several times to ensure total extraction and measuring the intensity of fluorescence in a fluorophotometer, using a standard prepared from a 3 g/l fluorescein solution.[28]

Significance of porphyrins in blood and urine

Normal red cells contain 40–520 μg/l of protoporphyrin and 0–40 μg/l of coproporphyrin.★[28] Increased amounts are present during the first few months of life and, at all ages, in iron-deficiency anaemia or latent iron deficiency, in lead poisoning, thalassaemia, some cases of sideroblastic anaemia and the anaemia of chronic infection.

Normally, a small amount of coproporphyrin is excreted in the urine (100–250 μg/day; mean in women 135 μg, in men 170 μg).[30] This is demonstrable by the qualitative test described above, the intensity of pink-red fluorescence being proportional to the concentration of coproporphyrin. The excretion of coproporphyrin is increased when erythropoiesis is hyperactive, e.g. in haemolytic anemias, polycythaemia and in pernicious anaemia, sideroblastic anemias etc. It is exceptionally high in lead poisoning and it is also high in liver disease; renal impairment results in diminished excretion.

Normally, porphobilinogen cannot be demonstrated in urine, and only traces of uroporphyrin (5–30 μg/day),[28] not detectable by the qualitative test described above, are present.

The increase in urinary coproporphyrin excretion occurring in the above conditions is known as 'porphyrinuria'. There is no increase in uroporphyrin excretion. The porphyrias, on the other hand, are a group of disorders associated with *abnormal* porphyrin metabolism. There are several forms of porphyria, each with a different clinical and biochemical manifestation.[16] Two are of

haematological importance, namely, congenital erythropoietic porphyria and erythropoietic protoporphyria. In the former, uroporphyrin and coproporphyrin are present in red cells and urine in increased amounts; in the latter, increased protoporphyrin is found in the red cells, but the urine is normal. In erythropoietic porphyria haemolytic anaemia may occur.

RECOGNITION AND MEASUREMENT OF ABNORMAL HAEMOGLOBIN PIGMENTS

Methaemoglobin (Hi), sulphaemoglobin (SHb) and carboxyhaemoglobin (HbCO) are of clinical importance, and each has a characteristic absorption spectrum demonstrable by simple spectroscopy or more definitively, by spectrophotometry. If the absorbance of a dilute solution of blood (e.g. 1 in 200) is measured at wavelengths between 400 and 700 nm, characteristic absorption spectra are obtained (Fig. 9.4). In practice, the abnormal substance represents usually only a fraction of the total Hb (except in coal-gas poisoning), and its identification and accurate measurement may be difficult. Hi can be measured more accurately than SHb.

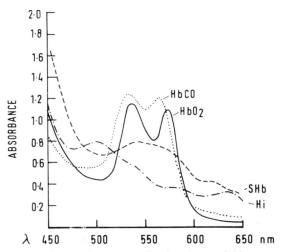

Fig. 9.4 Absorption spectra of various haemoglobin pigments. HbCO = carboxyhaemoglobin; HbO_2 = oxyhaemoglobin; SHb = sulphaemoglobin; Hi = methaemoglobin.

★ Protoporphyrin: 1 μg × 1.77 ≡ 1 nmol. Coproporphyrin: 1 μg × 1.527 ≡ 1 nmol.

Spectroscopic examination of blood for methaemoglobin and sulphaemoglobin

Method

Dilute blood 1 in 5 or 1 in 10 with water and then centrifuge. Examine the clear solution, preferably in daylight, using a hand spectroscope. It is important that the greatest possible depth or concentration of solution consistent with visibility should be examined and that a careful search should be made (with varying depths or concentrations of solution) for absorption bands in the red part of the spectrum at 620–630 nm. If bands are seen in the red, add a drop of yellow ammonium sulphide to the solution. A band due to Hi, but not that due to SHb, will disappear. For comparison, laked blood may be treated with a few drops of potassium ferricyanide (50 g/l) solution which will cause the formation of Hi. SHb may be prepared by adding to 10 ml of a 1 in 100 dilution of blood 0.1 ml of a 1 g/l solution of phenylhydrazine hydrochloride and a drop of water which had been previously saturated with hydrogen sulphide. The spectra of the unknown and the known pigments may then be compared in a reversion spectroscope. The absorption band in the red due to Hi is at 630 nm (cf methaemalbumin at 624 nm) (Fig. 9.2).

Hi and SHb are formed intracellularly; they are not found in plasma except under very exceptional circumstances, e.g. when their formation is associated with intravascular haemolysis.

Measurement of methaemoglobin in blood

Principle. Hi has a maximum absorption at 630 nm. When cyanide is added this absorption band disappears and the resulting change in absorbance is directly proportional to the concentration of Hi. Total Hb in the sample is then measured after complete conversion to HiCN by the addition of ferricyanide-cyanide reagent. The conversion will measure HbO_2 and Hi but not SHb. Thus, the presence of a large amount of SHb will result in an erroneously low measurement of total Hb.

The method described below is based on that of Evelyn and Malloy.[10] Turbidity of the haemolysate can be overcome by the addition of a non-ionic detergent such as Sterox SE or Nonidet P40.[36]

Reagents

> *Phosphate buffer.* 0.1 mol/l, pH 6.8.
> *Potassium cyanide.* 50 g/l.
> *Potassium ferricyanide.* 50 g/l.
> *Non-ionic detergent* (Sterox SE or Nonidet P40). 10 ml/l.

Method

Lyse 0.2 ml of blood in a solution containing 4 ml of buffer and 6 ml of detergent solution. Divide the lysate into two equal volumes (A and B). Measure the absorbance of A in a spectrophotometer at 630 nm (D_1). Add 1 drop of KCN solution and measure the absorbance again, after mixing (D_2). Add 1 drop of potassium ferricyanide solution to B, and after 5 min, measure the absorbance at the same wavelength (D_3). Then add 1 drop of KCN solution to B and after mixing make a final reading (D_4). All the measurements are made against a blank containing buffer and detergent in the same proportion as present in the sample.

Calculation

$$\text{Methaemoglobin (\%)} = \frac{D_1 - D_2}{D_3 - D_4} \times 100.$$

The test should be carried out within 1 h of collecting the blood. After dilution, the buffered lysate can be stored for up to 24 h at 2–4°C without significant auto-oxidation of Hb to Hi.

Screening method for determination of sulphaemoglobin in blood

Principle. An absorbance reading at 620 nm measures the sum of the absorbance of HbO_2 and SHb in any blood sample. In contrast to HbO_2, the absorption band due to SHb is unchanged by the addition of cyanide. The residual absorbance, as read at 620 nm, is therefore proportional to the concentration of SHb.

The absorbance of the HbO_2 alone at 620 nm can only be inferred from a reading at 578 nm, and a conversion factor[36] has to be determined experimentally for each instrument by determining A^{578}/A^{620} on a series of normal blood samples. The absorbance of SHb is obtained by subtracting the absorbance of the HbO_2 from that of the total Hb. This provides an approximation only, but it may be regarded as adequate for clinical purposes in the absence of a more reliable method.

Method

Mix 0.1 ml of blood with 10 ml of a 20 ml/l solution of a non-ionic detergent (Sterox SE or Nonidet P40). Record the absorbance (A) at 620 nm (total Hb). Add 1 drop of 50 g/l KCN and after standing for 5 min, record A at 620 nm and at 578 nm.

Calculation

$$\text{Sulphaemoglobin (SHb) (\%)} = 2 \times \frac{A^{620}\text{SHb}}{A^{620}\text{HbO}_2}$$

where

$$A^{620}\text{HbO}_2 = \frac{\text{Absorbance read at 578 nm}}{\text{Conversion factor}}$$

and $A^{620}\text{SHb} = A^{620}$ total Hb $- A^{620}$ HbO_2.

Significance of methaemoglobin and sulphaemoglobin in blood

Hi is present in small amounts in normal blood, and comprises 1–2% of the total Hb. Its concentration is very slightly higher in infants, especially in premature infants, than in older children and adults.[17] Excessive formation of Hi occurs as the result of oxidation of Hb by drugs and chemicals such as phenacetin, sulphonamides, aniline dyes, nitrates and nitrites etc.

The Hi produced by drugs is chemically normal and the pigment can be reconverted back to HbO_2 by reducing agents such as methylene blue.

Other (rare) types of methaemoglobinaemia are caused by inherited haemoglobin abnormalities (types of Hb M). The absorption spectra of the Hb Ms differ from that of normal Hi and they react slowly and incompletely with cyanide; their concentration cannot be estimated by the method of Evelyn and Malloy.[10]

Methaemoglobinaemia leads to cyanosis which becomes obvious with as little as 15g Hi per 1, i.e. 10%.

SHb is usually formed at the same time as Hi; it represents a further and irreversible stage in Hb degradation. It is present as a rule at a much lower concentration than is Hi.

Demonstration of carboxyhaemoglobin

Principle. HbO_2, but not HbCO, is reduced by sodium dithionite and the percentage of HbCO in a mixture can be determined by reference to a calibration graph.

Calibration graph

Dilute 0.1 ml of normal blood in 20 ml of 0.4 ml/l ammonia and divide into two parts. To each add 20 mg of sodium dithionite. Then bubble pure CO into one for 2 min, so as to provide a 100% solution of HbCO.

Add various volumes of the HbCO solution to the reduced Hb solution to provide a range of concentrations of HbCO. Within 10 min of adding the dithionite, measure the absorbance of each solution at 538 nm and 578 nm. Plot the quotient A^{538}/A^{578} on arithmetical graph paper against the % HbCO in each solution.

Method[35,36]

Dilute 0.1 ml of blood in 20 ml of 0.4 ml/l ammonia and add 20 mg of sodium dithionite. Measure the absorbance in a spectrophotometer at 538 nm and 578 nm within 10 min. Calculate the quotient A^{538}/A^{578} and read the % HbCO in the blood from the calibration curve[36] or calculate it from the equation[35]:

$$\% \text{ HbCO} = \left(2.44 \times \frac{A^{538}}{A^{578}}\right) - 2.68.$$

Significance of carboxyhaemoglobin in circulating blood

Carbon monoxide has an affinity for Hb c 200 times that of oxygen. This means that even low concentrations of CO rapidly lead to the formation of HbCO. From 0.2% to 0.5% of HbCO is present in normal blood and up to 3% in smokers.[36] A high concentration in blood causes tissue anoxia and may lead to death. Recovery can take place, as HbCO dissociates in the presence of high concentrations of oxygen.

IDENTIFICATION OF MYOGLOBIN IN URINE

The absorption spectra of myoglobin and Hb are similar, although not identical, and it is not possible to distinguish them readily by spectroscopy or even by spectrophotometry unless they are first separated by column chromatography.[4] The following is a simple screening test for identifying the presence of myoglobin in urine; it is based on the fact that Hb and myoglobin are precipitated in urine at different degrees of ammonium sulphate saturation. First, it is necessary to demonstrate by precipitation with sulphosalicylic acid that the pigment in the urine is a protein.

Method

Add 3 ml of a 30 g/l solution of sulphosalicylic acid to 1 ml of urine. Mix well and filter. If the pigment is a protein, it will be precipitated. (If the filtrate retains the abnormal colour, this must be due to a non-protein pigment, perhaps a porphyrin.) If the pigment has been shown to be a protein, add 2.8 g of ammonium sulphate to 5 ml of urine (≡80% saturation). Shake the mixture to dissolve the ammonium sulphate, then filter or centrifuge. In myoglobinuria the filtrate will be abnormally coloured; in haemoglobinuria the filtrate will be of normal colour and the precipitate coloured.

REFERENCES

[1] BERGMEYER, H. U. (1974). *Methods of Enzymatic Analysis*, 2nd edn. Academic Press, New York and London.

[2] BLODHEIM, S. H., MARGOLIASH, E. and SHAFRIR, E. (1958). A simple test for myohemoglobinuria (myoglobinuria). *Journal of American Medical Association*, **167**, 453.

[3] BRUS, I. and LEWIS, S. M. (1959). The haptoglobin content of serum in haemolytic anaemia. *British Journal of Haematology*, **5**, 348.

[4] CAMERON, B. F., AZZAM, S. A., KOTITE, L. and AWAD, E. S. (1965). Determination of myoglobin and hemoglobin. *Journal of Laboratory and Clinical Medicine*, **65**, 883.

[5] CHAPLIN, H. Jnr, CASSELL, M. and HANKS, G. E. (1961). The stability of the plasma hemoglobin level in the normal human subject. *Journal of Laboratory and Clinical Medicine*, **57**, 612.

[6] CHONG, G. C. and OWEN, J. A. (1967). Determination of methaemalbumin in plasma. *Journal of Clinical Pathology*, **20**, 211.

[7] CROSBY, W. H. and DAMESHEK, W. (1951). The significance of hemoglobinemia and associated hemosiderinuria, with particular reference to various types of hemolytic anemia. *Journal of Laboratory and Clinical Medicine*, **38**, 829.

[8] CROSBY, W. H. and FURTH, F. W. (1956). A modification of the benzidine method for measurement of hemoglobin in plasma and urine. *Blood*, **11**, 380.

[9] DACIE, J. V. (1960). *The Haemolytic Anaemias: Congenital and Acquired. Part I: The Congenital Anaemias*, 2nd edn., p. 15. Churchill, London.

[10] EVELYN, K. A. and MALLOY, H. T. (1938). Microdetermination of oxyhemoglobin, methemoglobin and sulfhemoglobin in a single sample of blood. *Journal of Biological Chemistry*, **126**, 655.

[11] FAIRLEY, N. H. and BROMFIELD, R. J. (1934). Laboratory studies in malaria and blackwater fever. Part III. A new blood pigment in blackwater fever and other biochemical observations. *Transactions of the Royal Society of Tropical Medicine and Hygiene*, **28**, 307.

[12] FERRIS, T. G., EASERLING, R. E., NELSON, K. J. and BUDD, R. E. (1966). Determination of serum-hemoglobin binding capacity and haptoglobin-type by acrylamide gel electrophoresis. *American Journal of Clinical Pathology*, **46**, 385.

[13] HANKS, G. E., CASSELL, M., RAV, R. N. and CHAPLIN, H. Jnr (1960). Further modification of the benzidine method for measurement of hemoglobin in plasma: definition of a new range of normal values. *Journal of Laboratory and Clinical Medicine*, **56**, 486.

[14] HANSTEIN, A. and MULLER-EBERHARD, U. (1968). Concentration of serum hemopexin in healthy children and adults and in those with a variety of hematological disorders. *Journal of Laboratory and Clinical Medicine*, **71**, 232.

[15] HEIDE, K., HAUPT, H., STÖRIKO, K. and SCHULTZE, H. E. (1964). On the heme-binding capacity of hemopexin. *Clinica Chimica Acta*, **10**, 460.

[16] KAPLAN, B. H. (1970). The control of heme synthesis. In *Regulation of Hematopoiesis*, Vol I, Ed. A. S. Gordon. Meredith Corporation, New York.

[17] KRAVITZ, H., ELEGANT, L. D., KAISER, E. and KAGAN, B. M. (1956). Methemoglobin values in premature and

mature infants and children. *American Journal of Diseases of Children*, **91**, 1.

[18] LAURELL, C.-B. and NYMAN, M. (1957). "Studies on the serum haptoglobin level in hemoglobinemia and its influence on renal excretion of hemoglobin." *Blood*, **12**, 493.

[19] LIJANA, R. C. and WILLIAMS, M. C. (1979). Tetramethyl benzidine—a substitute for benzidine in hemoglobin analysis. *Journal of Laboratory and Clinical Medicine*, **94**, 266.

[20] MIALE, J. B. (1977). *Laboratory Medicine: Hematology*, 5th edn., p. 1035. Mosby, St. Louis.

[21] MICHAELSSON, M., NOSSLIN, B. and SJÖLIN, S. (1965). Plasma bilirubin determination in the new born infant. A methodological study with special reference to the influence of haemolysis. *Paediatrica*, **35**, 925.

[22] MILLER, E. B., SINGER, K. and DAMESHEK, W. (1942). Use of the daily fecal output of urobilinogen and the hemolytic index in the measurement of hemolysis. *Archives of Internal Medicine*, **70**, 722.

[23] MOORE, G. L., LEDFORD, M. E. and MERYDITH, A. (1981). A micromodification of the Drabkin hemoglobin assay for measuring plasma hemoglobin in the range of 5 to 2000 mg/dl. *Biochemical Medicine*, **26**, 167.

[24] MULLER-EBERHARD, U. and CLEVE, H. (1963). Immunoelectrophoretic studies of the βl-haem-binding globin (haemopexin) in hereditary haemolytic disorders. *Nature (London)*, **197**, 602.

[25] MULLER-EBERHARD, U. (1970). Hemopexin. *New England Journal of Medicine*, **283**, 1090.

[26] NYMAN, M. (1959). Serum haptoglobin: methodological and clinical studies. *Scandinavian Journal of Clinical and Laboratory Investigation*, **11**, Suppl 39.

[27] RATCLIFF, A. P. and HARDWICKE, J. (1964). Estimation of serum haemoglobin-binding capacity (haptoglobin) on Sephadex G 100. *Journal of Clinical Pathology*, **17**, 676.

[28] RIMINGTON, C. (1971). Quantitative determination of porphobilinogen and porphyrins in urine and porphyrins in faeces and erythrocytes. *Association of Clinical Pathologists Broadsheet No.* **70**.

[29] SCHWARTZ, S., BERG, M. H., BOSSENMAIER, I. and DINSMORE, H. (1960). Determination of porphyrins in biological materials. *Methods of Biochemical Analysis*, **8**, 221.

[30] SCHWARTZ, S., HAWKINSON, V., COHEN, S. and WATSON, C. J. (1974). A micro-method for the quantitative determination of the urinary coproporphyrin isomers (I and III). *Journal of Biological Chemistry*, **168**, 133.

[31] SMITHIES, O. (1959). An improved procedure for starch-gel electrophoresis: further variations in the serum proteins of normal individuals. *Biochemical Journal*, **71**, 585.

[32] STANDEFER, J. C. and VANDERJOGT, D. (1977). Use of tetramethyl benzidine in plasma hemoglobin assay. *Clinical Chemistry*, **23**, 749.

[33] TISDALE, W. A., KLATSKIN, G. and KINSELLA, E. D. (1959). The significance of the direct-reacting fraction of serum bilirubin in hemolytic jaundice. *American Journal of Medicine*, **26**, 214.

[34] VALERI, C. R., BOND, J. C., FOWLER, K. and SOBUCKI, J. (1965). Quantitation of serum hemoglobin-binding capacity using cellulose acetate membrane electrophoresis. *Clinical Chemistry*, **11**, 581.

[35] VAN ASSENDELFT, O. W. (1970). *Spectrophotometry of Haemoglobin Derivatives*. Royal VanGorcum Ltd., Assen, The Netherlands.

[36] VAN KAMPEN, E. J. and ZULSTRA, W. G. (1965). Determination of hemoglobin and its derivatives. *Advances in Clinical Chemistry*, **8**, 141.

[37] VANZETTI, G. and VALENTE, D. (1965). A sensitive method for the determination of hemoglobin in plasma. *Clinica Chimica Acta*, **11**, 442.

[38] WOOTTON, I. D. P. (1974). *Micro-Analysis in Medical Biochemistry*, 5th edn. Churchill Livingstone, Edinburgh and London.

[39] WU, H. (1923). Studies on hemoglobin: ultra-method for determination of hemoglobin as peroxidase. *Biochemical Journal*, **2**, 189.

[40] YUNIS, J. J. (1969). *Biochemical Methods in Red-Cell Genetics*. Academic Press, New York and London.

10

Investigation of the hereditary haemolytic anaemias
(*Written in collaboration with E. C. Gordon-Smith*)

The various initial steps to be taken in the investigation of a patient suspected of having a haemolytic anaemia are outlined in Chapter 9 and the changes in red-cell morphology which may be found in haemolytic anaemias are illustrated in Chapter 5. In this chapter are described procedures useful in the investigation of patients thought to have haemolytic anaemias based on defects within the red-cell membrane or defective enzymes important in red-cell metabolism.

The technology required to identify precisely the defect in a particular instance of hereditary haemolytic anaemia has proliferated in recent years beyond the scope of most haematological laboratories. The precise identification of an enzyme defect, for example, depends upon the isolation and purification of the enzyme and the characterization of its kinetic and structural uniqueness. In a service laboratory it is sufficient to identify the general nature of the defect, whether it be in the membrane or the metabolic pathways of the red cell. With metabolic defects an attempt should be made, where possible, to pin-point the enzyme involved. Most of the enzyme assays have been standardized by the *International Committee for Standardization in Haematology* (ICSH).[10] A number of commercial kits are also available for the assay of various enzymes and for 2,3-diphosphoglycerate (2,3DPG). These tend to be rather expensive so the ICSH methods will be described here. In the first part of the chapter are described screening tests for spherocytosis, including hereditary spherocytosis (HS) and glucose-6-phosphate dehydrogenase (G6PD) deficiency. In the later sections specific enzyme assays are described and the measurement of 2,3DPG and reduced glutathione (GSH).

Osmotic fragility

Principle. The method to be described is based upon that of Parpart and co-workers.[35] Hypotonic saline buffered to pH 7.4 is used and the blood is added to the hypotonic solutions in the proportion of 1 to 100. The test is carred out at room temperature (15–25°C) and lysis is read photoelectrically.

Reagents

Prepare a stock solution of buffered sodium chloride (A.R.), osmotically equivalent to 100 g/l (1.71 mol/l) NaCl, as follows: dissolve NaCl, 90 g; Na_2NPO_4, 13.65 g* and $NaH_2PO_4 . 2H_2O$, 2.43 g in water and adjust the final volume to 1 l. This solution will keep for months without deterioration in a well stoppered bottle. In preparing hypotonic solutions for use it is convenient to make first a 10 g/l solution from the 100 g/l NaCl stock solution by dilution with water. Dilutions equivalent to 9.0, 7.5, 6.5, 6.0, 5.5, 5.0, 4.0, 3.5, 3.0, 2.0 and 1.0 g/l are convenient concentrations. Intermediate concentrations such as 4.75 and 5.25 g/l are useful in critical work and an additional 12.0 g/l dilution should be used for incubated samples.

It is convenient to make up 50 ml of each dilution. The solutions keep well at 4°C for some weeks but they should be discarded if moulds develop.

* or $Na_2HPO_2 . 2H_2O$, 17.115 g.

Method

Heparinized venous blood or defibrinated blood may be used: oxalated or citrated blood should be avoided because of the additional salts added to the blood. The test should be carried out within 2 h of collection but can be delayed for up to 6 h if the blood is kept at 4°C.

Add 50 μl volumes of the blood to be tested to 5 ml volumes of the range of hypotonic solutions and immediately mix by inverting several times. Allow the tubes to stand at room temperature for 30 min, then remix and centrifuge for 5 min at 1200–1500 **g**. Then compare the amount of lysis in each tube with that in the 100% lysis tube (1.0 g/l NaCl) using a photoelectric colorimeter with a yellow-green (e.g. Ilford 625) filter or a spectrophotometer at a wavelength setting of 540 nm. Use the supernatant from the 9.0 g/l NaCl tube as the blank or that from a 12 g/l NaCl tube if there is lysis in 9.0 g/l NaCl. Usually the supernatants can be poured by decantation into the colorimeter cell and with a good colorimeter as little as 1% lysis can be estimated. The concentration of Hb in the complete lysis tube should be such that the reading on the colorimeter scale does not exceed an absorbance of 0.5. If necessary, the supernatants may be diluted with an equal volume of 1.0g/l NaCl, or the blood to saline dilution may be made 1 to 200 at the start of the test.

Osmotic fragility after incubation at 37°C for 24 hours

Method

Defibrinated blood should be used, care being taken to ensure that sterlity is maintained. Incubate 1 ml or 2 ml volumes of blood in sterile 5 ml screw-capped bottles.

(It is useful to set up the samples in duplicate so that in the rare event of one bottle being infected, as shown by the Hb being markedly reduced, the whole experiment need not be spoiled.)

After 24 h, pool the contents of the duplicate bottles after thoroughly mixing the sedimented red cells in the overlying serum and estimate the fragility as previously described. As the fragility may be found to be markedly increased, set up additional hypotonic solutions containing 7.0 g/l and 8.0 g/l NaCl as well as a tube containing 9.0 g/l NaCl. In addition, use a solution equivalent to 12.0 g/l NaCl for sometimes, as in hereditary spherocytosis (HS), lysis may take place in 9.0 g/l NaCl: in this case use the supernatant of the tube containing 12.0 g/l NaCl as the blank in the colorimetric estimation.

The incubation fragility test is conveniently combined with the estimation of the amount of spontaneous autohaemolysis (see later).

Factors affecting osmotic-fragility tests

In carrying out osmotic-fragility tests by any method three variables capable of markedly affecting the results must be controlled, quite apart from the accuracy with which the saline solutions have been made up. These are:

1. The relative volumes of blood and saline.
2. The final pH of the blood in saline suspension.
3. The temperature at which the tests are carried out.

A proportion of 1 volume of blood to 100 or 200 volumes of saline is convenient because not only can the resultant haemolysis be read off directly in most colorimeters without further dilution but the concentration of blood is so small that the added plasma hardly affects the osmotic effect of the saline. When weak suspensions of blood in saline are used it is necessary to control the pH of the hypotonic solutions and it is for this reason that phosphate buffer is added to the saline in the present method. Even so, small differences will be found between the fragility of strictly venous blood and maximally aerated blood. For the most accurate results it is recommended that the blood should be mixed until bright red. Finally, for really accurate work the estimations should always be carried out at the same temperature, though for most purposes room temperature is sufficiently constant.

The extent of the effect of pH and temperature on osmotic fragility was well illustrated in the paper of Parpart and co-workers.[35] The effect of pH is more important: here a shift of 0.1 of a pH unit is equivalent to altering the saline concentration by 0.1 g/l, the fragility of the red cells being increased by a fall in pH. A rise in temperature decreases the fragility, a rise of 5°C being equivalent to an increase in saline concentration of about 0.1 g/l.

Lysis is virtually complete at the end of 30 min at 20°C and the hypotonic solutions may be centrifuged at the end of this time.

Further details of the factors which affect and control haemolysis of red cells in hypotonic solutions were given by Murphy.[34]

Recording the results of osmotic-fragility tests

Most workers have not been content to record merely the highest concentration of saline at which lysis is just detectable (initial lysis or minimum resistance) and the highest concentration of saline in which lysis appears to be complete (complete lysis or maximum resistance). It is useful also to record the concentration of saline causing 50% lysis, i.e. the median corpuscular fragility (MCF). The normal range of MCF at 20°C and pH 7.4 is 4.0–4.45 g/l (68–81 mmol/l) NaCl in fresh samples, 4.65–5.9 g/l (79–100 mmol/l) after incubation for 24 h.

When a range of hypotonic solutions has been used, a 'fragility curve' may be drawn by plotting the percentage of lysis in each tube against the corresponding concentration of salt solution. In normal subjects an almost symmetrical sigmoid curve results (Fig. 10.1). In disease, however, deviations from the normal type of curve may be found, e.g. curves with long tails due to a small proportion of very fragile cells.

Two other simple methods of recording the results quantitatively are available: the data may be plotted on probability paper or increment-haemolysis curves can be drawn (see below). Both methods emphasize heterogeneity of the cell population with respect to osmotic fragility. If the observed amounts of lysis of normal blood are plotted on the probability scale against concentrations of saline, an almost straight line can be drawn through the points, there being skewness only where lysis is becoming almost complete. This method enables the MCF to be read off with ease.

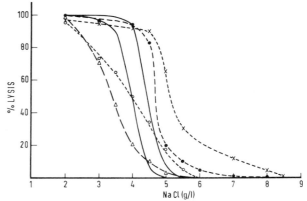

Fig. 10.1 Osmotic-fragility curves. Osmotic-fragility curves of patients suffering from: (a) sickle cell anaemia △-------△, (b) β-thalassaemia major ○-------○, (c) hereditary spherocytosis ●-------●, (d) 'idiopathic' warm auto-immune haemolytic anaemia X-------X. The normal range is indicated by the unbroken lines.

In disease, tailed curves result in varying degrees of skewness at the other end of the probability plot as well. In order to obtain increment-haemolysis curves, the differences in lysis between adjacent tubes are plotted against the corresponding saline concentrations. Definitely bimodal curves may be obtained during recovery from a haemolytic episode.[40]

Methods have been developed for measuring osmotic fragility by automatic procedures. The Fragiligraph* is an instrument in which red cells, diluted in isotonic NaCl solution are placed in a mirocuvette, two walls of which are made of dialysing membrane and surrounded by water.[17] The cells lyse as the salt concentration of the medium decreases and the degree of lysis is recorded automatically in the form of a fragility curve. This curve is not exactly the same as that derived by the traditional method, as it is a reflection of the effects of both hypotonicity and time of exposure. A method suitable for an AutoAnalyser has also been described.[22]

Significance of osmotic-fragility tests

The osmotic fragility of freshly taken red cells reflects their ability to take up water without lysis. This is determined by their volume to surface area

* Kalmedic Instruments Inc., 969 Park Avenue, New York 10028.

ratio. The ability of the normal red cell to withstand hypotonicity results from its biconcave shape which allows the cell to increase its volume by about 70% before the surface membrane is stretched: once this limit is reached lysis occurs.[27] Spherocytes have an increased volume to surface area ratio; their ability to take in water before stretching the surface membrane is thus more limited than normal and they are therefore particularly susceptible to osmotic lysis. The increase in osmotic fragility is a property of the spheroidal shape of the cell and is independent of the cause of the spherocytosis. Characteristically, osmotic fragility curves from patients with HS who have not been splenectomized show a 'tail' of very fragile cells. (Figs. 10.1 and 10.2). When plotted on probability paper the graph indicates two populations of cells, the very fragile and the normal or slightly fragile. After splenectomy the red cells are more homogeneous, the osmotic-fragility curve indicating a more continuous spectrum of cells, from fragile to normal.

Decreased osmotic fragility indicates the presence of unusually flattened red cells (leptocytes) in which the volume to surface area ratio is decreased. Such a change occurs in iron-deficiency anaemia and thalassaemia in which the red cells with a low MCH and MCV are unusually resistant to osmotic lysis (Fig. 10.1). Reticulocytes and red cells from splenectomized patients also tend to have a greater amount of membrane compared with normal cells and are osmotically resistant. In liver disease target cells may be produced by passive accumulation of lipid[15] and these cells, too, are resistant to osmotic lysis.

The osmotic fragility of red cells after incubation for 24 h at 37°C is also a reflection of their volume to surface area ratio but the factors which alter this ratio are more complicated than in fresh red cells. The increased osmotic fragility of normal red cells which occurs after incubation (Fig. 10.2) is mainly caused by swelling of the cells associated with an accumulation of sodium which exceeds loss of potassium. Such cation exchange is determined by the membrane properties of the red cell which control the passive flux of ions and the metabolic competence of the cell which determines the active pumping of cations against concentration gradients. During incubation for 24 h the metabolism of the red cell becomes stressed and the pumping

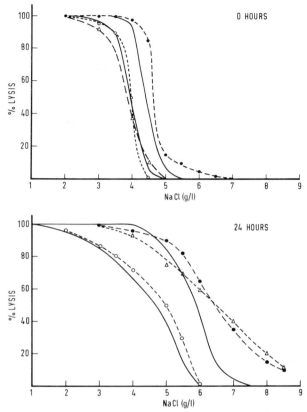

Fig. 10.2 Osmotic-fragility curves before and after incubating blood at 37°C for 24 hours. From patients suffering from: (a) hereditary spherocytosis ●-------●, (b) pyruvate-kinase deficiency △-------△ and (c) hereditary non-spherocytic haemolytic anaemia of undiagnosed type ○-------○. The normal range is indicated by the unbroken lines.

mechanisms tend to fail, one factor being a relative lack of glucose in the medium.

The osmotic fragility of red cells which have an abnormal membrane, such as those of HS and hereditary elliptocytosis (HE) increases abnormally after incubation (Fig. 10.2). The results with red cells with a glycolytic deficiency, such as those of pyruvate kinase (PK) deficiency, are variable. In severe deficiencies, osmotic fragility may increase substantially (Fig. 10.2) but in other cases the fragility is decreased due to a greater loss of potassium than gain of sodium. In thalassaemia major and minor, osmotic fragility is frequently markedly reduced after incubation, again due to a marked loss of potassium.[24] A similar, though usually less marked, change is seen in iron-deficiency anaemia.

Osmotic-fragility tests are therefore a useful indication of an abnormality of the red cell but the results, if abnormal, are not diagnostic of a specific disorder.

GLYCEROL LYSIS-TIME TESTS

The osmotic-fragility test is somewhat cumbersome and requires 2 ml or more of whole blood. It is thus not suitable for use in newborn babies nor as a population screening test. In 1974 Gottfried and Robertson introduced a glycerol lysis-time (GLT) test, a one-tube test, to measure the time taken for 50% haemolysis of a blood sample in a buffered hypotonic saline-glycerol mixture.[21] The original method had greater sensitivity in the osmotic resistant range but could also identify most patients with HS by a shorter GLT_{50}. Better identification of HS blood from normal was obtained by 24 h incubation of samples and by modifying the glycerol reagent.[20] Zanella and colleagues modified the original test further by decreasing the pH.[45] There is some loss of specificity for HS with the acidified compared with the original method but in practice this loss is unimportant.

Acidified glycerol lysis-time test[45]

Reagents

Phosphate buffered saline (PBS). Add 9 volumes of 9.0 g/l (154 mmol/l) NaCl to 1 volume of 100 mmol/l phosphate buffer (2 volumes of Na_2HPO_4, 14.9 g/l added to 1 volume of KH_2PO_4, 13.61 g/l). Adjust the pH to 6.85 ± 0.05 at room temperature (15–25°C). This adjustment must be accurate.

Glycerol reagent (300 mmol/l). Add 23 ml of glycerol (27.65 g A.R. grade) to 300 ml of PBS and bring the final volume of 1 l with water.

Method

Add 20 μl of whole blood, anticoagulated with EDTA, to 5.0 ml of PBS, pH 6.85. Mix the suspension carefully. Transfer 1.0 ml to a standard 4 ml cuvette of a spectrophotometer equipped with a linear-logarithmic recorder. Fix the wavelength at 625 nm and start the recorder. Add 2.0 ml of the glycerol reagent rapidly to the cuvette with a 2.0 ml syringe pipette. The rate of haemolysis is measured by the rate of fall of turbidity of the reaction mixture. The results are expressed as the time required for the optical density to fall to half the initial value ($AGLT_{50}$). The test can also be carried out using a colorimeter and stopwatch.

Results

Normal blood takes more than 1800 s (30 min) to reach the $AGLT_{50}$. The time taken is similar for blood from normal adults, newborn infants and cord samples. In patients with HS the range of the $AGLT_{50}$ is 25–150 s. A short $AGLT_{50}$ may also be found in chronic renal failure, chronic leukaemias, auto-immune haemolytic anaemia and in some pregnant women.

Significance of the AGLT

The glycerol in the hypotonic PBS slows the rate of entry of water molecules into the red cells so that the time taken for lysis may be conveniently measured. The same principles apply as with the osmotic-fragility test. Cells with a high volume to surface area ratio resist swelling for a shorter time than normal cells. This applies to all spherocytes, whether the spherocytosis is caused by HS or other mechanisms. The test is particularly useful in screening family members of patients with HS where morphological changes are too small to indicate clearly whether the disorder is present or not.

Autohaemolysis (spontaneous haemolysis developing in blood incubated at 37°C for 48 hours)

Method

Use sterile defibrinated blood and deliver four 1 ml or 2 ml samples into sterile 5 ml screw-capped bottles. Add to two of the bottles 50 or 100 μl of sterile 100 g/l glucose solution so as to provide a concentration of glucose in the blood of at least 30 mmol/l. Place the series of bottles in the incubator at 37°C. After 24 h invert the bottles gently six times to mix the contents.

After incubating for 48 h pool the contents of each pair of bottles. Remove a sample for the estimation of the PCV and centrifuge the remainder to obtain the supernatant serum.

Estimate the spontaneous lysis by means of a colorimeter or in a spectrophotometer at 625 nm. As a rule it is convenient to make a 1 in 10 dilution of the incubated serum in cyanide-ferricyanide (Drabkin's) solution, unless there is marked haemolysis when a 1 in 25 or 1 in 50 dilution is more suitable. A corresponding dilution of the pre-incubation serum is used as a blank and a 1 in 100 or 1 in 200 dilution of the whole blood in Drabkin's solution indicates the total amount of Hb present and serves as a standard.

Calculate the percentage lysis, allowing for the change in PCV resulting from the incubation as follows:[39]

$$\text{Lysis (\%)} = \frac{R_t}{R_o} \times \frac{D_o}{D_t} \times (1 - \text{PCV}_t) \times 100,$$

where, R_o = reading in colorimeter of diluted whole blood; R_t = reading in colorimeter of diluted serum at 48 h; PCV_t = packed cell volume at time T; D_o = dilution of whole blood (e.g. 1 in 200 = 0.005), and D_t = dilution of serum (e.g. 1 in 10 = 0.1).

The reading at time T is multiplied by $(1 - \text{PCV}_t)$ so as to give the concentration which would be found if the liberated haemoglobin was dissolved in whole blood, i.e. in both plasma and red-cell compartments, not in the plasma compartment alone.

Normal range of autohaemolysis[23]

Lysis at 48 h. Without added glucose 0.2–2.0%; with added glucose 0–0.9%.

The results obtained are sensitive to slight differences in technique and each laboratory should use a carefully standardized procedure and establish its own normal range. It is more accurate (although more time consuming) to measure lysis by a chemical method rather than by a direct photometric method, particularly if the amount of liberated haemoglobin is small.[23]

Significance of increased autohaemolysis

Little or no lysis takes place when normal blood is incubated for 24 h under sterile conditions and the amount present after 48 h is small.[39] If glucose is added so that it is present throughout the incubation the development of lysis is markedly slowed. The amount of autohaemolysis which occurs after 48 h with and without glucose is determined by the properties of the membrane and the metabolic competence of the red cell. In membrane disorders such as HS the rate of glucose consumption is increased to compensate for an increased cation leak through the membrane.[16] During the 48 h incubation glucose is therefore used up relatively rapidly so that energy production fails more quickly than normal unless glucose is added. This is one factor which contributes to the increased rate of autohaemolysis in HS. Usually, but not always, the addition of glucose to the blood decreases the rate of autohaemolysis in HS in about the same proportion as with normal blood (Fig. 10.3). This was referred to as Type-1 autohaemolysis.[39] When the utilization of glucose via the glycolytic pathway is impaired, as in PK deficiency, the rate of autohaemolysis at 48 h is usually increased and glucose fails to correct or may even aggravate lysis (Type-2 autohaemolysis, Fig. 10.4). A similar result may be seen in severe HS (Type B), but in the absence of spherocytosis failure of glucose to diminish autohaemolysis is a strong indication of a glycolytic block. Blood from patients with G6PD deficiency or other disorders of the pentose phosphate pathway may undergo a slight increase in autohaemolysis (without additional glucose) which is corrected by the addition of glucose. Commonly the result is normal but examination of the incubated blood may show an increase in methaemoglobin (Hi) (see below). Not all glycolytic enzyme deficiencies give a Type-II reaction so that a Type-I result does not exclude the possibility of such a defect.

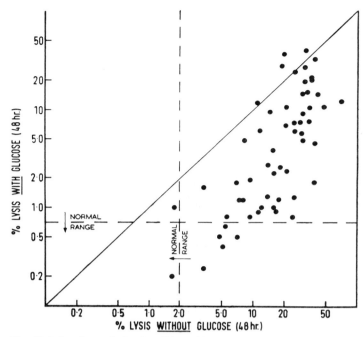

Fig. 10.3 Autohaemolysis after 48 hours' incubation at 37°C of sterile defibrinated blood derived from 57 patients suffering from hereditary spherocytosis, with and without the addition of glucose. Points lying near or on the diagonal line indicate that glucose had little or no effect on the rate of haemolysis (a Type-B result). (Reproduced from *The Hereditary Haemolytic Anaemias* by J. V. Dacie, Davidson Lecture, 1967. Publication No. 34 of the Royal College of Physicians of Edinburgh.)

In the acquired haemolytic anaemias the results of the autohaemolysis tests are variable and generally not very helpful in diagnosis. In the autoimmune haemolytic anaemias lysis may be increased in the absence of additional glucose but the effect of added glucose is unpredictable. In paroxysmal nocturnal haemoglobinuria (PNH) the autohaemolysis of aerated defibrinated blood is usually normal.

Autohaemolysis may be increased in haemolytic anaemias caused by oxidant drugs or when there are defects in the reducing power of the red cell. Heinz bodies and/or Hi will be detectable at the end of incubation. Normally red cells produce less than 4% Hi after 48 h incubation and Heinz bodies are not seen. Red cells containing an unstable haemoglobin also contain Heinz bodies at the end of the incubation period and increased amounts of Hi.

The nucleosides adenosine, guanosine and inosine, like glucose, diminish the rate of auto-haemolysis when added to blood. Remarkably, adenosine triphosphate (ATP) strikingly retards haemolysis in PK deficiency, although glucose itself is ineffective.[18] ATP does not pass the red-cell membrane.

The autohaemolysis test lacks specificity. This has drawn much criticism upon the test, including the suggestion that it has no place in the screening of blood for inherited defects.[7] The best way to detect metabolic defects in red cells is undoubtedly to measure glucose consumption, lactate production and the contribution to metabolism of the pentose phosphate pathway. These measurements are, unfortunatly, difficult and are likely to be undertaken only by specialized laboratories. The autohaemolysis test does provide some information about the metabolic competence of the red cells and helps to distinguish membrane defects from enzyme defects if the results of the tests are taken together with other observations such as morphology, inheritance and presence or absence of associ-

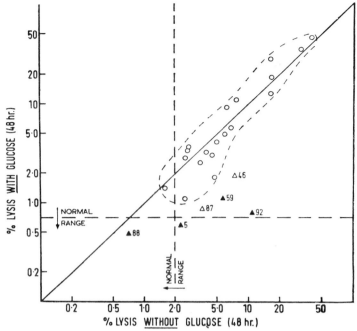

Fig. 10.4 Autohaemolysis after 48 hours' incubation at 37°C of sterile defibrinated blood derived from 19 patients suffering from pyruvate-kinase deficiency with and without the addition of glucose (hollow circles). Data from six other patients suffering from other types of hereditary non-spherocytic haemolytic anaemia have been added for comparison. Points lying near or on the diagonal line indicate that glucose had little or no effect on haemolysis. (For reference see Fig. 10.3).

ated clinical disorders. The autohaemolysis test will undoubtedly be abandoned as soon as a more suitable screening test becomes available.

DETECTION OF ENZYME DEFICIENCIES IN HEREDITARY HAEMOLYTIC ANAEMIAS

It should be possible for most haematological laboratories to identify the commoner enzyme deficiencies, i.e. of G6PD and PK and to indicate where the probable defect lies in the rarer disorders. Detailed investigation of the aberrant enzymes and of the metabolism of the abnormal cells is probably best done in specialized laboratories. Comprehensive accounts of methods available for studying red-cell metabolism are to be found in *Biochemical Methods in Red Cell Genetics* by Yunis (1969),[44] *Red Cell Metabolism, a Manual of Biochemical Methods*,

2nd edition by Beutler (1975)[6] and the ICSH recommendations.[10]

There are two stages in the diagnosis of red-cell enzyme defects: first, screening procedures and, secondly, specific enzyme assays. The simple non-specific screening procedures such as the osmotic-fragility and autohaemolysis tests, which have already been described, may indicate the presence of a metabolic disorder and simple biochemical tests are available to show whether the disorder is in the pentose phosphate or the Emden-Meyerhof pathways; these intermediate stages of glycolysis are illustrated in Fig. 10.5.

SCREENING TESTS FOR G6PD DEFICIENCY AND OTHER DEFECTS OF THE PENTOSE PHOSPHATE PATHWAY

Many variants of the red-cell enzyme, G6PD, have been detected and the methods used to identify

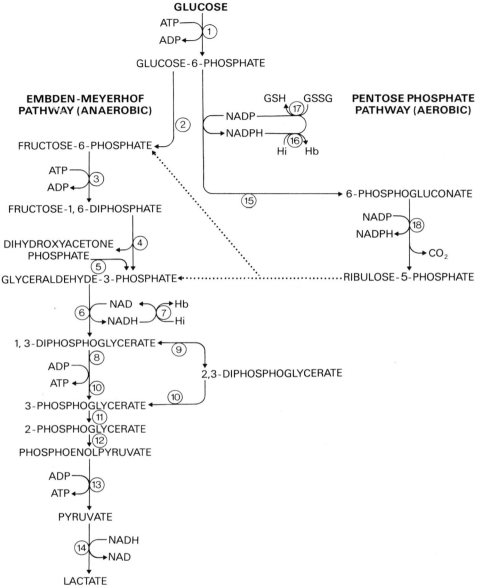

Fig. 10.5 Schematic representation of red-cell glycolytic pathways. The enzymes are indicated as follows:
(1) Hexokinase; (2) Glucosephosphate isomerase; (3) Phosphofructokinase; (4) Aldolase; (5) Triose phosphate isomerase; (8) Phosphoglycerate kinase; (9) Diphosphoglyceromutase; (10) Diphosphoglycerate phosphatase; (11) Phosphoglyceromutase; (12) Enolase; (13) Pyruvate kinase; (14) Lactate dehydrogenase; (15) Glucose-6-phosphate dehydrogenase; (16) NADPH-methemoglobin reductase; (17) Glutathione reductase; (18) 6-Phosphogluconate dehydrogenase. For explanation of abbreviations, see p. 176.

variants have been standardized.[43] Inheritance is sex-linked as the enzyme is controlled by one gene locus in the X chromosome. Variants which have deficient activity produce one of several types of clinical disorder. The two most common variants are the Mediterranean type which has very low activity and which may lead to favism, i.e. acute intravascular haemolysis following the ingestion of broad beans, and the A− type found in black populations in West Africa and the USA which leads to primaquine sensitivity. Both groups are susceptible to haemolysis produced by oxidant drugs and infections.

Much less frequently a chronic, non-spherocytic haemolytic anaemia is produced by rare variants of the enzyme. Severe neonatal jaundice with anaemia occurs in about 5% of patients who have major deficiencies of enzyme activity.

G6PD deficiency in hemizygous (male) or homozygous (female) individuals may be readily detected by screening tests but it is more difficult to detect heterozygous (female) carriers. Other defects of the pentose phosphate pathway (see p. 160) also lead to deficiency in the reducing power of the red cell. The clinical syndromes associated with these defects include intravascular haemolysis, with or without methaemoglobinaemia, in response to oxidative drugs.

G6PD catalyses the oxidation of glucose-6-phosphate (G6P) to 6-phosphogluconate (6PG) with the simultaneous reduction of nicotine-adenine dinucleotide phosphate ($NADP^+$) to reduced NADP (NADPH):

$$G6P + NADP^+ \underset{G6PD}{\rightleftharpoons} 6PG + NADPH.$$

In a second, linked, oxidative reaction 6PG is converted to ribulose-5-phosphate (Ru5P) and CO_2 with the linked reduction of a further molecule of $NADP^+$ to NADPH. The reaction is catalysed by 6PG dehydrogenase (6PGD):

$$6PG + NADP^+ \underset{G6PD}{\longrightarrow} Ru5P + CO_2 + NADPH.$$

The release of CO_2 drives the reaction to the right so that in practice the pathway is not reversible.

NADPH is an important reducing compound for the conversion of oxidized glutathione (GSSG) to glutathione (GSH) (see Fig. 10.5) and, under conditions of stress, the reconversion of Hi to Hb. Screening tests for G6PD deficiency depend upon the inability of cells from deficient subjects to convert an oxidized substrate to a reduced state. The substrates used may be the natural one of the enzyme, $NADP^+$, or other naturally occurring substrates linked by secondary reactions to the enzyme, for example GSSG or Hi or artificial dyes.

Which screening test is used in any particular laboratory will depend upon a number of factors such as cost, time required, temperature and humidity and availability of reagents. Two specific tests are described here.

Fluorescent screening test for G6PD deficiency

The method is that of Beutler and Mitchell,[8] modified on the recommendation of the ICSH.[11]

Principle. NADPH, generated in blood in the presence of G6PD, fluoresces under long-wave UV light.

Reagents

D-*Glucose-6-phosphate*, 10 mmol/l. Dissolve 305 mg of the disodium salt, or an equivalent amount of the potassium salt, in 100 ml of water.

$NADP^+$, 7.5 mmol/l. Dissolve 60 mg of $NADP^+$, disodium salt, in 10 ml of water.

Saponin. 750 mmol/l (10 g/l).

Tris-HCl buffer. pH 7.8 (see p. 436).

Oxidized glutathione (GSSG), 8 mmol/l. Dissolve 49 mg of GSSG in 10 ml of water.

Mix the reagents in the following proportion: 2 volumes of G6P; 1 volume of $NADP^+$; 2 volumes of saponin; 3 volumes of buffer; 1 volume of GSSG; 2 volumes of water. The combined reagent is stable at $-20°C$ for 2 or more years and for 2 months at least if kept at 4°C. Azide may be added to prevent growth by contaminants without loss of activity. 100 μl volumes of the reagent may be placed in appropriate small tubes and kept at $-20°C$ ready for use.

Method

Add 10 μl of whole blood, either anticoagulated (EDTA or heparin) or added before clotting to 100 μl of the reagent mixture and keep at room temperature (15–25°C). Deliver *c* 10 μl of the blood in the reaction mixture on to a Whatman No. 1 filter paper at the beginning of the reaction and after 5–10 min. A shorter interval may be appropriate at a high ambient temperature (*c* 25–30°C). Examine the spots under UV light. Set up control samples of normal blood and known G6PD-deficient blood at the same time.

If the samples are to be collected away from the laboratory, place about 10 μl of blood on Whatman No. 1 filter paper and allow it to dry. Cut out the disc of dried blood in the laboratory and add it to the reaction mixture.

The activity of the enzyme in anticoagulated (ACD) blood is stable for about 21 days at 4°C and about 5 days at 25°C.

Interpretation

Fluorescence is produced by NADPH formed from NADP$^+$ in the presence of G6PD. Some of the NADPH produced is oxidized by GSSG, but this reaction, catalyzed by glutathione reductase, is normally slower than the rate of NADPH production. Red cells with less than 20% of normal G6PD activity do not cause fluorescence.

The method is most useful for screening large numbers of individuals but many heterozygotes will be missed. False-positive results (inappropriate fluorescence) may occur if subjects with G6PD Type A− are examined shortly after a haemolytic crisis when the reticulocyte count is high. This problem may be overcome by examining the enzyme activity of the lowest layer of cells after centrifugation, i.e. of blood freed as far as possible of reticulocytes.

Methaemoglobin reduction test

The method was developed by Brewer et al in 1962.[13]

Reagents

Sodium nitrite. 180 mmol/l.
Dextrose, 280 mmol/l. Dissolve 5 g of A.R. dextrose and 1.25 g of NaNO$_2$ in 100 ml of water.
Methylene blue, 0.4 mmol/l. Dissolve 150 mg of methylthionine chloride (methylene blue chloride, Sigma) in 1 l of water.
Nile blue sulphate. 22 mg in 100 ml of water. This may be used as an alternative to methylene blue. It is the better reagent if the

test is to be combined with the Hi elution test (see p. 164).

The reagents may be used in a variety of ways to suit the convenience of the laboratory. A batch of tubes may be prepared in advance of use by mixing equal volumes of the reagents (sodium nitrite with methylene blue or Nile blue sulphate) and pipetting 0.2 ml of the combined reagent into individual glass tubes. Glass tubes must be used because plastic may adsorb some reagents. The contents of the tubes are allowed to evaporate to dryness at room temperature (15–25°C) or in an oven at a temperature not exceeding 37°C. The tubes must then be tightly stoppered. The reagent will keep for 6 months at room temperature. The reagents may, however, be used fresh, without drying.

Method

Use anticoagulated blood (heparin or ACD) and test the samples preferably within 1 h of collection. With blood from severely anaemic patients adjust the PCV to 0.40 ± 0.05. Add 2 ml of blood to the tube containing 0.2 ml of the combined reagent either freshly prepared or dried. Close the tube with a stopper and gently mix the contents by inverting it 15 times. Prepare control tubes by adding 2 ml of blood to a similar tube without reagents (normal reference tube) and to a tube containing 0.1 ml of sodium nitrite-dextrose mixture without methylene blue (positive reference tube). Incubate the samples at 37°C for 3 h.

If multiple samples are to be tested, the incubations should be started serially at 4 min intervals so that each sample can be incubated for exactly 3 h. After the incubation, pipette 0.1 ml volumes from the test sample, the normal reference tube and the positive reference tube into 10 ml of water in separate, clear glass test-tubes of identical diameter. Mix the contents gently. Compare the colours in the different tubes (see below).

Interpretation

Sodium nitrite converts Hb to Hi. When no methylene blue is added methaemoglobin persists, but incubation of the samples with methylene blue allows stimulation of the pentose phosphate pathway in subjects with normal G6PD levels. The Hi is reduced during the incubation period. In G6PD-deficient subjects the block in the pentose phosphate pathway prevents this reduction. Normal samples have a colour similar to that in the normal reference tube—a clear red. Blood from deficient subjects gives a brown colour similar to that in the positive reference tube. Heterozygotes give intermediate reactions.

The advantages of this method include cheapness, ready availability of reagents and independence of equipment apart from a water-bath. The major disadvantage is the time taken to perform the test, and the need to carry out the test within 1 h of collecting the blood samples.

Jacob and Jandl's ascorbate–cyanide screening test[28]

Principle. When sodium cyanide and sodium ascorbate are added to a sample of blood, catalase is inhibited by the cyanide and this allows H_2O_2 to be generated from the coupled oxidation of ascorbate and oxyHb (HbO_2). The H_2O_2 so generated will convert HbO_2 to hemichromes and Hi unless it is reduced by glutathione peroxidase. This reaction requires GSH as the proton donor. In G6PD-deficient cells the supply of GSH is decreased.

Reagents

Ascorbate. Dispense 10 mg of sodium ascorbate and 5 mg of glucose into a number of small tubes. The tubes are stoppered and may be stored indefinitely at $-20°C$.

Sodium Cyanide. Dissolve 500 mg of NaCN in 50 ml of water and add 20 ml of iso-osmotic phosphate buffer, pH 7.4. Neutralize the solution (to pH 7.0) with 2 mol/l HCl* and make up the volume to 100 ml with water. This solution is stable indefinitely at c 20°C.

* This should be carried out in a fume cupboard. To avoid liberation of cyanide gas the pH must not be allowed to fall below 7.0.

Cyanide solutions must never be pipetted using the mouth. To avoid liberation of cyanide gas the pH must not be allowed to fall below 7.0.

Method

Heparinized or EDTA, but not oxalated, whole blood is suitable. First aerate to a bright red colour by inverting the tubes so that blood and air mix. Then add 2 ml to a tube containing ascorbate and glucose and add 2 drops of cyanide solution. Incubate the mixture without a stopper in a water-bath at 37°C, and shake occasionally. Mix the suspension thoroughly after 2 h and again at 3–4 h, noting its colour on each occasion. The change in colour is not very great and the detection of the end-point of the test requires experience. The change is best appreciated by gently shaking the tubes and observing the colour of the film of blood on the side of the tubes. Normal blood remains red. Blood deficient in reducing power takes on a brownish hue.

As controls, samples of normal blood and known G6PD-deficient blood should be set up in parallel with the test sample(s).

Results

As already mentioned, the test is not specific for G6PD deficiency. However, G6PD-deficient blood becomes brown within 1–2 h while normal blood darkens slowly over several hours. Heterozygotes with intermediate levels of G6PD activity may (or may not) become brown within 2 h.

Positive reactions are found in GSH deficiency, glutathione reductase (GR) deficency and glutathione peroxidase (GPx) deficiency False positive results in newborn infants may be due to their relative deficiency of GPx.[30]

DETECTION OF G6PD HETEROZYGOTES

Females heterozygous for G6PD deficiency have two populations of cells, one with normal G6PD activity and the other deficient. This is the result of random suppression of one or other X chromosome in individual embryonic cells early in the development of the embryo. Cells which subsequently develop from each of these cells will have the characteristics of only the active X chromosome.[31] The total activity of G6PD in the blood depends upon the proportion of active and deficient cells and may vary from 20 to 80% of the normal. Screening tests fail to identify most heterozygotes. The deficient cells may, however, be identified in blood films by a cytochemical test (p. 113) and by an elution procedure based on the methaemoglobin reduction test.[19]

Methaemoglobin elution test for G6PD heterozygotes

Principle. HbO_2 cannot be eluted from red cells in the presence of H_2O_2 and cyanide because it retains peroxidatic activity. Hi is converted to HiCN by cyanide and this has no peroxidatic activity. This property has been adapted in a differential staining technique which will stain individual cells retaining HbO_2 in the methaemoglobin reduction test but will show Hi-containing cells as ghosts.[19]

Reagents

Potassium cyanide, 400 mmol/l. Dissolve 260 mg of KCN in 10 ml of water. Under no circumstances should this solution be pipetted by mouth.

Elution fluid. Mix 80 ml of ethanol (96% v/v), 16 ml of 200 mmol/l citric acid (3.84 g in 100 ml water) and 5 ml of H_2O_2 (30% v/v). The solution is only active for 1 day.

Staining fluid. Haematoxylin, 7.5 g/l in 96% (v/v) ethanol.

Counter stain. Aqueous erythrosin, 1 g/l or aqueous eosin, 20 g/l.

Method

Use the incubated samples from the reduction test (see above). For preference use samples incubated with Nile blue sulphate rather than methylene blue and oxygenate the samples during incubation, either by bubbling 95% O_2–5% CO_2 mixtures through them continuously or, equally adequately, by blowing expired air gently through the samples with a pipette from time to time. Add 20 μl of KCN solution to 1 ml of blood and mix gently. Make blood films on clean, dry glass slides. Dry the films quickly in air. Immerse the slides in the elution fluid and agitate them up and down for 1 min. Allow them to stand for a further 2 min. Wash the slides first in methanol and then in water for 30 s each. Stain the films for 2 min with haematoxylin, rinse in tap water, then restain with the erythrosin counterstain for 2 min. Rinse the slides in tap water and allow to dry in the air. Examine the films under the microscope and count the proportion of stained cells (normal) to ghosts (Hi cells).

Interpretation and comments

In females heterozygous for G6PD deficiency the proportion of G6PD-deficient (ghost) cells varies from case to case: while usually 40–60% of the cells are deficient, the proportion may be much less, and in extreme cases only about 7% are deficient. Apparently normal subjects may, in a few instances, have a small residue of Hi-containing cells after the Hi reduction test, but this rarely exceeds 5% of cells. Nearly all heterozygotes can be reliably detected if Nile blue sulphate is used and there is good oxygenation of the samples in the initial incubation. Nile blue sulphate increases the sensitivity of the test because the reduced form of the dye, which is produced in any normal cells that are present, diffuses less readily out of these cells than reduced methylene blue. There is, thus, less likely to be artefactual reduction of Hi in G6PD-deficient cells from inward diffusion of an extrinsic reducing compound. The test is fairly cumbersome but is useful for family studies.

RED-CELL ENZYME ASSAYS

The number of red-cell enzyme deficiencies which are known to cause haemolytic anaemia increases steadily. In practice, this means that, unless the deficiency is one of the common variants, like

G6PD or pyruvate kinase (PK) deficiency, multiple enzyme assays are needed to identify the defect. The methods for assaying each enzyme are almost as numerous as the variants themselves and for this reason the *International Committee for Standardization in Haematology* has produced simplified methods suitable for diagnostic purposes.[10] These methods are not necessarily the most appropriate for detailed study of the kinetic properties of enzymes but they are relatively simple to set up and should allow comparison of results between different laboratories.

General points of technique

Collection of blood samples

Blood samples may be anticoagulated with heparin (10 iu/ml blood), EDTA (1 mg/ml blood) or acid-citrate-dextrose (for formulae and volumes see p. 432). In any of these anti-coagulants all enzymes are stable for 6 days at 4°C and 24 h at 25°C, and with the exceptions of triose phosphate isomerase (TPI) and phosphofructokinase (PFK), enzyme activity is stable for 5 days at 25°C. Samples of blood should be transferred to central laboratories in tubes surrounded by wet ice (4°C). Frozen samples are unsuitable because the cells are lysed by freezing. Further details of enzyme stability are given by Beutler.[6] Approximately 1 ml of blood is required for each enzyme assay.

Separation of red cells from blood samples

White cells and platelets generally have higher enzyme activities than red cells. The activity of the enzyme in these cells may not be affected when it is deficient in red cells, for example in PK deficiency. It is, therefore, necessary to prepare red cells as free from contamination as possible. Various methods are suitable (ICSH)[10]; two are described below.

Washing of red cells

Centrifuge the anticoagulated blood at 1200–1500 *g* for 5 min and remove the plasma together with the buffy coat layer. Resuspend the cells in 9 g/l NaCl (saline) and repeat the procedure three times. This will remove about 80–90% of the white cells. In PK assays the remaining white cells may be sufficient to give misleading results, but this simple method is adequate in most instances when more complicated manoeuvres are impracticable.

Filtration through microcrystalline-cellulose mixtures

Preparation of column. Mix thoroughly together in ice-cold saline equal parts by weight of microcrystalline cellulose (Sigma Cell Co., mean size 50 μm) and α-cellulose (Sigma Chemical Co.) just before use. The slurry produced should be just thin enough to pour easily. Pour 4–5 ml of the slurry into a 5 ml plastic syringe clamped in the vertical position. Place a pea-sized piece of cotton wool over the outlet of the syringe. When the slurry has settled there should be a bed of the microcrystalline cellulose-α-cellulose mixture about 1.5 ml deep. The column should be made freshly for each batch of enzyme assays and used promptly.

Addition of blood. Add the washed cells to the column up to 2 ml at a time and wash the red cells through with c 1 ml of saline for each 1 ml of blood. At the end of this filtration pass a further 7 ml of saline through the column with gentle stirring. By this method about 99% of the white cells and about 90% of the platelets are removed. About 97% of the red cells are recovered and reticulocytes are not removed selectively. Wash the cells collected from the column twice in 10 volumes of ice-cold saline and finally resuspend them in the saline to give a c 50% suspension. Determine the red-cell count and PCV in a sample of the suspension.

The 2 ml column can separate 18 ml of ACD, 15 ml of heparinized or 8 ml of EDTA blood. Defibrinated blood, which does not contain platelets, can also be used.

Preparation of haemolysate

Mix 1 volume of the washed or filtered suspension with 9 volumes of a stabilizing solution. This consists of 2.7 mmol/l EDTA, pH 7.0, and 0.7 mmol/l 2-mercaptoethanol (100 mg of EDTA disodium salt and 5 μl of 2-mercaptoethanol in 100 ml of water); the pH is adjusted to 7.0 with HCl or NaOH.

Prepare the haemolysate by freeze-thawing. Rapid freezing is achieved using a dry-ice acetone bath or methanol which has been cooled to $-20°C$. Thawing is achieved in a water-bath at 25°C. The haemolysate is ready for use without further centrifugation. Dilutions, when necessary, are carried out in the stabilizing solution. The haemolysate should be prepared freshly for each batch of enzyme assays. Most enzymes in haemolysates are stable for 8 h at 4°C. G6PD activity falls off rather more rapidly.

Control samples. Control samples should always be assayed at the same time as the test samples even when a normal range for the various enzymes has been established. Take the control samples of blood at the same time as the test samples and treat them in the same way. Where possible, choose control samples with a similar reticulocyte count as the test blood. Alternatively, establish ranges of enzyme activity for blood samples with a high reticulocyte count and run a normal control each time.

Reaction buffer

The ICSH recommendation is for a tris-HCl/EDTA buffer which is appropriate for all the common enzymes assays. The buffer consists of 1 mmol/l tris-HCl and 5 mmol/l Na$_2$EDTA, the pH being adjusted to 8.0 with HCl.

Dissolve 15.75 g of tris-HCl and 186 mg of Na$_2$EDTA in water, adjust the pH to 8.0 with 1 mol/l HCl and bring the volume to 100 ml at 25°C.

Only two assays will be described in detail—those for G6PD and PK. However, the principles of these assays apply to all other enzyme assays. The assays are carried out in a spectrophotometer at a wavelength of 340 nm unless otherwise indicated. If a filter photometer is used 366 nm is a suitable wavelength. A final reaction mixture of 1.0 ml (or 3.0 ml) is suitable, the quantities given in the text

being for 1.0 ml reaction mixtures unless otherwise stated. All dilutions of auxillary enzymes are made in the stablizing solution and all working materials should be kept in an ice-bath until ready for use. The assays are carried out at a controlled temperature, 37°C being the most appropriate. Cuvettes loaded with the assay reagents should be pre-incubated at this temperature for 10 min before starting the reaction. In most cases the reaction is started by the addition of substrate.

G6PD ASSAY

The reactions involving G6PD have already been described (p. 160). The activity of the enzyme is measured in two steps. The conversion of NADP$^+$ to NADPH in the two reactions catalysed by G6PD and 6PGD is first measured. In a second assay the conversion of 6PG to Ru5P and of NADP$^+$ to NADPH, catalysed by 6PGD, is measured separately. Subtraction of the second assay result from the first overall reaction gives a measure of G6PD activity.

Method

Assay conditions. The assays are carried out at 37°C, the cuvettes containing the first five reagents being incubated for 10 min before starting the reaction by adding the substrates as shown in Table 10.1.

The change in optical density following the addition of the substrate is measured over the first 5 min of the reaction. The value of the blank is subtracted from the test reaction, either automatically if a double beam spectrophotometer is used or by calculation.

Calculation of enzyme activity

The activities of the enzymes in the haemolysate are calculated from the initial rate of change of NADPH accumulation:

G6PD activity in the lysate (in μmol/ml)

$$= \left(\Delta A/\text{min reaction 1} - \Delta A/\text{min reaction 2} \right)$$
$$\times \frac{10^3}{6.22},$$

Table 10.1 G6PD assay

	G6PD + 6PGD Reaction 1	6PG Reaction 2	Blank
Tris HCl EDTA buffer, pH 8.0	100 μl	100 μl	100 μl
MgCl$_2$, 100 mmol/l	100 μl	100 μl	100 μl
NADP, 10 mmol/l	20 μl	20 μl	20 μl
1 in 20 haemolysate	20 μl	20 μl	20 μl
Stabilizing solution	560 μl	660 μl	760 μl
start reaction by adding:			
G6P, 6 mmol/l	100 μl	—	—
6PG, 6 mmol/l	100 μl	100 μl	—

where 6.22 is the mmol extinction coefficient of NADPH at 340 nm (3.30 is the value at 366 nm) and 10^3 is the correction for various dilutions in the reaction mixture. Results are expressed per 10^{10} red cells, per ml red cells or per g Hb by the appropriate calculation from the known values of the washed red-cell suspension. Normal values should be determined for each laboratory.

G6PD is relatively stable and venous blood may be stored in ACD for up to 3 weeks at 4°C without loss of G6PD activity.

Normal values

The normal range for the combined reaction and for G6PD activity alone should be determined for each laboratory. If the ICSH method is used, values should not differ widely from those given by that panel. Results are expressed in enzyme units (eu) which are the μmoles of substrate converted per min at 37°C. These values are 12.1 ± 2.09 eu/g Hb for the combined reaction and 8.34 ± 1.59 eu/g Hb for G6PD when corrected for 6PGD activity.

IDENTIFICATION OF G6PD VARIANTS

There are many variants of G6PD in different populations with enzyme activity ranging from zero to 400–500% of normal activity. Since G6PD cannot be isolated, purified and its amino acid composition identified, classification and delineation of variants depend upon an investigation of their physical and chemical characteristics. Criteria were laid down by a WHO scientific group in 1967 for the minimum requirements for identification of such variants and these recommendations still stand.[43] The tests are carried out on male hemizygotes and are:

Red-cell G6PD activity;
Electrophoretic migration;
Michaelis constant (K_m) for G6P;
Relative rate of utilization of 2-deoxyG6P (2dG6P);
Thermal stability.

Additional tests include:
Determination of pH optima;
K_m for NADP;
Heat of activation;
Response to inhibitors;
Migration on chromatographic media.
The methods for these tests are detailed in the WHO Technical Report.[43]

PYRUVATE KINASE ASSAY

Many variants of PK have been described which have deficient enzyme activity in vivo.[32,33] In most cases deficient activity can be identified by simple enzyme assay. However, PK is a polymeric enzyme, subject to many allosteric controls. In some cases the maximum velocity (V_{max}) of the enzyme is normal or nearly so but at the low substrate concentrations found in vivo some enzyme variants have low activity, either because they have a low affinity for the substrate, phosphoenolpyruvate (PEP) (as measured by a high Michaelis constant, K_m, for PEP) or because they are not activated by important allosteric ligands, e.g. fructose-1,6-diphosphate (F1,6P). Some of these unusual variants can be identified by carrying out the enzyme assay at high, saturating, substrate concentrations and also at low substrate concentrations.[26] Functional PK deficiency can also be identified by finding high concentrations of the substrates immediately above the block in the glycolytic pathway, particularly 2,3DPG. (For measurement of 2,3DPG, see below.)

Method

The preparation of haemolysate, buffer and stabilizing solution are exactly the same as for the G6PD assay. In the PK assay it is particularly important to remove as many contaminating white cells and platelets as possible because these cells are generally unaffected by a deficiency affecting the red cells and contain high activities of PK. The principle of the assay is as follows:

$$PEP + ADP \xrightarrow{PK} pyruvate + ATP.$$

The pyruvate so formed is reduced to lactate in a reaction catalysed by lactate dehydrogenase with the conversion of NADH to NAD^+:

$$pyruvate + NADH \xrightarrow{LDH} lactate + NAD^+.$$

This indicator reaction is ensured by adding LDH to the reaction mixture and the PK activity is measured by the rate of fall of optical density at 340 nm (366 nm in a filter photometer).

The reaction conditions are established in a 1 ml cuvette at 37°C by adding all the reagents except the substrate PEP to the cuvette and incubating them at 37°C for 10 min before starting the reaction by the addition of the PEP. The amount of reagents to be added for low substrate conditions are shown in parenthesis.

Reagents

	Assay	Blank
Buffer: 1 mol/l tris-HCl with 5 mmol/l Na₂EDTA	100 μl	100 μl
KCl: 1 mmol/l	100 μl	100 μl
NADH: 10 mmol/l	20 μl	20 μl
ADP, neutralized: 15 mmol/l (6 mmol/l)	100 μl	—
LDH: 600 u/ml of stabilizing solution (p. 165)	10 μl	10 μl
1 in 20 haemolysate	20 μl	20 μl
Water	450 μl	550 μl
PEP: 50 mmol/l (2.5 mmol/l)	100 μl	100 μl

The change in absorbance (A) is measured over the first 5 min and the activity of the enzyme in μmoles NADH reduced/min/ml haemolysate is calculated as follows:

$$\frac{\Delta A/min}{6.22} \times 10,$$

where 6.22 is the mmol extinction coefficient of NADH at 340 nm (3.30 should be used if the measurements are made at 366 nm). The results can be expressed per 10^{10} red cells, per g Hb or per ml of packed cells, the appropriate value being derived from measurements made on the washed red-cell suspension.

Normal values

As with all enzyme assays, a normal range should be determined for each laboratory. Values should, however, not be widely different between laboratories if the ICSH methods are used. The normal range for PK activity at 37°C is 15.0 ± 1.99 eu/g Hb. At a low substrate (low S) concentration the normal activity is 14.9 ± 2.71% of that at the high substrate concentration.

Estimation of reduced glutathione (GSH)

Principle. The method described[9] is based on the development of a yellow colour when 5,5'-dithiobis (2-nitrobenzoic acid) (Ellman's reagent, DTNB) is added to sulphydryl compounds. The colour which develops is fairly stable for about 10 min and the reaction is little affected by variation in temperature.

The reaction is read at 412 nm. GSH in red cells is relatively stable and venous blood samples anticoagulated with ACD maintain GSH levels for up to 3 weeks at 4°C. GSH is slowly oxidized in solution, so only fresh lysates should be used for the assay.

Reagents

Lysing solution. Disodium EDTA, *1 g/l.*

Precipitating reagent. Metaphosphoric acid (sticks), 1.67 g; disodium EDTA 0.1 g; NaCl 30 g; water to 100 ml. Solution is more rapid if the reagents are added to boiling water and the volume made up after cooling. This solution is stable for at least 3 weeks at 4°C. If any NaCl remains undissolved the clear supernatant should be used.

Disodium hydrogen phosphate. 3 mmol/l: $Na_2HPO_4.12H_2O$, 107.5 g/l, or $Na_2HPO_4.2H_2O$, 53.4 g/l or anhydrous Na_2HPO_4, 42.6 g/l.

DTNB reagent. Dissolve 20 mg of DTNB in 100 ml of buffer, pH 8.0. Sodium citrate, 100 mmol/l (10 g/l) or tris/HCl, are suitable buffers. The solution is stable for up to 3 months at 4°C.

Glutathione standards. When standard curves are constructed, suitable dilutions are made from a 1.62 mmol/l (50 mg/dl) stock solution of GSH. The stock solution should be made freshly with degassed (boiled) water or saline for each run as GSH oxidizes slowly in solution.

Method

Add 0.2 ml of well mixed, anticoagulated blood, of which the PCV, red-cell count and haemoglobin have been determined, to 1.8 ml of lysing solution and allow to stand at room temperature for 5 min for lysis to be completed. Add 3 ml of precipitating solution, mix the solutions well and allow to stand for a further 5 min. After remixing, filter through a single thickness Whatman No. 42 filter paper.

Add 1 ml of clear filtrate to 4 ml of freshly made Na_2HPO_4 solution. Record the absorbance at 412 nm (A_1). Then add 0.5 ml of the DTNB reagent. The colour develops rapidly and remains stable for about 10 min. Read its development at 412 nm in a spectrophotometer or in a photometer with a suitable filter (A_2). A reagent blank is made using saline or plasma instead of whole blood.

Standard curves. If assays are carried out frequently, it is not necessary to construct standard curves for each batch. They are, however, essential initially to calibrate the apparatus used and should be done regularly to check the suitability of the reagents. Suitable dilutions of GSH are achieved by substituting 5, 10, 20 and 40 μl of the 1.62 mmol/l stock solution, made up to 0.2 ml with lysing solution, for the blood in the reaction.

Calculation

Determination of extinction coefficient (E). The molar extinction coefficient of the chromophore at 412 nm is 13 600. This only applies when a narrow band wavelength is available. When a broader wave band is used, the extinction coefficient is lower. The system may be calibrated by comparing the extinction absorbance in the test system (D_2) with that obtained in a spectrophotometer with a narrow band at 412 nm (D_1). The derived correction factor, E_1, is given by D_1/D_2 and is constant for the test system.

Calculation of GSH concentration

The amount of GSH in the cuvette sample (GSH_c) is given by:

$$\Delta A^{412} \times \frac{E_1}{E} \times 5.5 \ \mu mol.$$

The concentration of GSH in the whole blood sample is:

$$\frac{GSH_c \times 5}{0.2} \mu mol/ml.$$

The unit is often expressed in terms of mg/dl of red cells. The molecular weight of GSH is 307. Thus, GSH in mg/dl packed red cells is given by:

$$GSH_c \times \frac{5}{0.2} \times \frac{1}{PCV} \times 307 \times 100.$$

Normal range

The normal range may be expressed in a number of ways, e.g. $6.57 \pm 1.04 \ \mu mol/g$ Hb or $223 \pm 35 \ \mu mol/dl$ packed red cells or 69 ± 11 mg/dl packed cells.

The glutathione stability test

Principle. In normal subjects incubation of red cells with the oxidizing drug acetylphenyl-hydrazine has little effect on the GSH content, since the oxidation is reversed by the normal complement of reducing enzymes. By contrast, in G6PD-deficient subjects the content is significantly lowered.

Reagents

Acetylphenylhydrazine. Dissolve 100 mg in 1 ml of acetone. Transfer 0.05 ml volumes (containing 5 mg of acetylphenylhydrazine) by pipette to the bottom of 12 × 75 mm tubes. Dry the contents of the tubes in an incubator at 37°C, stopper with rubber bungs and store in the dark until used.

Method

Venous blood, anticoagulated with EDTA, heparin or ACD may be used; it may be freshly collected or previously stored at 4°C for up to 1 week. Add 1 ml to a tube containing acetyl-phenylhydrazine and place a further 1 ml in a similar tube not containing the chemical. Invert the tubes several times and then incubate them at 37°C. After 1 h mix the contents of the tubes once more and incubate the tubes for a further 1 h. At the end of this time determine and compare the GSH concentration in the test sample and in the control sample.

Interpretation

In normal adult subjects red-cell GSH is lowered by not more than 20% by incubation with acetyl-phenylhydrazine. In G6PD-deficient subjects it is lowered by more than this; in heterozygotes (females) the fall may amount to about 50% whilst in hemizygotes (males) the fall is often much greater and almost all may be lost.

GSH and GSH stability in infants

During the first few days after birth the red cells have a normal or high content of GSH. On the addition of acetylphenylhydrazine the GSH is unstable in both normal and G6PD-deficient infants. In normal infants, however, the instability can be corrected by the addition of glucose and by the time the normal infant is 3–4 days old the cells behave like adult cells.[30,46]

2,3-DIPHOSPHOGLYCERATE (2,3DPG)

The importance of the high concentration of 2,3DPG in the red cells of man was recognized at about the same time by Chanutin and Curnish[14] and Benesch and Benesch.[5] 2,3DPG affects the affinity of normal adult Hb for oxygen by binding with the tetramer and tending to keep it in the low affinity physical conformation.[1] The higher the concentration of 2,3DPG the greater the partial pressure of oxygen (pO_2) needed to produce the same oxygen saturation of a given Hb concentration. This effect is demonstrated by shifts in the oxygen dissociation curve produced by changes in 2,3DPG concentration (see p. 175).

Measurement of the concentration of 2,3DPG in red cells is also useful in identifying the probable site of an enzyme deficiency in the metabolic pathways of the cell. In general, enzyme defects cause an increase in the concentration of metabolic intermediates above the level of the block and a decrease in concentration below the block. Thus

2,3DPG is increased in PK deficiency and decreased in hexokinase deficiency. In most other disorders of the glycolytic pathways the 2,3DPG concentration is normal, because increased activity through the pentose phosphate pathway allows a normal flux of metabolites through the triose part of the glycolytic pathway.

Measurement of red cell 2,3DPG

Various methods have been used to assay 2,3DPG. Krimsky used the catalytic properties of 2,3DPG in the conversion of 3-phosphoglycerate (3PG) to 2-phosphoglycerate (2PG) by phosphoglycerate mutase (PGM).[29] At very low concentrations of the 2,3DPG the rate of conversion is proportional to the concentration of 2,3DPG. This method is, however, too cumbersome for the routine measurement of 2,3DPG. Rose and Liebowitz found that glycolate-2-phosphate increased the 2,3DPG phosphatase activity of phosphoglycerate mutase (PGM)[37] and a quantitative assay was evolved using these properties.

Principle. 2,3DPG is hydrolysed to 3PG by the phosphatase activity of PGM stimulated by glycolate-2-phosphate. This reaction is linked to the conversion of NADH to NAD$^+$ by glyceraldehyde-3-phosphate dehydrogenase (Ga3PD) and phosphoglycerate kinase (PGK):

$$2,3DPG \xrightarrow[\text{(glycolate-2-phosphate)}]{\text{2,3DPG phosphatase}} 3PG + Pi;$$

$$3PG + ATP \xrightarrow{PGK} 1,3DPG + ADP;$$

$$1,3DPG + NADH \xrightarrow{Ga3PD} Ga3P + Pi + NAD^+.$$

The fall in absorbance at 340 nm, as NADH is oxidized, is measured.

Method

Freshly drawn blood or heparinized blood may be used. If there is an unavoidable delay in starting the assay, blood (4 volumes) should be added to CPD anticoagulant (1 volume) and stored at 4°C. A control blood sample should be taken at the same time. 2,3DPG levels are stable for 48 h if the blood is stored in this way. The Hb, red-cell count and PCV should be measured on part of the sample. It is not necessary to remove white cells or platelets.

Deproteinization. Add 1 ml of blood to 3 ml of ice-cold 80 g/l trichloracetic acid (TCA) in a 10 ml conical centrifuge tube. Shake the tube vigorously, preferably on an automatic rotor mixer and then allow to stand for 5–10 min for complete deproteinization. The shaking is important, otherwise some of the precipitated protein will remain on the surface of the mixture. Centrifuge at about 1200 g for 5–10 min at 4°C to obtain a clear supernatant. The 2,3DPG in the supernatant is stable for 2–3 weeks when stored at 4°C.

Reagents

Triethanolamine Buffer, 0.2 mol/l, pH 7.6. Dissolve 9.3 g of triethanolamine HCl in c 200 ml of water; then add 5.0 g of disodium EDTA and 2.5 g of $MgSO_4.7H_2O$. Adjust the pH to 7.6 with 2 mol/l KOH (c 15 ml) and make up the volume to 250 ml with water.

ATP, sodium salt. 20 mg/ml; dissolved in buffer, this is stable for several months when frozen.

NADH, sodium salt. 10 mg/ml; this is relatively unstable and should be made freshly each day.

Glyceraldehyde-3-phosphate dehydrogenase. Crystalline suspension from rabbit muscle in ammonium sulphate (Sigma).

Phosphoglycerate kinase. Crystalline suspension from yeast in ammonium sulphate.

Phosphoglycerate mutase. Crystalline suspension from rabbit muscle in ammonium sulphate.

Glycolate-2-phosphate. D+, 2-phosphoglycolic acid (Sigma), 10 mg/ml. This is stable for several months when frozen.

Reaction

Deliver the reagents into a silica or high quality glass cuvette, with a 1 cm light path. The following quantities are for a 4 ml cuvette:

	Test	Blank
Triethanolamine buffer	2.50 ml	2.50 ml
ATP	100 μl	100 μl
NADH	100 μl	100 μl
Deproteinised extract	250 μl	—
Ga-3-PD	20 μl	20 μl
PGK	10 μl	10 μl
PGM	20 μl	20 μl
Water	—	250 μl
	3.00 ml	3.00 ml

Warm the mixtures at 25°C for 5 min and record the absorbance of both test and blank mixtures at 340 nm. Then start the reaction by the addition of 100 μl of glycolate-2-phosphate. Remeasure the absorbance (in 15 min) of the test and blank mixtures after completion of the reaction. Make further measurements after a further 5 min to make sure the reaction is complete. Only one blank is required for each batch of test samples.

Calculation

2,3DPG (μmol/ml blood)

$$= (\Delta A \text{ test} - \Delta A \text{ blank}) \times \frac{3.10}{6.22} \times 16$$

$$= (\Delta A \text{ test} - \Delta A \text{ blank}) \times 8$$

$$= D,$$

where 3.10 = the volume of reaction mixture, 6.22 = mmolar extinction coefficient of NADH at 340 nm and 16 = dilution of original blood sample (1 ml in 3.0 ml of TCA, 0.25 ml added to cuvette).

The results of 2,3DPG assays are best expressed in terms of Hb content or red-cell volume. Thus, if the result of the above calculation is represented by D, then:

$$D \times \frac{1000}{(Hb)} = 2,3DPG \text{ in } \mu\text{mol/g Hb or}$$

$$D \times \frac{1000}{(Hb)} \times \frac{64}{1000} = 2,3DPG \text{ in } \mu\text{mol/}\mu\text{mol Hb}$$

and

$$D \times \frac{1}{PCV} = 2,3DPG \text{ in } \mu\text{mol/ml (packed),} \\ \text{red cells}$$

where (Hb) = Hb in g/l of whole blood and 64 is the mol wt of Hb $\times 10^{-3}$. The molar ratio of 2,3DPG to Hb is about 0.75 : 1.

Normal range. 3.5–5.0 μmol/ml packed red cells or 8.5–15.9 μmol/g Hb. Each laboratory should determine its own normal range.

Significance of 2,3DPG concentration

An increase in 2,3DPG concentration is found in most conditions in which the arterial blood is undersaturated with oxygen and in most acquired anaemias. Decreased 2,3DPG levels occur in polycythaemia vera and in hypophosphataemic states. Acidosis, which shifts the oxygen dissociation curve to the right, causes a fall in 2,3DPG so that the oxygen dissociation curve of whole blood from patients with chronic acidosis (such as patients in diabetic coma or pre-coma) may have nearly normal dissociation curves. A rapid correction of the acidosis will lead to a major shift of the curve to the left, that is a marked increase in the affinity of Hb for oxygen, which may lead to tissue hypoxia. Caution should therefore be exercised in correcting acidosis.[1]

In PK deficiency 2,3DPG levels are 2–3 times normal. Increased 2,3DPG is also found when a PK enzyme with aberrant kinetics is present[32,33] which may give normal PK values under normal assay conditions (see above). In a rare variant of PK there is a high enzyme activity with low 2,3DPG. Such patients have erythrocytosis.

2,3DPG levels are generally slightly lower than normal in HS and this probably accounts for the slight erythrocytosis which is sometimes seen after splenectomy.

THE OXYGEN DISSOCIATION CURVE

The oxygen dissociation curve is the expression of the relationship between the partial pressure of oxygen and the saturation of Hb with oxygen. Details of this relationship and the physiological importance of changes in this relationship were worked out in detail at the beginning of this century by the great physiologists Hüfner, Bohr, Barcroft, Henderson and many others. Their work was summarized by Peters and Van Slyke in Quantitative Clinical Chemistry, Volume 1. The relevant chapters of this book have been reprinted[36] and it would be difficult to better their description of the importance of the oxygen dissociation curve:

The physiological value of hemoglobin as an oxygen carrier lies in the fact that its affinity for oxygen is so nicely balanced that in the lungs hemoglobin becomes 95–96 per cent oxygenated, while in the tissues and capillaries it can give up as much of the gas as is demanded. If the affinity were much less, complete oxygenation in the lungs could not be approached: if it were greater, the tissues would have difficulty in removing from the blood the oxygen they need. Because the affinity is adjusted as it is, both oxyhemoglobin and reduced hemoglobin exist in all parts of the circulation but in greatly varied proportions.[1]

MEASURING THE OXYGEN DISSOCIATION CURVE

Determination of the oxygen dissociation curve depends upon two measurements: the partial pressure of oxygen (pO_2) with which the blood is equilibrated, and the proportion of Hb which is saturated with oxygen. Methods for determining the dissociation curve fall into three main groups:

1. The pO_2 is set by the experimental conditions and the percent saturation of Hb is measured.

2. The percentage saturation is predetermined by mixing known proportions of oxygenated and deoxygenated blood and the pO_2 is measured .

3. The change in oxygen content of the blood is plotted continuously against pO_2 during oxygenation or deoxygenation and the percent saturation calculated.

The multiplicity of methods available for measuring the oxygen dissociation curve suggests that no method is ideal. The advantages and disadvantages of the various techniques have been reviewed.[4,41] The standard method with which new

methods are compared is the gasometric method of Van Slyke and Neill.[42] This method is slow and demands considerable expertise and is not suitable for most haematological laboratories. The method described below[38] is based on similar principles to that of Van Slyke and Neill but employs spectrophotometric measurement of reduced oxyhaemoglobin rather that direct gasometric measurement. The method may be used for suspensions of red cells as well as dilute Hb solutions.

Method

Principle. Oxygen at known pO_2 is added stepwise to a tonometer which contains a dilute suspension of red cells in which the Hb is completely deoxygenated. The Hb in the cells is equilibrated with the gas and the percent saturation is measured spectrophotometrically after each addition. Because the Hb concentration is low there is a negligible shift in the pO_2 in the gas phase after equilibration.

Apparatus

Tonometer-Cuvette. This is not available commercially but can be made in a glass-blowing workshop.*

A tonometer, 5 cm high by 5 cm maximum diameter, is made from Pyrex glass. To one end is fused a high vacuum stopcock† with a single side arm at right angles to the main axis of the apparatus. Small scratches should be made around the entry hole so that air can be admitted slowly. To the other end of the tonometer is fused, via a graded seal, a silica cuvette, 1 cm in light path and 4 ml in volume. Silica cuvettes should be used since the fusion process will distort ordinary glass cuvettes. The joints should be made to withstand pressures of at least 100 kPa (1 atmosphere). The whole apparatus (Fig. 10.6) should be no more than 20 cm high. The total volume of the tonometer and additions is measured. The

---

* As designed by Professor E. R. Huehns and colleagues at University College Hospital, London.
† Quickfit, high vacuum stopcock TH6 (Baird and Tatlock (London) Ltd), suitably modified, is appropriate.

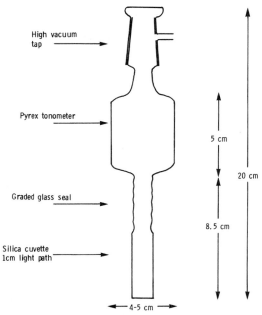

High vacuum
tap

Pyrex tonometer

5 cm

20 cm

Graded glass seal

8.5 cm

Silica cuvette
1cm light path

4-5 cm

Fig. 10.6 Apparatus used in determination of oxygen dissociation curve.

stopcock is greased with silicone grease, taking care that none gets into the apparatus.

Spectrophotometer. Double-beam spectrophotometer with modified cuvette housing (e.g. Pye-Unicam, S.P.8000).

High Vacuum pump.

Gas burette. Made from a graduated 3 ml pipette.

Reagents

Stock phosphate buffer, pH 7.43. 80 ml of 150 mmol/l Na_2HPO_4 and 20 ml of 150 mmol/l Na H_2PO_4.

Working Buffer. Add 1 volume of stock buffer to 4 volumes of 154 mmol/l (9 g/l) NaCl. The pH must be 7.43 ± 0.01.

Other phosphate buffers of suitable pH may be prepared for studying the Bohr effect.

Method

Weigh the freshly greased tonometer. Dilute 2–4 drops of heparinized blood in about 10 ml of working buffer and place in the tonometer

which is then evacuated via the side arm of the stopcock using a high vacuum pump. Close the stopcock and disconnect the tonometer from the pump and then rotate it horizontally in a water-bath at 37°C for 3 min. This allows equilibration between the gases in the blood and buffer and the vacuum. Repeat the evacuation and equilibration twice more to ensure complete deoxygenation of the Hb. After a further equilibration, dry the cuvette, wipe it clean and place it in the appropriate part of the spectrophotometer. After 30 s, to allow movement of red cells to stop, record the absorbance between 500 and 600 nm as a continuous spectrum. Then remove the tonometer from the spectrophotometer, dry the interior of the side arm, and attach the side arm to the gas burette. Let a known volume of air (about 2 ml) into the tonometer through the side arm, the exact amount of air being measured by movement of the mercury bubble and recorded. Again equilibrate the Hb with the gas in the tonometer by rotating the apparatus at 37°C for 3 min. Measure the absorbance over the same range once more after 30 s. Add further volumes of air in the same way and repeat the process after each addition. In this way a family of curves is built up until finally the stopcock is opened to the air and the Hb becomes fully saturated. Read the absorbance at 540, 560 and 576 nm from the tracings.

Finally weigh the tonometer and its contents.

Calculation

$$pO_2 \text{ (mmHg)} = \frac{\left(P - \dfrac{H \times SVP}{100}\right) \times 0.21}{V - v} \times A,$$

where P = atmospheric pressure in mm Hg*; H = relative humidity in percent; SVP = saturated vapour pressure at room temperature in mm Hg; 0.21 = fraction of O_2 in air; V = volume of tonometer in ml;

* × 0.133 kPa.

v = volume of contents in ml, and A = volume of air added in ml.

$$v = W_2 - W_1$$

where W_2 = weight of tonometer + contents and W_1 is weight of tonometer alone, assuming sp gr 1.0 for the blood/buffer suspension.

% saturation of Hb

$$= \frac{(A_{540} - A_{540}^{deoxy}) + (A_{560}^{deoxy})}{(A_{540}^{oxy} - A_{540}^{deoxy}) + (A_{560}^{deoxy} - A_{560}^{oxy})} \times 100$$

or

% saturation of Hb

$$= \frac{(A_{576} - A_{576}^{deoxy}) + (A_{560}^{deoxy} - A_{560})}{(A_{576}^{oxy} - A_{576}^{deoxy}) + (A_{560}^{deoxy} - A_{560}^{oxy})} \times 100,$$

where A_{540}, A_{560} and A_{576} are the absorbances of the partially saturated Hb at the appropriate wavelength and A^{deoxy} and A^{oxy} indicate the absorbance of the totally desaturated and totally oxygenated samples, respectively. The results are then plotted as a graph to obtain the full dissociation curve.

Assessment of the method

The method has the advantages that the curve can be determined on a small sample of blood and that it is relatively quick (about 45 min for a complete curve) and fairly simple. It is, too, a resonably inexpensive method, providing the spectrophotometer can be used for other purposes. The method is particularly suitable for determining the 'n' value of a Hb and calculating the Bohr effect. Its major disadvantage is that dilute suspensions of blood do not behave like whole blood and that the curve determined in this way gives no indication of what is happening in vivo to the $p_{50}O_2$. For these reasons it is useful for diagnostic work in identifying abnormal haemoglobins but it is not useful for research work which requires a knowledge of shifts in the oxygen affinity of blood in vivo.

Interpretation

Figure 10.7 shows the sigmoid nature of the oxygen dissociation curve of Hb A and the effect of hydrogen ions on the position of the curve. A shift of the curve to the right indicates decreased affinity of the Hb for oxygen and hence an increased tendency to give up oxygen to the tissues: a shift to the left indicates increased affinity and so an increased tendency for Hb to take up and retain oxygen. Hydrogen ions, 2,3DPG and some other organic phosphates such as ATP shift the curve to the right. The amount by which the curve is shifted may be expressed by the $p_{50}O_2$, i.e. the partial pressure of oxygen at which the haemoglobin is 50% saturated.

The oxygen affinity, as represented by the $p_{50}O_2$, is related to compensation in haemolytic anaemias.[3] 1 g of Hb can carry about 1.34 ml of O_2. Figure 10.8 shows the O_2 dissociation curves of Hb A and Hb S plotted according to the volume of oxygen contained in 1 l of blood when the Hb concentrations are 146 g/l and 80 g/l, respectively. The $p_{50}O_2$ of Hb A is given as 26.5 mm Hg

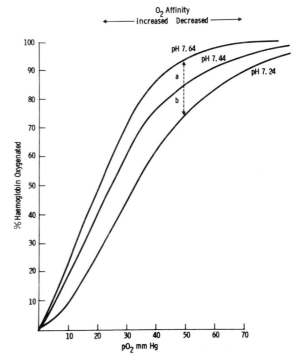

Fig. 10.7 The effect of pH upon the oxygen dissociation curve.

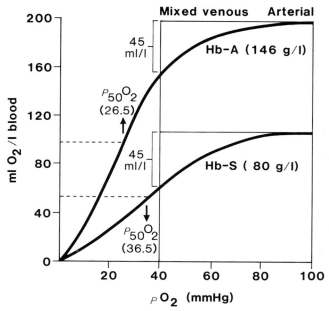

Fig. 10.8 The effect of O_2 affinity on O_2 delivery to tissues.

(3.5 kPa) and Hb S as 36.5 mm Hg (4.8 kPa). It will be seen that in the change from arterial to venous saturation the same volume of oxygen is given up despite the difference in Hb concentration. Patients with a high $p_{50}O_2$ achieve a stable Hb at a lower level than normal and this should be taken into account when planning transfusion for these patients.

The Bohr effect

Bohr et al described the effect of CO_2 on the oxygen dissociation curve.[12] An increase in CO_2 concentration produces a shift to the right, i.e. a decrease in oxygen affinity. It was soon realised that this effect was mainly due to changes in pH, although CO_2 itself has some direct effect. The Bohr effect is given a numerical value, $\Delta \log p_{50}O_2/\Delta pH$, where $\Delta \log p_{50}O_2$ is the change in $p_{50}O_2$ produced by a change in pH (ΔpH). The normal value of the Bohr effect at physiological pH and temperature is about 0.45.

Hill's constant

Hill thought that there was a constant ('n') which represented the number of molecules of oxygen which would be combined with 1 molecule of Hb.[25] Experiment showed that the value was 2.6 rather than the expected 4. The explanation for this lies in the effect of binding 1 molecule of oxygen by Hb on the affinity for binding further oxygen molecules by Hb, the so called allosteric effect of haem-haem interaction: 'n' is a measure of this effect and the calculation of the 'n' value helps in identifying abnormal haemoglobins,[2] the molecular abnormality of which leads to abnormal haem-haem interaction.

Abbreviations used in this chapter

ADP, AMP, ATP	Adenosine di-, mono- or tri-phosphate
ALD	Aldolase
DHAP	Dihydroxyacetone phosphate
1,3DPG; 2,3DPG	1,3- or 2,3-Diphosphoglycerate
DPGM	Diphosphoglycerate mutase
2,3DPGPase	2,3-Diphosphoglycerate phosphatase
DTNB	5,5'-Dithiobis(2-nitrobenzoic acid) (Ellman's reagent)
En	Enolase

F1,6P	Fructose-1,6-diphosphate
F6P	Fructose-6-phosphate
Ga3P	Glyceraldehyde-3-phosphate
Ga3PD	Glyceraldehyde-3-phosphate dehydrogenase
G6P	Glucose-6-phosphate
2DG6P	2-Deoxyglucose-6-phosphate
G6PD	Glucose-6-phosphate dehydrogenase
GPI	Glucose phosphate isomerase
GPx	Glutathione peroxidase
GR	Glutathione reductase
GSH	Reduced glutathione
GSSG	Oxidized glutathione
Hx	Hexokinase
LAC	Lactate
LDH	Lactate dehydrogenase
NAD^+, NADH	Nicotine adenine dinucleotide,
$NADP^+$, NADPH	Nicotine adenine dinucleotide phosphate
Pi	Inorganic phosphate
PEP	Phosphoenolpyruvate
PFK	Phosphofructokinase
6PG	6-Phosphogluconate
6PGD	6-Phosphogluconate dehydrogenase
3PG, 2PG	3-(or 2-) Phosphoglycerate
PGK	Phosphoglycerate kinase
PGM	Phosphoglyceromutase
PK	Pyruvate kinase
Ru5P	Ribulose-5-phosphate
TPI	Triose phosphate isomerase

REFERENCES

[1] ALBERTI, K. G. M. M., DARLEY, J. H., EMERSON, P. M. and HOCKADAY, T. D. R. (1972). 2,3-diphosphoglycerate and tissue oxygenation in uncontrolled diabetes mellitus. *Lancet*, ii, 391.
[2] BELLINGHAM, A. J. (1972). The physiological significance of the Hill parameter 'n'. *Scandinavian Journal of Haematology*, 9, 552.
[3] BELLINGHAM, A. J. and HUEHNS, E. R. (1968). Compensation in haemolytic anaemias caused by abnormal haemoglobins. *Nature (London)*, 218, 924.

[4] BELLINGHAM, A. J. and LENFANT, C. (1971). Hb affinity for O_2 determined by O_2-Hb dissociation analyser and mixing technique. *Journal of Applied Physiology*, 30, 903.
[5] BENESCH, R. and BENESCH, R. E. (1967). The effect of organic phosphates from the human erythrocyte on the allosteric properties of haemoglobin. *Biochemical and Biophysical Research Communications*, 26, 162.
[6] BEUTLER, E. (1975). *Red cell Metabolism. A Manual of Biochemical Methods* 2nd edn. Grune and Stratton, New York.
[7] BEUTLER, E. (1978). Why has the autohemolysis test not gone the way of the cephalin flocculation test? *Blood*, 51, 109.
[8] BEUTLER, E. and MITCHELL, M. (1968). Special modification of the fluorescent screening method for glucose-6-phosphate dehydrogenase deficiency. *Blood*, 32, 816.
[9] BEUTLER, E., DURON, O. and KELLY, B. (1963). Improved method for the determination of blood glutathione. *Journal of Laboratory and Clinical Medicine*, 61, 882.
[10] BEUTLER, E., BLUME, K. G., KAPLAN, J. C., LÖHR, G. W., RAMOT, B. and VALENTINE, W. N. (1977). International Committee for standardization in haematology: recommended methods for red-cell enzyme analysis. *British Journal of Haematology*, 35, 331.
[11] BEUTLER, E., BLUME, K. G., KAPLAN, J. C., LÖHR, G. W., RAMOT, B. and VALENTINE, W. N. (1979). International Committee for standardization in haematology: recommended screening test for glucose-6-phosphate dehydrogenase (G-6-PD) deficiency. *British Journal of Haematology*, 43, 465.
[12] BOHR, C., HASSELBACH, K. and KROGH, A. (1904). Ueber einen in biologischer Beziehung wichtigen Einfluss, den die Kohlensäurespannung des Blutes auf dessen Sauerstoffbindungübt. *Skandinavisches Archiv für Physiologie*, 16, 402.
[13] BREWER, G. J., TARLOV, A. R. and ALVING, A. S. (1962). The methemoglobin reduction test for primaquine-type sensitivity of erythrocytes. A simplified procedure for detecting a specific hypersusceptibility to drug hemolysis. *Journal of the American Medical Association*, 180, 386.
[14] CHANUTIN, A. and CURNISH, R. R. (1967). Effect of organic and inorganic phosphates on the oxygen equilibrium of human erythrocytes. *Archives of Biochemistry and Biophysics*, 121, 96.
[15] COOPER, R. A. (1970). Lipids of human red cell membrane: normal composition and variability in disease. *Seminars in Hematology*, 7, 296.
[16] DACIE, J. V. (1960). *The Haemolytic Anaemias: Congenital and Acquired. Part I: The Congenital Anaemias*, 2nd edn., p. 42. Churchill, London.
[17] DANON, D. (1963). A rapid micromethod for recording red cell osmotic fragility by continuous decrease of salt concentration. *Journal of Clinical Pathology*, 16, 377.
[18] DE GRUCHY, G. C., SANTAMARIA, J. N., PARSONS I. C. and CRAWFORD, H. (1960). Nonspherocytic congenital hemolytic anemia. *Blood*, 16, 1271.
[19] GALL, J. C., BREWER, G. J. and DERN, R. J. (1965). Studies of glucose-6-phosphate dehydrogenase activity of individual erythrocytes: the methemoglobin-elution test for identification of females heterozygous for G6PD deficiency. *American Journal of Human Genetics*, 17, 359.
[20] GOTTFRIED, E. L. and ROBERTSON, N. A. (1974). Glycerol lysis time of incubated erythrocytes in the diagnosis of hereditary spherocytosis. *Journal of Laboratory and Clinical Medicine*, 84, 746.
[21] GOTTFRIED, E. L. arid ROBERTSON, N. A. (1974). Glycerol

lysis time as a screening test for erythrocyte disorders. *Journal of Laboratory and Clinical Medicine*, **83**, 323.

22 GOWDY, J. and KONEMAN, E. W. (1967). Erythrocyte osmotic fragility adapted to the AutoAnalyser. *American Journal of Clinical Pathology*, **47**, 682.

23 GRIMES, A. J., LEETS, I. and DACIE, J. V. (1968). The autohaemolysis test: appraisal of the method for the diagnosis of pyruvate kinase deficiency and the effect of pH and additives. *British Journal of Haematology*, **14**, 309.

24 GUNN, R. B., SILVERS, D. N. and ROSSE, W. F. (1972). Potassium permeability in β-thalassaemia minor red blood cells. *Journal of Clinical Investigation*, **51**, 1043

25 HILL, A. V. (1910). The possible effect of the aggregation of the molecules of haemoglobin on its dissociation curves. *Journal of Physiology*, **40**, 4.

26 International committee for standardization in haematology. (1979). Recommended methods for the characterisation of red cell pyruvate kinase variants. *British Journal of Haematology*, **43**, 275.

27 JACOB, H. S. and JANDL, J. H. (1964). Increased cell membrane permeability in the pathogenesis of hereditary spherocytosis. *Journal of Clinical Investigation*, **43**, 1704.

28 JACOB, H. S. and JANDL, J. H. (1966). A simple visual screening test for glucose-6-phosphate dehydrogenase deficiency employing ascorbate and cyanide. *New England Journal of Medicine*, **274**, 1162.

29 KRIMSKY, I. (1965). D-2,3-Diphosphoglycerate. In *Methods of Enzymatic Analysis*. Ed. H. U. Bergmeyer, p. 238. Academic Press, New York and London.

30 LUBIN, B. H. and OSKI, F. A. (1967). An evaluation of screening procedures for red cell glucose-6-phosphate dehydrogenase deficiency in the newborn infant. *Journal of Pediatrics*, **70**, 788.

31 LYON, M. F. (1961). Gene action in the X-chromosomes of the mouse. (Mus musculus L.). *Nature (London)*, **190**, 372.

32 MIWA, S., FUJII, H., TAKEGAWA, S., NAKATSUJI, T., YAMATO, K., ISHIDA, Y. and NINOMIYA, N. (1980). Seven pyruvate kinase variants characterised by the ICSH recommended methods. *British Journal of Haematology*, **45**, 575.

33 MIWA, S., NAKASHIMA, K., ARIYOSHI, K., SHINOHARA, K., ODA, E. and TANAKA, T. (1975). Four new pyruvate kinase (PK) variants and a classical PK deficiency. *British Journal of Haematology*, **29**, 157.

34 MURPHY, J. R., (1967). The influence of pH and temperature on some physical properties of normal erythrocytes and erythrocytes from patients with hereditary spherocytosis. *Journal of Laboratory and Clinical Medicine*, **69**, 758.

35 PARPART, A. K., LORENZ, P. B., PARPART, E. R., GREGG, J. R. and CHASE, A. M. (1947). The osmotic resistance (fragility) of human red cells. *Journal of Clinical Investigation*, **26**, 636.

36 PETERS, J. P. and VAN SLYKE, D. D. (1931). Hemoglobin and oxygen. In *Quantitative Clinical Chemistry, Vol. I, Interpretations*, p. 525. Williams and Wilkins, Baltimore.

37 ROSE, Z. B. and LIEBOWITZ, J. (1970). Direct determination of 2,3-diphosphoglycerate. *Annals of Biochemistry and Experimental Medicine*, **35**, 177.

38 ROSSI-FANELLI, A. and ANTONINI, É. (1958). Studies on the oxygen and carbon monoxide equilibria of human myoglobin. *Archives of Biochemistry and Biophysics*, **77**, 478.

39 SELWYN, J. G. and DACIE, J. V. (1954). Autohemolysis and other changes resulting from the incubation in vitro of red cells from patients with congenital hemolytic anemia. *Blood*, **9**, 414.

40 SUESS, J., LIMENTANI, D., DAMESHEK, W. and DOLLOFF, M. J. (1948). A quantitative method for the determination and charting of the erythrocyte hypotonic fragility. *Blood*, **3**, 1290.

41 TORRANCE, J. D. and LENFANT, C., (1969–70). Methods for determination of O_2 dissociation curves, including Bohr effect. *Respiration Physiology*, **8**, 127.

42 VAN SLYKE, D. D. and NEILL, J. M. (1924). The determination of gases in blood and other solutions by vacuum extraction and manometric measurement. *Journal of Biological Chemistry*, **61**, 523.

43 World Health Organization Scientific Group (1967). Standardization of procedures for the study of glucose-6-phosphate dehydrogenase. *Technical Report Series*, No. 366. WHO, Geneva.

44 YUNIS, J. J. (1969). *Biochemical Methods in Red Cell Genetics*, Academic Press, New York.

45 ZANELLA, A., IZZO, C., REBULLA, P., ZANUSO, F., PERRONI, L. and SIRCHIA, G. (1980). Acidified glycerol lysis test: a screening test for spherocytosis. *British Journal of Haematology*, **45**, 481.

46 ZINKHAM, W. H. (1959). An in-vitro abnormality of glutathione metabolism in erythrocytes from normal newborns: mechanism and clinical significance. *Pediatrics*, **23**, 18.

11

Investigation of the haemoglobinopathies
(Written in collaboration with J. M. White and Beverley A. Frost)

When it is suspected that a patient is suffering from a haemoglobinopathy, the clinical history and ethnic group, family history, the physical findings and the blood picture provide important information. However, for a definitive diagnosis, an abnormal Hb and/or the laboratory features of thalassaemia have to be demonstrated.

The *International Committee for Standardization in Haematology (ICSH) Expert Panel on Abnormal Haemoglobins and Thalassaemia* have proposed a recommended procedure for the identification of haemoglobinopathies.[31,32] The proposals have been incorporated in the recommendations in this chapter.

The laboratory investigation should be carried out in several stages:

1. *Preliminary tests*
   a. Blood count and film.
   b. Zone electrophoresis of Hb at an alkaline pH on cellulose acetate.
   c. Tests for sickling and/or solubility.
   d. Quantitative estimation of Hb A_2.
   e. Quantitative and qualitative distribution of Hb F.
2. *Identification of abnormal haemoglobins*
   If indicated, further electrophoresis techniques to identify abnormal Hbs:
   a. Phosphate buffer cellulose acetate electrophoresis.
   b. Citrate agar gel electrophoresis.
   c. Starch gel electrophoresis.
   d. Starch block electrophoresis.
   e. Globin chain separation at pH 6.0 and 8.9.
   f. Isoelectric focussing.
3. *Special tests for*
   a. Unstable haemoglobins.
   b. Hb Ms.

c. Altered affinity Hbs.
4. *Globin chain synthesis rates*
In cases of thalassaemia where the diagnosis is difficult, determination of the rate of $\alpha:\beta$ globin chain synthesis.
5. *Chromatography, fingerprinting, amino-acid sequencing*
Readers are referred to Lehmann and Huntsman.[17]

COLLECTION OF BLOOD AND PREPARATION OF HAEMOLYSATES

Blood can be collected into any anticoagulant, but if the samples have to be transported, ACD is the most suitable.

For routine analysis wash the red cells three times in 9.0 g/l NaCl (saline) and then lyse them by adding to the packed cells 2 volumes of water and 1 volume of toluene or carbon tetrachloride (CCl_4). Both of these solutions are toxic and should be used with care. Mouth pipetting must be avoided. After shaking in a mechanical agitator, centrifuge the mixture at 3000 rpm (1200 *g*) for 30 min and pipette off the clear Hb solution. Preferably, however, since organic solvents precipitate unstable Hbs and free globin chains, better results are obtained by lysing the cells in 2 volumes of water (without toluene) and centrifuging at 20 000 rpm (18 000 *g*) at 4°C for 20 min.

In a routine laboratory, if many samples are to be analysed, a practical rapid alternative is to lyse the once-washed packed cells with a few drops of a solution containing 20 g/l saponin plus 10 g/l KCN. However, this type of haemolysate does not keep for more than 1–2 days at 4°C or at room temperature, as it tends to gel.

Storing specimens prepared by either procedure at −20°C is satisfactory only for a few weeks, but lysates can be stored indefinitely in liquid nitrogen.

PRELIMINARY TESTS

Blood count and film

A full blood count, including red-cell count, haemoglobin level, mean cell volume and mean cell haemoglobin, provide valuable information in the diagnosis of both α and β thalassaemias, whilst examination of blood films may show characteristic red-cell changes, e.g. target cells with Hb C and sickle cells with Hb S.

Cellulose acetate electrophoresis at alkaline pH

For routine work, the best method for separating abnormal Hbs is by electrophoresis on cellulose acetate membrane. This method is simple and generally satisfactory for distinguishing the common types of Hb. Various buffers can be used for Hb electrophoresis at an alkaline pH, with a continuous or discontinuous system.

Continuous buffer system

Tris-EDTA-borate, pH 8.9. Tris-(hydroxymethyl)-aminomethane 14.4 g; EDTA (disodium salt) 1.5 g; boric acid 0.9 g; water to 1 l.

Discontinuous buffer system

Tris-EDTA-borate, pH 9.1 (anode chamber). Tris-(hydroxymethyl)-aminomethane 25.1 g; EDTA (disodium salt) 2.5 g; boric acid 1.9 g; water to 1 l.

Barbitone, pH 8.6 (cathode chamber). Sodium diethyl barbiturate 25.75 g; barbitone (diethyl barbituric acid) 4.6 g; thiomersal (preservative) 0.25 g; water to 5.1.

Method

Soak cellulose acetate membrane strips* in the buffer used (a mixture of equal volumes of the two buffers in the discontinuous system) and, after blotting, place them across the bridges of the electrophoresis tank. Secure the strips using wicks of Whatman No. 1 filter paper, soaked in buffer.

Apply the haemolysate near to the cathode bridge. A variety of applicators are available commercially, or a fine pen or fine capillary tube may be used.

Then carry out electrophoresis at 200–300 V (approximately 1 mA/cm width of strip). Separation should be complete within 30 min. Then stain the strips for c 2 min in 0.2% ponceau S in 3% trichloracetic acid. Remove excess stain with 7% acetic acid, made up in tap water.

The relative electrophoretic mobility of some Hbs at pH 8.9 are shown in Fig. 11.1.

Control preparation

It is advisable to electrophorese a known control sample with each electrophoresis.

The following method is recommended for preparing a control haemolysate containing Hbs A, F, S and C:
1. Obtain the following fresh blood samples (in any anticoagulant): AC; SS; F (cord blood).
2. Wash the cells three times with saline. Lyse the cells with a half volume of water and add 1 volume of CCl_4. Mix vigorously and then centrifuge for 10 min at 3000 rpm (1200 g).
3. Add a few drops of 0.3 mol/l KCN (2 g/dl) to the haemolysate to stabilize the Hb as cyanmethaemoglobin (HiCN).
4. Adjust the Hb concentrations of the haemolysates with water to within 20 g/l; ideally between 120–140 g/l.
5. Mix equal volumes of the three haemolysates.
6. Check the mixture by electrophoresis.

* e.g. Celagram II: Shandon Southern, Runcorn, Cheshire; Seprapore III: Gelman Hawksley Ltd, Lancing, Sussex.

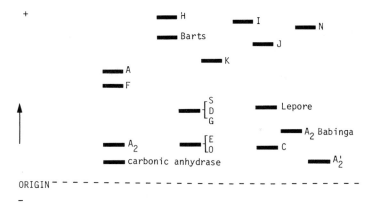

Fig. 11.1 **Relative mobilities of some abnormal haemoglobins on cellulose acetate.** Tris buffer, pH 8.9 (Adapted from Ref. 22).

7. Dispense in 0.5 ml volumes. If stored at 4°C they should be stable for several weeks; however, if stored in liquid nitrogen they should be stable for several months.

TESTS FOR Hb S

Tests to detect the presence of Hb S depend on the decreased solubility of the abnormal Hb at low oxygen tensions.

Sickling in whole blood

The sickling phenomenon may be simply demonstrated in a thin wet film of blood sealed between slide and cover-glass by means of a petroleum jelly-paraffin wax mixture. Sickling develops in the various types of sickle-cell disease and also in Hb S trait. In homozygous Hb S disease (or Hb SC disease or Hb S/β-thalassaemia) marked sickling is usually visible after incubation for 1 h or less at 37°C and filamentous forms are conspicuous (Fig. 11.2). In Hb S trait the process is slower and the changes are less severe (Fig. 11.3) and incubation for as long as 12 h may be necessary for the changes to develop. They can, however, be hastened by the addition of reducing agents to the blood, e.g. sodium dithionite (see below).

Method using reducing agent[13]

Reagents
(A) Sodium dithionite ($Na_2S_2O_4$), 0.114 mol/l: 19.85 g/l. Prepare freshly just before use.
(B) Disodium hydrogen phosphate (Na_2HPO_4), 0.114 mol/l: 16.2 g/l. For use, mix 2 volumes of A with 3 volumes of B to obtain a final pH of *c* 6.8.

Add 5 drops of the freshly prepared reagent to 1 drop of anticoagulated blood on a slide. Cover immediately with a cover-glass and seal with petroleum jelly-paraffin wax mixture. Sickling takes place almost immediately in Hb-S disease and should be obvious in Hb-S trait within 1 h.

Qualitative solubility test[12]

Hb solubility tests provide a rapid method for the detection of Hb S. They are particularly useful for tentatively discriminating between Hb S homozygotes and Hb S with Hb A or an abnormal Hb or thalassaemia. It is, however, inadvisable to give an opinion on the exact genotype of the patient (e.g. Hb AS, SS or SC) without confirmation by electrophoresis.

Reagents

Phosphate buffer, pH 7.1. Potassium dihydrogen phosphate (KH_2PO_4) 33.78 g, dipotas-

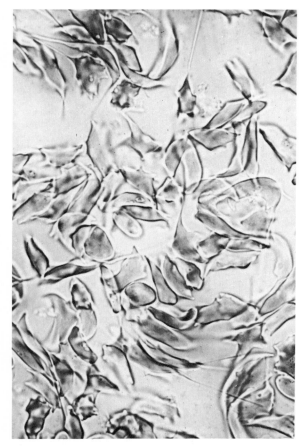

Fig. 11.2 Photomicrograph of sickled red cells. Sealed preparation of blood; Hb SS. Fully sickled filamentous forms predominate. ×900.

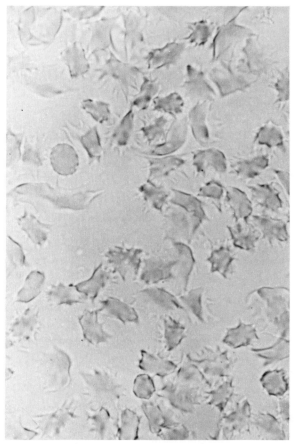

Fig. 11.3 Photomicrograph of sickled red cells. Hb AS. A similar preparation to that shown in Fig. 11.2. 'Holly leaf' sickling is shown. ×900.

sium hydrogen phosphate (K$_2$HPO$_4$) 59.33 g, white saponin 2.5 g, water to 250 ml.

Working solution. Dissolve 0.1 g of sodium dithionite in 10 ml of buffer just prior to use.

Method

Using a Pasteur pipette, add 4 drops of whole blood to 2 ml of the working solution in a round-bottomed glass tube (e.g. 90 × 10 mm). After mixing thoroughly, centrifuge the tube at 1200 *g* for 5 min. Allow the centrifuge to stop without braking and remove the tube carefully without disturbing its contents. The appearances are shown in Fig. 11.4.

Hb S forms a red precipitate at the top and soluble Hb, if present, gives a red colour to the solution beneath this precipitate. In Hb SS the subnatant solution is colourless or pink if substantial amounts of Hb F are present (see below). All other Hbs (e.g. A, C, D, G) yield red solutions. It may be possible to distinguish between Hb S/β-thalassaemia (in which there are small amounts of Hb A) and Hb AS, and also between Hb SS and Hb SC or Hb SD, which give single bands on routine electrophoresis at pH 8.9 or 8.6. Hb F does not precipitate and gives a pink tinge to the subnatant solutions; in patients who are Hb SS and have substantial amounts of Hb F, the amount of colour is usually much less than in Hb S/β-thalassaemia or Hb AS.

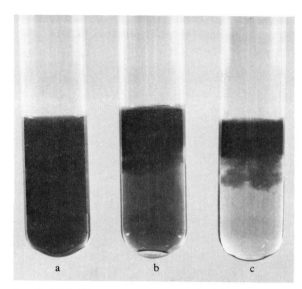

Fig. 11.4 Solubility tests for demonstrating Hb S. (a) Hb A; (b) Hb AS; (c) Hb SS.

Commercial kits

Several commercial kits* for the rapid detection of Hb S, based on the Hb's insolubility, are now available. They are useful, but not more so than the solubility test described above.

Possible causes of false-positive results are hyperproteinaemia and an unstable haemoglobinopathy, giving rise to Heinz bodies in red cells, especially after splenectomy.[12]

ESTIMATION OF Hb A$_2$

The *International Committee for Standardization in Haematology* has made recommendations for two methods suitable for Hb A$_2$ estimation.[33] The first uses separation of Hb A$_2$ by electrophoresis on cellulose acetate membrane, based on the method of Marengo-Rowe.[20] The second method is the microcolumn technique of Efremov et al.[8] The microcolumn method is simpler and more precise, but the electrophoretic method pro-

vides a useful screen for the presence of some abnormal Hbs; it is more suitable for the laboratory performing tests only intermittently.

Electrophoresis

Reagent

Buffer, 0.13 mol/l tris-EDTA-borate, pH 9.1. Tris-(hydroxymethyl)-aminomethane 82.5g; EDTA (disodium salt) 7.8 g; boric acid 4.6 g; water to 5 l.

Method

Soak two cellulose acetate strips per sample in buffer and blot. Place the strips across the bridges of the tank. Secure with buffer-soaked filter paper wicks.

Apply approximately 10 μl of a haemolysate (approximately 10 g/dl) between the cathode bridge and mid-point of the strip, leaving not less than a 0.5 cm gap at each side of the strip. A glass capillary tube is a suitable applicator. Apply 200 V until there is a clear separation, which normally takes place within 60–100 min. Then cut out the Hb A and Hb A$_2$ zones and elute them in 20 ml and 4 ml, respectively, of buffer, for a minimum of 30 min. Set up a normal control with each batch of samples.

Read the absorbance (A) at 413 nm and determine the percentage of Hb A$_2$ by the equation below. Treat a Hb-free piece of cellulose acetate similarly, and use as a blank.

Calculation

$$\% \text{ Hb A}_2 = \frac{A^{413}\text{HbA}_2}{(A^{413}\text{HbA} \times 5) + A^{413}\text{HbA}_2} \times 100.$$

Normal range. 1.8–3.5%.

Micro-column chromatography[8]

Reagents

Stock buffer, 1.0 mol/l tris. Tris-(hydroxymethyl)-aminomethane 121.1 g; water to 1 l.

---

* S-Test, Mercia Diagnostics Ltd.; Sickledex, Ortho Diagnostics Ltd.; Sicklequick, General Diagnostics Ltd.

Working buffers, 0.05 mol/l tris-HCl, pH 8.5, 8.3 and 7.0. For each buffer add to 200 mg of KCN 100 ml of stock 1.0 mol/l tris buffer, and make up with water to 2 l. Adjust the pH with concentrated HCl. Columns should be prepared in Pasteur pipettes using a pre-swollen microgranular anion exchange resin, Whatman DE 52 (diethylaminoethyl cellulose).

To prepare the slurry, add 10 g of DE 52 to 200 ml of tris/HCl buffer, pH 8.5. Mix gently for a few min, then adjust the pH of the thoroughly suspended resin to 8.5 with concentrated HCl. Allow the resin to settle, remove the supernatant and resuspend the resin in a further 200 ml of pH 8.5 buffer. Check that the pH is steady at 8.5, which it normally is in *c* 10 min. Then allow the resin to settle and remove enough of the buffer so that the settled resin comprises about half the total volume.

Set up disposable Pasteur pipettes with short stems vertically in stands. Place either a 3 mm glass bead or a very small piece of cotton wool in the tapered part of the pipette to act as a base for the column. If cotton wool is used, it should not be packed tightly and should be moistened with pH 8.5 buffer. Fill the pipette with thoroughly resuspended slurry allowing the column to pack under gravity to a height of about 6 cm.

Dilute 1 drop of haemolysate with 5 drops of pH 8.5 buffer. When all the excess buffer has drained from the column, gently apply the Hb solution to the top of the column, and allow a few minutes for it to be adsorbed on to the resin. Then apply buffer at pH 8.3 gently to the column with a piece of polythene tubing attached to the top of the pipette acting as a reservoir. About 9 ml of pH 8.3 buffer should be used to elute the Hb A_2 band, the greater part of which should elute between 4 and 6 ml. Collect the eluate in a 10 ml flask or cylinder and make up the volume to 10 ml with the pH 8.3 buffer.

Then elute the remaining Hb A, using 10 ml of pH 7.0 buffer; collect the eluate and make up the volume to 25 ml with pH 7.0 buffer. If, at any stage, the flow through the column stops, it should be discarded.

Read the absorbance of the eluted Hbs at 413 nm against a blank of pH 8.3 buffer.

Calculation

Calculate the % Hb A_2 as follows:

$$\% \text{ Hb } A_2 = \frac{A^{413}HbA_2}{(A^{413}HbA \times 2.5) + A^{413}HbA_2} \times 100.$$

Each laboratory should determine its own normal range for this method, but this should be very close to that for Hb A_2 estimation by electrophoresis (1.8–3.5%).

Significance

The percentage of Hb A_2 is usually raised in β-thalassaemia, range 4.0–7.0%; and in the β unstable haemoglobinopathies.[30] However, in some types of thalassaemia, i.e. $\beta\delta$-thalassaemia, the Hb A_2 percentage is normal or low. It is also normal or low in α-thalassaemia trait and is usually low in Hb H disease. In acquired disorders, too, the Hb A_2 percentage may be altered: e.g. raised in pernicious anaemia;[15] lowered in iron-deficiency anaemia,[15] sideroblastic anaemia[29] and aplastic anaemia.[23] More than 8–10% 'Hb A_2' suggests the presence of another Hb.

Hb E does not separate from Hb A_2 by any technique described in this chapter; however, when present it usually comprises more than 25% of the total Hb. Hb E can be separated from Hb C by column chromatography.[22] Hb C will also elute with Hb A_2. This normally exceeds 35% of the total, and can be identified by citrate agar gel electrophoresis.

ESTIMATION OF Hb F

Hb F may be estimated by several methods, all of which are based on its resistance to denaturation at alkaline pH.

For small amounts of Hb F the method of Betke et al[1] is most reliable, whilst for levels of over 50%, and in cord blood, the method of Jonxis and Visser[14] is preferable.

Method of Betke et al[1]

Prepare a cyanmethaemoglobin (HiCN) solution by adding 0.2 ml of red-cell lysate or 0.1 ml of washed packed red cells to 4 ml of Drabkin's solution (p. 28)*.

To 2.8 ml of the HiCN solution add 0.2 ml of 1.2 mol/l NaOH; mix thoroughly and leave for exactly 2 min at room temperature (18–25°C). Then add 2.0 ml of saturated ammonium sulphate; mix thoroughly. Allow to stand for 10 min. Filter through a Whatman No. 42 filter paper.

Make a 25% standard by adding 0.7 ml of the HiCN solution to 4.3 ml of Drabkin's solution. Read the absorbance of both test and standard at 540 nm.

Calculate the percentage of Hb F as follows:

$$\% \text{ Hb F} = \frac{A^{540}\text{test} \times 25}{A^{540}\text{standard}}.$$

Method of Jonxis and Visser[14]

Add 0.1 ml of blood or haemolysate (approximately 100 g/l) to 10 ml of water; then add 2 drops of 10% NH_4OH solution. Measure the absorbance at 576 nm (A_B). Then add 0.1 ml of the same blood or lysate to 10 ml of 0.06 mol/l NaOH; add 2 drops of 10% NH_4OH solution at room temperature. Mix thoroughly and measure the absorbance every min for 15 min (A_T). Then place the solution at 37°C for 15 min, cool to room temperature and measure the absorbance (A_E). The ratio $A_B : A_E$ should be constant.

Calculate the percentage of undenatured Hb at each minute:

$$\frac{A_T^{576} - A_E^{576}}{A_B^{576} - A_E^{576}} \times 100.$$

Then plot the percentage on the logarithmic scale of semi-logarithmic paper, against time. This should produce a straight line from

* The reagents used should not contain any detergent as this can reduce the resistance of Hb F to alkali denaturation, leading to falsely low results.

which the original amount of Hb F, i.e. that at zero time, can be found by extrapolation.

Significance

In infants aged 1 yr the level of Hb F should not be more than 1%. The normal range for adults is 0.5–0.8%.

Increased levels are found in many disorders, notably in β-thalassaemia trait and sickle-cell disease. But any haematological condition, congenital or acquired, may be associated with a slight increase.

Distribution of Hb F in red cells

If the percentage of Hb F is elevated, its distribution in the red cells may be elucidated by means of a cytochemical method (see p. 111). The method is valuable, for it distinguishes the 'classical' African type of HPFH*, in which all the red cells contain about the same amount of Hb F, from other causes of a raised Hb F (e.g. β-thalassaemia), in which the amount in each cell varies greatly. However, it should be noted that in some of the HPFH disorders which result in high levels, the Hb F is unequally distributed throughout the red cells.[6] Peripheral blood films can be examined by fluorescence microscopy after staining with anti-γ chain immunofluorescent antibody. Hb F can be demonstrated in this way (p. 112) but the technique affords no advantages over the cytochemical method.

DEMONSTRATION OF Hb H INCLUSIONS

When a patient has red-cell indices suggestive of thalassaemia, namely a low MCH and a high red-cell count, but does not have a raised Hb A_2 or Hb F level, and is not iron deficient, then α-thalassaemia may be suspected. This can be diagnosed by measurement of globin chain sythesis (see p. 189).

Demonstration of Hb H inclusions confirms the diagnosis of α-thalassaemia, but it cannot be excluded by failure to observe the inclusions.

* Hereditary persistance of fetal haemoglobin.

Method

Mix 2 volumes of whole blood with 1 volume of 1% New methylene blue in saline. Then incubate at 37°C for 1 h. Make a film of the suspension and when dry examine microscopically unfixed, using a 2 mm objective as for a reticulocyte count.

Significance

In Hb H disease, many cells will develop inclusions but in α-1-thalassaemia trait, only occasional cells (1 in 1000 to 1 in 5000) contain inclusions and these may not be found even after searching for 5–10 min. This test is therefore of very limited value in the diagnosis of α-thalassaemia trait. False positives can be induced by over-incubation, i.e. for more than 1 h. The relative value of this test has been examined in different ethnic groups.[34]

IDENTIFICATION OF ABNORMAL HAEMOGLOBINS

When an abnormal haemoglobin has been demonstrated by Hb electrophoresis at an alkaline pH on cellulose acetate membrane, other electrophoretic techniques may be useful in making a presumptive identification. It is useful to measure the percentage of a variant Hb, and this can usually be done using the buffer and procedure recommended on p. 183 for Hb A_2 estimation by electrophoresis. The elution volume should be adjusted according to the proportion of the variant being investigated.

Of the fast-moving variants, Hb Barts and Hb H can be distinguished by their movement on cellulose acetate membrane with a phosphate buffer at pH 7.0. Variants moving in a similar manner to Hb S, but with a negative solubility test, can be separated from Hb S on citrate agar gel electrophoresis at pH 6.0. This technique is useful when investigating double heterozygotes, e.g. Hb SD or Hb SG; it can also be used to distinguish Hb E, Hb C and Hb O, which move similarly at an alkaline pH on cellulose acetate, and also to separate Hb A from Hb F. This is particularly useful as an aid to the diagnosis of abnormal Hbs in cord blood, and to detect small amounts of Hb A in thalassaemia.

Globin-chain separation at both acid and alkaline pH is a useful technique for identifying the abnormal chain and is simple to perform using Cellogel cellulose acetate strips*.

Starch gel electrophoresis is a very sensitive method which gives good results.

Phosphate buffer electrophoresis, pH 7.0

Hb H and Hb Barts can be distinguished from other fast-moving variants by their movement towards the anode when using cellulose acetate membrane with phosphate buffer, pH 7.0

Buffer

0.1 mol/l phosphate, pH 7.0.
   Stock solutions. (a) $NaH_2PO_4.H_2O$ 27.6 g; water to 1 l; (b) Na_2HPO_4 anhydrous, 28.4 g; water to 1 l.
   Working buffer. 39 ml (a) + 61 ml (b); bring to 200 ml with water.

Method

Soak cellulose acetate strips in buffer, blot and place across the bridges. Apply the haemolysate at the centre of the strip and carry out electrophoresis at 150 V for c 1 h.
   The amount of Hb H or Hb Barts can be estimated by eluting the Hb bands in measured volumes of water (see method for Hb A_2, p. 183).

Citrate agar-gel electrophoresis, pH 6.0[19]

Stock citrate buffer. Sodium citrate 147 g; water 600 ml. Adjust the pH to 6.0 with 50% citric acid and then make the volume to 1 l with water.
   Working buffer. Dilute the stock buffer 1 in 10 for preparation of the gel and for use in the chambers.

* Whatman, Cambridge.

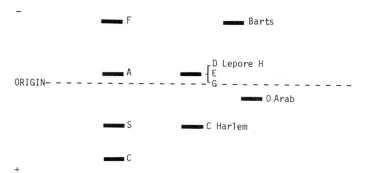

Fig. 11.5 Relative mobilities of some abnormal haemoglobins on agar gel.
Citrate buffer, pH 6.0 (Adapted from Ref. 22).

Method

Make a 1% agar solution by adding 1 g of Difco Bacto-Agar* to 100 ml of working buffer and melt in a boiling water-bath. Keep unused stock and working buffer at 4°C.

Smear a few drops of hot agar over glass slides, 7.5 cm × 10 cm, and dry on a hot plate for 5 min. Place the pre-coated slides on a level surface and pipette approximately 9 ml of hot agar on to each one and spread it to cover the slide evenly. Allow to set before moving the slide. A plastic film, Gelbond†, may be used as an alternative to the glass slides and has proved very satisfactory in use and is easy to store.

Dilute the haemolysates to be tested to 10–30 g Hb/l, matching their Hb content closely to that of control samples. For detection of minor Hb components, as in cord blood, a 100 g/l haemolysate is preferable. Samples may be applied using a commercial applicator, e.g. Shandon Multi-Applicator. Load the applicator plate wells with a drop of diluted lysate, prime the applicator and gently place the applicator on to the agar, without cutting the gel surface. Leave the applicator in contact with the gel for c 15 s.

Prepare the tank with cold buffer and filter paper wicks, and place the slides, agar side down, on to the wicks. Apply a constant current of 50 mA. Separation should be complete within approximately 1 h.

* Bacto-Agar, Difco Laboratories.
† Miles Laboratories Ltd.

Stain the agar gel with Ponceau S or bromophenol blue, either before or after drying the agar in an 80°C oven or on a hot plate. Pour off the stain after 20 min, and wash off excess stain with water.

Stains

Bromophenol blue. Dissolve 100 mg of bromophenol blue in 1 l of water containing 10 ml of glacial acetic acid.

Ponceau S. 20 g/l in 30 g/l trichloracetic acid.

The relative mobilities of some Hbs on agar gel are shown in Fig. 11.5

Starch-gel electrophoresis

This is a very sensitive method for the detection of abnormal Hbs. Starch-gel trays are now commercially available for both horizontal and vertical systems, and they can be made very cheaply from Perspex (Fig. 11.6). The vertical system is to be preferred as the bands, especially minor ones, are better resolved.

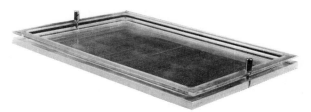

Fig. 11.6 Perspex tray for starch gel electrophoresis.

Buffers

Continuous tris buffer system, pH 8.6, 0.08 mol/l. Tris-(hydroxymethyl)-aminomethane 110.0 g; EDTA 5.85 g; boric acid 30.9 g; water to 1 l.

Dilute the buffer 1 in 20 for making gels, 1 in 5 for the anodal chamber and 1 in 7 for the cathodal chamber.

This is the most useful continuous buffer for routine work.

Discontinuous tris and sodium borate buffer system, pH 8.5, 0.045 mol/l. *Gels*: tris-(hydroxymethyl)-aminomethane 49.5 g; citric acid 5.0 g; water to 5 l. *Chambers*: boric acid 92.5 g; 10 mol/l NaOH 25.0 g; water to 5 l.

This buffer system has the advantage that minor Hb components are resolved more easily. However, major components tend to diffuse and the gels are less easy to handle.

Phosphate, pH 7.1, 5.4 mmol/l.[9] Titrate 0.04 mol/l disodium hydrogen phosphate to pH 7.1 with syrupy phosphoric acid. Dilute 40 ml of the buffer with 300 ml of water.

The undiluted buffer is used for the electrode chambers and the diluted buffer is used for the gel. Separation takes about 4 h. This buffer is the most satisfactory one available for demonstrating Hb Barts and Hb H, especially when they are present in low concentrations.

Method

Make up hydrolysed starch (Connaught Laboratories) in buffer at a concentration of about 90–120 g/l. The volume should be more than sufficient to fill the tray. Thoroughly shake the mixture in a 1 l Erlenmeyer flask and heat over a flame, continuously shaking, until the gel becomes translucent. Remove the dissolved air by applying a vacuum to the side arm of the flask, and in this way a mixture containing only small bubbles will be obtained. Excessive degassing should be avoided as this can result in dry gels. Pour the molten gel into the tray, allowing some to overflow the sides. After cooling, cut slots of 1 cm length through the gel with a razor. Soak filter papers of similar size in haemolysates (20–40 g/l), insert into the slots and leave in position. Place the gel mould in the two buffer chambers with strips of Whatman No. 3 paper, four layers thick, soaked in the buffer, at either end. Cover the system with a thin sheet of polythene and a glass plate, secured with elastic bands. Carry out electrophoresis for 2 h at 30 mA, or overnight at 8 mA. Remove the top section and slice the gel in half longitudinally with a cheese wire. Then stain one-half with a protein stain, such as amido black, or with a Hb stain such as orthotolidine (see below).

Stains

Amido black stain. Diluent: glacial acetic acid 200 ml; methanol 900 ml; water 900 ml. Add 0.8 g of amido black to 1 l of the diluent.

Pour the stain over the gel and leave for 5 min. Then wash the gel with several changes of the diluent. The stained gel will keep indefinitely if sealed under Cellophane.

Orthotolidine. Orthotolidine 0.5 g; sodium nitroprusside 1 g; glacial acetic acid 50 ml.

Add a sufficient volume of the solution to cover the gel completely. Then add 30% hydrogen peroxide (100 vol) (5 ml/l stain) and leave the mixture until the desired intensity of staining is obtained, usually in 5 min. Then wash the gel several times with water. The stain is more readily retained if the gel is kept at 4°C.

Starch block electrophoresis[16]

This medium provides a sensitive method for separating Hbs but the process is time-consuming and unsuitable for routine use. It can be used for the estimation of Hb A or for the separation and estimation of other Hb variants.

Buffers

Barbitone, pH 8.9. Sodium diethylbarbiturate 10.3 g; diethylbarbituric acid 0.92 g; water to 1 l.

This is the most suitable for routine use, e.g. for the separation of Hb S from Hb C and for the isolation of Hb A$_2$.

Phosphate, pH 7.0. Titrate 0.04 mol/l disodium hydrogen phosphate to pH 7.0 with syrupy phosphoric acid.

This buffer is recommended for the separation and estimation of Hb Barts and Hb H. Migration is rapid and separation is adequate in 8–12 h at 30–40 mA and 250 V.

Method

Wash potato starch four times in the appropriate buffer and pour the mixture into trays, 25 × 30 × 0.5 cm, containing three thicknesses of Whatman No. 3 paper which have been soaked in the buffer and placed in the trays with half left outside to make contact with the buffer. Soak up excess buffer with large sheets of filter paper until the starch is just moist when pressed. Cut slits measuring 1 cm into the block, one-third of the way from the cathode and pipette in the haemolysate (Hb *c* 100 g/l). Each slit should hold about 1 ml. Cover the whole with a sheet of polythene and a thick glass plate and secure with thick clamps on either side. Carry out electrophoresis at 4°C and, using barbitone buffer, continue this for 18 h at 30 mA and 250 V. Inspect the bands by trans-illumination and cut out fractions if desired. Elute the Hb by allowing the fractions to stand in barbitone buffer at 4°C. Filter the eluate through a sintered glass funnel.

GLOBIN CHAIN ANALYSIS

This is an extremely useful procedure for determining which of the globin chains is involved in an abnormal Hb. Three methods are available for separating globin chains: two are electrophoretic, using starch gel and cellulose acetate gel, respectively, and are suitable for routine procedures; the third is chromatographic and, being more complicated, is less suitable as a routine procedure.

However, it is relatively easy to perform and has other practical applications.

Preparation of globin

Lyse washed red cells in 4 volumes of water and remove the stroma by centrifugation at *c* 1500 *g* for 20 min. Then add the clear lysate drop by drop, with thorough mixing after each drop, to at least 20 volumes of acid-acetone mixture (acetone 98 volumes, conc. HCl 2 volumes) kept at −20°C. Separate the white, flocculent precipitate which forms immediately by centrifugation at *c* 100 *g* for 2–3 min and wash first in acetone (cooled to −20°C) and then in ether. The globin should then be dried in air or, preferably, in a stream of nitrogen.

Separation in Cellogel*

Globin chain separation can be carried out at acid and alkaline pH, and the differences in mobility under these conditions can give a good indication of the identity of a variant haemoglobin.

Alkaline buffer

Barbitone buffer, pH 8.6. Sodium diethyl barbiturate 51.5 g; barbitone (diethyl barbituric acid) 9.2 g; thiomersal (preservative) 0.5 g; water to 5 l. For use, add 240 g of urea to 400 ml of buffer.

Acid buffer

Tris-EDTA-borate-citrate, pH 6.0. Tris 10.2 g; EDTA 0.6 g; borate 3.2 g; water to 1 l. For use, add 240 g of urea to 400 ml of buffer and adjust to pH 6.0 with saturated citric acid.

Dissolve 10 mg of globin, prepared as above, in 0.5 ml of a 2-mercaptoethanol in urea solution, prepared by dissolving 12.0 g of urea in water, adding 0.5 ml of 2-mercaptoethanol, then diluting to 15 ml with water.

Alternatively, the following quick method may be used for the preparation of the globin

* Whatman, Cambridge.

sample. The method appears to present no disadvantages.

Mix 20 μl of haemolysate, 20 μl of the urea buffer and 20 μl of 2-mercaptoethanol in a small glass tube. Allow to stand for 30 min. (This mixture is stable up to 4 h.)

At the same time, soak the Cellogel strip in urea buffer and place with the penetrable surface, as indicated by the manufacturer, uppermost on to the bridges. Secure with soaked filter paper strips. Apply the sample across the strip in a thin line with a pen nib about 2 cm from the anode. Control samples should be set up with each test sample. Apply a constant voltage (200 V) across the strip. Separation of globin chains will be complete within $1\frac{1}{2}$–2 h.

It should be noted that when the quick sample preparation method is used, the coloured haem component of the mixture will migrate rapidly along the strip into the anode buffer, within about 15 min. The globin component is colourless.

Stain the strip with Ponceau S and remove the excess stain by immersion in 7% (v/v) acetic acid for 10 min, with two changes of acetic acid. Then immerse the Cellogel strip in absolute methanol for 1 min, and subsequently in a clearing solution (87 ml of methanol, 12 ml of glacial acetic acid, 1 ml of glycerol) for 2 min. Place the strip on a glass plate and warm at 50–60°C on a hot plate until the strip is dry and translucent. It can then be peeled off the glass and stored at room temperature.

Separation of globin chains on starch gel[4]

Barbitone buffer. Dissolve 18.4 g of diethyl-barbituric acid in 500 ml of boiling water; add 60 ml of 1 mol/l NaOH and make up the volume to 1 l with water. Adjust the pH to 8.0 with 1 mol/l NaOH.

Method

Prepare gels by adding about 100 g of starch to 300 ml of barbitone buffer containing 180 g of urea. Warm the mixture at 70°C for 5–10 min, constantly shaking, and then pour into the gel mould, as described on p. 00.

Dissolve 1–3 mg of globin in 0.1 ml of urea-barbitone buffer containing 2-mercaptoethanol (50 μl/5 ml of buffer). Then centrifuge the solution and apply the supernatant to the gel. Fill the buffer chambers with urea-barbitone buffer (containing 2-mercaptoethanol). Carry out electrophoresis at 4°C for 22 h at 33–45 mA and 250 V. Finally, stain the gels with amido black, in the usual way (see p. 188).

Interpretation of results

The direction of migration of the globin chains in globin separation is from the anode to the cathode, whilst in electrophoresis at an alkaline pH on cellulose acetate whole Hbs migrate from the cathode to the anode. If the mobility of a whole Hb is known on electrophoresis at pH 8.6, then abnormal α and β chains can be differentiated. If an abnormal Hb moves *faster* than Hb A on electrophoresis at an alkaline pH, the abnormal chain will migrate on globin separation more slowly than its normal counterpart. The α chains move faster than the β chains and migrate nearer to the cathode. Thus, an Hb which migrates rapidly on electrophoresis at an alkaline pH due to an abnormal α chain will produce a *slow-moving* band of α chains on globin separation, which will migrate between the normal α and β chains. Under the same circumstances, a *fast-moving* Hb due to an abnormal β chain will produce a *slow-moving* band of β chains migrating behind the normal β chain.

The relative mobilities of various α chain and β chain mutant Hbs are shown in Figs. 11.7 and 11.8.

SEPARATION OF GLOBIN CHAINS BY CHROMATOGRAPHY[5]

This technique gives excellent quantitative separation of normal and abnormal globin chains, and it can be used to separate an abnormal chain in milligram quantities before further analysis by fingerprinting. Also, if the red cells from which the

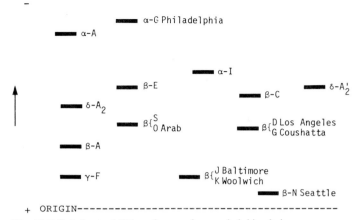

Fig. 11.7 Relative mobilities of some abnormal globin chains.
Urea-tris-EDTA-borate-citrate buffer, pH 6.0 (Adapted from
Ref. 22).

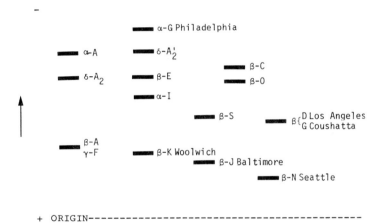

Fig. 11.8 Relative mobilities of some abnormal globin chains.
Urea-barbitone buffer, pH 8.6 (Adapted from Ref. 22).

Hb was derived have previously been incubated
with a radioactive amino acid, the technique can be
used for measuring the relative rates of chain
synthesis.

Materials

Urea solution (8 mol/l). Dissolve 62 g of
urea (Merck)* in 600 ml of water and bring to
a final volume of 1300 ml with continuous
stirring. Deionize the solution by passing it
down a column, 9 cm high and 5 cm in diameter, of the resin Duolite DM-F*.

Starting buffer. Dissolve 0.5 g of disodium
hydrogen phosphate (Na_2HPO_4) in 700 ml of

the urea solution and adjust the pH to 6.4 with
a few drops of orthophosphoric acid. If the pH
falls too low, it can be raised with a few drops
of concentrated NaOH. Add 80 mg of Cleland's reagent (dithiothreitol*).

Final buffer. Dissolve 2.2 g of disodium hydrogen phosphate (Na_2HPO_4) in 300 ml of the
starting buffer and adjust the pH to 6.4 with
orthophosphoric acid. Add 30 mg of Cleland's
reagent.

Method

Dissolve 40 mg of globin in 5 ml of the starting buffer. Then dialyse the solution in a

* BDH Ltd, Poole, England.

* Sigma Chemical Co. Ltd., Poole, England.

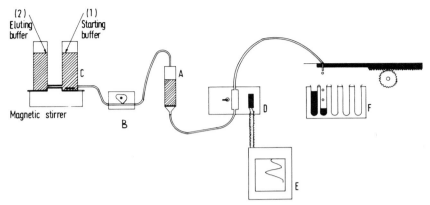

Fig. 11.9 Diagram of apparatus for chromatographic separation of globin chains.
A, chromatography column; B, peristaltic pump; C, gradient mixer; D, detector unit;
E, recorder; F, fraction collector.

Visking tube (8/32) against 200 ml of the starting buffer for 2 h, with one change of buffer after the first hour. Add 10 mg of carboxymethylcellulose (Whatman CM23) to 100 ml of the starting buffer and after 10 min pour the slurry into a glass tube 15 mm in diameter, so as to give a column 10 cm in height.

Then apply the dialysed globin to the column, which should now be connected up to a peristaltic pump and washed for 30 min with starting buffer until the non-haem proteins have eluted. They will produce a sharp narrow peak on a recording spectrophotometer. When the absorbance has returned to the base line, remove the connecting clamp between cylinder A and D (Fig. 11.9) and continue the pumping at 0.4 ml/min. Then carry out the chain elution using 250 ml of the starting buffer and 250 ml of the final buffer. The continuous mixture of the two will result in a linear Na_2HPO_4 gradient; as the buffer is pumped out of the starting buffer cylinder the same volume of final buffer is drawn into it from the other chamber, and the mixture is constantly mixed by the magnetic stirrer. Elution continues until the last chain (α chain) has completely eluted, normally after 250–300 ml of the buffer have passed through the column.

Interpretation

The chains elute in the order: γ, β, α. If an abnormal chain is more negatively charged than normal, it will elute from the column before the normal chain. For identification, collect the eluate by means of a fraction collector and measure the absorbance of the contained chains at 280 nm in a spectrophotometer. The α chain has a lower absorbance than the β chain.

Globin chain synthesis rates: Determination of the relative rates of α and β chain synthesis

Reagents

Krebs-Ringer-Phosphate (KRP) (see below). *Stock solutions.*
1. *NaCl, 1.5 mol/l*: 87.66 g NaCl in 1 l of deionized water.
2. *Phosphate buffer*, pH 7.4: (I) 0.1 mol/l $NaH_2PO_4 \cdot 2H_2O$: 15.6 g in 1 l. (II) 0.1 mol/l $Na_2HPO_4 \cdot 2H_2O$: 17.8 g in 1 l. Add 19 parts (e.g. 28.5 ml) of (I) to 81 parts (e.g. 121.5 ml) of (II); adjust the pH to 7.4 with either NaOH, if too low, or orthophosphoric acid, if too high.
3. *KCl, 0.15 mol/l*: 5.6 g of KCl dissolved in 500 ml of water.
4. *MgSO₄, 0.15 mol/l*: 2.7 g of $MgSO_4 \cdot 7H_2O$ dissolved in 100 ml of water.
5. *CaCl₂, 0.11 mol/l*: 1.62 g of $CaCl_2 \cdot 2H_2O$ dissolved in 100 ml of water.

To make KRP for use. Make up 100 ml of 1.5 mol/l NaCl (solution 1) to 1 l with water. Add 120 ml of phosphate buffer, pH 7.4 (solution 2), 40 ml of 0.15 mol/l KCl (solution 3),

10 ml of 0.15 mol/l MgSO$_4$ (solution 4) and 10 ml of 0.11 mol/l CaCl$_2$ (solution 5). Stir carefully to avoid precipitation. Adjust the pH to 7.4 with 1 mol/l NaOH. Check the osmolarity with an osmometer and adjust with 1.5 mol/l NaCl or water, if necessary, to obtain a reading of 280–300 m-osmoles.

Incubation medium (dialysed AB plasma)

Obtain 300 ml of AB plasma (preferably Rh−ve). Remove the free amino acids by dialysis, as follows:

Boil about 1 m of Visking tubing (size 20/30) in water for 10 min; do not allow to dry. Cut in two; tie two knots at one end of each piece and fill each piece with plasma, tying the other end of each piece with two knots. Dialyse in KRP the two prepared pieces of tubing in a cold room at 4°C. Change the KRP twice, as follows:

Dialysis 1: for 1 h only.

Dialysis 2: for minimum of 4 h, maximum of 12 h.

Dialysis 3: for minimum of 12 h, maximum of 48 h.

Note that the calcium in the KRP will cause a small amount of fibrin deposition in the plasma. Remove this by filtering the dialysed plasma through nylon mesh. Measure the volume and add 6 mg/ml of glucose. Then add 1.33 ml of leucine-free amino acid mixture to 100 ml of plasma, stir well and deliver 5-ml volumes into glass bottles. Label them 'leu-free medium' (LFM) and store them at −20°C. Deliver the remainder of the dialysed plasma into 50-ml plastic bottles, label as 'dialysed plasma + glu (no AA)', with date, and store at −20°C or, if possible, at −80°C. The pH of this incubation mixture falls when it has frozen. When thawed, measure the pH and adjust to 7.4 with 0.1 mol/l NaOH.

Amino acid (AA) mixture (Leucine-free media)

Make up a 20 mmol/l solution of each amino acid (AA) in water (10 ml should be adequate). When an amino acid is available only as a mixture of D and L forms, use twice the calculated amount. Store these stock solutions at 4°C.

To obtain a solution lacking a particular amino acid, mix 1 ml of each of the stock solutions, omitting the particular amino acid not required. The composition of single amino acid (AA) stock solutions is given in Table 11.1.

Table 11.1 Composition of single amino acid (AA) stock solutions

Amino acid	Mol wt	Wt (mg) for 10 ml of a 20 mmol/l solution
Alanine	68	13.6
*Arginine	174 + 2H$_2$O = 210	42.0
Aspartic acid	133	26.6
*Asparagine	132 + H$_2$O = 150	30.0
*Cysteine	121 + 2H$_2$O = 157	31.4
Glutamic acid	147	29.0
Glutamine	146	28.0
Glycine	75	15.0
Histidine	155	31.0
Iso-leucine	131	26.2
*Lysine	146 + 2H$_2$O = 182	33.6
Methionine	149	29.0
Phenylalanine	165	33.0
Proline	115	23.0
Serine	105	21.0
Threonine	119	22.8
Tryptophan	204	40.8
Tyrosine	181	36.2
Valine	57	11.4

* These amino acids come in the hydrated form.

Add to the ready-made incubation medium the leucine-free AA solution in the proportion of 1.33 ml of AA solution to 100 ml of dialysed plasma.

Labelling globin chains

Take 10 ml of venous blood into ACD and centrifuge at c 5000 rpm (4000 **g**) for 20 min. Remove the plasma and resuspend the cells in an equal volume of KRP solution and recentrifuge. Repeat this three times. If the reticulocyte count is <5%, transfer the packed cells from the final washing to siliconed centrifuge tubes with screw caps, place in an angle-head superspeed rotor and centrifuge at 120 000 **g** (40 000 rpm) for 1 h. Remove the tubes gently, remove the plasma and take 0.5–1 ml of the top layer of the cells. The number of reticulocytes should have increased by a factor of 5.

Wash the cells three times with KRP at 4°C. Add c 100 μCi of ^{3}H-leucine* in 100 μl of KRP to 0.5–1 ml of packed cells and 1 ml of leucine-free medium. Incubate at 37° for 2 h. 1 mCi of ^{3}H-leucine/ml can be obtained from Amersham in a vial. The contents are dried under a stream of N_2 and then re-suspended in 1 ml of KRP.

Normally, for adult red cells, as opposed to antenatal work using fetal cells, 1 mCi of ^{3}H-leucine is used and the cells are preferably reticulocyte-enriched, as described above, by high-speed centrifugation before incubation with the isotope. After the incubation, wash the cells three times with 9 g/l NaCl at 4°C. Either freeze and process the haemolysate later or make globin immediately, as described above. Separate the chains, as described on p. 190.

Collecting and eluting the fractions

Collect 6 c 1-ml fractions per 14 min (flow rate 0.4 ml/min), and after c 20 fractions have been collected and the absorbance base line is stable, start the gradient and continue eluting for 16 h, collecting in all c 70 fractions, monitoring the absorbance with a recording spectrophotometer.

Counting

Pipette a 0.15 ml volume from each fraction, the optical density of which is already recorded, into a vial containing 4 ml of a scintillation fluid. Mix the contents thoroughly, using a vortex mixer. (Several scintillation fluids are available; a suitable one is Instagel†.)

Each vial should be counted in a liquid scintillation counter for 1, 5 or 10 min each, depending on the radioactivity. The relative rate of synthesis of each chain is determined

* Amersham Radiochemical, Code TRK 170.
† Packard, Caversham, Berks.

as a ratio:

$$\frac{\text{Total } \alpha\text{-chain counts}}{\text{Total } \beta\text{-chain counts}}.$$

Typical results are given in Table 11.2. A schematic diagram of the apparatus required is shown in Fig. 11.9.

Table 11.2 Typical results for the α-chain to β-chain ratio as obtained by liquid scintillation counting

	α : β ratio
Normal	0.95–1.05
β-thalassaemia trait	1.4–1.7
Thalassaemia major	>20
Hb H disease	0.25
α-thalassaemia-1	0.5–0.6
α-thalassaemia-2	0.75–0.9

DETECTION OF AN UNSTABLE HAEMOGLOBIN

The clinical and haematological features of this group of disorders were reviewed by White and Dacie.[30] Laboratory diagnosis depends on the demonstration of a Hb which is abnormally sensitive to precipitation by heat or by isopropanol. The results of the autohaemolysis test and starch-gel electrophoresis may, however, suggest the diagnosis.

Autohaemolysis test

If an unstable Hb is present, the serum may appear brown or opaque after incubation for 48 h. This would be due to the presence of methaemoglobin (Hi) and Heinz bodies, and numerous Heinz bodies will be seen if the incubated red cells are stained with methyl violet. Normal cells do not form Heinz bodies under these conditions.

Starch-gel electrophoresis at pH 8.6

In some unstable haemoglobinopathies haem-depleted components may be seen which migrate in the position of Hb S or just in front of Hb A_2; and, in addition, free α chains may migrate to the cathode.

Heat-instability test[7]

This should be carried out on fresh blood samples in any anticoagulant. A control blood sample must always be tested at the same time, and if it is not possible to have a fresh blood sample from the patient, a control sample of the same age must be tested.

Lyse 1 ml of washed red cells with 5 ml of water and add 5 ml of 0.15 mol/l tris-HCl buffer, pH 7.4 (p. 436). Remove the stroma by centrifugation at c 1500 g for 20 min. Then transfer 5 ml of the lysate to a glass test tube, which should then be heated at 50°C for up to 60 min. Examine the tube periodically for turbidity and fine flocculation. A precipitate which is easily visible to the naked eye will be formed if a heat-unstable Hb is present. Slight precipitation is of doubtful significance and, if present, the test should be repeated. In any case, the result from the patient's blood must be carefully compared with that of the normal control.

If a precipitate is present, centrifuge the suspension. Then dilute equal volumes of the clear supernatant and of the original (unheated) haemolysate 1 in 20 in cyanide-ferricyanide (modified Drabkin's) reagent (p. 28) and read their absorbance at 280 nm:

% unstable Hb

$$= \frac{A^{280} \text{ of unheated sample} - A^{280} \text{ of heated sample}}{A^{280} \text{ of unheated sample}} \times 100.$$

Isopropanol precipitation test[3]

Prepare a haemolysate (c 100 g Hb per l) from packed washed red cells by lysing them in 1.5 volumes of water. Remove the stroma by centrifugation at c 1500 g for 20 min. Prepare isopropanol buffer by adding isopropanol, 17% by volume, to 0.1 mol/l tris/HCl buffer,

pH 7.4 (p. 436). The isopropanol buffer can be kept for several weeks if well stoppered and stored at 4°C.

Place two 10–15 mm diameter glass tubes, each containing 2 ml of isopropanol buffer, in a water-bath at 37°C. After about 5 min, add 0.2 ml of fresh control normal haemolysate to one tube and 0.2 ml of test haemolysate to the other. Stopper the tubes, mix by inversion and replace in the water-bath. Examine after 5, 20 and 30 min.

The normal Hb control solution will remain clear for 30–40 min, whereas, in the presence of an unstable Hb, a precipitate will form within 5 min, becoming flocculent by 20 min. Haemoglobins such as Hb E and Hb H, which are slightly unstable, will give a slight precipitate at 20 min. This test is therefore useful for discriminating between Hb C and Hb E, as Hb C is stable.

Comparison of the heat-instability and isopropanol tests

Both tests seem to be equally sensitive. The heat-instability test has the disadvantage that it requires a water-bath adjusted to 50°C. However, the isopropopanol test, although carried out at 37°C, has the disadvantage that Hb F starts to precipitate in about 15 min and 'false-positive' results may thus be obtained if the Hb F content of the blood is raised.

DETECTION OF HAEMOGLOBIN M

Several types of Hb M are known which differ from methaemoglobin A (Hi A) and also, in subtle ways, from each other; indeed, each type has its own special characteristics. They can be distinguished from Hi A by spectroscopy and also by electrophoresis.

Spectral analysis of Hb M

Each type of Hb M has its own distinct spectrum. Hi A has two absorption maxima, at

498 nm and 630 nm, whilst the maxima of the Hb Ms are shifted to slightly lower wavelengths. The maxima for oxyHb are 540 and 576 nm, whilst deoxyHb has one peak at 555 nm. Also, when potassium cyanide (KCN) is added to Hi A, the conversion to HiCN is fast and complete, whilst the reaction of the Hb Ms with KCN is slower, and complete conversion is not always achieved.

Preparation of methaemoglobin A

Lyse washed red cells with water to give a concentration of about 1 g Hb per l. Then convert the Hb to Hi by the addition of 5 µl of 0.1 mol/l potassium ferricyanide per ml of lysate. Leave for 10 min at room temperature (18–25°C). Then record the spectrum of Hi A on an automatic scanning spectrophotometer.

Then scan the spectrum of a water lysate of the suspected Hb M. If a Hb M is present, the spectrum will reflect the admixture of Hb A with the Hb M. If the spectrophotometer is set to a fixed wavelength of 630 nm, then conversion of Hi to HiCN can be followed by the addition of 50 µl of 1 mol/l KCN per ml of lysate. The spectrum of one Hb M is shown in Fig. 11.10.

Electrophoretic separation of Hb Ms

If a Hb M is suspected, prepare a lysate without KCN, thus avoiding any conversion to HiCN. Compare the sample against Hb A and Hi A. Some Hb Ms can be separated on alkaline electrophoresis, on which Hi A runs slightly cathodally to Hb A. Clearer results can be obtained by starch gel electrophoresis in phosphate buffer at pH 7.1. Prepare Hi A as for spectral analysis, but at a concentration of 20 g/l.

Stock buffer, pH 7.1. Disodium hydrogen phosphate (Na$_2$HPO$_4$) 13.3 g; potassium dihydrogen phosphate (KH$_2$PO$_4$) 2.15 g; water to 2 l.

Working buffer. Stock buffer 60 ml; water to 300 ml.

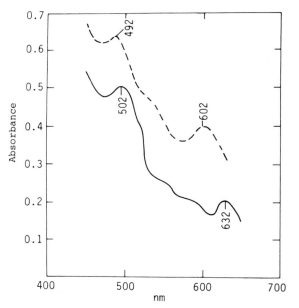

Fig. 11.10 Absorption maxima of methaemoglobins in the range 450–650 nm. —— Normal methaemoglobin; ---- Hb M Saskatoon. (Reference 17, by kind permission of the authors and the publishers).

Method

Starch should be mixed with the working buffer and the gel prepared as described on p. 188. Fill the electrode compartments of the system with undiluted stock buffer and then carry out electrophoresis. Hb Ms migrate more slowly than Hi A.

Altered affinity haemoglobins

Electrophoresis techniques may or may not be helpful, depending on whether the amino acid substitution has involved a charge change.

The most important investigation is the measurement of the oxygen dissociation curve (p. 172). The most significant finding is a decreased Hill's constant ('n' value), since this can only come about by a change in the structure of Hb. The p_{50} may be either increased or decreased. It has to be borne in mind that the p_{50} alone may be modified by other factors, e.g. by the high concentration of 2,3DPG in pyruvate kinase deficiency.

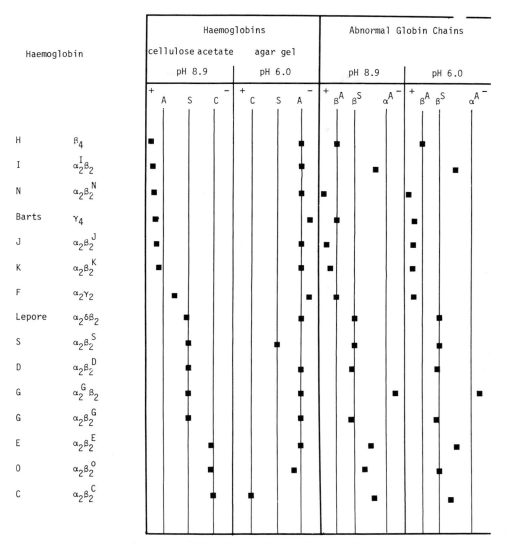

Fig. 11.11 Comparison of relative mobilities of some abnormal haemoglobins by various methods (adapted from Ref. 32). The positions of Hb A, Hb S and Hb C and their corresponding chains are indicated by the vertical lines.

SUGGESTED USE OF ELECTROPHORETIC TECHNIQUES IN THE ANALYSIS OF HAEMOGLOBINS

1. *Routine analysis*
   Cellulose acetate: tris buffer, pH 8.9, or tris/barbitone (discontinuous) buffer, pH 9.1/8.6.
2. *Demonstration and estimation of Hb A_2*

   a. Cellulose acetate: tris buffer, pH 9.1.
   b. Microcolumn chromatography.
3. *Demonstration and estimation of Hb Barts and Hb H*
   Cellulose acetate: phosphate buffer, pH 7.0.
4. *Separation of Hb S from Hb D and Hb G*
   Agar gel: citrate buffer, pH 6.0.
5. *Separation of Hb C from Hb E and Hb O*
   a. Agar gel: citrate buffer, pH 6.0.
   b. Isopropanol stability test.

6. *Separation of Hb I from Hb H*
Cellulose acetate: phosphate buffer, pH 7.0.

7. *Identification of variant chains*
Globin-chain separation at pH 8.6 and pH 6.0.

The relative mobilities of some abnormal haemoglobins by various methods are shown in Fig. 11.11.

REFERENCES

[1] BETKE, K., MARTI, H. R. and SCHLICHT, I. (1959). Estimation of small percentages of foetal haemoglobin. *Nature (London)*, **184**, 1877.

[2] BOYER, S. H., FAINER, D. C. and NAUGHTON. M. A. (1963). Myoglobin inherited structural variation in man. *Science*, **140**, 1228.

[3] CARRELL, R. W. and KAY, R. (1972). A simple method for the detection of unstable haemoglobins. *British Journal of Haematology*, **23**, 615.

[4] CHERNOFF, A. I. and PETTIT, N. M. Jnr (1964). The amino acid composition of haemoglobin: III. Qualitative method for identifying abnormalities of the polypeptide chains of haemoglobin. *Blood*, **24**, 750.

[5] CLEGG, J. B., NAUGHTON, M. A. and WEATHERALL, D. J. (1966). Abnormal human haemoglobins: separation and characterisation of α and β chains by chromatography and the determination of two new variants, Hb Chesapeake and Hb J (Bangkok). *Journal of Molecular Biology*, **19**, 91.

[6] CLEGG, J. B. and WEATHERALL, D. J. (1976). Molecular basis of thalassaemia. *British Medical Bulletin*, **32**, 262.

[7] DACIE, J. V., GRIMES, A. J., MEISLER, A., STEINGOLD, L., HEMSTED, E. H., BEAVEN, G. H. and WHITE, J. C. (1969). Hereditary Heinz-body anaemia. A report of studies on five patients with mild anaemia. *British Journal of Haematology*, **10**, 338.

[8] EFREMOV, C. D., HUISMAN, T. H. J., BOWMAN, K., WRIGHTSTONE, R. N. and SCHROEDER, W. A. (1974). Microchromatography of hemoglobins. II. A rapid method for the determination of hemoglobin A_2. *Journal of Laboratory and Clinical Medicine*, **83**, 657.

[9] GAMMACK, D. B., HUEHNS, E. R., LEHMANN, H. and SHOOTER, E. M. (1961). The abnormal polypeptide chains in a number of haemoglobin variants. *Acta Genetica et Statistica Medica*, **11**, 1.

[10] GERALD, P. G. (1966). 'The methemoglobinemias' in *Metabolic Basis of Inherited Disease*, Eds. J. B. Stanbury, J. B. Wyngaarden and D. S. Fredrickson, p. 1069. McGraw-Hill, New York.

[11] GRAHAM, J. L. and GRUNBAUM, B. W. (1963). A rapid method for microelectrophoresis and quantitation of hemoglobin on cellulose acetate. American Journal of Clinical Pathology, 39, 567.

[12] HUNTSMAN, R. G., BARCLAY, G. P. T., CANNING, D. M. and DAWSON, G. I. (1970). A rapid whole blood solubility test to differentiate the sickle-cell trait from sickle-cell anaemia. *Journal of Clinical Pathology*, **23**, 781.

[13] ITANO, H. A. and PAULING, L. (1949). A rapid diagnostic test for sickle cell anemia. *Blood*, **4**, 66.

[14] JONXIS, J. H. F. and VISSER, H. K. A. (1956). Determination of low percentages of fetal hemoglobin in blood of normal children. *American Medical Association Journal of Diseases of Children*, **92**, 588.

[15] JOSEPHSON, A. M., MASRI, M. S., SINGER, L., DWORKIN, D., and SINGER, K. (1958). Starch block electrophoretic studies on human hemoglobin solutions. II. Results in cord blood, thalassemia and other hematologic disorders: comparison with Tiselius electrophoresis. *Blood*, **13**, 543.

[16] KUNKEL, H. G., CEPPELLINI, R., MÜLLER-EBERHARD, U. and WOLF, J. (1957). Observations on the minor basic hemoglobin component in the blood of normal individuals and patients with thalassemia. *Journal of Clinical Investigation*. **36**, 1615.

[17] LEHMANN, H. and HUNTSMAN, R. G. (1974). *Man's Haemoglobins*. 2nd edn. North-Holland Publishing Company, Amsterdam.

[18] LINGREL, J. B. and BORSOOK, H. (1963). A comparison of amino acid incorporation in the hemoglobin and ribosomes of marrow erythroid cells and circulating reticulocytes of severely anemic rabbits. *Biochemistry*, **2**, 309.

[19] MARDER, V. J. and CONLEY, C. L. (1959). Electrophoresis of hemoglobin on agar gels: frequency of hemoglobin D in a negro population. *Bulletin of the Johns Hopkins Hospital*, **105**, 77.

[20] MARENGO-ROWE, A. J. (1965). Rapid electrophoresis and quantitation of haemoglobins on cellulose acetate. *Journal of Clinical Pathology*, **18**, 790.

[21] POULIK, M. D. (1957). Starch gel electrophoresis in a discontinuous system of buffers. *Nature* (London), **180**, 1477.

[22] SCHMIDT, R. M. and BROSIOUS, E. M. (1976). *Basic laboratory methods of hemoglobinopathy detection*. US Dept. of Health, Education and Welfare Publication No. (CDC) 77-8266. Center for Disease Control, Atlanta.

[23] SHEPARD, M. K., WEATHERALL, D. J. and CONLEY, C. L. (1962). Semi-quantitative estimation of the distribution of fetal hemoglobin in red cell populations. *Bulletin of the Johns Hopkins Hospital*, **110**, 293.

[24] SINGER, K., CHERNOFF, A. I. and SINGER, L. (1951). Studies on abnormal hemoglobins: I. Their demonstrations in sickle cell anemia and other hematologic disorders by means of alkali denaturation. *Blood*, **6**, 413.

[25] SMITHIES, O. (1959). An improved procedure for starch-gel electrophoresis: further variations in the serum proteins of normal individuals. *Biochemical Journal*, **71**, 585.

[26] WEATHERALL, D. J. and CLEGG, J. B. (1981). *The Thalassaemia Syndromes*, 3rd edn. Blackwell Scientific Publications, Oxford.

[27] WEATHERALL, D. J., GILLIES, H. M., CLEGG, J. B., BLANKSON, J. A., MUSTAPHA, D., BOI-DOKU, F. S. and CHAUNHURY, D. A. (1971). Preliminary surveys for the prevalence of the thalassaemia genes in some African populations. *Annals of Tropical Medicine and Parasitology*, **65**, 253.

[28] WHITE, J. M. (1976). The unstable haemoglobins. *British Medical Bulletin*, **32**, 219.

[29] WHITE, J. M., BRAIN, M. C. and ALI, M. A. M. (1971). Globin synthesis in sideroblastic anaemia. I. α and β peptide chain synthesis. *British Journal of Haematology*, **20**, 263.

[30] WHITE, J. M. and DACIE, J. V. (1971). The unstable haemoglobins—molecular and clinical features. *Progress in Hematology*, **7**, 69.

[31] International committee for standardization in hematology (1978). Recommendations of a system for identifying abnormal hemoglobins. *Blood*, **52**, 1065.

[32] International committee for standardization in hematology (1978). Simple electrophoretic system for presumptive identifications of abnormal hemoglobins. *Blood*, **52**, 1058.

[33] International committee for standardization in haematology (1978). Recommendations for selected methods for quantitative estimation of Hb A_2 and for Hb A_2 reference preparation. *British Journal of Haematology*, **38**, 573.

[34] WALFORD, D. M. and DEACON, R. (1976). Alpha-thalassaemia trait in various racial groups in the United Kingdom. Characterization of a variant of alpha-thalassaemia in Indians. *British Journal of Haematology*, **34**, 193.

12

Laboratory methods used in the investigation of paroxysmal nocturnal haemoglobinuria (PNH)

Paroxysmal nocturnal haemoglobinuria is an acquired disorder in which the patient's red cells are abnormally sensitive to lysis by normal constituents of plasma. In its classical form it is characterized by haemoglobinuria during sleep (nocturnal haemoglobinuria), jaundice and haemosiderinuria. Not uncommonly, however, PNH presents as an obscure anaemia without obvious evidence of intravascular haemolysis or develops in a patient suffering apparently from aplastic anaemia or more rarely from myelosclerosis or leukaemia.[8,12,31]

PNH red cells are unusually susceptible to lysis by complement.[11,28] This can be demonstrated in vitro by a variety of tests, e.g. the acidified-serum (Ham),[11,16] sucrose,[14,16] thrombin,[7] cold-antibody lysis,[9] inulin[4] and cobra-venom[17] tests. In the acidified-serum, inulin and cobra-venom tests, complement is activated via the alternative (Pillemer) pathway, while in the cold-antibody test, and probably the thrombin test, complement is activated by the classical sequence initiated through antigen–antibody interaction. In the sucrose lysis test a low ionic strength is thought to lead to the binding of IgG molecules non-specifically to the cell membrane and to the subsequent activation of complement via the classical sequence. In addition, the alternative pathway appears to be activated.[20] In each test PNH cells undergo lysis because of their greatly increased sensitivity to lysis by complement.

Minor degrees of increased lysis may be observed in the cold-antibody lysis and sucrose tests with the red cells from a variety of dyserythropoietic anaemias, e.g. aplastic anaemia, megaloblastic anaemia and myelosclerosis.[5,18] Weak positive results in these tests have thus to be interpreted with care. PNH red cells, however, almost always undergo major amounts of lysis in these tests which thus have considerable value as screening procedures. A positive acidified-serum test is probably specific for the PNH red-cell abnormality and the cobra-venom test can also be carried out in such a way as to make positive tests specific for PNH.[17] A characteristic feature of positive tests for PNH is that not all the patient's cells undergo lysis, even if the conditions of the test are made optimal for lysis (Fig. 12.1). This implies that only a proportion of any patient's PNH red-cell population is hypersensitive to lysis by complement. This population varies from patient to patient, and there is a direct relationship between the proportion of red cells that can be lysed (in any of the diagnostic tests) and the severity of in-vivo haemolysis.

The phenomenon of some red cells being sensitive to complement lysis and some insensitive was studied quantitatively by Rosse and Dacie who obtained two-component complement sensitivity curves in a series of PNH patients.[28] Later, Rosse and his co-workers reported that in some cases three populations of red cells could be demonstrated:[25,26,27]

1. Very sensitive (Type-III) cells, 10–15 times as sensitive as normal cells.

2. Cells of medium sensitivity (Type-II), 3–5 times as sensitive as normal cells.

3. Cells of normal sensitivity (Type-I).

In vivo, the proportion of Type-III cells parallels the severity of the patient's illness, and it is these Type-III cells which are lysed in the acidified-serum test. In the sucrose and cold-antibody lysis tests, however, both Type-III and Type-II cells undergo lysis. Both types of cells bind on more complement component C3 than normal, but with Type-III cells there is, in addition, increased sensi-

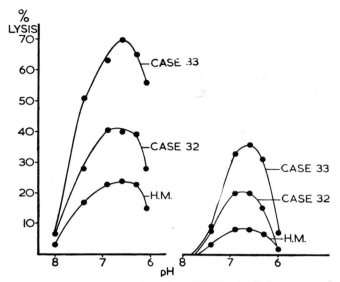

Fig. 12.1 Effect of pH on lysis in vitro of PNH red cells by human sera. The red cells of three patients (Cases 32, 33 and H.M. of different sensitivity) were used, and two fresh normal sera, one serum being more potent than the other.

tivity to the terminal complement components C5b–C9.[24] It is this double mechanism of increased sensitivity which makes Type-III cells so hypersensitive to complement lysis.

PNH is a clonal disorder of stem cells[23] and it is possible to demonstrate that the granulocytes and platelets are hypersensitive to complement lysis in appropriate immune systems.[1] Remarkably, too, it has been found that a variety of chemicals, in particular sulphydryl compounds, can act on normal red cells in vitro so as to increase their complement sensitivity. In this way PNH-like red cells can be created in the laboratory and can be used as useful reagents (p. 205).

Acidified-serum test (Ham test)

Principle. The patient's red cells are exposed at 37°C to the action of normal or the patient's own serum suitably acidified to the optimum pH for lysis (pH 6.5–7.0) (Fig. 12.1).

The patient's red cells can be obtained from defibrinated, heparinized, oxalated, citrated or EDTA blood, and the test can be satisfactorily carried out even on cells which have been stored at 4°C for up to 2–3 weeks in ACD solution or in Alsever's solution, if kept sterile. The patient's serum is best obtained by defibrination, for if in PNH it is obtained from blood allowed to clot in the ordinary way at 37°C or at room temperature it will almost certainly be found to be markedly lysed. Normal serum should similarly be obtained by defibrination, but serum derived from blood allowed to clot spontaneously at room temperature or at 37°C can be used. Normal serum known to be strongly lytic to PNH red cells is to be preferred to patient's serum, the lytic potentiality of which is unknown. However, if the test is positive using normal serum it is important, particularly if the patient appears not to be suffering from overt intravascular haemolysis, to obtain a positive result using the *patient's* serum, in order to exclude HEMPAS (see below).

The variability between the sera of individuals in their capacity to lyse PNH red cells is shown in Fig. 12.1. The activity of a single individual's serum also varies from time to time[32] and it is always important to include in any test, as a positive control, a sample of known PNH cells or artificially created 'PNH-like' cells (see p. 205).

The sera should be used fresh, i.e. within a few hours of collection. Their lytic potency is retained for several months at $-70°C$, but at $4°C$ and even at $-20°C$ they deteriorate within a few days.

Method

Deliver 0.5 ml samples of fresh normal serum, group AB or ABO-compatible with the patient's blood, into six (three pairs) of 75×12 mm glass tubes. Place two tubes at $56°C$ for 10–30 min in order to inactivate complement. Keep the other two pairs of tubes at room temperature and add to the serum in two of the tubes one-tenth volumes (0.05 ml) of 0.2 mol/l HCl. Add similar volumes of acid subsequently to the inactivated serum samples. Then place all the tubes in a $37°C$ water-bath.

While the serum samples are being dealt with, wash samples of the patient's red cells and of normal red cells (compatible with the normal serum) twice in 9.0 g/l NaCl (saline) and prepare 50% suspensions in saline. Then add one-tenth volumes of each of these cell suspensions (0.05 ml) to single tubes containing unacidified fresh serum, acidified fresh serum and acidified inactivated serum, respectively (Table 12.1). Mix the contents carefully and leave the tubes at $37°C$. Centrifuge them after about 1 h.

Add 0.05 ml of each cell suspension to 0.55 ml of water so as to prepare a standard for subsequent quantitative measurement of lysis and retain 0.5 ml of serum for use as a blank. For the measurement of lysis, deliver 0.3 ml volumes of the test serum supernatants, the blank serum and the lysed cell suspension equivalent to 100% lysis into 5 ml of 0.4 ml/l ammonia or Drabkin's reagent. Measure the lysis in a photoelectric colorimeter using a yellow-green (e.g. Ilford 625) filter or in a spectrophotometer at a wavelength of 540 nm.

If the test cells are from a case of PNH, they will undergo definite, although, as already mentioned, incomplete lysis in the acidified serum. Very much less lysis, or even no lysis at all, will be visible in the unacidified serum. No lysis will be brought about by the acidified inactivated serum. The normal control sample of cells should not undergo lysis in any of the three tubes.

In PNH 10–50% lysis is usually obtained, when lysis is measured as liberated haemoglobin. Exceptionally, there may be as much as 80% lysis or as little as 5%.

The red cells of patients who have been transfused undergo less lysis, because the normal transfused cells, despite circulation in the patient, behave normally. In PNH, it is characteristic that a young cell (reticulocyte-rich) population, such as the upper red-cell layer obtained by centrifugation, undergoes more lysis than the red cells derived from mixed whole blood.

Significance of the acidified-serum test

A positive acidified-serum test, carried out with proper controls, denotes the PNH abnormality (or

Table 12.1 The acidified-serum test

Reagents	Test (ml)			Controls (ml)		
	1	2	3	4	5	6
Fresh normal serum	0.5	0.5	0	0.5	0.5	0
Heat-inactivated normal serum	0	0	0.5	0	0	0.5
0.2 mol/l HCl	0	0.05	0.05	0	0.05	0.05
50% patient's red cells	0.05	0.05	0.05	0	0	0
50% normal red cells	0	0	0	0.05	0.05	0.05
Lysis (in a positive test)	Trace (2%)	+++ (30%)	—	—	—	—

abnormalities), and unless the test is positive PNH cannot be diagnosed. The only other disorder which at first sight may appear to give a clear-cut positive test is a rare congenital dyserythropoietic anaemia, CDA Type II or HEMPAS.[6,34] In contrast to PNH, however, HEMPAS red cells undergo lysis in only a proportion (about 30%) of normal sera; moreover, they do *not* undergo lysis in the patient's own acidified serum and the sucrose lysis test is negative. In HEMPAS, lysis appears to be due to the presence on the red cells of an unusual antigen which reacts with a complement-fixing IgM antibody ('anti-HEMPAS') present in many normal sera.[34]

Heating at 56°C inactivates the lytic system and, if there is lysis in inactivated serum, the test cannot be considered positive. Markedly spherocytic red cells or effete normal red cells may lyse in acidified serum, probably due to the lowered pH, and such cells may lyse, too, in acidified inactivated serum.

It must be stressed that PNH red cells are not unduly sensitive to lysis by a lowered pH per se. The addition of the acid adjusts the pH of the serum-cell mixture to the optimum for the activity of the lytic system. As is shown in Fig. 12.1, it is possible to construct pH–lysis curves, if different concentrations of acid are used. The optimum pH for lysis is between pH 6.5 and 7.0 (measurements made after the addition of the red cells to the serum).

THROMBIN TEST

Crosby observed that PNH red cells underwent more lysis in acidified serum if thrombin was added.[7] He suggested that this reaction might be a useful test for PNH. Much of the effect seems to be due to anti-human-red-cell antibodies present in varying amounts in commercial preparations of thrombin,[3] or to the presence of complement components. In practice, the thrombin test is seldom if ever positive when the simple acidified-serum test is completely negative.

COBRA-VENOM TEST[17]

In this test complement is activated via the alternative pathway by the addition to serum of partially purified cobra venom. In Kabakçi, Rosse and Logue's hands the percentage of lysis of a series of PNH red-cell samples was almost identical with the PNH 'sensitive-cell' percentage as determined by the complement lysis sensitivity test.[17] The parallelism between the results of the cobra-venom test and the acidified-serum test was less close. Lysis was only observed in patients thought on other grounds to have PNH and the results in patients with myeloproliferative disorders or aplastic anaemia were strictly negative.

The cobra-venom test seems likely to prove to be useful and reliable in the diagnosis of PNH. As, however, cobra venom contains factors, probably phospholipases, which lyse normal red cells in the absence of serum, the test has the disadvantage that the factor in the venom activating C3 proactivator in serum has to be separated from the crude venom by column chromatography before it can be used. Details were given by Kabakçi et al.[17]

SCREENING TESTS FOR PNH

'Heat resistance test'[15]

Allow blood to clot at 37°C and inspect for spontaneous lysis. A positive test is not specific for PNH although, characteristically, PNH blood lyses rapidly and markedly, i.e. haemoglobin can be seen diffusing from the clot into the serum as soon as the clot has retracted. Exceptionally, in patients with autoimmune haemolytic anaemia in whom there is very marked spherocytosis, the clot may undergo almost as rapid lysis.

Inulin Test[4]

Place 1 drop (50 μl) of inulin (100 g/l in saline) in one of two 75 × 10 mm glass tubes. Deliver 3 ml of freshly collected blood into each of the tubes, which are then stoppered, gently mixed and allowed to stand at 37°C for at least 30–45 min until the clot has retracted. Then centrifuge the tubes and inspect the supernatant serum for lysis. Lysis in the inulin-containing tube with less lysis (or no lysis) in the control tube comprises a positive test. A control test using normal blood should always be put up at the same time. There should be no lysis or no difference in lysis between the two tubes of the control.

'Cold-antibody lysis' test

The greatly increased sensitivity of PNH red cells to complement can be dramatically demonstrated if the cells are suspended in dilutions of a high-titre cold agglutinin (anti-I) in the presence of fresh human serum complement.[9] Using suitable dilutions of the reagents, PNH red cells undergo marked lysis whereas normal red cells undergo little or no lysis. This reaction, the basis of the cold-antibody lysis test, is, however, not quite specific for PNH as the red cells from some patients with various types of dyserythropoietic anaemia may undergo minor, or rarely moderate, amounts of lysis.[18]

An anti-I serum is required (titre at 4°C, >8000), which when used unacidified fails to lyse at room temperature most normal human red cells, i.e. a typical anti-I serum from a patient suffering from the cold-haemagglutinin disease. Such sera keep their properties for years if frozen at −20°C. The serum should be distributed in 0.5–1.0 ml volumes in a number of tubes to avoid repeated thawing and freezing.

Method

Make a 1 in 50 or 1 in 100 dilution of the anti-I serum in undiluted fresh normal group AB or ABO-compatible serum. Deliver two 0.5 ml volumes of the serum into 75 × 12 mm tubes and add 0.5 ml volumes of a 5% suspension of washed normal and test (? PNH) red cells to the serum samples, respectively. Add a further 0.5 ml volume of the washed test cells to a tube containing 0.5 ml of saline to serve as a standard for the quantitative measurement of lysis. Retain 0.5 ml of the serum mixture as a blank. After 1 h at room temperature centrifuge the two tubes containing the serum-cell suspensions, and add 0.3 ml volumes of their supernatants to 5 ml of 0.4 ml/l ammonia or Drabkin's reagent. Measure lysis in a photoelectric colorimeter using a yellow-green (e.g. Ilford 625) filter or in a spectrophotometer at a wavelength of 540 nm. Add 0.3 ml of the diluted red-cell suspension to a further 5 ml of the diluent to give a standard for 100% lysis.

If a powerfully complement-fixing (i.e. lytic) anti-serum is available, a very sensitive anti-I lysis test can be carried out using diluted human AB serum as complement. This is the basis of the complement lysis sensitivity test and the less elaborate 'four-tube complement lysis sensitivity' test.[28] These tests are probably more specific for PNH than is the original and very simple cold-antibody lysis test.

Sucrose lysis test[13,14,16]

An iso-osmotic solution of sucrose (92.4 g/l) is required. This can be stored at 4°C for up to 2–3 weeks.

For the test, set up two tubes, one containing 0.05 ml of fresh normal group AB or ABO-compatible serum diluted in 0.85 ml of sucrose solution, and the other 0.05 ml of serum diluted in 0.85 ml of saline. Add to each tube 0.1 ml of a 50% suspension of washed red cells. After incubation at 37°C for 30 min, centrifuge the tubes and examine for lysis. If lysis is visible in the sucrose-containing tube, measure this in a photoelectric colorimeter, using the tube containing saline as a blank and a tube containing 0.1 ml of the red-cell suspension in 0.9 ml of 0.4 ml/l ammonia in place of the sucrose-serum mixture as a standard for 100% lysis.

Interpretation

The sucrose lysis test is based on the fact that red cells adsorb complement components from serum at low ionic concentrations.[20,22] PNH cells, because of their great sensitivity will undergo lysis but normal red cells do not. The red cells from some cases of leukaemia[5] or myelosclerosis[33] may undergo a small amount of lysis, almost always <10%; in such cases the acidified-serum test is usually negative and PNH should not be diagnosed. In PNH, lysis varies from 10% to 80%, but exceptionally may be as little as 5%. Sucrose lysis and acidified-serum lysis[19] of PNH red cells are fairly closely correlated. The sucrose lysis test is typically negative in HEMPAS (see p. 203).

PNH-LIKE RED CELLS

By treating normal red cells with certain chemicals it is possible to increase their complement sensitivity so that they take on many of the characteristics of PNH cells.[29] The chemicals include sulphydryl compounds such as L-cysteine, reduced glutathione (GSH) and 2-aminoethyl*iso*thiouronium bromide (AET). AET is especially useful, and AET cells can be used conveniently as a positive control for in-vitro lysis tests for PNH.[32]

Preparation of AET cells[30]

Prepare an 8 g/l solution of AET and adjust its pH to 8.0 with 5 mol/l NaOH. Collect normal blood into ACD and wash it twice in 9 g/l NaCl (saline). Add 1 volume of the packed cells to 4 volumes of the AET solution in a 75 × 12 mm glass tube which is then stoppered. Mix the contents gently and place the tube at 37°C for 10–20 min. (According to Jenkins, the optimal time of incubation varies from red cell sample to red cell sample.[16]) Then wash the cells repeatedly with large volumes of saline until the supernatant is colourless. The red cells are now ready for use.

RED-CELL ACETYLCHOLINESTERASE (AChE) IN PNH

Red-cell AChE activity is often diminished in PNH.[2,10,21] It seems likely that the activity of the enzyme is zero in sensitive (Type-III) PNH red cells, but because only a proportion, often a minority, of the red cells are abnormal in PNH, a lowered red-cell AChE activity may not be demonstrable in whole blood.[21] AChE assay has, therefore, only limited diagnostic value. The significance of the lowered AChE activity of the PNH red cell and its relation to lysis, if any, is not known. The AChE activity of AET cells is reduced but, in contrast to PNH, the reduced activity is not correlated with lysis in acidified serum or sucrose.[29]

Assay of acetylcholinesterase (AChE) activity

In the 4th edition of this book (p. 506), Michel's electrometric method was described. An alternative method depends on the release by AChE of sulphydryl (SH) groups from a substrate of acetylthiocholine.[35] The SH groups react with 5,5'-dithiobis-(2-nitrobenzoic acid) to give a yellow colour which can be measured spectrophotometrically. AChE activity is expressed in u/ml of packed red cells, the unit being the amount of enzyme converting 1 μmol of substrate per min. The following technique, based on Weber's method,[35] is simple and reliable.

Reagents

Buffer. 0.05 mol/l phosphate buffer in saline, pH 7.2.

Substrate. 0.031 mol/l acetylthiocholine iodide (available from Boehringer as 0.156 mol/l; this stock should be diluted 1 in 5 for use).

DTNB Reagent. 0.25 mmol/l 5,5'-dithiobis-(2-nitrobenzoic acid) in 0.05 mol/l phosphate buffer, pH 7.2

Method[35]

Defibrinated, heparinized, EDTA or ACD blood can be used. AChE is relatively stable and blood can be kept for at least 3 days at 20°C without apparent loss of activity.

Determine the PCV of the blood to be tested. Place 0.1 ml of blood in a 100 × 12 mm tube and wash it three times in 9 g/l NaCl (saline). Remove the last supernatant as completely as possible. Resuspend the red cells in 10 ml of buffer. Dilute 1 ml of this suspension with 4 ml of buffer and, after mixing, pipette 1 ml into a silica cuvette (1 cm optical pathway) containing 2 ml of DTNB reagent. Leave the cuvette for 3 min at 30°C and then add 0.1 ml of substrate. Mix the suspension and measure the absorbance in a spectrophotometer at a wavelength of 412 nm or in a photoelectric colorimeter with a blue (e.g. Ilford 622) filter. Make readings every 1 min for 6 min, against a blank of 2.1 ml of DTNB reagent and 1 ml of cell suspension. Remix the contents of the cuvette prior to each reading. Calculate the mean change in absorbance per 1 min (ΔA/min). Set up a control test to correct for non-enzymatic hydrolysis using buffer instead of red-cell suspension. Deduct the ΔA/min of the control from the ΔA/min of the test solution. This effect is relatively small, however, and need not be taken into account in routine diagnostic tests.

Calculation

AChE activity (u/l of red cells) is given by:

$$\frac{\Delta A/\text{min}}{\text{PCV}} \times \frac{500 \times 10^3 \times 3.1}{13.6 \times d}$$

$$= \frac{\Delta A/\text{min}}{\text{PCV}} \times 114 \times 10^3,$$

where ΔA/min = absorbance change per min at 412 nm, 500 = blood dilution factor, 10^3 = factor converting ml to l, 3.1 = volume of reacting solution, 13.6 = micromolar extinction coefficient of DTNB at 412 nm, and d = depth of optical pathway in cm (= 1 cm).

Normal range. 8–13 $\times 10^3$ u/l.

REFERENCES

[1] ASTER, R. H. and ENRIGHT, S. E. (1969). A platelet and granulocyte membrane defect in paroxysmal nocturnal hemoglobinuria: usefulness for the detection of platelet antibodies. *Journal of Clinical Investigation*, **48**, 1199.

[2] AUDITORE, J. V. and HARTMANN, R. C. (1959). Paroxysmal nocturnal hemoglobinuria: II. Erythrocyte acetylcholinesterase defect. *American Journal of Medicine*, **27**, 401.

[3] BLUM, S. F. and GARDNER, F. H. (1967). Paroxysmal nocturnal hemoglobinuria. Mechanism of the enhancement of hemolysis by bovine thrombin. *Blood*, **30**, 352.

[4] BRUBAKER, L. H., SCHABERG, D. R., JEFFERSON, D. H. and MENGEL, C.E. (1973). A potential rapid screening test for paroxysmal nocturnal hemoglobinuria. *New England Journal of Medicine*, **288**, 1059.

[5] CATOVSKY, D., LEWIS, S. M. and SHERMAN, D. (1971). Erythrocyte sensitivity to *in-vitro* lysis in leukaemia. *British Journal of Haematology*, **21**, 541.

[6] CROOKSTON, J. H., CROOKSTON, M. C., BURNIE, K. L., FRANCOMBE, W. H., DACIE, J. V., DAVIS, J. A. and LEWIS, S. M. (1969). Hereditary erythroblastic multinuclearity associated with a positive acidified-serum test: a type of congenital dyserythropoietic anaemia. *British Journal of Haematology*, **17**, 11.

[7] CROSBY, W. H. (1950). Paroxysmal nocturnal hemoglobinuria. A specific test for the disease based on the ability of thrombin to activate the hemolytic factor. *Blood*, **5**, 843.

[8] DACIE, J. V. and Lewis, S. M. (1972). Paroxysmal nocturnal haemoglobinuria: clinical manifestations, haematology and nature of the disease. *Series Haematologica*, **5**, 3.

[9] DACIE, J. V., LEWIS, S. M. and TILLS, D. (1960). Comparative sensitivity of the erythrocytes in paroxysmal nocturnal haemoglobinuria to haemolysis by acidified normal serum and by a high-titre cold antibody. *British Journal of Haematology*, **6**, 362.

[10] DE SANDRE, G. and GHIOTTO, G. (1958). Über die Bedeutung der Acetylcholinesterase der Erythrocyten. *Helvetica Medica Acta*, **25**, 235.

[11] HAM, T. H. and DINGLE, J. H. (1939). Studies on destruction of red blood cells. II. Chronic hemolytic anemia with paroxysmal nocturnal hemoglobinuria: certain immunological aspects of the hemolytic mechanism with special reference to serum complement. *Journal of Clinical Investigation*, **18**, 657.

[12] HANSEN, N. E. and KILLMAN, S.-A. (1968). Paroxysmal nocturnal haemoglobinuria. A clinical study. *Acta Medica Scandinavia*, **184**, 525.

[13] HARTMANN, R. C. and JENKINS, D. E. Jnr (1966). The 'sugar water' test for paroxysmal nocturnal hemoglobinuria. *New England Journal of Medicine*, **275**, 155.

[14] HARTMANN, R. C., JENKINS, D. E. Jnr and ARNOLD, A. B. (1970). Diagnostic specificity of sucrose hemolysis test for paroxysmal nocturnal hemoglobinuria. *Blood*, **35**, 462.

[15] HEGGLIN, R. and MAIER, C. (1944). The 'heat resistance' of erythrocytes. A specific test for the recognition of Marchiafava's anemia. *American Journal of Medical Sciences*, **207**, 624.

[16] JENKINS, D. E. Jnr (1979). Paroxysmal nocturnal hemoglobinuria hemolytic systems. In *A Seminar on Laboratory Management of Hemolysis*, p. 45–49. American Association of Blood Banks, Washington.

[17] KABAKCI, T., ROSSE, W. F. and LOGUE, G. L. (1972). The lysis of paroxysmal nocturnal haemoglobinuria red cells by serum and cobra factor. *British Journal of Haematology*, **23**, 693.

[18] LEWIS, S. M., DACIE, J. V. and TILLS, D. (1961). Comparison of the sensitivity to agglutination and haemolysis by a high-titre cold antibody of the erythrocytes of normal subjects and of patients with a variety of blood diseases including paroxysmal nocturnal haemoglobinuria. *British Journal of Haematology*, **7**, 64.

[19] LEWIS, S. M. and SIRCHIA, G. (1972). PNH: disease or defect? *British Journal of Haematology*, **23** (Suppl.), 71

[20] LOGUE, G. L., ROSSE, W. F. and ADAMS, J. P. (1973). Mechanisms of immune lysis of red blood cells in vitro. I. Paroxysmal nocturnal hemoglobinuria cells. *Journal of Clinical Investigation*, **52**, 1129.

[21] METZ, J., BRADLOW, B. A., LEWIS, S. M. and DACIE, J. V. (1960). The acetylcholinesterase activity of the erythrocytes in paroxysmal nocturnal haemoglobinuria in relation to the severity of the disease. *British Journal of Haematology*, **6**, 372.

[22] MOLLISON, P. H. and POLLEY, M. J. (1964). Uptake of γ-globulin and complement by red cells exposed to serum at low ionic strength. *Nature (London)*, **203**, 535.

[23] ONI, S. B., OSUNKOYA, B. O. and LUZZATTO, L. (1970). Paroxysmal nocturnal hemoglobinuria: evidence for monoclonal origin of abnormal red cells. *Blood*, **36**, 145.

[24] PARKMAN, C. H., ROSENFIELD, S. I., JENKINS, D. E. Jnr, THIEM, P. A. and LEDDY, J. P. (1979). Complement lysis of human erythrocytes. Differing susceptibility of two types of paroxysmal nocturnal hemoglobinuria cells to C5,6–9. *Journal of Clinical Investigation*, **64**, 428.

[25] ROSSE, W. F. (1972). The complement sensitivity of PNH cells. *Series Haematologica*, **5**, 101.

[26] ROSSE, W. F. (1973). Variations in the red cells in paroxysmal nocturnal haemoglobinuria. *British Journal of Haematology*, **24**, 327.

[27] ROSSE, W. F., ADAMS, J. P. and THORPE, A. M. (1974). The population of cells in paroxysmal nocturnal haemoglobinuria of intermediate sensitivity to complement lysis: significance and mechanism of increased immune lysis. *British Journal of Haematology*, **28**, 281.

[28] ROSSE, W. F. and DACIE, J. V. (1966). Immune lysis of normal human and paroxysmal nocturnal hemoglobinuria (PNH) red blood cells. I. The sensitivity of PNH red cells to lysis by complement and specific antibody. *Journal of Clinical Investigation*, **45**, 736.

[29] SIRCHIA, G. and FERRONE, S. (1972). "The laboratory substitutes of the red cell of paroxysmal nocturnal haemoglobinuria (PNH): PNH-like red cells." *Series Haematologica*, **5**, 137.

[30] SIRCHIA, G., FERRONE, S. and MERCURIALI, F. (1965). The action of two sulfhydryl compounds on normal human red cells. Relationship to red cells of paroxysmal nocturnal hemoglobinuria. *Blood* **25**, 502.

[31] SIRCHIA, G. and LEWIS, S. M. (1975). Paroxysmal nocturnal haemoglobinuria. *Clinics in Haematology*, **4**, 199.

[32] SIRCHIA, G., MARUBINI, E., MERCURIALI, F. and FERRONE, S. (1973). Study of two *in vitro* diagnostic tests for paroxysmal nocturnal haemoglobinuria. *British Journal of Haematology*, **24**, 751.

[33] STRATTON, F. and EVANS, D. I. K. (1967). Lysis of P.N.H. cells in solutions of low ionic strength. *British Journal of Haematology*, **13**, 862.

[34] VERWILGHEN, R. L., LEWIS, S. M., DACIE, J. V., CROOKSTON, J. H. and CROOKSTON, M. C. (1973). HEMPAS: Congenital dyserythropoietic anaemia (Type II). *Quarterly Journal of Medicine*, **42**, 257.

[35] WEBER, H. (1966). Rasche und einfache Ultramikromethode zur Bestimmung der serumcholinesterase. *Deutsche Medizinische Wochenschrift*, **91**, 1927.

13

Investigation of the haemostatic mechanism
(Written in collaboration with W. R. Pitney and M. Brozovic)

HAEMOSTATIC PLUG FORMATION

The spontaneous arrest of bleeding from a severed blood vessel is due to the formation of an impervious seal produced from the constituents of the blood at the site of injury. This haemostatic plug forms within a few minutes of trauma and is a complicated process involving vascular responses, platelet aggregation and activation of the blood coagulation mechanism. Reactions within these various components of haemostasis occur simultaneously and are mutually dependent. Defective haemostatic plug formation is manifested by spontaneous haemorrhage or abnormal bleeding following trauma or surgical intervention. Before considering the manner in which the haemostatic mechanism may be investigated, it is appropriate to discuss briefly the physiology of normal haemostasis.

Role of the blood vessel

Vessels with muscular coats contract following injury, thus assisting haemostatic plug formation by reducing blood flow. Vasoconstriction occurs, however, even in the microcirculation in vessels without smooth muscle cells. The mechanism appears to be humoral and it is probably due to the release of a vasoconstrictor substance from platelets during the process of platelet adhesion and aggregation.[7] This substance, thromboxane A_2, will be considered further in the section on platelets. The stimulus to haemostatic plug formation is damage to the vascular endothelium. The endothelial cell thus plays an active role in haemostasis; it synthesizes and secretes at least three substances which are involved in the formation and localization of the haemostatic plug. These are von Willebrand factor, prostacyclin and plasminogen activator. Von Willebrand factor (VIII:WF) is part of a molecular complex which also possesses factor VIII clotting activity.[2] It is involved in the adhesion of platelets to subendothelium and lack of this protein is the cause of the prolonged bleeding time in von Willebrand's disease. Prostacyclin (PGI_2) is synthesized from arachidonic acid in the endothelial cells; it is a powerful inhibitor of platelet aggregation[13] and prevents platelet deposition on normal vascular endothelium. It may help to localize the haemostatic plug to the site of vessel wall damage. Plasminogen activator is the enzyme which converts plasminogen to plasmin which in turn lyses fibrin.[4] Release of this enzyme is stimulated by vessel wall damage, and this property of the endothelial cell also assists in localizing the haemostatic plug. Exposed subendothelium provides a surface for platelet adhesion and also activates the blood coagulation mechanism with eventual production of fibrin which reinforces the plug.

Platelet–vessel wall interaction

The primary haemostatic plug is composed essentially of a mass of aggregated platelets held together by fibrin. Normal platelets have the propensity to adhere to vascular subendothelium, and platelet adhesion is the first recognized step when the formation of haemostatic plugs is studied in the experimental animal. Platelet adhesion at the site of vessel wall injury is followed by the appearance of a mass of aggregated platelets which occludes the lumen of the vessel and arrests blood flow. Within a short time, fibrin is seen at the periphery and in the

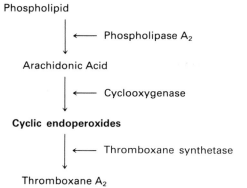

Phospholipid

$\longleftarrow$ Phospholipase A_2

Arachidonic Acid

$\longleftarrow$ Cyclooxygenase

Cyclic endoperoxides

$\longleftarrow$ Thromboxane synthetase

Thromboxane A_2

Fig. 13.1 Formation of thromboxane A_2 from phospholipid in the platelet membrane.

Table 13.1 Nomenclature of blood coagulation factors

Factor	Synonym or description
I	Fibrinogen (FI seldom used)
II	Prothrombin (FII seldom used)
V	Proaccelerin, labile factor
VII	Proconvertin, stable factor
VIII:C	FVIII coagulant activity, antihaemophilic factor (AHF)
VIII:WF	FVIII activity which corrects prolonged bleeding time in von Willebrand's disease. Ristocetin cofactor activity?
VIIIR:Ag	Protein precipitated by specific rabbit antiserum
IX	Christmas factor, plasma thromboplastin component (PTC)
X	Stuart-Prower factor
XI	Plasma thromboplastin antecedent
XII	Hageman factor, contact factor
XIII	Fibrin-stabilizing factor (FSF), transamidase
Prekallikrein	Fletcher factor
HMW (high molecular weight) kininogen	Fitzgerald factor

interstices of the platelet aggregates and the platelets become degranulated and finally structureless on microscopy.

The physiological stimulus to platelet aggregation appears to be exposure of the platelet membrane to collagen fibrils in the subendothelium or to adenosine diphosphate (ADP) liberated from adherent platelets.

Collagen, ADP, thrombin, adrenaline and serotonin may all induce platelet aggregation by activating the enzyme phospholipase A_2 in the platelet membrane, thereby causing the conversion of membrane phospholipid to a number of fatty acids, including arachidonic acid (Fig. 13.1). Arachidonic acid is converted by the platelet enzyme cyclooxygenase to cyclic endoperoxides which are further converted by the enzyme thromboxane synthetase to thromboxane A_2. Thromboxane A_2 is a powerful inducer of platelet aggregation and its production also causes the release of ADP from the dense granules of the platelet. This acts as a trigger for further platelet aggregation.

BLOOD COAGULATION[5]

The role of blood coagulation in haemostatic plug formation, although obviously important, is not fully understood. Haemostatic plugs are composed mainly of aggregated platelets, but fibrin is necessary to stabilize the plug and bind it to the vessel wall. Fibrin is the end-result of blood coagulation and its appearance in the plugs indicates that thrombin has been generated locally. Patients with deficiencies of coagulation factors and those receiving heparin may form haemostatic plugs in the normal time, but the plugs tend to be unstable and rebleeding commonly occurs if they are disturbed.

Plasma contains at least ten proteins directly involved in blood coagulation, and two further proteins involved in the kallikrein–kinin system participate in the kinetics of the coagulation mechanism. Most coagulation factors are referred to by Roman numerals assigned to them by the International Committee for Nomenclature of Blood Clotting Factors, but fibrinogen and prothrombin are usually referred to by their proper names and not as factors I and II, respectively.[9] The numeral classification is shown in Table 13.1 alongside some of the commonly used synonyms. Clotting factors act either as substrates (zymogens) which under the influence of enzymes are themselves converted into active enzymes or they act as cofactors in complexes formed with enzyme and substrate. The enzymatic form of a coagulation factor is denoted by the suffix 'a' after the numeral.

Blood contains within itself all the constituents necessary for clotting, which readily occurs when shed blood comes into contact with a foreign surface. The process is known as the intrinsic

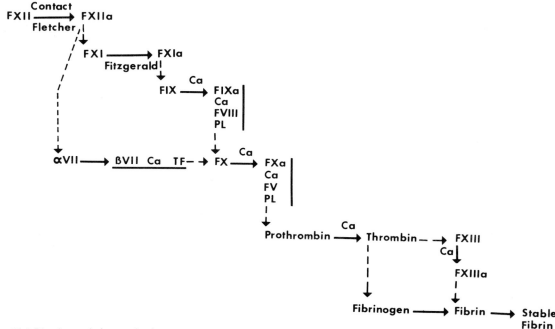

Fig. 13.2 Blood coagulation mechanism.

coagulation mechanism. Blood clotting is accelerated when extracts of various tissues (thromboplastins) are added and this process is known as the extrinsic coagulation mechanism. The extrinsic mechanism bypasses the initial time-consuming reactions of the intrinsic mechanism, but both mechanisms have a final common pathway. The distinction between the intrinsic and the extrinsic coagulation mechanisms is not as clear-cut as previously thought, and activation of the intrinsic mechanism also activates the extrinsic mechanism by an action of factor XIIa on factor VII. Both mechanisms may be studied separately in the laboratory, but they are integrated in the scheme of blood coagulation shown in Fig. 13.2.

The essential features of this scheme are that factor XII is converted into an active enzyme (fXIIa) by contact with a foreign surface and the reaction is accelerated in the presence of prekallikrein (Fletcher factor). Contact activation is delayed if blood is allowed to clot in plastic or siliconized-glass tubes and it is accelerated by the presence of foreign surfaces such as glass beads or kaolin. Factor XIIa converts factor XI into factor XIa, the reaction being facilitated by a high molecular-weight kininogen (Fitzgerald factor). Calcium ions

are not required up to this stage of coagulation. Factor XIIa also converts the single chain factor VII molecule (αVII) to a double chain molecule (βVII) with many times more activity. Factor XIa in the presence of calcium ions converts factor IX to factor IXa, which in turn complexes with factor VIII:C and phospholipid to convert factor X to factor Xa. Factor X may also be activated by a complex of βVII, calcium ions and thromboplastin. Factor Xa complexes with factor V, calcium ions and phospholipid to convert prothrombin to thrombin. The main action of thrombin is to split fibrinopeptides A and B from the respective Aα and Bβ chains of fibrinogen to produce fibrin monomer which undergoes polymerization to form a visible clot. Thrombin also converts factor XIII into an activated form in the presence of calcium ions. Factor XIIIa cross-links the γ and, to the lesser extent, the α chains of fibrin to produce a fibrin which is more stable and more resistant to the lytic action of plasmin.

Properties of coagulation factors

A list of important properties is shown in Table 13.2. Differences in stability, utilization during

Table 13.2 Some properties of coagulation factors

Factor	Molecular weight	Electrophoretic mobility	Plasma concentration	Adsorbed by	Presence in serum	Vitamin K dependent	Temp. and time for precipitation	Stability at 37°C
I (fibrinogen)	340 000	β-globulin	1.5–4.0 g/l	—	absent	No	56°C/10 min	Yes
II (prothrombin)	72 000	α-globulin	100–150 mg/l	Al(OH)$_3$	trace to <10%	Yes	56°C/10 min	Yes
V	250 000	β-globulin	c 10 mg/l	—	absent	No	56°C/3 min	No
VII	45 000	α-globulin	c 0.5 mg/l	Al(OH)$_3$	present	Yes	56°C/5 min	Yes
VIII: C	c 300 000	?	?	—	absent	No	56°C/5 min	No
VIII: WF	polymers up to 20 × 10^6	β-globulin	c 10–15 mg/l	—	present	No	65°C/10 min	Yes
IX	55 000	α_1-globulin	4–7 mg/l	Al(OH)$_3$	present	Yes	56°C/10 min	Yes
X	55 000	α_1-globulin	c 5 mg/l	Al(OH)$_3$	present	Yes	56°C/20 min	Yes
XI	200 000	γ-globulin	c 5 mg/l	Celite	present	No	60°C/10 min	No
XII	80 000	β-globulin	c 20 mg/l	glass	present	No	65°C/10 min	Yes
XIII	320 000	β-globulin	10 mg/l	—	trace to <10%	No	56°C/20 min	Yes

clotting and adsorption characteristics enable partial separation of clotting factors in plasma and provide a basis for the preparation of laboratory reagents. Plasma which has been stored at 37°C serves as a reagent which is deficient in factor V and VIII:C. Citrated plasma absorbed with aluminium hydroxide is deficient in factors II, VII, IX and X, while serum contains factors VII, IX, X, XI and XII. Plasma taken from patients 48 h after commencing oral anticoagulants shows an isolated factor VII deficiency. After about a week's therapy, there is a proportional decrease in concentrations of factors II, VII, IX and X.

Localization of the haemostatic plug

Blood coagulation is an autocatalytic process culminating in a rapid generation of thrombin after a considerable period of delay during which contact activation and activation of factor X take place. There is evidence that thrombin, once formed, catalyzes its own production by accelerating some of the intermediate steps in the clotting process. During normal haemostasis, thrombin is formed

locally within the vascular system at the site of injury. It is essential that thrombin production be restricted to this site; if allowed to disperse and remain active in the general circulation, it would cause diffuse intravascular clotting. A number of mechanisms ensure localization of the haemostatic process. Clotting factor interactions and thrombin generation occur more efficiently on the surface of platelets where phospholipid (platelet factor 3) facilitates the spatial relationship of the proteins prior to interaction. Thrombin generation tends to be confined to the region of the platelet aggregate. Thrombin is also absorbed readily by fibrin which is being formed in the same locality. Activated clotting factors such as factor IXa, factor Xa and thrombin, as well as factors V and VIII, which are able to disperse from the immediate area of plug formation are rapidly complexed to and inactivated by the naturally-occurring plasma inhibitor of serine proteases, antithrombin III,[19] and protein C.[23]

Antithrombin III is an α_2 globulin with a molecular weight of about 64 000 daltons (plasma concentration: 0.25–0.4 g/l); it is identical with the substance in plasma known as heparin co-factor. Other naturally occurring inhibitors of coagulation include α_2 macroglobulin and α_1 antitrypsin, but these are of minor importance.

Protein C is a vitamin-K dependent plasma protein with anticoagulant and profibrinolytic activities.[22,23] Its functional activity depends on its phospholipid and calcium binding properties. Limited proteolysis by thrombin converts protein C into the active enzyme; this in turn interacts with an endothelial surface cofactor, thrombomodulin,[24] and rapidly inactivates factors V and VIII, and inhibits prothrombin activation.

THE NORMAL FIBRINOLYTIC MECHANISM

The role of fibrinolysis in normal haemostasis is uncertain. The essential purpose of fibrinolysis is to digest and solubilize fibrin, thus restoring patency to occluded vessels. In the presence of systemic hyperactivity of the fibrinolytic system, haemostatic plugs break down and rebleeding occurs. It might be inferred that fibrinolysis is not a helpful mechanism in primary haemostasis. However, fibrinolysis may be important in localizing the plugs and in the eventual recanalization of the injured vessel. Fibrinolysis occurs through the action of the proteolytic enzyme, plasmin, which attacks fibrin to produce a soluble product, fragment X. Further degradation of fragment X produces lower molecular-weight fragments Y and D. Fragment Y is finally degraded to another fragment D and fragment E. Thus one mole of fibrin produces two moles of fragment D and one mole of fragment E. These fragments are called fibrin degradation products (FDP). They retain the antigenic determinants of fibrinogen and react with antifibrinogen antisera, but during the process of formation further antigens are exposed which enable production of a specific antiserum against fragments D and E. Plasmin is formed by the action of a proteolytic enzyme, plasminogen activator, on an inactive β globulin precursor, plasminogen (Fig. 13.3). Plasminogen activator is found in many tissues and is secreted into the blood by vascular endothelial cells. It is probably also formed in the blood from a precursor protein,

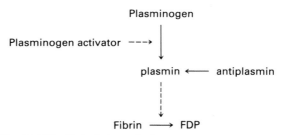

Fig. 13.3 The fibrinolytic mechanism.

proactivator, and factor XIIa is involved in this conversion. The various forms of plasminogen activator in the blood and tissues are immunologically distinct. There is a naturally-occurring plasmin inhibitor in the α_2 globulin fraction of plasma, α_2 antiplasmin. This inhibitor, with a molecular weight of 65 000–70 000 daltons, binds preferentially and rapidly to plasmin to form a complex with neoantigenic determinants.[3] Using an appropriate antiserum, the complex may be detected in the blood in hyperfibrinolytic states. Other plasmin inhibitors are α_2 macroglobulin, antithrombin III and inter-α-inhibitor. Inhibitors to plasminogen activators (anti-activators) may also exist but these have not been characterized adequately.

INVESTIGATION OF THE HAEMOSTATIC MECHANISM

Haemostasis may be deranged in the following circumstances:

1. A deficiency or defect of coagulation factors, either congenital or acquired.
2. The presence in the blood of inhibitors to the action of coagulation factors.
3. Excessive fibrinolysis.
4. Thrombocytopenia.
5. Platelet dysfunction.
6. A combination of some of the above defects.

An investigation of the haemostatic mechanism is always warranted in any patient who bleeds spontaneously or who shows excessive bleeding after trauma or surgical procedures. In general, there are two stages in the investigation of such a patient:

1. The establishment of the presence of an abnormality.

2. The definition, and perhaps quantitative assay, of the abnormality. The first stage in diagnosis can be achieved by screening tests; the second stage needs more specific (and usually more elaborate and time-consuming) tests.

Laboratory investigation is necessary, also, in any patient who is to undergo an operation and in whom either the past history, the family history and the nature of the disease process or the type of operation suggests that abnormal bleeding may occur.

Finally, the laboratory may be involved in the control of therapy in patients with known haemorrhagic disorders. The aim of therapy is to correct the haemostatic defect and to maintain adequate haemostasis. Quantitative assays of coagulation factors are often necessary for this type of control.

It is apparent that patients may bleed because of defects in blood coagulation or in platelets or as the result of excessive fibrinolysis. It is also true that for each group of defects some laboratory tests are particularly appropriate. However, the history of the patient, the type of bleeding or the circumstances under which bleeding occurs will modify the laboratory approach to the individual patient. Furthermore, some clinical situations require urgent laboratory diagnosis whereas in others a more leisurely, formal and comprehensive assessment of the haemostatic process is feasible. It is not practical to devise a scheme of investigation which will be useful under all circumstances.

Screening tests of haemostasis

These are non-specific tests designed to assess overall haemostatic function and which are useful for the screening of patients who may have a bleeding disorder. Unfortunately, screening tests, while relatively simple, lack sensitivity; and it does not necessarily follow that a patient has a normal haemostatic mechanism if the results of the tests to be described are all normal. Attention must be paid to the history and clinical findings to decide whether further more specific tests are also needed.

The following screening sequence is recommended: first of all carry out a bleeding time, partial thromboplastin time with kaolin, one-stage prothrombin time, thrombin time, platelet count and examination of a stained blood film. If the results of these tests are normal and the history is, nevertheless, strongly suggestive of a bleeding disorder, calculate the prothrombin consumption and carry out a capillary resistance test. If an abnormality is detected in the partial thromboplastin or one-stage prothrombin time, or both, undertake mixing experiments and tests for the presence of an inhibitor.

The bleeding time

Principle. A standard incision is made on the volar surface of the forearm and the time for which the incision bleeds is measured. Cessation of bleeding indicates the formation of haemostatic plugs which in turn are dependent upon an adequate number of platelets and the ability of the platelets to adhere to subendothelium and to form aggregates.

Standardized template method[12]

Place a sphygmomanometer cuff around the patient's arm above the elbow and inflate to 40 mmHg throughout the test. Clean the volar surface of the forearm with 70% ethanol and chose an area of skin which is devoid of visible superficial veins. Press a sterile metal template with a linear slit 11 mm long firmly against the skin and use a scalpel blade with a guard so arranged that the tip of the blade protrudes 1 mm through the template slit. In this way make an incision 9 mm long and 1 mm deep. Modifications of the template and blade are available commercially.*

Blot off gently but completely with filter paper, at 15 s intervals, the blood exuding from the linear cut. When bleeding has ceased, carefully oppose the edges of the incision and apply an adhesive strip to lessen the risk of keloid formation and an unsightly scar. It was proposed initially that the test be

* e.g. Simplate (General Diagnostics), Thrombolette (Boehringer).

performed in triplicate and the results averaged. It is usual in practice, however, to report the result of a single test.

Normal range. 2.5–9.5 min.

Ivy's method[10]

The test is similar to the template method, but instead of a standardized incision, two separate punctures 5–10 cm apart are made in quick succession using a disposable lancet. The B-D Microlance (Becton, Dickinson Ltd.) which has a cutting depth of 2.5 mm and width just over 1.0 mm is suitable; it can be inserted to its maximum depth without fear of penetrating too deeply. A source of inaccuracy with Ivy's method is a tendency for the puncture wound to close before bleeding has ceased.

Normal range with Ivy's method. 2–7 min; the upper limit, however, varies, depending on the size of the incision.

Significance of the bleeding time

The bleeding time is often prolonged in thrombocytopenia, but correlation between the degree of prolongation and the platelet count is poor. A prolonged bleeding time is more likely when the low platelet count is due to defective marrow production than to increased platelet destruction. In the latter situation, the circulating platelets tend to be larger (younger) and more reactive than normal.

A prolonged bleeding time is usual in von Willebrand's disease due to defective adhesion of platelets to subendothelium. In patients with congenital or acquired platelet dysfunction, the bleeding time may be prolonged due to inability of the platelets to form aggregates normally. A common cause of acquired platelet dysfunction is aspirin ingestion; 1 g may result in prolongation of the bleeding time up to 20 min,[12] and as little as 300 mg may affect the bleeding time. Patients should be instructed not to take any drugs, if possible, for a week before testing.

Although the bleeding time is usually normal in patients with coagulation defects, the haemostatic plugs are unstable and rebleeding commonly occurs if the scab is removed.

Test of capillary resistance

A test which has been widely applied in the investigation of the haemorrhagic disorders is the capillary resistance test (Hess's Test). In principle this test consists of inflating a sphygmomanometer cuff placed round the arm and inspecting the volar surface of the forearm below the elbow and the area about the wrist for petechiae after a standard period of inflation. The test, unfortunately, suffers from being comparatively crude and from often being carried out in an unstandardized way.

To carry out the test maintain the pressure of the cuff at 80 mmHg for 5 min and look for petechiae after a further 5 min. In health, very few petechiae should be produced; in thrombocytopenia, numerous petechiae become visible. The test may be positive even though the bleeding time is normal. Presumably in such cases the capillaries fail to withstand an increase in pressure although the mechanisms which arrest the bleeding from a breach in the vessel wall without increase in pressure are intact.

WHOLE-BLOOD COAGULATION TIME TEST

This test is rarely used nowadays. For details see previous editions of this book.

GENERAL NOTES ON COAGULATION TECHNIQUES

Blood coagulation techniques appear deceptively easy, basic tests requiring apparatus no more complicated than a water-bath, test tubes, pipettes and a stop-watch or automatic clot timer. Although the methodology is fairly simple to master, accurate results are not possible unless particular attention is given to the proper collection and processing of blood samples, the selection and preparation of reagents and the necessity for appropriate control specimens.

Collection of venous blood

Venous blood samples should be obtained whenever possible; indeed, they are essential for most tests. By using the appropriate expertise available in paediatric departments, it is usually possible to obtain venous blood from infants and young children and even from neonates. It is practical to perform a limited number of tests on capillary blood, but it would certainly be unwise to make a firm diagnosis of a congenital bleeding disorder such as haemophilia unless a satisfactory venous sample was available. For a discussion of capillary blood tests, see Stuart et al.[21]

The patient should preferably come to the laboratory for tests for haemostasis. When this is not practicable, the samples should be brought to the laboratory as soon as possible, and if tests for fibrinolysis are required, the tube containing the patient's blood must be immersed in crushed ice at the patient's bedside. The patient should not be taking non-steroidal anti-inflammatory drugs and should be fasting, if platelet aggregation tests are to be performed, since turbid plasma obscures the changes in optical density associated with platelet aggregation. For tests of fibrinolysis, it is essential that the patient be rested for at least 15 min before blood is withdrawn. The investigation should be planned before the blood is collected so that the appropriate containers are on hand and the total amount of blood required is known.

Withdraw blood without undue venous stasis and without frothing into a plastic syringe fitted with a short needle of 19 or 20 SWG. The venepuncture must be a 'clean' one and, if there is any difficulty, take a new syringe and needle and try another vein. Distribute the blood into tubes as follows, after detaching the needle from the syringe:

1. Add an appropriate quantity of blood to 32 g/l trisodium citrate in the proportion of 9 volumes of blood to 1 volume of citrate in a plastic tube or tubes and mix gently by inversion after covering with a plastic cap. Place the tubes containing the citrated samples obtained for screening procedures, factor assays and fibrinolysis tests in crushed ice and transport them as quickly as possible to the laboratory. Separate the plasma by centrifugation, as described on p. 216, without delay. Citrated blood for platelet aggregation tests should remain in capped tubes at room temperature.

2. Take an appropriate amount of blood into a tube containing dried EDTA so that a platelet count can be carried out and blood films made.

3. Collect clotted blood at this stage so that serum will be available if required later in the investigation. For this purpose place 3–4 ml of blood in a 75 × 12 mm glass test-tube, and keep at 37°C in a water-bath. If this is to be used for a prothrombin-consumption test, note the whole-blood clotting time and start a stop-watch, so that the serum can be separated at exactly 1 h after clotting.

Control blood samples

Obtain blood from a normal subject and treat as 1 and 3 above. Process and test the samples at the same time as those of the patient.

Equipment

Water-baths set at 37°C should have a tolerance of no more than ±0.5°C as temperature markedly affects the speed of clotting reactions. A water-bath with plastic or glass slides is preferable and some type of cross-illumination helps in determining the exact time of appearance of fibrin. At least three or four stop-watches are necessary for a laboratory doing anything more than basic coagulation tests. Disposable Pasteur pipettes marked at 0.1 ml and automatic pipettes which deliver 0.1 ml and 0.2 ml volumes are replacing the straight 0.1 and 0.2 ml pipettes with flanged tops in many laboratories.

A number of instruments are available which record automatically the end-point in coagulation tests, most of them using either an electromechanical or a photoelectric principle. At least 10 different types of auto-mated instruments to record clotting times are in use in Britain. They reduce observer error and enable several tests to be performed concurrently, but in a national study of prothrombin time techniques, they did not eliminate local technique variables or reduce inter-laboratory error.[16] These instruments are of value where large numbers of tests are performed, but they have only limited applica-tion in a small laboratory.

All plasma or serum samples, or reagents derived from them, should be kept in plastic or siliconized glass tubes until required and those reagents to be used in a day's tests should be placed conveniently at hand in melting ice. However, with a few deliberate exceptions, actual clotting tests are carried out at 37°C in plain glass tubes of standard size, namely, 10 mm or 12 mm external dia-meter. It is essential that all glassware be chemically clean and absolutely free from traces of detergents. Ideally, the cleaning of glassware used in coagulation tests should be the responsibility of one individual and should be handled separately from the routine laboratory glassware. Alternatively, disposable glassware can be used.

PROTHROMBIN TIME

The introduction by Quick of the measurement of the clotting time of plasma after the addition of brain extract can be seen in retrospect to be a landmark in the study of blood coagulation and the haemorrhagic disorders. Introduced originally as a test for prothrombin activity—hence the name—the test is now known to measure in addition, and more importantly, factors V, VII and X. It is also relatively sensitive to the presence of heparin in the blood and hypofibrinogenaemia.

The test in its various modifications can be used as an important screening test for deficiencies of the above-mentioned factors occurring spontaneously in disease or produced as the result of the adminis-tration of anticoagulant drugs such as coumarin and indanedione.

In this section on screening tests a method based on the original technique of Quick will be described.[18] Although an inaccurate title, the term 'prothrombin time' is so firmly established that it seems pointless to advocate the use of a more accurately descriptive term such as 'brain-thromboplastin time.'

Prothrombin time by the Quick one-stage method

Principle. A potent preparation of human or rabbit brain emulsion is added to citrated plasma. The mixture is then recalcified and the clotting time estimated.

Reagents

Patient's and control plasma samples. Cen-trifuge citrated blood without delay at 1200–1500 *g* for 15 min. Then remove the super-natant plasma and place it in a clean glass tube.

If the test is not carried out at once, the sample should be placed at 4°C where it may remain for several hours. A delay of more than 6 h is undesirable and specimens so kept usually show a shortening of their prothrom-bin time by several seconds. This phe-nomenon is due to activation of kallikrein in the cold and conversion of the α form of factor VII to the more active β form. If the specimen is visibly haemolyzed it should be discarded.

Human brain emulsion. An extract of ace-tone-dried brain is widely used (for prepara-tion, see Appendix, p. 433).

Suspend 0.03 g of the dry brain powder in 5 ml of 9 g/l NaCl (saline) and warm at 37°C for 15–30 min, with occasional shaking. The coarse particles are allowed to sediment and the opalescent supernatant is used for the test.

Ideally, a new tube for brain powder should be used every time a batch of tests is per-formed, but the saline suspension may be kept for a day or two at 4°C without deteriora-tion, or longer if frozen at −20°C.

It is convenient to make up large batches of brain powder; if suitably stored (see p. 433), human brain powder retains its potency for many months.

Many laboratories in Britain use a phenol-saline suspension of human brain known as the British Comparative Thromboplastin* as a working reagent for prothrombin time tests. This material is produced in large volumes without significant variation in sensitivity between batches.

Rabbit brain emulsion. A number of commercial rabbit brain preparations, as well as preparations containing rabbit brain and calcium chloride, are available. Rabbit brain thromboplastin is not as sensitive as human brain to factor-VII deficiency, and these preparations usually give faster clotting times with deficient plasma samples. However, the commercial preparations are usually satisfactory for the investigation of patients with bleeding disorders. In all instances, the manufacturer's instructions should be followed.

Calcium chloride. 0.025 mol/l calcium chloride may be prepared conveniently from a commercial molar solution.

Method

Deliver 0.1 ml of plasma into the bottom of a 75 × 10 mm glass test-tube placed in a water-bath at 37°C and add 0.1 ml of brain suspension to it. After a delay of about 1 min, add 0.1 ml of warmed 0.025 mol/l calcium chloride and mix the contents of the tube carefully. Start a stop-watch and hold the tube with its lower end submerged. Tilt the tube continuously but gently from the vertical to just short of the horizontal so that its contents can be observed for the first signs of clotting. A fibrin clot developing within a second marks the end-point. A shielded horizontal source of light should be arranged to provide effective lighting of the sample being tested. Repeat the test at least once for each specimen and record the mean time. Include at least one normal control plasma sample in each batch of tests.

* Available from the National Reference Laboratory for Anticoagulant Reagents and Control, Withington Hospital, Manchester.

Normal range. (Quick method): 10–14 s. It has been repeatedly demonstrated that the normal values obtained in any laboratory depend upon exactly how the test is carried out. In particular, the values observed with normal and pathological plasma samples depend greatly on the source and type of brain thromboplastin used. Each laboratory has to establish its own normal range.

Significance of an abnormal prothrombin time

The prothrombin time test is a non-specific indicator of the extrinsic blood coagulation mechanism. As already mentioned, deficiencies of prothrombin and factors, V, VII and X give rise to a prolonged time, as well as the presence of heparin in the blood and hypofibrinogenaemia.

The common causes of a long one-stage time are:

1. Therapy with coumarin or indanedione drugs.
2. Obstructive jaundice.
3. Haemorrhagic disease of the newborn.
4. Liver disease.

   Less common causes are:

5. Heparin therapy.
6. Loss of clotting proteins from the blood via the kidneys in renal disease, e.g. in nephrotic syndromes.
7. Congenital deficiency of one or more of factors II, V, VII or X.
8. Fibrinogen deficiency.
9. Malabsorption states (vitamin K deficiency).

There are, too, a number of common artefactual causes which should be considered if a long time is not expected. These include the following:

1. Faulty collection of the specimen, resulting in partial clotting and serum being tested instead of plasma.

2. An excess of citrate or insufficient blood so that there is an incorrect volume of citrate in relation to the blood.

3. An unsuitable anticoagulant, such as EDTA, used in collecting the sample.

4. An unduly high PCV, so that there is less plasma than normal per unit volume of blood and consequently an excess of anticoagulant.

5. Technical errors, such as a hole in the tube containing calcium chloride, the water-bath set at an incorrect temperature or a faulty thromboplastin reagent.

If an artefactual cause of an increased time is suspected, a normal control plasma should be tested, the patient's blood sample should be checked for small clots and a further sample obtained, if necessary. If the PCV of the blood is high, the effect of adding 0.05 mol/l calcium chloride in place of 0.025 mol/l calcium chloride should be tried.

Prothrombin time using Russell's viper venom

Principle. Russell's viper venom in the presence of calcium converts factor X to factor Xa; factor VII is not involved in the reaction.

Reagents

Patient's and control plasma samples. As for the the Quick one-stage method.
Russell's viper venom/cephalin reagent (Diagen*). The material is freeze-dried and when reconstituted with 6.0 ml of water contains Russell's viper venom at a dilution of 1 in 150 000 and cephalin at optimal concentration.
Calcium chloride. 0.025 mol/l calcium chloride.

Method

The test is performed in the same manner as the Quick one-stage method, but the viper venom reagent is used instead of brain suspension.

Normal range. 11–13 s.

Significance

A prolonged prothrombin time using brain suspension, but a normal time with Russell's viper venom, indicates factor VII deficiency.

---

* Diagnostic Reagents Ltd., Thame, Oxon.

Thrombin time of plasma

Principle. Thrombin is added to the plasma and the clotting time measured. The thrombin time is affected by the concentration and reactability of fibrinogen, and by the presence of inhibitory substances. The clotting time and the appearance of the clot are equally informative.

Reagents

Bovine or human thrombin is used, freshly diluted in a plastic tube to a concentration of about 10 NIH units per ml. Suitable sources of thrombin are:
1. Fibrindex (Ortho), each ampoule containing 50 NIH units of freeze-dried human thrombin, which should be reconstituted with 1 ml of 9 g/l NaCl (saline).
2. Thrombin Topical (Parke, Davis & Co.), which is distributed in bottles containing 5000 NIH units of freeze-dried bovine thrombin.

The latter may be reconstituted with saline to 50 NIH units per ml and stored frozen in plastic vials, but it slowly loses its potency even at −20°C.

Method

Place 0.2 ml of normal plasma in a 75 × 12 mm glass tube in the water-bath at 37°C and blow in 0.1 ml of thrombin. Measure the clotting time and observe the nature of the clot. Adjust the concentration of thrombin, if necessary, so that normal plasma gives a clotting time of 10 ± 1 s. Repeat the procedure using the test plasma.

The concentration of thrombin can be reduced by dilution in buffered saline (Appendix, p. 435) to give a control time of 15–18 s (usually about 20–25 units of thrombin/ml). This makes the thrombin time more sensitive to defects of polymerization and to the presence of inhibitory substances. A prolongation of the clotting time to 20 s or more is considered abnormal. Clotting times with diluted thrombin are not as reproducible as with concentrated thrombin, and a variation of 1–2 s in duplicates is not uncommon.

When the result is abnormal, repeat the tests, adding 0.1 ml of protamine solution (10 mg/100 ml of buffered saline) to the plasma samples before the thrombin. A normal clotting time and a firm clot in the test sample indicates that heparin or FDP were interfering with the thrombin–fibrinogen reaction. A delayed clotting time and a poor clot in the test with protamine indicate fibrinogen depletion, an abnormal fibrinogen or an abnormal plasma globulin, and further tests should be performed.

Thrombin time using Reptilase or ancrod

Reptilase-R*, a purified thrombin-like snake-venom enzyme from *Bothrops atrox* and ancrod (Arvin),[†] a similar enzyme from *Agkistrodon rhodostoma* may be used to replace thrombin in the thrombin clotting time test. The test is performed exactly as described for thrombin. These snake-venom enzymes are not inhibited by heparin, so that a prolonged thrombin time and a normal Reptilase time is diagnostic of the presence of heparin in the plasma.[6] The Reptilase time is less prolonged than the thrombin time in the presence of fibrinogen/fibrin degradation products (FDP), but is more prolonged than the thrombin time in patients with congenital dysfibrinogenaemia.

Significance of an abnormal thrombin time

The commonest causes of a prolonged thrombin time are the presence of heparin, fibrinogen/fibrin degradation products, or depletion of fibrinogen. In chronic liver disease the thrombin time is often prolonged and the clots are transparent and bulky. The defect is caused by abnormalities of fibrin polymerization. Abnormal polymerization is also the cause of a long thrombin time in some congeni-

tal dysfibrinogenaemias and in multiple myeloma. The thrombin time is usually a few seconds longer in plasma from newborn infants than in normal adult plasma.

Partial thromoboplastin time with kaolin (PTTK)[11,17]

This test is also known as the Activated Partial Thromboplastin Time (APTT) and the Kaolin-Cephalin Clotting Time (KCCT).

Principle. Platelet-poor plasma is pre-incubated with an activating agent so that the time-consuming reactions associated with the contact phase of coagulation are completed before the addition of calcium. Phospholipid is supplied to replace platelet factor 3 activity. There are many modifications of the test using commercial preparations of phospholipid of animal or plant origin or combined reagents of phospholipid and activator. Activating agents include kaolin, ellagic acid, micronized silica and colloidal celite. The optimal times for the pre-incubation of plasma with activator vary with the different preparations. The method described here employs kaolin as activator and Manchester lyophilized reagent* as phospholipid. A chloroform extract of acetone-dried brain, prepared as suggested by Bell and Alton[1], has also been used.

Reagents

Plasma. Citrated normal and test plasma samples. Separate the plasma by centrifugation at 1200–1500 *g* for 15 min and keep at 4°C until tested, but for not longer than 2 h.

Kaolin. Suspend kaolin BP in barbitone buffer, pH 7.4, at a concentration of 5 g/l. It is stable at room temperature indefinitely.

Phospholipid. Manchester lyophilized reagent.* Many other reagents exist, containing different phospholipids. None is clealy superior to the others, at least for the diagnosis of mild haemophilia,[15] and the laboratory

---

* Pentapharm Ltd., Basel.
[†] Berk Pharmaceuticals Ltd. Station Road, Shalford, Guildford, Surrey.

* Available from National Reference Laboratory for Anticoagulant Reagents and Control, Withington Hospital, Manchester.

should use the reagent it is familiar with. The preparation of platelet substitute (Bell and Alton) and Inosithin are described in the Appendix, p 434.

Calcium. 0.025 mol/l calcium chloride.

Method

Mix equal volumes of the diluted phospholipid solution and the kaolin suspension and leave in a glass tube in the water-bath at 37°C.

Place in a 75 × 12 mm glass tube in the water-bath 0.1 ml of normal or test plasma, and follow this with 0.2 ml of the well-shaken kaolin phospholipid mixture. Start a stop-watch and leave the plasma-kaolin-phospholipid mixture at 37°C with occasional shaking. Exactly 10 min later, add 0.1 ml of pre-warmed calcium chloride and start a second stop-watch. Record the time taken for the mixture to clot.

Repeat the test at least once with both normal and patient's plasma. The end-point is usually quite distinct and the clots are well seen due to the presence of the kaolin. It is possible to do four tests at 2 min intervals if sufficient stop-watches are available.

Normal range. 35–43 s. A result which is consistently 7 s or more greater than the normal control should be considered abnormal.

Significance of the partial thromboplastin time test

The test is used widely as a sensitive, quick and practical way to demonstrate defects of coagulation in the intrinsic pathway. It is of course a non-specific test, the PTTK being prolonged in deficiencies of factors XII, XI, X, IX, VIII, V or II. A normal result is obtained with factor VII deficient plasma. The test is used frequently to monitor heparin therapy and coagulation factor replacement therapy and it may be modified to detect the presence of circulating anticoagulants. Shorter than normal times have been reported in hypercoagulable states. The test is most useful in the detection of haemophilia A ('haemophilia') and haemophilia B (Christmas disease), and all but the mildest grades should give abnormal results. It will not, however, distinguish between factor-VIII and factor-IX deficiency.

The normal range depends upon the technique, and laboratories should determine their own ranges, particularly if commercial reagents are used. A number of comparative studies have demonstrated that different commercial reagents vary in their sensitivity to factor-VIII and factor-IX deficiency and to the coagulation defect induced by heparin therapy.[8,14,20] Automated methods usually give shorter times than manual methods.[16] Manufacturers' instructions should be followed if commercial reagents are used. In general, the partial thromboplastin time is not prolonged unless the concentration of the deficient coagulation factor is <20% of the normal (or <20 iu/dl for factor VIII:C[15]).

Mixing experiments

If an abnormality is detected with the prothrombin time test or the partial thromboplastin time test further information on the nature of the defect may usually be obtained by mixing experiments. The test plasma is mixed with either normal plasma or plasma with a known coagulation defect and the test is repeated, noting the degree of correction, if any.

If the abnormality is a prolonged prothrombin time, the following reagents are useful for mixing experiments:

1. *Aluminium-hydroxide-adsorbed normal plasma.* Place 0.9 ml of normal plasma in a 75 × 12 mm glass tube in the water-bath at 37°C and add 0.1 ml of aluminium hydroxide gel (alumina). See Appendix (p. 433) for details of preparation of alumina. Shake the mixture and leave for 2 min at 37°C and then centrifuge. The prothrombin time of the adsorbed plasma should be >60 s. Adsorbed plasma is deficient in factors II, VII and X, but contains factor V.

2. *'Aged plasma'.* This is oxalated plasma which has been incubated at 37°C for 48 h. It is deficient in factor V, but contains factors II, VII and X.

3. *Coumarin plasma.* Plasma from a patient commenced on warfarin therapy 48–72 h previously; it is deficient in factor VII only. Plas-

Table 13.3 Mixing experiments

Prothrombin time test of plasma partially corrected by addition of:

Normal plasma	Adsorbed plasma	Aged plasma	48–72 h coumarin plasma	Interpretation
Yes	Yes	No	Yes	Factor V deficiency
Yes	No	Yes	No	Factor VII deficiency
Yes	No	Yes	Yes	Factor II or X deficiency
Yes	Yes	Yes	Yes	Fibrinogen deficiency
No	No	No	No	Anticoagulant present

ma from a patient on warfarin for a week or more is deficient in factors II, VII and X.

The above factor-deficient plasmas may be obtained commercially if not readily available.

4. *Normal plasma.*

Method

Measure the prothrombin times of mixtures of 4 volumes of test plasma and 1 volume of the reagents 1, 2, 3 and 4. The results may be interpreted by reference to Table 13.3.

An abnormality due to factor-VIII deficiency is corrected by the addition to test plasma of normal plasma or factor-IX deficient plasma but not factor-VIII deficient plasma. Factor IX deficiency is corrected by normal plasma and factor-VIII deficient plasma, but not factor IX-deficient plasma. Failure to correct the abnormality with normal plasma indicates the presence of an anticoagulant.

Prothrombin-consumption test

Principle. During normal coagulation, thrombin production (and prothrombin utilization) continues after the blood or plasma has clotted. If the serum is tested 1 h after coagulation, it will be found that practically all the prothrombin has been 'consumed'. If there is a deficiency of any of the factors required for the coagulation of blood or plasma in glass, prothrombin will be incompletely consumed and more than normal will be present in the serum 1 h after coagulation. This is so even if the blood or plasma itself clots in the normal time.

Reagents

Citrated Plasma.

Serum. Separate the serum from clotted blood 1 h after coagulation has taken place in a plain glass tube placed at 37°C in a water-bath. 1 h after coagulation is selected as a standard time to carry out the test. If the actual estimation cannot be carried out 1 h after clotting, separate the serum after 1 h and citrate it with a one-ninth volume of 32 g/l sodium citrate so as to inhibit further conversion of prothrombin.

Human or rabbit brain suspension. See p. 216.

Calcium. 0.025 mol/l calcium chloride.

Human or bovine fibrinogen. 1.5–2.0 g/l.

Method

Place sufficient calcium chloride solution and fibrinogen in the water-bath at 37°C before the actual test is started. Then deliver 0.1 ml of plasma into a 75 × 12 mm glass tube and add 0.1 ml of brain emulsion. After waiting a minute or so for the plasma and thromboplastin to warm, add 0.1 ml of the calcium chloride solution to the mixture and start a stop-watch. After exactly 60 s, add 0.2 ml of the fibrinogen solution to the tube containing the recalcified plasma. Record the clotting time of the fibrinogen.

There is one difficulty in the test: at a time after the recalcification of the plasma corresponding with the prothrombin time the plasma will clot. The clot has to be removed on a wooden swab-stick before the fibrinogen is added. (It is convenient to put the swab-stick in the tube at the start of the experiment.)

Table 13.4 Interpretation of screening tests

PTTK	Prothrombin Time	Thrombin Time	PCI	Interpretation
Abn	N	N	Abn	Deficiency of FXII, XI, IX or VIII; FVIII inhibitor.
Abn	Abn	N	*	Deficiency of FX, V or II; could be multiple deficiencies, e.g. FX, IX, VII and II.
N	Abn	N	*	FVII deficiency; repeat prothrombin time using Russell's viper venom.
Abn	Abn	Abn	*	Disseminated intravascular coagulation; heparin in blood (Reptilase time should be normal, if heparin); fibrinogen abnormality.
N	N	N	Abn	Thrombocytopenia or platelet dysfunction; check platelet count and bleeding time.

* The prothrombin-consumption index is not a practical test when the prothrombin time is prolonged.
N = normal; Abn = abnormal.

Repeat the test in exactly the same way using serum instead of plasma. Naturally, in this instance, there will be no clot to remove before the fibrinogen is added, except perhaps in severe haemophiliacs.

Reporting results

The relationship between the plasma and serum clotting times is expressed as an index; i.e. the prothrombin-consumption index (PCI):

$$\frac{\text{plasma clotting time}}{\text{serum clotting time}} \times 100.$$

This method of reporting suffers from the fact that *low* percentages are normal, whilst a value of 100% is grossly abnormal. For this reason some workers are content to record simply the clotting time using serum as the 'serum prothrombin time' or 'serum prothrombin activity'.

Normal range of prothrombin-consumption index (PCI). 0–30% (serum prothrombin time >30 s). As the amount of prothrombin consumed is affected by the way the blood is allowed to clot, each laboratory should establish its own range of normal values.

Significance of an abnormal PCI

The prothrombin-consumption index is a non-specific test of clotting efficiency. It is sensitive not only to defects in the coagulation cascade, but also to platelet abnormalities, such as thrombocytopenia or platelet dysfunction. In some cases it is the only abnormality detected on screening and serves as an indicator that further tests such as coagulation factor assays or platelet function tests should be carried out.

SUMMARY OF SCREENING TESTS

The measurement of bleeding time and capillary resistance, the platelet count, prothrombin time, prothrombin-consumption index, thrombin time and partial thromboplastin time with kaolin together provide useful and practical information for the exclusion of a bleeding disorder. If all results are normal, it is most unlikely that a serious bleeding disorder has been missed. A single abnormal result should not be considered without reference to the results of the other tests in the screening procedure. Table 13.4 shows some well-recognized patterns of results with the partial thromboplastin time with kaolin, prothrombin time, thrombin time and prothrombin-consumption index. Interpretation of the probable haemostatic defect indicates the further investigations which should be performed. These will often involve quantitative assay of one or more coagulation factors or an investigation of platelet function.

REFERENCES

[1] BELL, W. N. and ALTON, H. G. (1954). A brain extract as a substitute for platelet suspensions in the thromboplastin generation test. *Nature (London)*, **174**, 880.

[2] BLOOM, A. L. (1977). Physiology of Factor VIII. In *Recent Advances in Blood Coagulation*, Ed. Poller, L., Vol. 2, p. 141–181. Churchill Livingstone, Edinburgh.

[3] COLLEN, D. (1976). Identification and some properties of a new fast reacting plasmin inhibitor in human plasma. *European Journal of Biochemistry*, **69**, 209.

[4] DAVIDSON, J. F. (1977). Recent advances in fibrinolysis. In *Recent Advances in Blood Coagulation*, Ed. Poller, L., Vol. 2, p. 91–122. Churchill Livingstone, Edinburgh.

[5] ESNOUF, M. P. (1977). Biochemistry of blood coagulation. *British Medical Bulletin*, **33**, 213.

[6] FUNK, C., GMÜR, J., HEROLD, R. and STRAUB, P. W. (1971). Reptilase-R—a new reagent in blood coagulation. *British Journal of Haematology*, **21**, 43.

[7] HAMBERG, M., SVENSSON, J. and SAMUELSSON, B. (1975). Thromboxanes: a new group of biologically active compounds derived from prostaglandin endoperoxides. *Proceedings of the National Academy of Science*, U.S.A. **72**, 2994.

[8] HOFFMANN, J. J. M. L. and MEULENDIJK, P. N. (1978). Comparison of reagents for determining the activated partial thromboplastin time. *Thrombosis and Haemostasis*, **39**, 640.

[9] International Committee for the Nomenclature of Blood Clotting Factors (1962). Nomenclature of blood-clotting factors. *British Medical Journal*, **i**, 465.

[10] IVY, A. C., NELSON, D. and BUCHER, G. (1940). The standardization of certain factors in the cutaneous 'venostasis' bleeding time technique. *Journal of Laboratory and Clinical Medicine*, **26**, 1812.

[11] MACPHERSON, J. C. and HARDISTY, R. M. (1961). A modified thromboplastin screening test. *Thrombosis et Diathesis Haemorrhagica*, **6**, 492.

[12] MIELKE; C. H., KANESHIRO, M. M., MAHER, I. A., WEINER, J. M. and RAPAPORT, S. I. (1969). The standardized Ivy bleeding time and its prolongation by aspirin. *Blood*, **34**, 204.

[13] MONCADA, S., GRYGLEWSKI, R., BUNTING, S. and VANE, J. R. (1976). An enzyme isolated from arteries transforms prostaglandin endoperoxides to an unstable substance that inhibits aggregation. *Nature (London)*, **263**, 663.

[14] MORIN, R. J. and WILLOUGHBY, D. (1975). Comparison of several activated partial thromboplastin time methods. *American Journal of Clinical Pathology*, **64**, 241.

[15] O'BRIEN, P. F., NORTH, W. R. S. and INGRAM, G. I. C. (1981). The diagnosis of mild haemophilia by the partial thromboplastin time test. WFH/ICTH study of the Manchester method. *Thrombosis and Haemostasis*, **45**, 162.

[16] POLLER, L., THOMSON, J. M. and YEE, K. F. (1978). Automated versus manual techniques for the prothrombin time: results of proficiency assessment studies. *British Journal of Haematology*, **38**, 391.

[17] PROCTOR, R. R. and RAPAPORT, S. I. (1961). The partial thromboplastin time with kaolin. A simple screening test for first stage plasma clotting factor deficiencies. *American Journal of Clinical Pathology*, **36**, 212.

[18] QUICK, A. J. (1942). The Hemorrhagic Diseases and the Physiology of Hemostasis. Thomas, Illinois.

[19] ROSENBERG, R. D. (1975). Actions and interactions of antithrombin and heparin. *New England Journal of Medicine*, **292**, 146.

[20] SHAPIRO, G. A., HUNTZINGER, S. W. and WILSON, J. E. (1977). Variation among commercial activated partial thromboplastin time reagents in response to heparin. *American Journal of Clinical Pathology*, **67**, 477.

[21] STUART, J., PICKEN, A. M., BREEZE, G. R. and WOOD, B. S. B. (1973). Capillary-blood coagulation profile in the newborn. *Lancet*, **ii**, 1467.

[22] KISIEL, W. (1979). Human protein C. Isolation, characterization and mechanism of activation of α-thrombin. *Journal of Clinical Investigation*, **564**, 761.

[23] MARLAR, R. A., KLEISS, A. and GRIFFIN, J. H. (1982). Mechanism of action of human activated protein C thrombin dependent anticoagulant enzyme. *Blood*, **59**, 1067.

[24] ESMON C. T. and OWEN, W. G. (1981). Identification of an endothelial cell cofactor for thrombin catalysed activation of protein C. *Proceedings of the National Academy of Science*, U.S.A., **78**, 2249.

14

Quantitative assay of coagulation factors
(Written in collaboration with W. R. Pitney and M. Brozovic)

Assay of the plasma concentrations of coagulation factors is frequently necessary:

1. To establish the diagnosis of a bleeding disorder.
2. To assess its severity.
3. To monitor replacement therapy.
4. To detect the carrier state in families where one or more members are affected with a congenital bleeding disorder.

Diagnosis

Although the nature of an abnormality detected by screening tests may be established by mixing experiments using the prothrombin time or partial thromboplastin time with kaolin (p. 219), it is often simpler to proceed directly to the assay of relevant coagulation factors. For example, a prolonged PTTK with a normal prothrombin time in the absence of a circulating anticoagulant is an indication for assay of factors VIII and IX (and, if these results are normal, of factors XI and XII as well).

Assessment of severity

Most congenital bleeding disorders are graded mild, moderate or severe on a combination of clinical findings and assay of the deficient factor. In fact, there is usually a good correlation between the factor assay and the severity of bleeding. For instance, the risk of spontaneous haemarthrosis is negligible in a haemophiliac who has a plasma-factor VIII concentration >4% of normal, whereas the risk is great with a value <1%. Knowledge of the plasma-factor concentration is almost essential prior to counselling the patient concerning permissible physical activity and life style.

Replacement therapy

Assays are required for monitoring replacement therapy in patients with coagulation disorders who are subjected to dental extractions or surgical procedures. There is now considerable information available concerning the level of each factor which enables the haemostatic mechanism to function adequately. In general, the aim of replacement therapy is to keep the concentration of the deficient factor above this minimum level until the risk of haemorrhage has passed. Assays are also essential to determine the potency of concentrates used in replacement therapy, so that the therapeutic dose can be calculated.

Detection of carrier state

Symptomless relatives of patients with congenital bleeding disorders frequently request advice concerning the likelihood that they may transmit the disorder to their offspring. A knowledge of the pattern of inheritance may be sufficient to reassure some individuals. However, where the inheritance pattern indicates a possibility that the relative is a symptomless carrier, assays are essential before appropriate counselling can be undertaken.

APPROPRIATE METHOD OF ASSAY

An individual may have a deficiency of a coagulation factor either because of impaired synthesis or because a variant of a molecule is synthesized which is deficient in clotting activity. In both instances, assays based on clotting tests will be low, but where a variant molecule is synthesized, an immunological assay for the concentration of antigenic protein may be normal. Immunological assay, as well as clotting assay, is particularly relevant in the assay of factor VIII.

Patients with von Willebrand's disease usually synthesize reduced amounts of a functionally normal factor VIII, whereas haemophiliacs synthesize normal amounts of a clotting factor without coagulant activity.[18,42,62] Immunological assays are useful also in detecting the female carrier of haemophilia, in whom there is a marked discrepancy between immunological and biological factor VIII activity.[7,18]

For biological assays of most coagulation factors there is usually one 'best' method, which, with some modifications, is used by a majority of laboratories. Special considerations apply to the assays of factor VIII procoagulant activity (FVIII:C) and factor X. Factor VIII:C may be assayed by either a one-stage method based on the partial thromboplastin time or a two-stage method based on the thromboplastin generation test.[9] There are discrepancies between the results of one-stage and two-stage assays, particularly with plasma samples from patients with liver disease,[52] in intravascular coagulation[44] and with normal plasma samples analysed against a standard consisting of factor VIII concentrate.[4] The cause of these discrepancies is not clear and it is uncertain which of the two assay methods gives the more reliable answer, although the two-stage assay has been reported to correlate better with the immunological assay of factor VIII related antigen (FVIIIR:Ag).[22]

Biological assays for factor X using Russell's viper venom cephalin reagent (see p. 232) may occasionally give a normal result, when similar assays using brain extract acting through the intrinsic mechanism (see p. 230) are low.[26,47] It is apparent that factor X deficiency involves a number of different molecular abnormalities.

The parallel line bioassay of coagulation factors

If two materials containing the same coagulation factor are assayed in a specific coagulation assay in a range of dilutions, and the clotting times are plotted against the dilutions of plasma on graph paper a curved line is obtained; if the plot is drawn on double log paper, a sigmoid curve with a

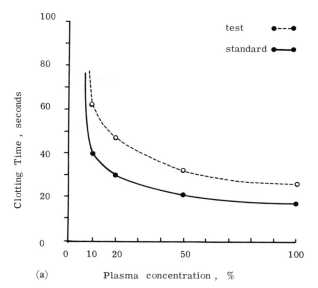

(a)

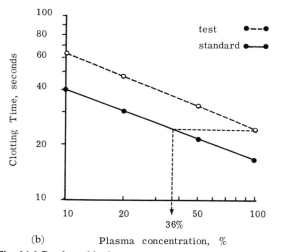

(b)

Fig. 14.1 Prothrombin time test.
(a) Clotting times obtained with 2-fold dilutions of factor VII-deficient plasma (test) and normal plasma (standard) plotted on linear (ordinary) graph paper.
(b) The same data plotted on double-log graph paper. Two parallel straight lines are obtained. The horizontal shift of the test line from the standard line represents the difference in potency; in this case the potency of the test plasma is 36% of the standard.

straight middle section is obtained (Fig. 14.1). If the dilutions of test and standard are chosen carefully, two straight parallel lines can be drawn. The horizontal distance between the two lines represents the difference in potency ('strength' or concentration) of the factor assayed. If the test line is to the right of the standard it contains less factor than the standard; if to the left, it contains more.[5]

When setting up and performing parallel line assays, a number of measures must be taken to ensure that the assay is valid and reliable. Firstly, the dilutions of test and standard should be chosen so that the coagulation times obtained lie on the linear portion of the dose response curve. For example, when assaying factor VIII:C by one-stage assay, dilutions giving times of 50–100 s are chosen, if the blank clotting time is over 150 s (p. 232). At least two, and preferably three or more dilutions are tested to give the best graphical or mathematical solution.

The results can be worked out graphically or mathematically. If the graphical solution is used, mean values for clotting times are plotted against the dilutions on double log paper. The dilutions are converted to decimals; the lowest dilution of the standard is considered 100% or 1.0 to enable direct reading from the concentration axis (see Table 14.1 and Fig. 14.1). Best fit lines are drawn through each set of the points (Fig. 14.1). Non-parallel or grossly curved lines indicate an invalid assay and should be discarded. To obtain the actual potency of the test sample in terms of the standard, a horizontal line is drawn through both dose response lines to cut the test sample line where it crosses 1.0 (100%). A vertical line is then dropped on to the concentration axis and the relative potency of the test sample read directly off the concentration scale.

Mathematical solutions are better than graphical ones, as they provide exact criteria for parallelism and curvature. Computer or calculator programmes can be used to calculate the results.[16,61]

Reproducibility and inter-laboratory variations

The ideal assay would involve a simple, rapid technique, not requiring costly reagents, with a high degree of reproducibility on multiple testing of the one sample and a small variation in results when assays of the same sample are performed in different laboratories. Biological assays are far from ideal in all of these respects. Individual factor VIII:C assays in the one laboratory have a CV of 10–20%, and greater precision can only be achieved by repeated estimations.[29] Factor VIII:C

assays performed on the same sample by experienced technologists using their own reagents showed a precision ranging from 6 to 19%,[30] most of the variability being accounted for by differences between reagents.

Even the comparatively simple prothrombin time test, which is the basis of some clotting factor assays, shows considerable inter-laboratory variation. A group of hospitals using the same plasma and thromboplastin reported results with a CV of up to 18% from the mean.[36] Reliable and reproducible results are more likely to be achieved when clotting-factor assays are performed frequently by personnel experienced in the techniques and using reliable reagents. Nevertheless, the degree of accuracy required in clotting-factor assays is related to the clinical situation and the technologist in the small laboratory who is called upon to perform assays infrequently should not feel that no attempt should be made. A considerable error in the assay for factor VIII:C is unlikely to be important if the assay is performed for the diagnosis of haemophilia. Accuracy is much more essential, however, when assays are used to monitor replacement therapy or to detect the carrier state. These types of assays are best performed at Haemophilia Centres.

Standards for coagulation factor assays

The concentration of some coagulation factors may vary as much as four-fold in different normal plasma samples and it is not sufficient to use plasma from any one person to represent 100% clotting activity. A normal plasma pool, if obtained from sufficient donors, it likely to have a mean concentration of coagulation factors which is close to 100%. A laboratory standard may be prepared as follows:

Collect venous blood samples from a number of donors (see below) adding 9 volumes of blood to 1 volume of 32 g/l sodium citrate. Centrifuge without delay at 1200–1500 *g* for 15 min. Remove the supernatant plasma samples without disturbing the buffy coats and pool in a plastic container. Distribute 1.0 ml volumes into plastic vials which are then capped. Store frozen, preferably at −70°C. If storage at this temperature is not available, the standards may be stored at $-20°C$, but loss of potency is likely to be more rapid.

Within limits, large pools are preferable, but the size depends on the volume of assay work performed in the laboratory. Most pools are made from between 6 and 40 donors. The donors should be fasting, if possible, and it is preferable to include roughly equal numbers of both sexes over the age range of 20–60 years. Women taking oral contraceptives should not contribute to a standard pool.

Laboratories such as Haemophilia Centres, which perform frequent assays, should regularly check the activity of the laboratory standard against a standard in international units (iu), such as the British Standard for Blood Coagulation factor VIII Plasma, Human, obtainable from the National Institute for Biological Standards and Control, Holly Hill, Hampstead, London NW3 6RB. These working standards are freeze-dried preparations of plasma or concentrated material which have been calibrated against a WHO international standard. In laboratory standards thus calibrated, factor VIII:C concentration is expressed as iu/dl.

Commercial standards are also available for the assay of a number of coagulation factors. These consist of either freeze-dried plasma or concentrate which has been calibrated by the manufacturer against WHO international standards, provided for this purpose also by the National Institute for Biological Standards and Control. Commercially available standards are more conveniently used by small laboratories which perform assays infrequently. Commercial standards should be stored and processed as recommended by the manufacturer.

Participation in quality control schemes is of major importance for all laboratories carrying out coagulation assays.

Immunological assays

The increasing sophistication of plasma fractionation procedures in recent years has led to the production of purified coagulation factors. Such purified proteins may be used to raise appropriate antisera in laboratory animals; these antisera have the capacity to precipitate when they react in vitro with the corresponding antigen. Commercial antisera are available for most of the coagulation factors and they provide a new dimension to the investigation of coagulation-factor disorders. Antigen may be measured by immunodiffusion, immunoelectrophoresis or radioimmunoassay. The most practical application for immunological assays is the measurement of FVIIIR:Ag in haemophilia, von Willebrand's disease and in suspected carriers of the haemophilia gene. Adequate standards are essential for quantitative assay by immunological methods; they may be national, as the already described British Standard for factor VIII, commercial, or a locally collected normal plasma pool.

Assays using synthetic substrates (chromogenic assays)

Thrombin, factor Xa and plasmin are all serine proteases with relatively high substrate specificities. Various amino acid sequences have a high affinity for these proteases, and synthetic substrates based on the amino acid sequence in the natural substrates are available and can be used in assay systems. The synthetic substrates are tri- and tetra-peptides in which the chromophore, p-nitroaniline, is attached to the N-terminal amino acid. When the substrate reacts with the specific protease, the chromophore is released with a significant change in the absorbance spectrum. The rate at which p-nitroaniline is released may be measured photometrically at 405 nm and the reaction can be followed on a chart recorder (initial rate method) or after stopping the reaction at a specified time (end-point method).

Chromogenic substrates have been developed for the measurement of thrombin, factor Xa, plasmin, antithrombin III and heparin as well as for urokinase and plasma kallikrein. The measurement of antithrombin III has found the greatest clinical acceptance and will be described on p. 240. It should be remembered that the available substrates are not completely specific for individual proteases and some cross-reactivity remains a problem. The development of more highly specific substrates with good solubility and high affinity for individual proteases, together with advances in automation, promises to simplify techniques and reduce the time required for many coagulation-factor assays. Whether chromogenic assays will largely replace clotting assays is uncertain; it is still not definite that there is always good correlation between the results in the two types of assay.

With the exception of fibrinogen, all coagulation factors may be assayed by methods based on the prothrombin time or partial thromboplastin time. In this section, representative assays will be described in detail and modifications required for other assays will be indicated.

ESTIMATION OF FIBRINOGEN (FACTOR I)

Quantitative method modified from Ratnoff and Menzie[50]

Principle. Fibrinogen in plasma is converted into fibrin by the action of thrombin. The fibrin is collected on glass beads, washed, boiled with sodium hydroxide and its tyrosine content estimated, using Folin-Ciocalteu phenol reagent.

Reagents

Plasma. Add 4.5 ml of blood to 0.5 ml of 32 g/l sodium citrate and 0.5 ml of 100 mg/ml epsilon amino-caproic acid (EACA) in 9 g/l NaCl (saline). The EACA is used to prevent degradation of fibrinogen in vitro by excessive fibrinolysis which may be present in conditions associated with low fibrinogen concentrations. Centrifuge the blood at 1200–1500 *g* for 15 min and pipette off the supernatant plasma.

Glass beads. 0.5 mm diameter glass beads are suitable. Wash them with chromic acid, rinse and dry before use.

Thrombin. Bovine Topical Thrombin (Parke-Davis) at a concentration of 1000 NIH units per ml is suitable.

Folin-Ciocalteu phenol reagent.

Tyrosine standard. Dissolve 200 mg of DL-tyrosine in 1 l of 0.1 mol/l HCl. This gives a

stock solution of 0.2 mg/ml which is stable if kept at 4°C.

Method

Place 1 g of glass beads in each of two 15 ml conical centrifuge tubes and add 10 ml of saline to each. Add 0.2 ml of plasma by pipette to each tube (0.5 ml, if the fibrinogen value is expected to be low). Mix the contents of the tubes by inversion and add 0.05 ml of thrombin. Mix the contents of the tubes again and slowly invert them several times until a clot forms around the beads. Then allow the tubes to stand for at least 20 min; they may be left at this stage overnight in the refrigerator. Then gently invert the tubes and centrifuge them at 1200–1500 *g* for 15 min. Remove the supernatant by pipette, leaving the fibrin enmeshed on the glass beads. Take care that small pieces of fibrin are not lost.

Wash the fibrin three times with saline, centrifuging the tubes at 1200–1500 *g* for 15 min between washes. Finally, remove all the saline and add 1.0 ml of 2.5 mol/l (100 g/l) NaOH to the fibrin enmeshed on the beads. Cover the tubes with metal caps (Oxoid) and place in a boiling water-bath for 15 min. Then cool them and add 7.0 ml of water to each. After mixing, transfer the contents of each tube to 150 × 16 mm tubes. Then add 3.0 ml of 1.9 mol/l (200 g/l) sodium carbonate and, after mixing, add 1.0 ml of Folin-Ciocalteu reagent. Allow the tubes to stand for 20 min for the blue colour to develop.

Standard solution. Prepare the standard solution by mixing together in a 150 × 16 mm tube the following reagents: tyrosine standard 0.2 ml, 2.5 mol/l (100 g/l) NaOH 1.0 ml, water 6.8 ml, 1.9 mol/l (200 g/l) sodium carbonate 3 ml, Folin-Ciocalteu reagent 1.0 ml.

Blanks. Two blanks are required, one to read with the test samples and one to read with the standard solution. Prepare the test blank by adding 1.0 ml of 2.5 mol/l NaOH to glass beads in a centrifuge tube and placing the tube in a boiling water-bath for 15 min. When cool, add 7.0 ml of water and transfer the contents to a 150 × 16 mm tube. Then add 3.0 ml of 1.9 mol/l sodium carbonate and 1.0 ml of Folin-Ciocalteu reagent.

Prepare the standard blank in the same way as the standard solution except that the tyrosine is omitted and the volume of water is 7.0 ml.

Reading results and calculations

Read the results in a spectrophotometer at a wavelength of 650 nm using a 1 cm light path in glass cuvettes. Average the readings of the duplicate samples.

If 0.2 ml of plasma is used, the concentration of fibrinogen (g/l) is given by:

$$\frac{A^{650} \text{ test solution}}{A^{650} \text{ standard}} \times \frac{234^*}{100}.$$

If 0.5 ml of plasma is used, the concentration is given by

$$\frac{A^{650} \text{ test solution}}{A^{650} \text{ standard}} \times \frac{93.6^*}{100}.$$

Normal range: 2.0–4.0 g/l.

It is not usually necessary to correct for the dilution of whole blood due to the addition of citrate and EACA.

Notes on fibrinogen assay

The Ratnoff and Menzie method measures fibrinogen as thrombin-clottable protein. Although a standard method, it is time consuming and not very practical if a result is required urgently. The

---

* A factor of 11.7 is used in the calculation to convert liberated tyrosine to fibrinogen. The concentration of fibrinogen in g/l is given by the formula:

$$\frac{A^{650} \text{ test solution}}{A^{650} \text{ standard}} \times \text{volume of tyrosine standard (ml)}$$

$$\times \text{ concentration of tyrosine standard (g/l)}$$

$$\times \frac{1}{\text{volume of plasma(ml)}} \times 11.7.$$

The volume of tyrosine standard is 0.2 ml and the concentration 0.2 g/l.

method also underestimates the fibrinogen concentration if fibrinogen degradation products or soluble complexes of fibrinogen with fibrin monomer are present in the blood. A low result will be recorded in patients with dysfibrinogenaemia in whom the plasma fibrinogen is structurally abnormal, but present in normal concentration. Other methods of measuring fibrinogen include heat precipitation,[43] salt precipitation,[23] a modified thrombin clotting time,[14] thrombin-clot turbidity[20] and immunological methods.

A rapid method of fibrinogen assay[14]

Principle. The clotting time of plasma after the addition of thrombin in excess is proportional to the concentration of fibrinogen.

Reagents

Plasma. Citrated plasma from the patient and a normal subject.

Thrombin. Bovine Topical Thrombin (Parke-Davis). Dissolve the powder in saline to give a final concentration of c 250 NIH units per ml. The diluted thrombin may be stored frozen in plastic vials at −20°C.

Barbitone buffered saline, pH 7.4. See Appendix for method of preparation, p. 436.

Fibrinogen. Human fibrinogen (Kabi). Dissolve 40 mg in 100 ml of barbitone buffered saline to give a concentration of 0.4 g/l.

Method

Dilute the fibrinogen solution further with buffered saline to obtain solutions of 0.1, 0.2 and 0.3 g/l. Place in one of four 75 × 12 mm glass tubes in a water-bath 0.2 ml of each fibrinogen solution, ranging from 0.1 to 0.4 g/l. Next, blow 0.2 ml of thrombin into each tube in turn and record the clotting times of the mixtures. Repeat the procedure and calculate the mean clotting times for each concentration of fibrinogen. Plot the clotting times against the fibrinogen concentrations on double log paper when a straight line should be obtained.

Dilute the patient's and the normal plasma samples 1 in 10 with barbitone buffered saline. To 0.2 ml of each plasma dilution add 0.2 ml of thrombin and record the clotting times. Repeat the test and average the times. Read off the concentrations of fibrinogen corresponding to the clotting times from the standard graph and multiply by the dilution (×10) to give the fibrinogen concentrations of the plasma samples. It is usually not necessary to correct for the dilution of whole blood due to the addition of citrate. If the test plasma dilution gives clotting times which do not fall in the range 0.1–0.4 g/l of fibrinogen, make appropriate new dilutions and repeat the test.

Because the clot often may not be readily seen, a coagulometer is valuable in detecting the end-point.

An even more simple and rapid semi-quantitative assay may be performed by comparing the thrombin clotting times of dilutions of normal plasma and test plasma, and expressing the ratio of dilutions giving the same clotting times as the fibrinogen titre.

Semi-quantitative assay of fibrinogen[57]

Principle. Serial dilutions of both normal and test plasma samples are clotted with thrombin. The highest dilutions in which fibrin clots can be observed are compared. The tests should be carried out with dilutions (a) in saline, (b) in saline containing EACA (to prevent fibrinolysis) and (c) in saline containing protamine sulphate (to overcome the inhibitory effect of split-products of fibrinogen and fibrin, if present). In emergencies, however, dilutions in saline alone usually give the required information.

Reagents

Citrated plasma. From the patient and a control.

Thrombin. Fibrindex (Ortho) is suitable; reconstitute an ampoule containing 50 NIH units with 2 ml of saline before use.

Epsilon aminocaproic acid (EACA; 6 aminohexanoic acid*) : 1 mg/ml in saline.

Protamine sulphate. 400 mg/l in saline.

Method

Set up three sets of seven 75 × 12 mm glass tubes for the normal and the test plasma samples. Into each tube of the first set place 0.5 ml of saline; into each tube of the second set 0.5 ml of EACA in saline; into the first tube of the third set 0.5 ml of protamine sulphate in saline, and into the other six tubes 0.5 ml of saline.

Add 0.5 ml of plasma to the first tube of each set; mix the contents of the tube and transfer 0.5 ml to the second tube, and so on, so as to give final concentrations of plasma from 1 in 2 to 1 in 128. Add 0.1 ml volumes of thrombin to each tube and mix well with the plasma dilutions.

Place the tubes at 37°C and leave undisturbed for 15 min; then inspect them for the presence or absence of fibrin.

Interpretation

Normally, fibrin clots will be seen in all the plasma dilutions up to 1 in 128. In severe hypofibrinogenaemia, no clots will be found in any dilution and in partial states of depletion they will be found only in the first 1–3 tubes. If excessive fibrinolysis is present, the fibrin clots will be visible in the tubes containing EACA to a greater dilution than in the tubes containing saline alone. If split products of fibrin or fibrinogen are present in the plasma, fibrin clots will be visible in the tubes containing protamine to a greater dilution than in the tubes containing saline alone.

ASSAYS BASED ON THE PROTHROMBIN TIME (PROTHROMBIN, FACTORS V, VII AND X)

Principle. The one-stage prothrombin time of plasma is sensitive to deficiencies of factors

* e.g. BDH or Sigma.

Table 14.1 Conversion of plasma dilutions into concentration for the parallel line assay

Type and factor to be assayed	Dilution of standard	Concentration %
One-stage factor VIII or IX	1 in 10, 1 in 50, 1 in 100 or	100, 20, 10
	1 in 10, 1 in 40, 1 in 160	100, 25, 12.5
Two-stage factor VIII	1 in 40, 1 in 80, 1 in 160	100, 50, 25
Factor X	1 in 10, 1 in 100, 1 in 1000	100, 10, 1
Factor V, VII, II	1 in 5, 1 in 25, 1 in 125 or	100, 20, 4
	1 in 3, 1 in 9, 1 in 27	100, 33, 11

VII, X, V, fibrinogen and prothrombin. Freeze-dried samples of human plasma with deficiencies of prothrombin, factor V or factor VII are available commercially. These preparations contain not more than 1% of the deficient factor but adequate concentrations of the other factors necessary for the prothrombin-time test. Assays are based on a comparison of the degree of correction of the long prothrombin time of the factor-deficient plasma after the addition of dilutions of the test plasma or a standard plasma pool. The prothrombin-time estimations are carried out in the usual manner using brain thromboplastin and added calcium chloride.

In the case of factor X, a commercial reagent is available consisting of freeze-dried charcoal-filtered ox plasma. This reagent is deficient in both factors VII and X, but if the prothrombin-time tests are performed using Russell's viper venom, factor VII deficiency does not influence the result and the reagent can be used for a specific assay for factor X.

Assays of factors II (prothrombin), V and VII

Reagents

Factor-deficient plasma. Appropriate factor-deficient plasma from a patient or a freeze-dried commercial reagent*. If commercial freeze-dried plasma is used, follow the instructions of the manufacturer to reconstitute and use the method recommended for the assay.

* e.g. Behringwerke; Immuno; Dade.

Barbitone buffered saline. See Appendix.
Thromboplastin. Either human or rabbit brain thromboplastin may be used.
Calcium chloride. A 0.025 mol/l solution is used.
Standard plasma. See p. 226.

Method

Prepare dilutions of standard and test plasma 1 in 10, 1 in 50 and 1 in 100 in buffered saline. The three dilutions of each are tested simultaneously in the following way: mix 0.1 ml of standard plasma dilution, 0.1 ml of deficient plasma and 0.1 ml of thromboplastin in a glass tube and place in a water-bath. Allow 30 s to warm to 37°C. Add 0.1 ml of the $CaCl_2$ solution and record the clotting time for each tube. Repeat the same procedure on the same three dilutions of the standard plasma and another factor-deficient plasma; then continue with the test plasma dilutions in the same way. Record the mean clotting time with each dilution.

Plot clotting times against dilutions on double log paper; read the results off the graph (Fig. 14.1, Table 14.1).

Alternative methods for the assay of factor II, V and VII are available. The venom of the Taipan viper (*Oxyuranus scutellatus*) is able to convert prothrombin directly to thrombin in the absence of any of the known clotting factors. It may be used as a specific reagent for a one-stage assay of *prothrombin.*[19]

Factor V-deficient plasma may be prepared by incubating oxalated normal plasma at 37°C for 3 days under sterile conditions. The plasma is obtained from blood mixed with a one-ninth volume of 14 g/l potassium oxalate. The aged plasma may be stored at −20°C until required. Alternative sources of factor-VII-deficient plasma include plasma obtained from a patient about 48 h after commencing warfarin therapy and plasma from a colony of Beagle dogs with a congenital deficiency of factor VII.[24]

Assay of factor X[64]

Principle. The adsorption of plasma with any of a number of inorganic adsorbents prolongs the prothrombin time using brain extract because variable amounts of factors II, VII and X are removed. Russell's viper venom is insensitive to factor VII deficiency and if venom is used instead of brain extract, prolongation of the prothrombin time reflects deficiency of factors II and X. By careful adsorption of ox plasma with charcoal, sufficient prothrombin (factor II) is left in the plasma to make it a sensitive substrate plasma for the measurement of factor X. Prothrombin times using Russell's viper venom are then performed on mixtures of the adsorbed ox plasma with dilutions of normal and test plasma.

Reagents

Factor X substrate plasma (Diagen)*. The material is freeze-dried as supplied. Reconstitute with 0.3 ml of water.

Russell's viper venom/cephalin reagent (Diagen)*. This is also freeze-dried and when reconstituted with 6.0 ml of water contains Russell's viper venom at a dilution of 1 in 150 000 and cephalin at optimum concentration.

Normal and test plasma. Make 1 in 10, 1 in 100 and 1 in 1000 dilutions in buffered saline, pH 7.4.

Calcium. 0.025 mol/l calcium chloride.

---

* Diagnostic Reagents Ltd., Thame, Oxon.

Method

Place in a 75 × 12 mm glass tube at 37°C 0.1 ml of substrate plasma, 0.1 ml of a dilution of normal or test plasma and 0.1 ml of Russell's viper venom/cephalin reagent. After exactly 30 s blow in 0.1 ml of calcium chloride and record the clotting time of the mixture. Repeat the procedure with the other dilutions of normal and test plasma. Perform each determination in duplicate.

The clotting times when plotted against the concentration of plasma should give a straight line on double-log paper. Lines are drawn for both the normal and test plasma samples and these should be parallel. The factor X concentration of the test plasma may be read off such a graph, by comparing the test plasma figures with the normal figures.

ASSAYS BASED ON THE PARTIAL THROMBOPLASTIN TIME (FACTORS VIII, IX, XI AND XII)

Principle. Freeze-dried samples of human or bovine plasma deficient in factor VIII, factor IX, factor XI or factor XII are available commercially. These samples contain not more than 1% of the deficient factor but adequate concentrations of the other factors necessary for the partial thromboplastin time test (PTTK). Assays are based on a comparison of the degree of correction of the prolonged PTTK of the factor-deficient plasma after the addition of dilutions of the test plasma or of a standard plasma pool. The one-stage assay for factor VIII:C will be described in detail, but similar principles apply to the assay of factors IX, XI and XII.

Factor VIII assay[27]

Reagents

Factor VIII:C-deficient plasma. If using a commercial reagent, the freeze-dried plasma should be reconstituted according to the manufacturer's instructions. If suitable haemophilic plasma is available, this may be stored at −20°C in 1 ml volumes in plastic containers for periods up to 1 month. The plasma should have a PTTK of 150 s or more and no inhibitor should be present.

Standard plasma. As for other assays (see p. 226), prepare 1 in 10, 1 in 20 and 1 in 100 dilutions of the standard plasma in barbitone buffered saline. Standard plasma calibrated against a standard with an established factor VIII:C content in international units (iu) per dl should be used whenever possible.

Test plasma. Prepare 1 in 5, 1 in 10 and 1 in 20 dilutions. When assaying factor VIII concentrate, 1 in 20, 1 in 100 and 1 in 200 dilutions are suitable.

Phospholipid. Either Bell and Alton's phospholipid or a number of commercial reagents may be used. If Inosithin is used, a 1 in 10 dilution in barbitone buffered saline of the 1% stock solution (see p. 434) is suitable.

Calcium. 0.025 mol/l calcium chloride.

Kaolin. Kaolin BP, 5 g/l, in barbitone buffered saline.

Method

Pipette 0.1 ml of factor VIII:C-deficient plasma, 0.1 ml of standard or test plasma dilution, 0.1 ml of phospholipid and 0.1 ml of kaolin into a 75 × 12 mm glass tube and incubate for exactly 10 min at 37°C with occasional shaking. Then add 0.1 ml of calcium chloride and start a second stop-watch at the moment of the addition of the calcium chloride. Record the clotting time of the mixture. Repeat the procedure with all the standard and test plasma dilutions (Table 14.2). Using five stopwatches, it is possible to have four mixtures incubating at 2 min intervals, thus reducing the overall time of the assay considerably.

The clotting times of the mixtures containing dilutions of standard plasma should fall on a straight line when plotted on double-log paper against concentrations of factor VIII:C. The line given by the clotting times of the dilutions of the test plasma should parallel that given by the standard plasma. In the assay illustrated in Table 14.2 the factor VIII:C

Table 14.2 Result of a factor VIII assay based on the partial thromboplastin time

Dilution of standard plasma	Clotting time (s)	Dilution of test plasma	Clotting time (s)
1 in 10	76	1 in 5	86
1 in 20	86	1 in 10	98
1 in 100	110	1 in 20	110

concentration of the test plasma was 20% of the standard.

If the standard plasma is calibrated in terms of international units (iu), the factor VIII:C content of the test plasma can also be expressed in iu/dl. For example, if the standard plasma has 65 iu factor VIII:C/dl, the test plasma will have 20% of 65 iu/dl, that is 13 iu/dl.

Factor VIII assay based on the thromboplastin generation test[9,48]

Principle. Thromboplastin generation tests are carried out using reagents grossly deficient in factor VIII, but containing all the other clotting factors in normal proportions. The effect of adding dilutions of patient's plasma to the system as a source of factor VIII is compared with that produced by adding dilutions of a standard normal plasma.

Reagents

Factor V reagent. Two factor V preparations will be described. One is available commercially and is prepared from bovine plasma; the other is prepared from haemophilic plasma.

1. *Bovine factor V (Diagen)*.* This is a freeze-dried preparation of factor V without factor VIII activity. The unopened vials should be stored at −20°C. Reconstitute the contents of the vial with 1.0 ml of water, and dilute the solution further to 20 ml with barbitone buffered saline, pH 7.4. Distribute the solution in tubes in volumes sufficient for a day's use and

* Diagnostic Reagents Ltd., Thame, Oxon.

store at −20°C. It can be kept for up to 1 month at −20°C without appreciable loss of activity.

2. *Adsorbed haemophilic plasma.* Plasma from a severe haemophiliac is a good source of factor V free from factor VIII. It is essential that the FVIII content of the plasma should be less than 1% and that tests for inhibitors should be negative. Distribute platelet-poor citrated haemophilic plasma in 0.9 ml volumes in small plastic tubes and store at −20°C; such samples are usually satisfactory for about 1 month. Before the actual test, mix a 0.9 ml volume with 0.1 ml of aluminium hydroxide gel ('alumina') and carry out the adsorption, as described on p. 220. Dilute the adsorbed plasma 1 in 5 with barbitone buffer before use.

Normal serum. It is preferable to use a pool consisting of four to six normal sera. Allow about 4 ml of blood from each donor to clot at 37°C in glass tubes containing beads. Invert the tubes once or twice during clotting to make sure that contact activation is optimal. Then leave the clotted specimens at 37°C for 4 h and separate the serum by centrifugation. Pool the serum samples and leave at 4°C overnight. Then dilute the pooled serum 1 in 10 in barbitone buffered saline and distribute in glass tubes in volumes sufficient for a day's use. The diluted serum, if stored at −20°C, can be used for up to 1 month.

Phospholipid. Bell and Alton's phospholipid (p. 434) or Inosithin may be used. The latter is usually used at a concentration of 0.2 mg/ml. Inosithin tends to give somewhat longer substrate clotting times than brain phospholipid, and this is an advantage in this test.

Standard factor VIII. Either a standard plasma pool or a commercial factor VIII:C standard may be used. Thaw the standard plasma at 37°C, inverting the tube several times to make sure that any cold-precipitable material goes back into solution. Then adsorb it with 'alumina' and prepare dilutions from 1 in 40 to 1 in 640 in barbitone buffered saline. A convenient way of doing this is to take five glass tubes and to add 7.8 ml of saline to the first, 1.0 ml to the second, 3.0 ml to the third, 7.0 ml to the fourth and 7.5 ml to the fifth. Pipette 0.2 ml of adsorbed standard plasma into the

first tube and mix by inversion (giving a 1 in 40 dilution). Then pipette 1.0 ml volumes from the first tube into the second, third and fourth tubes, and a 0.5 ml volume into the fifth tube, giving 1 in 80, 160, 320 and 640 dilutions, respectively.

Test plasma. Adsorb the citrated plasma with 'alumina' and make appropriate dilutions. If the factor-VIII:C concentration is expected to be about normal, 1 in 80, 1 in 160 and 1 in 320 dilutions are suitable, but for plasma samples with low factor VIII:C concentrations use 1 in 10, 1 in 20 and 1 in 40 dilutions.

Substrate plasma. Use citrated normal plasma obtained by centrifugation at 2000–3000 *g* for 5–10 min. This must be prepared on the day of the test.

Calcium chloride. 0.025 mol/l calcium chloride.

Keep all reagents at 4°C in a refrigerator or in ice-water on the bench until actually used.

Method

Up to eight dilutions of the standard or test plasma may be tested concurrently. Place into a series of 75 × 12 mm tubes in the back row of a rack in a water-bath 0.1 ml volumes of substrate plasma, and into another series of tubes in the front row of the rack, pipette 0.1 ml volumes of factor V reagent, diluted serum, phospholipid and standard or test plasma dilution (or buffered saline blank), respectively. After allowing the contents of the tubes to warm to 37°C, add 0.1 ml of calcium chloride to the first tube and start a stop-watch. At 1 min intervals, add calcium chloride to successive tubes, so that after 7 min the calcium chloride has been added to all eight tubes. At exactly 8 min, pipette a 0.1 ml volume from the first tube and, together with 0.1 ml of calcium chloride, add it to a tube containing substrate plasma. Start a second stop-watch (preferably foot-operated) and record the time taken for the substrate plasma to clot.

Repeat the above procedure at 1 min intervals so that each mixture is sub-sampled after

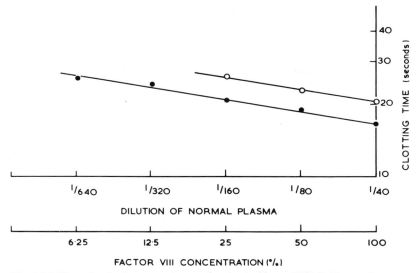

Fig. 14.2 Thromboplastin-generation test for assay of factor VIII:C. The graphs illustrate the substrate clotting times of the standard plasma (●) and test plasma (○) at various dilutions. A 1 in 40 dilution of the standard has been given a value of 100%. In this example, the Factor VIII:C in the test plasma is 25%.

8 min incubation. If a series of plasma samples are being assayed, test the standard dilutions at the beginning and again at the end of the assays to show that there has been no 'drift' in clotting times.

Calculation

Plot the substrate clotting times given by the various dilutions of standard and test plasma against the dilution of plasma on double-log paper (Fig. 14.2). The points should approximate to straight lines. The line drawn through the points given by the test plasma dilutions should be parallel to one drawn through points given by the standards. If the 1 in 40 dilution of the standard plasma is given a value of 100% factor VIII:C, then the factor VIII:C concentration of the test sample can be read off the graph directly (Fig. 14.2).

Estimation of factor VIII antigen (FVIIIR : Ag)[58,63]

Principle. Factor VIII antigen is measured using a heterologous precipitating antiserum and quantitative immunoelectrophoresis.[34]

Reagents

Barbitone buffer. pH 8.6, ionic strength 0.05. Dissolve 103 g of sodium diethyl barbiturate and 20 g of diethyl barbituric acid in water and make up to 10 l with water.

Test Plasma. Citrated plasma is used.

Standards. Calibrated commercial or national standards (such as the Blood Coagulation Factor VIII, Plasma, Human; obtainable from the National Institute for Biological Standards and Control, Holly Hill, Hampstead, London NW3 6RB) should be used, or a normal plasma pool stored deep-frozen in 0.2–0.3 ml volumes and calibrated against other standards. The standard plasma is used undiluted, and diluted 1 in 2 and 1 in 4 in barbitone buffer.

Factor VIII antiserum. An antiserum from rabbits immunized with purified human factor VIII is used. Commercial preparations (e.g. Behringwerke) are available.

Agarose. Indubiose (L'Industrie Biologique Francaise) or other suitable preparation.

Immunoelectrophoresis plates. c 70 × 63 mm. The size is not critical, but the plate should be wide enough to allow 12 wells 3 mm in diameter to be punched into the gel which is to cover the plate. The plates are smeared with 1.5% agarose in water, allowed to dry overnight at room temperature and subsequently stored at 4°C.

Punch. To make 3 mm holes in the gel.

Stain. Coomassie Brilliant Blue, 1%, in a solvent consisting of absolute ethanol 9 volumes, water 9 volumes, and glacial acetic acid 1 volume is suitable. The solvent, without the stain, is used also for de-staining the gels.

Electrophoresis tank, power pack and wicks. Standard laboratory equipment.

Method

Add sufficient agarose to a flask containing barbitone buffer in a boiling water-bath to make a 1% solution. After the dissolved agarose has cooled to 50–56°C transfer 8 ml to a test tube containing 30 μl of factor-VIII antiserum. Mix the contents and pour on to the immunoelectrophoretic plate to form a gel about 1 mm deep. It may be helpful, but it is not essential, to use a mould to assist in obtaining gel of the correct depth. A second immunoelectrophoresis plate placed on top of the mould ensures that the depth of the gel is uniform.

After 5–10 min, when the gel has set, punch 12 wells 3 mm in diameter in a straight line across the width of the gel, about 1 cm from one edge. Remove the punched-out sections of the gel by gentle suction, using a 2.6 mm suction needle. The gel is now ready to accept the test and standard materials.

Add to each pair of wells duplicate 5-μl volumes of the appropriate plasma or plasma dilution. The normal plasma pool is tested undiluted and at 1 in 2 and 1 in 4 dilutions, so that each plate is sufficient for three test samples in duplicate. Position filter paper wicks carefully to connect the gel with electrode troughs filled with barbitone buffer. Complete the circuit with the well positioned at the cathode and electrophorese for 15–20 h at a consistent current of 10 mA.

After completion of the electrophoresis, remove the plate and wash out the wells with water. Lay the moist filter paper on top of the gel followed by several layers of dry filter paper and add a flat weight of about 1 kg. Exert pressure for 10 min to express superfluous fluid and then dry the gel with a warm air current until it is flat and shiny.

Immerse the dried gel in the stain for 15 min and then wash it in the solvent and finally in water. Then allow it to dry in the air at room temperature. The distance of the migration is determined by direct measurement from the top of the well to the apex of the precipitin 'rocket'.

Calculation

Measure the rocket heights in mm to the nearest 0.25 mm. Construct a graph on double-log paper by plotting the heights reached by the standard plasma pool undiluted and diluted 1 in 2 and 1 in 4 against their FVIIIR:Ag concentrations, expressed as 100%, 50% and 25% of normal, respectively.

Read off the concentration of FVIIIR:Ag in the test plasma directly from the graph.

Comment

The optimal concentration of antiserum in the gel is determined by trial and error. Too much antiserum gives rockets of insufficient length for precision whereas too little antiserum gives rockets which stain too faintly for reliable measurement. The measurement of FVIIIR:Ag is important in the detection of the haemophilic carrier and in the diagnosis of von Willebrand's disease. In the latter condition, measurement of FVIII:WF (ristocetin co-factor, see p. 252) is also necessary. Measurement of the various factor-VIII activities should always be performed on samples of the same test plasma.

Measurement of factor VIII inhibitors[28]

Inhibitors which occur in the plasma of haemophiliacs and occasionally in patients with previously normal haemostasis may be detected by mixing experiments in which equal volumes of patient and normal plasma are incubated at 37°C. An inhibitor is suspected if the PTTK of the mixture is prolonged significantly when compared to that of a mixture of normal plasma and buffered saline incubated for a similar period of time. Such tests should be performed at regular intervals in all severe haemophiliacs, for the development of an inhibitor complicates the patient's management. It is desirable to estimate the potency of an inhibitor, when present, as a guide to the clinical progress of the patient and the likely benefit of replacement therapy.

Principle. Test plasma, diluted if necessary, is incubated with a standard plasma containing 100% factor VIII:C. The decrease in factor VIII:C concentration of the incubation mixture is expressed quantitatively as Bethesda units/ml inhibitor activity of the test plasma.

Reagents

Citrated test plasma. See p. 215.
Normal plasma pool. See p. 226.
Imidazole buffered saline. 0.05 mol/l, pH 7.4. See Appendix, p. 435.
Reagents for factor VIII:C assay. Either a one-stage or a two-stage method may be used (see p. 232).

Method

Incubate equal volumes of test plasma and normal plasma at 37°C for 2 h in a stoppered glass tube, and incubate a control mixture of equal volumes of buffer and normal plasma concurrently. At the end of 2 h, assay both mixtures for factor VIII:C content. If the factor VIII:C concentration of the mixture of test plasma and normal plasma is <25% of that of the mixture of buffer and normal plasma, repeat the test using an appropriate dilution of test plasma in buffer in the incubation mixture with normal plasma.

Calculation

Record the ratio of factor VIII:C concentration in the mixture of the test plasma and normal

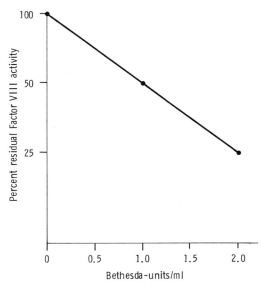

Fig. 14.3 Measurement of factor VIII inhibitor. Relationship between factor VIII:C activity in a standard plasma and the inhibitor activity of a test plasma. At 50% inhibition the test plasma contains 1 Bethesda inhibitor unit/ml.

plasma to that in the mixture of the normal plasma and buffer, and express as a percentage. A value of 100% (i.e. both mixtures have the same factor VIII:C content) indicates that no inhibitor is demonstrable. A value of 50% has been accepted by definition to indicate that the test plasma contains 1.0 Bethesda inhibitor units per ml. Other percentage values may be converted into inhibitor units by reference to the graph shown in Fig. 14.3, where percentage on a log scale is plotted against units on a linear scale. If the test plasma requires dilution to obtain a result which can be read off this graph, use the appropriate multiplication factor in the final calculation.

Comment

This method may not detect some weak, but clinically significant, inhibitors in haemophiliacs. The kinetics of different inhibitors vary and the definition of potency in units is not very precise. Nevertheless, the above method, which has gained wide acceptance, provides a uniform technique to enable a comparison of the results obtained in different laboratories. The allocation of a certain number of Bethesda inhibitor units to a test plasma does not imply that any specific number of factor VIII:C units infused into the patient will neutralize the circulating inhibitor.

Assay of factor XIII[38]

Accurate measurement of plasma factor XIII concentration can be achieved by measuring plasma transamidase activity, but the available methods are too complicated for routine clinical use. For practical purposes, the qualitative assay described below is sufficient to diagnose a congenital deficiency.

Principle. Factor XIII is activated during the clotting of blood from an inactive precursor. Calcium ions and thrombin are necessary for this activiation. Activated factor XIII stabilizes the fibrin clot, by a process of transamidation. The stable clot is insoluble in 5 mol/l urea whereas clots from plasma deficient in factor XIII are soluble.

Reagents

Plasma. Citrated plasma from patient and control subject.
Calcium. 0.025 mol/l calcium chloride.
Urea. 5 mol/l urea (300 g/l).

Method

Place 0.2 ml of the test and control plasma samples in 75 × 12 mm glass tubes and add 0.2 ml of calcium chloride to each tube. Incubate the tubes for 30 min at 37°C. Then add 3.0 ml of 5 mol/l urea and shake the clots up in the urea solution. Leave the tubes overnight at room temperature and inspect the clots the next day.

If factor XIII is present in the plasma, the clot in the test sample will still be present. A positive control, i.e. an urea-soluble clot, can be produced by adding 0.2 ml of thrombin (20 NIH units/ml) to 0.2 ml of EDTA plasma. Such a clot is soluble in urea because of lack of the free calcium ions which are needed for the action of factor XIII.

THE LABORATORY DIAGNOSIS OF DISSEMINATED INTRAVASCULAR COAGULATION[49,57]

The syndrome of disseminated intravascular coagulation (DIC) may result from either of two mechanisms. The presence of procoagulant material in the circulation may trigger the blood coagulation process or widespread vascular damage may cause multiple fibrin-platelet thrombi in the microcirculation. In either situation, consumption of coagulation factors and platelets leads to haemorrhage which is aggravated by the presence in the blood of fibrinogen/fibrin degradation products (FDP) which themselves have an anticoagulant effect. Furthermore, fibrin deposition in the microcirculation may cause impairment of organ function as well as damage to red cells, resulting in microangiopathic haemolytic anaemia.

In the acute defibrination syndrome, there is usually little difficulty in diagnosis. The blood may fail to clot or a small piece of fibrin may appear in the clotting tube; if the tube is agitated, the fibrin may be dislodged and lost amongst the red cells, thus giving an erroneous impression that fibrinolysis has taken place. If there is doubt concerning the size of the clot, the contents of the clotting tubes should be poured gently into a Petri dish where the clot may be observed more readily.

In subacute or chronic states of intravascular coagulation, severe depletion of fibrinogen may not occur and the clot size may not be obviously abnormal. This is particularly likely to be the case when hyperfibrinogenaemia was present before the episode of defibrination, e.g. in pregnancy, carcinoma and infections. In such situations, a number of investigations may be necessary to confirm the diagnosis. These can be performed conveniently in the following order:

Screening tests

1. One-stage prothrombin time.
2. Partial thromboplastin time with kaolin.
3. Thrombin clotting time.
4. Platelet count.
5. Blood film.

The one-stage prothrombin time and the partial thromboplastin time are prolonged due to consumption of coagulation factors. The thrombin clotting time is prolonged from fibrinogen deficiency and from the presence of fibrinogen/fibrin degradation products.

Thrombocytopenia is present and the blood film may show evidence of microangiopathic haemolytic anaemia.

More elaborate tests

1. Detection of FDP (see p. 244).
2. Screening test for fibrin monomers (see p. 239).
3. Euglobulin clot lysis time (see p. 242).
4. Quantitative assays for fibrinogen and blood coagulation factors, especially factors V and VIII:C.
5. Plasma antithrombin III assay (see p. 240).

Interpretation of tests for disseminated intravascular coagulation

The diagnosis of DIC in a situation other than acute defibrination may be difficult and requires the correct interpretation of the results of a number of tests. Difficulties in diagnosis may occur in patients who have had severe haemorrhage resulting in depletion of clotting factors and platelets, in patients with liver disease in whom the synthesis of a number of clotting factors may be deficient, in patients with a hyperfibrinolytic state and in patients with acute thrombocytopenia due to other causes. There is no single test the result of which is conclusive for DIC. Increased concentrations of FDP may result from lysis of both intravascular and extravascular fibrin, from excessive fibrinolysis digesting circulating fibrinogen, or from failure of the kidney to excrete or liver to clear products being produced normally.

Tests for FDP may be positive, too, in extensive haematoma formation, in venous thrombosis with or without pulmonary embolism, in hyperfibrinolytic states and in renal failure. Soluble fibrin monomers complexed to fibrinogen or FDP may also be detected in thrombosis, hyperfibrinolysis and severe infections.

The euglobulin clot lysis time is characteristically normal in DIC and markedly shortened in systemic fibrinolysis. However, a spuriously short time may be observed in DIC if the plasma fibrinogen is low, and a normal time in systemic fibrinolysis if the blood has been depleted of plasminogen. Coagulation factors may be reduced through bleeding or defective synthesis as well as by excessive consumption. Although the plasma antithrombin III concentration is reduced in DIC due to complexing with thrombin, it is also low in a number of other conditions, including liver disease, heparin therapy and congenital antithrombin III deficiency. Thrombocytopenia is a constant finding in DIC, and the diagnosis should not be made in the presence of a normal platelet count.

Screening test for fibrin monomers[11,37]

Principle. When thrombin acts on fibrinogen, some of the monomers do not polymerize but give rise to soluble complexes with plasma fibrinogen and FDP. These complexes can be dissociated in vitro by ethanol or protamine sulphate.

Reagents

Citrated test plasma.

Positive control. Prepare this by adding 0.1 ml of thrombin (0.2 NIH units/ml) to 0.9 ml of normal citrated plasma and incubating at 37°C for 30 min. Fibrin threads that form during the incubation period are removed by centrifugation.

Protamine sulphate. 1% (10 g/l).

Ethanol. 50% (v/v) in water.

Methods

Protamine sulphate test. Add 0.05 ml of protamine sulphate to 1 ml of citrated test plasma or 1 ml of positive control in 75 × 12 mm tubes pre-warmed to 37°C. Allow the mixtures to stand at 37°C for 3 min. A positive result is indicated by the formation of a feathery fibrin network or fine fibrin threads. The presence of amorphous material only is a negative result.

Ethanol gelation test. Add 0.15 ml of ethanol to 0.5 ml of citrated test plasma or positive control in 75 × 12 mm tubes at room temperature. After gentle agitation, inspect the tubes at 1 min intervals. A positive result is the formation of a definite gel within 3 min.

MEASUREMENT OF ANTITHROMBIN III

Antithrombin III is identical with the substance known as heparin cofactor. It inhibits a number of serine proteases including factors XIa, IXa, Xa, thrombin and plasmin[53] It may be measured using a coagulation test in tubes or in agarose gel,[8] by an immunological technique[22] or by a chromogenic substrate assay.[1] Coagulation assays are relatively complex; a laboratory which does not regularly perform them may find that the results are not always reproducible. For a laboratory doing only occasional antithrombin III estimations, chromogenic assay is the best choice. The results of immunological tests are rarely available on the same day; and a proportion of congenitally deficient patients have normal immunoreactive antithrombin III despite low biological activity.[55]

Chromogenic assay of antithrombin III[1]

Principle. Antithrombin III in patients' plasma is bound to heparin in vitro. The complex antithrombin III:heparin reacts with excess thrombin. The amount of thrombin bound is determined by the concentration of antithrombin III in plasma. Free, excess, thrombin is measured using a thrombin-specific substrate.

Reagents

Patient's citrated platelet-poor plasma. Use a commercially available kit* containing buffer, heparin, thrombin and thrombin-specific peptide.

---

* E.g. Coatest, Antithrombin III kit, Kabivitrum, Kabi Pharmaceutical Ltd., Builton House, 54–58 Uxbridge Road, London; or Antithrombin III kit, BCL Coagulation Diagnostics, Bell Lane, Lewis, East Sussex.

Method

Follow the manufacturer's instructions. Measure the colour change in a spectrophotometer at a wavelength of 405 nm.

Calculation

Read off the values from a standard curve prepared at the same time, according to the manufacturer's directions.

Normal range. The values may be expressed as inhibitor units (normal 11–14 u/ml), percent of normal plasma pool (80–125%) or as g/l (normal 0.2–0.4 g/l).

Immunological measurement of antithrombin III[22]

Principle. Among the immunological methods to estimate antithrombin III, radial immunodiffusion and rocket-electrophoresis are the most popular. In the immunodiffusion technique the antigen is allowed to diffuse radially into agarose containing a monospecific antiserum; after 48 h the area of the resulting precipitin rings is measured. Although it is possible for a laboratory to prepare immunodiffusion plates, it is more convenient to obtain them from commercial sources. Alternatively, the rocket-electrophoresis of Laurell can be applied. The advantage of the latter technique is that the results are obtained in a much shorter period of time.

Reagents

M-Partigen-antithrombin III immunodiffusion plates (Behringwerke). Each plate contains monospecific rabbit antiserum in an agar gel layer ready for immediate use. Each plate contains 12 numbered wells, allowing nine test samples and three dilutions of a standard to be tested. Follow the manufacturers instructions carefully.

Electro-immunodiffusion (Laurell rocket technique). The same conditions as described for the determination of the factor VIII R:Ag (see p. 235) can be applied. Antiserum to antithrombin III is commercially available (e.g. Behringwerke). The only difference from the factor VIII R:Ag assay is the antiserum concentration in the gel, which should be 0.7% with a test plasma dilution of 1 in 4. The remaining procedure is identical with that described for factor VIII R:Ag.

Protein standard plasma (Beringwerke). Lyophilized standard plasma with a designated concentration of antithrombin III in mg/dl (or g/l) is available. The use of this standard enables a numerical result to be obtained. Dissolve the contents of the vial in exactly 0.5 ml of water. Use the standard plasma, undiluted and at dilutions of 1 in 2 and 1 in 4 in 9 g/l saline, for immunodiffusion as well as for the rocket technique.

Standard plasma pool. See p. 226. A standard plasma diluted 1 in 2, 1 in 4 and 1 in 8 can replace the protein standard plasma, but the results of the antithrombin III measurement are then obtained as a percentage of the standard normal pool. Do not refreeze the standard plasma pool after it has been thawed.

Test plasma. Use citrated plasma. It may be frozen at −20°C or lower, but thawed once only for testing.

Calculation

When immunodiffusion plates are used, plot the squares of the diameters of the precipitin rings obtained with the three standard preparations against concentrations on linear graph paper. Read the concentration of antithrombin III in test plasma off the graph, multiplying the value obtained by the dilution factor.

The evaluation of electro-immunodiffusion plates is identical to that described for factor VIII R:Ag.

Normal range. 0.22–0.39 g/l (80–120%).

DEMONSTRATION OF INHIBITORS IN SYSTEMIC LUPUS ERYTHEMATOSUS (SLE) (THE LUPUS INHIBITOR)[21,35]

The nature of the inhibitor found not uncommonly in the plasma of patients with SLE has been the subject of much investigation. It appears to react during blood coagulation with the complex formed between factor Xa, factor V, calcium and phospholipid and so impedes the conversion of prothrombin to thrombin. The lupus inhibitor has an immediate action and incubation with normal plasma does not cause a progressive increase in any clotting time test beyond that obtained on immediate mixing. Although sometimes the cause of bleeding, it may be symptomless or even associated with venous thrombosis.[39]

The following are the classical abnormalities in clotting tests in blood from patients with a lupus inhibitor. The PTTK of the test plasma is prolonged and the presence of an inhibitor can be demonstrated by mixing experiments using the PTTK. If the PTTK of plasma is measured without the addition of phospholipid, the abnormality in the plasma becomes more obvious. The one-stage prothrombin time using brain extract may be normal or prolonged. If normal, the test should be repeated using a diluted brain extract (1 in 2 or 1 in 4 in buffered saline, pH 7.4.) when a prolongation compared to normal is observed. The one-stage prothrombin time is prolonged using Russell's viper venom/cephalin reagent as a source of thromboplastin and the prolongation becomes more obvious if the test is repeated without the cephalin component of the reagent. The plasma prothrombin concentration is normal when measured with Taipan snake venom reagent. Routine factor assays may give apparently low values due to the presence of the inhibitor in the reaction mixtures. The following test is recommended for the demonstration of 'SLE inhibitor' characteristics.

Test for the 'SLE inhibitor'[3]

Principle. The 'SLE inhibitor' is not absorbed by Al $(OH)_3$ and withstands heating at 56°C. It will also prolong the PTTK of normal plasma after these treatments.

Reagents

Citrated plasma. From the patient and a control subject (p. 215).

Aluminium hydroxide. $Al(OH)_3$ gel (p. 433).

Calcium. $CaCl_2$, 0.05 mol/l.

Method

Mix 0.4 ml of the patient's plasma sample in a glass tube and control plasma in another tube with 0.1 ml of diluted Al(OH)₃ reagent, incubate for 3 min at 37°C and remove the Al(OH)₃ by centrifugation. Heat the supernatants at 56°C for 30 min, then centrifuge to remove precipitated fibrinogen.

Set up PTTK tests by placing in four clotting tubes 0.1 ml, respectively, of the control plasma, the patient's plasma and Al(OH)₃-treated control and patient's plasma, and adding to each sample the phospholipid and kaolin suspension. Then carry out the PTTK as described on p. 219. Run duplicate tests in reverse order.

Interpretation

If the patient's Al(OH)₃-treated plasma takes longer to clot than the control treated plasma by 10 s or more, the characteristics of the 'SLE inhibitor' will have been demonstrated.

ASSESSMENT OF THE FIBRINOLYTIC SYSTEM

The fibrinolytic system can be over-activated resulting in a hyperfibrinolytic state with bleeding manifestations or it can be insufficiently active and hypofibrinolysis may contribute to or cause a thrombotic disorder or tendency.[17] Clinical assessment of these two extremes of fibrinolysis is occasionally required.

Hyperfibrinolysis

Hyperfibrinolysis is almost always a secondary event associated with DIC. The patient usually has acute haemostatic failure (p. 238) with multiple abnormalities, and it is rarely necessary to establish the presence of hyperfibrinolysis as an emergency. The measurement of FDP concentration, euglobulin lysis time and time of lysis of a fibrin plate are useful confirmatory tests.

Hyperfibrinolysis is only exceptionally a primary condition. It should be suspected if the platelet count remains consistently normal in the presence of acute defibrination, as demonstrated by a low fibrinogen concentration, high FDP levels and rapid euglobulin lysis time. Hyperfibrinolysis may be induced by thrombolytic therapy, but detailed laboratory assessment is required only if acute haemostatic failure ensues. Recently, a congenital deficiency of α_2 antiplasmin has been described;[31] such patients present with life-long histories of bleeding, and the diagnosis is established by measuring the α_2 antiplasmin concentration using a chromogenic or radioimmune assay. Commercial kits for chromogenic assay are available (See footnote on p. 240).

Hypofibrinolysis

Certain patients with recurrent venous thrombosis, arterial disease, vasculitis or connective tissue disorder have been shown to be deficient in normal fibrinolysis. Tests used to detect this 'hypofibrinolysis', e.g. the euglobulin lysis time and whole-blood dilute clot lysis time, are all based on the detection of the plasminogen activator in blood. The venous occlusion test may be a useful confirmatory investigation (see p. 243). The significance of these tests for detection of defective fibrinolysis remains, however, uncertain.

Euglobulin clot lysis time[59]

Principle. When plasma is diluted and acidified, the precipitate which forms contains plasminogen activator, plasminogen and fibrinogen. The natural inhibitors of fibrinolysis are not precipitated. The precipitate is redissolved, the fibrinogen is clotted with thrombin and the time for clot lysis is estimated. The test measures predominantly plasminogen activator activity.

Method

Mix venous blood with a one-ninth volume of 32 g/l sodium citrate in a plastic tube and place the tube in crushed ice until processed, even if there is likely to be a delay of only a few minutes. As soon as possible, and always within 30 min from the time of collecting the blood, centrifuge the sample at 4°C at 1200–1500 g for 5 min. Next, pipette 1 ml of supernatant plasma into 15 ml of water in a 50 ml conical flask. Then pass a stream of carbon dioxide over the surface of the plasma-water mixture for 3 min, rotating the flask manually. The tip of the tube emitting carbon dioxide should be c 1 cm above the fluid. The euglobulin fraction is rendered insoluble by the fall in pH and appears as a white cloud.

Divide the contents of the flask between two centrifuge tubes and centrifuge at 1200–1500 g for 2 min. Discard the supernatants and invert the tubes, wipe their walls dry with cotton wool on a stick and dissolve the precipitate in each tube in 0.5 ml of barbitone buffered saline, pH 7.4. A glass rod or applicator stick facilitates this procedure. Place two 0.3 ml volumes in 75 × 12 mm tubes and add 1 drop (25 μl) of thrombin solution (200 NIH units per ml). Cover the tubes with a plastic film, incubate at 37°C and observe for clot lysis.

Normal range. 90–240 min.

The major causes of variation in the results of different workers are failure to use a low temperature technique throughout until the time of addition of thrombin, the use of various anticoagulants at different concentrations and the type of buffer used. With a strictly controlled technique, results are reproducible.

The euglobulin clot lysis time is shortened by exercise and the patient should be recumbent and at rest for 15 min before blood is withdrawn. The time is shortened also by prolonged venous occlusion and blood should thus be withdrawn for the test without the use of a tourniquet if possible, or, if a tourniquet is necessary, it should be applied lightly for no longer than 30 s. The shortening of the euglobulin clot lysis time following venous occlusion is referred to as 'fibrinolytic capacity'.[51] The normal response to venous occlusion is de-

ficient in some patients with an increased risk of thrombosis.

Venous occlusion test

To carry out a venous occlusion test, withdraw blood from the arm without venous stasis and then inflate a sphygmomanometer cuff to a pressure midway between the systolic and diastolic blood pressures on the other arm and maintain at this pressure for a standard period of time (see below). Withdraw blood from below the blood pressure cuff immediately before deflation for measurement of the euglobulin clot lysis time and comparison with the clot lysis time of the sample withdrawn before the venous occlusion.

The period of venous occlusion recommended by different workers has varied from 20 min[51] to 10 min[56] and 5 min[60]. Venous occlusion is, however, painful and most patients will not tolerate the procedure for more than 5 min.

LYSIS OF FIBRIN PLATES[2,40]

Lysis of the euglobulin clot depends upon adequate concentrations of plasminogen and fibrinogen. After active fibrinolysis plasminogen values may be low and a normal or prolonged time may result, even in the presence of increased activator activity. If the fibrinogen concentration is low, a weak clot will form and its rapid disappearance may suggest increased activator activity when this is, in fact, normal. To overcome these difficulties, the euglobulin fraction may be placed on a fibrin plate which contains adequate amounts of plasminogen and fibrin and the area of lysis determined.

Principle. Most commercially available preparations of bovine or human fibrinogen are contaminated with plasminogen. Fibrinogen is clotted with thrombin and the plasma or euglobulin fraction under test is allowed to react with the clot. If plasminogen activator is present in the sample, the plasminogen in the fibrin clot will be converted into plasmin and lysis of fibrin will occur.

Reagents

Bovine or human fibrinogen (Kabi).

Thrombin Topical (Parke Davis). 50 NIH units/ml in 9 g/l NaCl.

Plates. Use 9-cm glass or plastic Petri-dishes. Clean the dishes in chromic acid for 24 h, then thoroughly rinse them in tap water and finally in distilled water. Detergent should not be used in cleaning the dishes as traces may cause lysis of fibrin. The clean plates need not be sterilized.

Calcium. 0.025 mol/l calcium chloride.

Dextran. 6% in 50 g/l glucose (Dextraven for intravenous administration).

Citrated platelet-poor plasma and euglobulin fraction. Prepare the plasma and euglobulin fraction with the same precautions as in the euglobulin clot lysis test.

Preparation of the plates. Dissolve 200 mg of fibrinogen powder in 60 ml of barbitone buffer (see p. 435) in a flask. Add 20 ml of calcium chloride and 20 ml of dextran to make the final volume up to 100 ml. This is sufficient for nine plates.

The Petri dishes must be placed on a level surface to ensure that the fibrin will be of an even depth. Pipette 10 ml of fibrinogen solution into each dish and add 0.3 ml of thrombin. Mix the contents by swirling for 20 s. When the fibrinogen has clotted, cover the dishes with lids fitted with filter paper and leave them undisturbed for 30 min before storing. They may be kept at 4°C for 3–4 days before use.

Method

Place 1 drop (25 μl) of plasma or euglobulin fraction toward the centre of each half of a fibrin plate, replace the lid and incubate the dish at 37°C for 24 h. Set up the tests in duplicate.

Interpretation

Measure the area of lysis in two directions at right angles to each other, and multiply the measurements. Plasma samples from normal persons at rest usually produce areas of lysis on unheated plates of <100 mm^2, while the euglobulin fraction from normal plasma may produce lysis up to 200 mm^2.

The major disadvantage of this test is the short period during which the plates may be stored before they become sloppy and unusable. The consistency and storage life of the plates may be improved by the addition of agarose solution.[10] Wells may be punched in such agarose/fibrin plates and a measured volume of the sample to be tested may be inserted. However, agarose-strengthened plates do not appear to be as sensitive as the plates described above for plasminogen-activator assay.

DETECTION OF FIBRINOGEN/FIBRIN DEGRADATION PRODUCTS (FDP)

The measurement of the products of plasmin digestion of fibrinogen or fibrin provides an indirect test for fibrinolysis. FDP may be demonstrated readily in the blood in both systemic fibrinolysis and in local fibrinolysis associated with the intravascular deposition of fibrin. FDP occur in trace amounts in the blood of healthy children and adults, presumably as a result of physiological fibrinolytic activity. The levels are higher in women during menstruation, especially in those with menorrhagia.[6] Increased concentrations have also been reported in hepatic cirrhosis, venous thrombosis and pulmonary embolism and in various types of renal failures.[12,54] In patients with renal homografts, a rising concentration of FDP in the urine may be associated with impending rejection of the graft.[13]

FDP can be detected in several ways. They interfere with the thrombin–fibrinogen reaction and cause a prolongation of the thrombin clotting time of plasma (see p. 218). Serum containing FDP induces rapid clumping of staphylococci. However, the most sensitive methods are immunological.

Table 14.3 More complex tests of the fibrinolytic system

Component of fibrinolytic system to be assayed	Technique
Plasminogen	Caseinolytic assay (see 5th edn.)
	Chromogenic assay (S-2251, Kabi)[32]
Plasma-plasminogen activators	Chromogenic substrate assay (S-2251, Kabi)[33]
Factor XII-dependent activators	Assay with kaolin[45]
Vessel-wall plasminogen activators	Histochemistry[46]
FDP (plasmin-specific)	Radio-immune assay of plasma fibrinopeptide B[65]
α_2 antiplasmin	Chromogenic assay (Coatest, Kabi)[1]
	Radioimmune assay (antiserum available from Nordic Immunological Laboratories, Tilburg, the Netherlands)[15]
α_2 macroglobulin	Immune assay (Laurell)[34]

Latex agglutination* method for FDP[25]

Principle. A suspension of latex particles in buffer is sensitized with specific antibodies to the purified FDP fragments D and E. The suspension is mixed on a glass slide with a serum or urine dilution. Aggregation indicates the presence of FDP in the sample. By testing the unknown sample at different dilutions, a semi-quantitative assay can be performed.

Reagents

Thrombo–Wellcotest Kit (Wellcome Reagents Ltd, Beckenham, Kent).

Method

Place 2 ml of venous blood in an FDP sample collection tube and mix immediately and thoroughly by inversion several times. These tubes contain thrombin to ensure rapid clotting and a proteolytic inhibitor to prevent in vitro fibrinolysis. Allow the tube to stand at 37°C until clot retraction commences; then centrifuge it and withdraw clear serum for testing.

Make 1 in 5 and 1 in 20 dilutions of serum in the glycine buffer provided with the kit. Mix 1 drop of each serum dilution on a glass slide with 1 drop of latex suspension; rock the slide gently for a maximum of 2 min while looking for macroscopic aggregation.

* Although generally termed 'agglutination', the reaction is better described as aggregation.

Urine is tested in a similar manner to serum. Place 2 ml in an FDP sample collection tube and allow it to stand at 37°C for at least 30 min. Then filter the urine through a glass fibre disc (Whatman GF/B) and test undiluted and diluted 1 in 5.

Interpretation

Serum. Aggregation with a 1 in 5 dilution of serum indicates a concentration of FDP in the original serum in excess of 10 μg/ml. Aggregation with a 1 in 20 dilution indicates an FDP level in excess of 40 μg/ml.

Urine. Aggregation with undiluted urine indicates an FDP concentration in excess of 2 μg/ml, while aggregation with the 1 in 5 dilution represents a concentration in excess of 10 μg/ml.

Results with the latex method correlate closely with the tanned red-cell method. The latex test has the advantages of convenience and simplicity and results may be obtained rapidly. It is very suitable for use in laboratories where tests for FDP are not performed regularly. The haemagglutination inhibition immuno-assay[41] is more difficult to perform than the latex agglutination method, but it is more suitable for use if a precise quantitative assay for FDP is required. The method was described in the Fifth Edition of this book.

OTHER TESTS OF THE FIBRINOLYTIC SYSTEM

Some specialized laboratories may wish to carry out more complex tests for research purposes or to investigate a special case. A list of such tests is given in Table 14.3.

REFERENCES

[1] ABILDGAARD, U., LIE, M. and ØDEGÅRD, O. R. (1977). Antithrombin (heparin cofactor) assay with 'new' chromogenic substrates (S-2238 and chromozym-TH). *Thrombosis Research*, **11**, 549.

[2] ASTRUP, T. and MULLERTZ, S. (1952). Fibrin plate method for estimating fibrinolytic activity. *Archives of Biochemistry*, **40**, 346.

[3] AUSTEN, D. E. C. and RHYMES, L. L. (1975). *A Laboratory Manual of Blood Coagulation*, p. 75. Blackwell Scientific Publications, Oxford.

[4] BARROWCLIFFE, T. W. and KIRKWOOD, T. B. L. (1978). An international collaborative assay of Factor VIII clotting activity. *Thrombosis and Haemostasis*, **40**, 260.

[5] BARROWCLIFFE, T. W. and KIRKWOOD, T. B. L. (1981). Principle of bioassay of haemostatic components. In *Haemostasis and Thrombosis*. Eds. A. L. Bloom and D. P. Thomas, p. 832. Churchill Livingstone, Edinburgh.

[6] BASU, H. K. (1970). Fibrin degradation products in sera of women with normal menstruation and menorrhagia. *British Medical Journal*, **i**, 74.

[7] BENNETT, B. and RATNOFF, O. D. (1973). Detection of the carrier state for classic hemophilia. *New England Journal of Medicine*, **288**, 342.

[8] BICK, R. L., KOVACS, I. and FEKETE, L. F. (1976). A new two-stage functional assay for antithrombin-III (heparin cofactor): clinical and laboratory evaluation. *Thrombosis Research*, **8**, 745.

[9] BIGGS, R., EVELING, J. and RICHARDS, G. (1955). The assay of antihaemophilic-globulin activity. *British Journal of Haematology*, **1**, 20.

[10] BISHOP, R., EKERT, H., GILCHRIST, G., SHANBROM, E. and FEKETE, L. (1970). The preparation and evaluation of a standardized fibrin plate for the assessment of fibrinolytic activity. *Thrombosis et Diathesis Haemorrhagica*, **23**, 202.

[11] BREEN, F. A. Jnr and TULLIS, J. L. (1968). Ethanol gelation: a rapid screening test for intravascular coagulation. *Annals of Internal Medicine*, **69**, 1197.

[12] BRIGGS, J. D., PRENTICE, C. R. M., HUTTON, M. M., KENNEDY, A. C. and McNICOL, G. P. (1972). Serum and urine fibrinogen–fibrin-related antigen (F. R.-antigen) levels in renal disease. *British Medical Journal*, **iv**, 82.

[13] CLARKSON, A. R., MORTON, J. B. and CASH, J. D. (1970). Urinary fibrin/fibrinogen degradation products after renal homotransplantation. *Lancet*, **ii**, 1220.

[14] CLAUSS, A. (1957). Rapid physiological coagulation method in determination of fibrinogen. *Acta Haematologica (Basel)*, **17**, 237.

[15] COLLEN, D. (1976). Identification and some properties of a new fast reacting plasmin inhibitor in human plasma. *European Journal of Biochemistry*, **69**, 209.

[16] COUNTS, R. B. and HAYS, J. E. (1979). A computer program for analysis of clotting factor assays and other parallel line bioassays. *American Journal of Hematology*, **71**, 167.

[17] DAVIDSON, J. F. and WALKER, I. D. (1981). Assessment of the fibrinolytic system. In *Haemostasis and Thrombosis*. Eds. A. L. Bloom and D. P. Thomas, p. 796. Churchill Livingstone, Edinburgh.

[18] DENSON, K. W. E. (1973). The detection of factor-VIII-like antigen in haemophilic carriers and in patients with raised levels of biological active factor VIII. *British Journal of Haematology*, **24**, 451.

[19] DENSON, K. W. E., BORRETT, R. and BIGGS, R. (1971). The specific assay of prothrombin using the Taipan snake venom. *British Journal of Haematology*, **21**, 219.

[20] ELLIS, B. C. and STRANSKY, A. (1961). A quick and accurate method for the determination of fibrinogen in plasma. *Journal of Laboratory and Clinical Medicine*, **58**, 477.

[21] EXNER, T., RICKARD, K. A. and KRONENBERG, H. (1975). Studies on phospholipids in the action of a lupus coagulation inhibitor. *Pathology*, **7**, 319.

[22] FAGERHOL, M. K. and ABILDGAARD, U. (1970). Immunological studies on human antithrombin III. Influence of age, sex and use of oral contraceptives on serum concentration. *Scandinavian Journal of Haematology*, **7**, 10.

[23] FOWELL, A. H. (1955). Turbidimetric method of fibrinogen assay. *American Journal of Clinical Pathology*, **25**, 340.

[24] GARNER, R. and CONNING, D. M. (1970). The assay of human factor VII by means of a modified factor VII deficient dog plasma. *British Journal of Haematology*, **18**, 57.

[25] GARVEY, M. B. and BLACK, J. M. (1972). The detection of fibrinogen/fibrin degradation products by means of a new antibody-coated latex particle. *Journal of Clinical Pathology*, **25**, 680.

[26] GIROLAMI, A., NICOLINI, R., FURLANI, E. and BAREGGI, G. (1973). Abnormal factor X (Factor X Friuli) coagulation disorder. *Acta Haematologica (Basel)*, **49**, 114.

[27] HARDISTY, R. M. and MACPHERSON, J. C. (1962). A one-stage Factor VIII (antihaemophilic globulin) assay and its use on venous and capillary plasma. *Thrombosis et Diathesis Haemorrhagica*, **7**, 215.

[28] KASPER, C. (1975). A more uniform measurement of Factor VIII inhibitors. *Thrombosis et Diathesis Haemorrhagica*, **34**, 869.

[29] KIRKWOOD, T. B. L. and BARROWCLIFFE, T. W. (1978). Discrepancy between one-stage and two-stage assays of Factor VIII coagulant activity. *British Journal of Haematology*, **39**, 147.

[30] KIRKWOOD, T. B. L., RIZZA, C. R., SNAPE, T. J., RHYMES, I. L. and AUSTEN, D. E. G. (1977). Identification of sources of inter-laboratory variation in Factor VIII assay. *British Journal of Haematology*, **37**, 559.

[31] KOIE, K., KAMIYA, T., OGATA, K. and TAKAMATSU, J. (1978). α_2-plasmin-inhibitor deficiency (Miyasato disease). *Lancet*, **ii**, 1334.

[32] KUOS, M. and FRIBERGER, P. (1979). Methods for plasminogen determination in human plasma and for streptokinase standardization. In *Progress in Chemical Fibrinolysis and Thrombolysis*, vol. 4. Eds. J. F. Davidson, V. Cepelak, M. M. Samama and P. C. Desnoyer, p. 154. Churchill Livingstone, Edinburgh.

[33] LATALLO, Z. S., TEISSEYRE, E. and LOPACINK, S. (1970). Assessment of plasma fibrinolytic system with use of chromogenic substrate. *Haemostasis (Basel)*, **7**, 150.

[34] LAURELL, C.-B. (1966). Quantitative estimation of proteins by electrophoresis in agarose gel containing antibodies. *Analytical Biochemistry*, **15**, 45.

[35] LECHNER, K. (1974). Acquired inhibitors in nonhemophilic patients. *Haemostasis*, **3**, 65.

[36] LECK, I., GOWLAND, E. and POLLER, L. (1974). The variability of measurements of the prothrombin time ratio in the National Quality Control Trials: a follow-up study. *British Journal of Haematology*, **28**, 601.

[37] LIPINSKI, B., WEGRZYNOWICZ, Z., BUDZYNSKI, A. Z., ZOPEC, M., LATALLO, Z. S. and KOWALSKI, E. (1967).

Soluble unclottable complexes formed in the presence of fibrinogen degradation products (FDP) during the fibrinogen-fibrin conversion and their potential significance in pathology. *Thrombosis et Diathesis Haemorrhagica*, **17**, 65.

[38] LOSOWKSY, M. S. and MILOSZEWSKI, K. J. A. (1977). Factor XIII. *British Journal of Haematology*, **37**, 1.

[39] MANOHARAN, A., GIBSON, L., RUSH, B. and FEERY, B. J. (1977). Recurrent venous thrombosis with a 'lupus' coagulation inhibitor in the absence of systemic lupus. *Australian and New Zealand Journal of Medicine*, **7**, 422.

[40] MARSH, N. A. and AROCHA-PINANGO, C. L. (1972). Evaluation of the fibrin plate method for estimating plasminogen activators. *Thrombosis et Diathesis Haemorrhagica*, **28**, 75.

[41] MERSKEY, C., LALEZARI, P. and JOHNSON, A. J. (1969). A rapid, simple, sensitive method for measuring fibrinolytic split products in human serum. *Proceedings of the Society for Experimental Biology and Medicine*, **131**, 871.

[42] MEYER, D., LAVERGNE, J.-M., LARRIEU, M.-J. and JOSSO, F. (1972). Cross-reacting material in congenital Factor VIII deficiencies (Hemophilia A and von Willebrand's disease). *Thrombosis Research*, **1**, 183.

[43] MILLAR, H. R., SIMPSON, J. G. and STALKER, A. L. (1971). An evaluation of the heat precipitation method for plasma fibrinogen estimation. *Journal of Clinical Pathology*, **24**, 827.

[44] NIEMETZ, J. and NOSSEL, H. L. (1969). Activated coagulation factors: in-vivo and in-vitro studies. *British Journal of Haematology*, **16**, 337.

[45] OGSTON, D. (1976). Assays of factor XII dependent pathway. In *Progress in Chemical Fibrinolysis and Thrombolysis*, Vol. 2. Eds. J. F. Davidson, M. M. Samama and P. C. Desnoyer, p.37. Raven Press, New York.

[46] PANDOLFI, M., BJERNSTAD, A. and NILSSEN, I. M. (1972). Technical remarks on the microscopic demonstration of tissue plasminogen. *Thrombosis et Diathesis Haemorrhagica*, **27**, 88.

[47] PARKIN, J. D., MADARAS, F., SWEET, B. and CASTALDI, P. A. (1974). A further inherited variant of coagulation Factor X. *Australian and New Zealand Journal of Medicine*, **4**, 561.

[48] PITNEY, W. R. (1956). The assay of antihaemophilic globulin (AHG) in plasma. *British Journal of Haematology*, **2**, 250.

[49] PITNEY, W. R. (1971). Disseminated intravascular coagulation. *Seminars in Hematology*, **8**, 65.

[50] RATNOFF, O. D. and MENZIE, C. (1951). A new method for the determination of fibrinogen in small samples of plasma. *Journal of Laboratory and Clinical Medicine*, **37**, 316.

[51] ROBERTSON, B. R., PANDOLFI, M. and NILSSON, I. M. (1972). 'Fibrinolytic capacity' in healthy volunteers at different ages as studied by standardized venous occlusion of arms and legs. *Acta Medica Scandinavica*, **191**, 199.

[52] ROGERS, J. S. and EYSTER, M. E. (1976). Relationship of Factor VIII-like antigen (VIII AGN) and clot promoting activity (VIII AHF) as measured by one- and two-stage assays in patients with liver disease. *British Journal of Haematology*, **34**, 655.

[53] ROSENBERG, R. D. (1975). Actions and interactions of antithrombin and heparin. *New England Journal of Medicine*, **292**, 146.

[54] RUCKLEY, C. V., DAS, P. C., LEITCH, A. G., DONALDSON, A. A., COPLAND, W. A., REDPATH, A. T., SCOTT, P. and CASH, J. D. (1970). Serum fibrin/fibrinogen degradation products associated with postoperative pulmonary embolus and venous thrombosis. *British Medical Journal*, **iv**, 395.

[55] SAS, G., BLASKÓ, G., BÁNHEGYI, D., JÁKÓ, J. and PÁLOS, L. A. (1974). Abnormal antithrombin III (antithrombin III 'Budapest') as a cause of a familial thrombophilia. *Thrombosis et Diathesis Haemorrhagica*, **32**, 105.

[56] SHAPER, A. G., MARSH, N. A., PATEL, I. and KATER, F. (1975). Response of fibrinolytic activity to venous occlusion. *British Medical Journal*, **iii**, 571.

[57] SHARP, A. A., HOWIE, B., BIGGS, R. and METHUEN, D. T. (1958). Defibrination syndrome in pregnancy: value of various diagnostic tests. *Lancet*, **ii**, 1309.

[58] SHOA'I, I., LAVERGNE, J. M., ARDAILLOU, N., OBERT, B., ALA, F. and MEYER, D. (1977). Heterogeneity of von Willebrand's disease: Study of 40 Iranian cases. *British Journal of Haematology*, **37**, 67.

[59] VON KAULLA, K. N. (1963). *Chemistry of Thrombolysis: Human Fibrinolytic Enzymes*. Thomas, Illinois.

[60] WALKER, I. D., DAVIDSON, J. F. and HUTTON, I. (1976). 'Fibrinolytic potential.' The response to a 5 minute venous occlusion test. *Thrombosis Research*, **8**, 629.

[61] WILLIAMS, K. M., DAVIDSON, J. M. F. and INGRAM, G. I. C. (1975). A computer program for the analysis of parallel line bioassays of clotting factors. *British Journal of Haematology*, **31**, 13.

[62] ZIMMERMAN, T. S., RATNOFF, O. D. and POWELL, A. E. (1971). Immunologic differentiation of classic hemophilia (factor VIII deficiency) and von Willebrand's disease. *Journal of Clinical Investigation*, **50**, 244.

[63] ZIMMERMAN, T. S., HOYER, L. W., DICKSON, L. and EDINGTON, T. S. (1975). Determination of the von Willebrand's disease antigen (factor VIII-related antigen) in plasma by quantitative immunoelectrophoresis. *Journal of Laboratory and Clinical Medicine*, **86**, 152.

[64] DENSON, K. W. (1961). The specific assay of Prower-Stuart Factor and Factor VII. *Acta Haematologica (Basel)*, **25**, 105.

[65] NOSSEL, H. L. WASSER, J., KAPLANG, K. L., LaGAMMA, K. F., YUDELMAN, I. and CANFIELD, E. (1979). Sequence of fibrinogen proteolysis and platelet release after intrauterine infusion of hypertonic saline. *Journal of Clinical Investigation*, **64**, 1371.

15

Investigation of platelet function
(Written in collaboration with W. R. Pitney and M. Brozovic)

Abnormal bleeding may be due to thrombocytopenia or to platelet dysfunction. In the latter disorder, the platelets are usually present in normal numbers but are either unable to adhere to subendothelium or to form aggregates.

Thrombocytopenia may be suspected from examination of the blood film and confirmed by a platelet count (see p. 43). If the platelet count is sufficiently low, the tourniquet test will be positive, there will be defective clot retraction and the bleeding time will be prolonged. The prothrombin consumption test will be abnormal also. The level of platelet count which is associated with spontaneous bleeding and bruising is variable. Some patients experience excessive bleeding when the platelet count is less than $80 \times 10^9/l$; others do not bleed with counts as low as $20 \times 10^9/l$.

Platelet dysfunction in the presence of a normal platelet count is more difficult to investigate. Again, the bleeding time, tourniquet test and prothrombin consumption test may be abnormal. In the rare congenital disorder known as the Bernard-Soulier syndrome, large, bizarre platelets may be observed in blood films.[9] Defective clot reaction may be seen in thrombasthenia (Glanzmann's disease), another rare congenital disorder. Usually, however, clot retraction is normal in disorders of platelet function and the platelets appear normal in blood films.

Adhesion of platelets to subendothelium may be studied directly in an experimental model.[38] Adhesion requires the presence of a plasma factor (factor VIII:WF), and the impaired haemostatic plug formation in von Willebrand's disease is not due to an intrinsic platelet defect but to a lack of this plasma factor (VIII:WF). A specific platelet membrane receptor is involved in the interaction between platelets, factor VIII:WF and subendothe-

lium. An abnormality of this receptor appears to be the basic defect in the Bernard-Soulier syndrome, which is characterized by inability of platelets to adhere to subendothelium.[9] Factor VIII:WF is probably identical with the plasma factor necessary for the occurrence of platelet aggregation in the presence of the antibiotic, ristocetin (Ristocetin Co-factor or factor VIII:RiCoF). An impaired response in platelet aggregation to ristocetin occurs in both von Willebrand's disease and the Bernard-Soulier syndrome.[31] An analysis of the aggregation response to ristocetin in these conditions avoids the necessity for more complex observations on platelet adhesion to subendothelium.

Physiological platelet aggregation commences with interaction between stimuli and membrane receptors and is mediated by activation of the cyclic endoperoxide pathway. Disorders of platelet function may arise from membrane abnormalities or from defects in the pathway.[13] Thrombasthenia is associated with a membrane abnormality which makes the platelet unresponsive to physiological stimuli; thrombasthenic platelets aggregate normally, however, with ristocetin.[40] Deficiency of the platelet enzymes, cyclo-oxygenase and thromboxane synthetase result in impaired production of thromboxane A_2 within the platelet and defective release of adenosine diphosphate (ADP) from the dense bodies.[25,41] A normal platelet release reaction is necessary for platelet aggregation to occur in response to dilute concentrations of collagen and for a second-wave aggregation response to adrenaline. Although platelets with defective release aggregate normally with strong concentrations of ADP, they fail to give a biphasic response or they undergo reversible aggregation when exposed to weak ADP concentrations. Platelet aggregation is impaired also in response to arachidonic acid in defects of the

Table 15.1 Platelet aggregation responses

Disorder	'Strong' ADP	Collagen	Adrenaline	Ristocetin	Arachidonic acid (Na salt)
Thrombasthenia	Abn	Abn	Abn	N[†]	Abn
Bernard-Soulier syndrome	N	N	N	Abn	N
von Willebrand's disease	N	N	N	Abn*	N
Cyclo-oxygenase or thromboxane synthetase deficiency	N	Abn	Abn	N	Abn
Storage pool disease	N	Abn	Abn	N	N
'Aspirin defect'	N	Abn	Abn	N[†]	Abn

N = normal aggregation; Abn = impaired aggregation.
* The finding of a normal aggregation response to ristocetin does not exclude the diagnosis of von Willebrand's disease. In the presence of other suggestive evidence, plasma should be assayed for factor VIII:WF.
[†] The ristocetin response may be impaired.[20]

cyclic endoperoxide pathway.[34] Similar platelet abnormalities associated with an impaired release reaction are observed following the ingestion of aspirin and other non-steroidal anti-inflammatory compounds which inhibit platelet cyclo-oxygenase.[35]

'Storage pool disease' depends upon another type of platelet abnormality which results in defective aggregation.[15,18] This abnormality is associated with a deficiency of the ADP that is normally stored in the dense bodies of the platelets and which is released during the release reaction. Platelet aggregation responses are, in general, similar to those observed with defects of the release reaction. However, the platelets of storage pool disease aggregate normally with arachidonic acid.[20]

There are other, less clearly defined, congenital disorders of platelet function which result in abnormal bleeding. In addition to drug ingestion, acquired platelet dysfunction may be associated with diseases such as renal failure[11] and myeloproliferative disorders.[19] Table 15.1 summarizes the result of platelet aggregation tests in a number of disorders of platelet function and in von Willebrand's disease.

PLATELET AGGREGATION[6,30]

The study of platelet aggregation responses to a number of stimuli is an essential part of the investigation of any patient with suspected plate-let dysfunction. Necessary equipment for platelet aggregometry includes an instrument known as a platelet aggregometer and a chart recorder. Platelet-rich plasma is placed in a plastic tube, warmed to 37°C in the heating block of the instrument and stirred by means of a small bar magnet or mechanical stirrer. Light transmission through the plasma is monitored continuously on a chart recorder. The addition of an aggregating agent results in the formation of increasingly larger platelet aggregates with a corresponding decrease in optical density. The change in optical density is recorded as a tracing by the chart recorder.

There are some basic requirements for successful platelet aggregometry. It is essential to obtain platelet-rich plasma from citrated venous blood collected into plastic tubes. The tubes must be capped to prevent loss of carbon dioxide from the blood with a resulting change in pH. The blood and platelet-rich plasma should be kept at room temperature during processing, since prior cooling inhibits the platelet aggregating response. It is preferable to test plasma from a fasting patient so as to avoid the opacity due to lipaemia which may partially obscure the changes in optical density due to platelet aggregation. It is essential that the patient does not take anti-inflammatory drugs for a week before testing and, since so many proprietary preparations contain aspirin, it is a wise precaution to test a specimen of urine for the presence of salicylates before performing platelet aggregation tests. Aggregating agents should be added in small volumes and they must be of known potency. Control tests using platelet-rich plasma from a subject known to give good aggregation responses are essential.

Platelet aggregation test

Reagents

Test and control platelet-rich plasma. Centrifuge citrated venous blood at room temperature (18–25°C) at 150–200 **g** for 10–15 min. Dilute the platelet-rich plasma with platelet-poor plasma to obtain a platelet count of *c* $250 \times 10^9/l$. The plasma may be left at room temperature in plastic stoppered tubes for up to 2 h before testing without influencing the results.

The volume of blood required for platelet aggregation tests depends upon the number of tests to be performed and the volume required for each test, the latter varying with the type of platelet aggregometer. For example, eight aggregation tests (see below) each using 0.9 ml of platelet-rich plasma, require 7.2 ml of plasma, and it would be advisable to withdraw 30 ml of blood to be certain that sufficient plasma was available.

ADP. Adenosine diphosphate, sodium salt, anhydrous (e.g. Sigma, BDH). Dissolve 4.93 mg of trisodium salt or 4.71 mg of disodium salt in 10 ml of saline, pH 6.8. This makes a 1 mmol/l stock solution; freeze in 0.5 ml volumes in stoppered plastic tubes and store deep frozen until use. For platelet aggregation testing, prepare 100 μmol/l, 50 μmol/l, 25 μmol/l and 10 μmol/l solutions in saline (see Table 15.2).

Collagen. Hormon-Chemie, München. This is a 1 mg/ml stock solution. Store at 4°C. For use, dilute in the buffer supplied to obtain 40 μg/ml and 20 μg/ml concentrations (see Table 15.2).

Adrenaline. 1-epinephrine bitartarate (Sigma). Dissolve 3.33 mg in 10 ml of glass-distilled or de-ionized water containing 0.1 % sodium metabisulphite, pH 3.5, to prepare a 1 mmol/l stock solution. Freeze in 0.5 ml volumes and store deep frozen. For use, prepare 20 and 200 μmol/l solutions in 0.1% sodium metabisulphite (see Table 15.2).

Ristocetin sulphate. H. Lunbeck & Co., Copenhagen. Each vial contains 100 mg of ristocetin. Dissolve in 5 ml of saline, freeze in 0.5 ml volumes and store frozen until required. For use, prepare 15 mg/ml, 12 mg/ml and 10 mg/ml solutions (see Table 15.2).

Arachidonic acid. Na-salt, 99% pure (Sigma). Dissolve 4.10 mg in 25 ml of 0.1 mol/l Na_2CO_3 to prepare a 0.50 mmol/l stock solution. Freeze in 0.5 ml volumes and store deep frozen until use. Use undiluted.

Table 15.2 Platelet aggregation test: dilutions used with various aggregating agents

Aggregating agent	Stock solution		Working dilutions		Final concentration, when 1 volume is added to 9 volumes of PRP
	Diluent	Concentration	Diluent	Concentration	
ADP	saline	1 mmol/1	saline	100 μmol/l	10 μmol/l
				50 μmol/l	5 μmol/l
				25 μmol/l*	2.5 μmol/l*
				10 μmol/l	1.0 μmol/l
Collagen		1 mg/ml	buffer†	40 μg/ml*	4 μg/ml*
				20 μg/ml	2 μg/ml
Adrenaline	0.1% sodium metabisulphite	1 mmol/l	0.1% sodium metabisulphite	200 μmol/l*	20 μmol/l*
				20 μmol/l	2 μmol/l
Ristocetin	saline	20 mg/ml	saline	15 mg/ml	1.5 mg/ml
				12 mg/ml*	1.2 mg/ml*
				10 mg/ml	1.0 mg/ml
Arachidonic acid (Na salt)	0.1 mol/l Na_2Co_3	0.50 mmol/l	use undiluted		50 μmol/l

* If only enough plasma is available for a single test, the starred concentration should be used.
† As supplied by Hormon-Chemie, München.

Method

The aggregometer incorporates a heating block which maintains a temperature of 37°C. It should be switched on 30 min before tests are performed. Pipette into a plastic tube the appropriate volume of plasma, e.g. 0.9 ml with a platelet count of approximately $250 \times 10^9/l$, and place the tube in the heating block. After 1 min to allow for warming, insert a motor-driven stirrer into the plasma and switch on the motor. Adjust the speed of the stirrer to that which gives optimal platelet aggregation when strong ADP is added to normal plasma; it is usually between 800 and 1100 rpm. Adjust the absorbance of the swirling plasma to 0.40 and adjust the chart recorder so that the difference in absorbance between platelet-rich and platelet-poor plasma causes the pen to traverse most of the width of the paper.

Spontaneous platelet aggregation may be observed in some platelet-rich plasma samples if stirred for 5–10 min in the absence of an aggregating agent. It is usual to test a sample of plasma for spontaneous aggregation as well as for aggregation after the addition of aggregating agents, e.g. ADP, adrenaline, collagen, ristocetin and sodium arachidonate (Table 15.2). Test both the patient's and the control plasma, and in each case observe the aggregation curve for up to 3 min.

Interpretation

In normal plasma there is no spontaneous aggregation and a single wave of aggregation is produced by a final concentration of 10 μmol/l ADP. Responses are somewhat variable with the weaker ADP concentrations. Commonly, there is biphasic aggregation at 2.5 μmol/l and 5 μmol/l concentrations and reversible aggregation at 1 μmol/l concentration. Biphasic aggregation is observed with adrenaline at final concentrations between 2 and 20 μmol/l. A single phase of aggregation is observed after a lag period with 4 μg/ml collagen. Monophasic aggregation is observed with 1.2 mg/ml ristocetin and 50 μmol/l sodium arachidonate (Fig. 15.1).

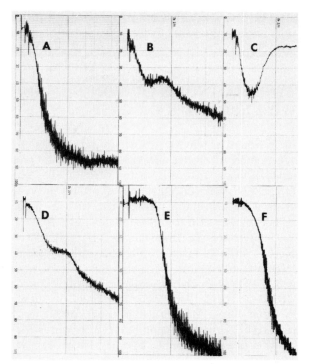

Fig. 15.1 Normal platelet aggregation responses. The time interval between the thick vertical lines is 2 min. A, ADP final concentration 5 μmol/l; B, ADP 2.5 μmol/l; C, ADP 1 μmol/l; D, adrenaline 20 μmol/l; E, collagen 4 μg/ml; F, sodium arachidonate 50 μmol/l. Ristocetin is not shown but would give a curve similar to F.

The aggregation response may be analyzed in more detail. The degree of aggregation may be measured as the change in optical density recorded as a percentage of the difference in optical density between platelet-rich and platelet-poor plasma. The lag phase may be measured as the time interval between the addition of the aggregating agent and the commencement of aggregation; it is relevant to an analysis of the response to collagen. The slope of aggregation response may be measured in degrees at the steepest portion of the aggregation curve. These measurements may be useful when studying hypercoagulability or the effects of platelet-inhibiting drugs.

Spontaneous platelet aggregation and increased responses to aggregating agents have been described in a number of conditions, including diabetes mellitus,[29] hyperlipidaemia,[10] transient cerebral ischaemic attacks,[36] angina pectoris, myocardial infarction and venous thrombosis.[42]

THE DIAGNOSIS OF VON WILLEBRAND'S DISEASE

As indicated previously, ristocetin induces platelet aggregation in normal plasma because of the presence of factor VIII:WF (factor VIII:RiCoF). The factor VIII:WF concentration of plasma may be assayed by a technique which depends upon the ability of ristocetin to induce platelet aggregation. An analysis of the three factor VIII activities— factor VIII:C, factor VIIIR:Ag and factor VIII:WF are indicated for the diagnosis of both von Willebrand's disease and haemophilia A (factor VIII deficiency). The classical findings are shown in Table 15.3. Although it is usual for all three factor VIII activities to be reduced in von Willebrand's disease, variable findings have been recorded and it may be more appropriate to refer to this disorder as the von Willebrand syndrome.[38]

Assay of factor VIII:WF (ristocetin co-factor assay)[27,28,33]

Principle. Washed platelets do not aggregate with ristocetin unless normal plasma is added as a source of factor VIII:WF. Their aggregation with ristocetin follows a dose-response curve depending upon the amount of plasma added. Normal platelets fixed with formaldehyde are as effective as fresh platelets in their response to ristocetin.[27,28]

Reagents

Citrated test plasma. This may be tested either fresh or after storage at −20°C.
Standard plasma pool. See p. 226.
EDTA, disodium salt, pH 6.8. See p. 433.
Formalin-treated platelets. Citrated blood from a normal individual or from therapeutic venesection in a patient with a normal platelet count can be used. ACD or CPD solution from the donor bag is ejected through the taking

Table 15.3 Factor VIII activities in haemophilia and von Willebrand's disease

	FVIII:C	FVIIIR:Ag	FVIII:WF
Haemophilia	reduced	normal	normal
von Willebrand's disease	reduced	reduced*	reduced

* May be normal or even increased. An abnormal pattern can be demonstrated on crossed immunoelectrophoresis.[6]

needle and replaced by the equivalent volume of 32 g/l (109 mmol/l) sodium citrate. It is convenient to collect *c* 500 ml of blood.

Centrifuge the citrated blood at about 300 **g** for 15 min at room temperature (18–25°C). Separate platelet-rich plasma (PRP). To 9 volumes of the PRP add 1 volume of EDTA. Incubate at 37°C for 1 h to reverse the effect of ADP released during the preparation. Add an equal volume of 2% formalin in 9 g/l NaCl (saline) and keep at 4°C for 1 h. Then centrifuge it at 200 **g** for 10 min at 4°C. Decant the supernatant and recentrifuge it at 250 **g** for 20 min at 4°C. Discard this supernatant and resuspend the platelet sediment in chilled (4°C) saline. Wash the platelets twice more. After the final wash, resuspend the platelets in 0.05% sodium azide in saline. Adjust the platelet count to $300–500 \times 10^9/l$. The suspension may be stored for 1 month at 4°C.

Buffer for plasma dilutions. Barbitone buffer, pH 7.4, containing 40 mg/ml of bovine serum albumin.
Ristocetin. 10 mg/ml.

Method

Make serial dilutions of the standard and test plasma in the albumin-buffer mixture, ranging from 1 in 2 to 1 in 64. Place 5 volumes (e.g. 0.25 ml) of the platelet suspension in the aggregometer tube followed by 4 volumes (e.g. 0.2 ml) of the undiluted plasma or plasma dilution. After allowing for warming in the heating block of the aggregometer add 1 volume (e.g. 0.05 ml) of ristocetin, and switch on the stirrer. The final concentration of ristocetin in the mixture is *c* 1 mg/ml.

Obtain platelet aggregation curves for both undiluted normal and test plasma for all the plasma dilutions. Measure the maximum amplitude in divisions of graph paper at 3 min after addition of the ristocetin for each dilution. To prepare a standard graph, plot the measurements against the dilutions of normal plasma on double-log graph paper. Then extrapolate the measurements of the test plasma and express the potency of test plasma as a proportion of the standard. Values below 40% are abnormal.

Normal range. 40–200%.

Platelet factor 3 availability[14]

Principle. The recalcification time of platelet-rich plasma is considerably shortened if the plasma is incubated with kaolin prior to the addition of calcium. Kaolin causes aggregation of platelets with subsequent availability of phospholipid which facilitates the reactions involving activated factor X, factor V and prothrombin.

Reagents

Platelet-rich normal and test plasma. Collect blood into citrate in plastic tubes. Centrifuge the citrated blood at 150–200 *g* for 10–15 min. Remove the plasma samples with siliconized pipettes and place in plastic tubes. Carry out platelet counts and dilute the samples with their own platelet-poor plasma, if necessary, to produce platelet counts of *c* 250 × 10⁹/l.

Platelet-poor normal and test plasma. Collect blood into citrate in plastic tubes. Centrifuge the blood samples at 1200–1500 *g* for 15 min.

Kaolin Levis. 5 mg/ml (see p. 219).

Calcium. 0.025 mol/l calcium chloride.

Method

Add 0.1 ml of the platelet-rich test plasma to 0.1 ml of platelet-poor normal plasma in a 75 × 12 mm glass tube held at 37°C in a water-bath. Add 0.2 ml of kaolin and start a stop-watch. Incubate the mixture for 20 min with occasional shaking and then add 0.2 ml of calcium chloride and record the clotting time with a second stop-watch. Repeat the procedure with a mixture of 0.1 ml of the platelet-poor test plasma and 0.1 ml of the platelet-rich normal plasma.

Interpretation

The two mixtures differ only in the platelets they contain and the clotting times should not differ by more than 2 or 3 s. A prolongation of the clotting time of the mixture containing the test platelets compared to that containing the normal platelets is evidence of reduced platelet factor 3 availability. It is desirable too, to measure the clotting times of mixtures of the platelet-rich and platelet-poor samples of the test plasma and normal plasma, respectively. In practice the whole series of mixtures (in duplicate) can be tested in one procedure by adding kaolin to the tubes at 1 min intervals.

It is claimed that this test can be made more sensitive by reducing the concentration of platelets in the mixture of platelet-rich and platelet-poor plasma. In one such modification, the clotting time of a 1 in 10 dilution of the patient's platelet-rich plasma in normal platelet-poor plasma is compared to that of a similar dilution of normal platelet-rich plasma in normal platelet-poor plasma.[32]

Platelet retention in glass-bead filters

When blood anticoagulated with citrate or heparin is passed through a column of minute glass beads*, some platelets remain trapped in the column. The percentage of retained platelets may be calculated by performing platelet counts on the blood sample before passage through the column and on the blood issuing from the column. Platelet retention is probably due both to platelet adhesion to glass and to platelet aggregates forming in the column which become trapped by the beads. With a carefully standardized technique, reduced platelet retention may be demonstrated in platelet dysfunction and in von Willebrand's disease,[8] while increased retention has been reported in conditions associated with

---

* Average diameter 0.5 mm (No. 7). Jencons Ltd., Hemel Hempstead Herts.

thrombosis.[5,7] Factors which influence platelet retention are the size of the glass beads, the degree of packing, the length of the column, the type of plastic used, the rate of blood flow and its PCV. Criticisms of the test are the wide normal range of results, poor discriminatory power between normal and abnormal blood samples and lack of reproducibility. The test is unlikely to provide diagnostic information which is not obtainable by other tests of platelet function and it is now seldom used. A method employing citrated blood was described in the fifth edition of this book (p. 386).

INVESTIGATION OF SUSPECTED DRUG INDUCED THROMBOCYTOPENIA

Numerous drugs have been associated with thrombocytopenia; quinine, quinidine, gold salts and sulphonamide derivatives are most commonly implicated. The most likely mechanism appears to be the formation of immune complexes of drug and anti-drug antibody which attach non-specifically to the platelet membrane. The platelets carrying the immune complexes are rapidly cleared by the reticulo-endothelial system and the platelet count falls to very low levels.

Once the patient is sensitized, the onset of purpura and thrombocytopenia is rapid, usually within 24 h of ingestion of the drug. Gold salts are an exception and thrombocytopenia may occur several months after the last injection. Diagnosis is usually suspected on the basis of drug history and the abrupt onset of bleeding. It is often, however, difficult to ascertain which drug is responsible. Many in vitro tests have been used, including ^{51}Cr release,[12] platelet factor 3 release[22] and complement fixation,[3] as well as the measurement of clot retraction and the platelet agglutination test described in the 5th edition of this book (p. 393–394). In vitro tests are frequently negative when drugs other than quinine or quinidine are implicated. The challenge of patients with a suspected drug may be very dangerous and must be undertaken with great care, and only if considered essential to establish a diagnosis.

MEASUREMENT OF PLATELET LIFE-SPAN

Principle. The procedure for measuring platelet life-span is broadly similar to that for red-cell survival (see p. 297). There is no satisfactory cohort label and for most studies[51] Cr or di-*iso*propyl phosphofluoridate (DFP) labelled with ^{32}P or ^{3}H have been used.[1,2,4,26] DFP has the advantage of labelling the platelets in vivo but has the disadvantage that red cells and leucocytes are labelled simultaneously and there is reutilization of the label as the platelets are destroyed. The use of ^{51}Cr as an in vivo label was originally hampered by the rapid initial disappearance of many of the labelled platelets from the circulation, as they were damaged by the labelling procedure. Technical modifications, especially a reduction in pH by the use of ACD anticoagulant,[4] have, however, largely overcome the problem of damage to the cells during labelling. The efficiency of the labelling has also been increased, so that it is now possible to study survival of autologous platelets even when the platelet count is $50 \times 10^9/l$ or less.[21] Recently [111]In (indium prepared as hydroxyquinolone[37]) has been found to be equally satisfactory;[4,10] this isotope has the added advantage that its high fraction of gamma emission makes it especially suitable for studying the distribution of the labelled platelets in the body by scanning or surface counting.[16,17]

In both methods platelet-rich plasma is separated from the whole blood collected into ACD and labelled with the isotope. The labelled platelet suspension is injected intravenously. The decline in radioactivity of circulating platelets is measured from venous samples over the next few days.

Standard method using [51]Cr[21]

On the basis of the patient's weight and platelet count, decide on the appropriate volume of blood (200–500 ml) to be collected. For every 100 ml of blood deliver 15 ml of NIH-A ACD (p. 432) into a sterile transfusion bag pack (with two satellite bags attached).

Take the blood into the bag, and then centrifuge the bag at 300 *g* for 15 min. Transfer the supernatant platelet-rich plasma (PRP) into the first satellite bag with the help of a plasma extractor. Add *c* 5 ml of ACD per 100 ml of PRP, then centrifuge the PRP at 1500 *g* for 15 min. Transfer all but 5 ml of the supernatant platelet-poor plasma (PPP) into the second satellite bag without disturbing the platelet pellet. Then resuspend the platelets by repeated gentle inversion of the bag.

Add 2 μCi of ^{51}Cr-sodium chromate per kg body weight to the platelet suspension. Leave undisturbed at room temperature for 30 min. Return all but 40 ml of the PPP from the second satellite bag. Then centrifuge the pack at 1500 *g* for 15 min. Carefully remove and discard the PPP from the first satellite bag without disturbing the platelet pellet. Transfer *c* 20 ml of non-radioactive PPP from the second satellite bag into the first. Gently resuspend the platelets. The suspension of platelets is now ready for the preparation of a standard and re-injection.

Retain *c* 1 ml of the suspension of labelled platelets as a standard for isotope measurement, and for determining the number of platelets in the injected material. Take up the remainder into a syringe. To measure the volume of platelet suspension injected, weigh the syringe before and after the injection.

Following the injection of the labelled platelets, obtain venous blood specimens after 30 min and 2 h and then at daily intervals. When the survival of the platelets is expected to be short, collect more specimens on the first day; it may be unnecessary to continue beyond 2–3 days. Collect daily specimens at the same time of day. On each occasion take 10–20 ml of blood into a syringe containing 0.2 ml of 100 g/l EDTA per 10 ml of blood. Carry out a platelet count on a part of the sample and dilute the remainder with an equal volume of 9 g/l NaCl (saline). Centrifuge the mixture at 300 *g* for 10 min and transfer the PRP to a counting tube. Add another volume of saline to the packed red cells, repeat the centrifugation and add the PRP to the same counting tube. Determine the

platelet count in a sample and measure the remaining volume precisely. Centrifuge the PRP at 2000 *g* for 30 min; then remove and discard the supernatant without disturbing the platelet pellet.

Prepare a standard by adding 0.1 ml of the original suspension to 2 ml of 10 g/l ammonium oxalate. Centrifuge at 2000 *g* for 30 min. Remove the supernatant without disturbing the platelet pellet. Resuspend in a volume equal to that of the blood samples. Measure the radioactivity in the samples and the standard in a gamma-ray scintillation counter.

To estimate platelet survival divide the platelet radioactivity in each blood sample by the platelet count to obtain radioactive counts per 10^9 platelets. Give the highest figure after injection a value of 100% and record the subsequent measurements as a percentage of this value (see below). The percentage recovery of the injected platelet radioactivity can be estimated from knowledge of the total radioactivity of the injected suspension (obtained from the radioactivity of the standard and an estimation of the blood volume, p. 281).

Method using ^{111}In[16]

Collect 42.5 ml of blood into a 50 ml syringe containing 7.5 ml of NIH-A ACD (p. 432). Transfer into sterile polypropylene centrifuge tubes. Centrifuge at *c* 200 *g* for 10 min. Transfer the platelet-rich plasma (PRP) into a sterile centrifuge tube and centrifuge at 1000 *g* for 10 min. Transfer the supernatant platelet-poor plasma (PPP) into a sterile container. Add to the platelet button 2–3 ml of ACD diluted 1 in 200 in 9 g/l NaCl (saline). Gently resuspend and transfer into one tube. Add about 100 μCi* of ^{111}In oxine (p. 283), drop by drop with gentle shaking. Stand at room temperature (18–25°C) for 10 min. Gently remove the supernatant PPP without disturbing the platelet button. Resuspend in 5–10 ml of PPP and re-inject. Collect specimens of blood (5 ml in EDTA) at the same times as for the ^{51}Cr

---

* A higher dose (300–500 μCi) is required for surface counting or quantitative scanning.

method. Measure the radioactivity in 1–2 ml of each sample of whole blood. Record their radioactivity as a percentage of that of the 30-min sample.

Calculation

Prepare a graph by plotting the radioactivity in cpm per 10^9 platelets against time after injection. The platelet life-span is estimated from the survival curve as for red-cell survival (see p. 300).

On the supposition that platelet survival curves are exponential, the mean platelet life-span can be calculated from the formula:

$$\text{Mean life-span} = \frac{T_{50}{}^{51}Cr}{\log_e 2} = \frac{T_{50}{}^{51}Cr}{0.69},$$

where T_{50} is the time taken for the platelet radioactivity to fall to 50% of its initial value. Normal platelet life-span is however, linear rather than exponential.

Normal range. 8–10 days.

The method of calculation described above is adequate when the reduction in platelet survival is marked, as in most clinical situations. When more precise assessment and analysis of the shape of the survival curve is required, more complex procedures must be carried out. *The International Committee for Standardization in Haematology* has published computer programs for obtaining estimates of mean platelet survival based on a number of different theoretical models.[21]

Platelet survival in disease

In idiopathic thrombocytopenia purpura (ITP) platelet life-span is considerably reduced, often to a few hours, and the measurement may have diagnostic and prognostic importance. In thrombocytopenia due to defective production of platelets the life-span should be normal provided that excessive platelets are not being lost by bleeding during the course of the study. In thrombocytopenia associated with splenomegaly the recovery of injected labelled platelets is low but their survival is usually almost normal. This is thought to indicate the existence of a large pool of platelets in the spleen which is freely interchangeable with the circulating platelets. Surface counting of radioactivity over the spleen and liver in ^{51}Cr studies has given inconsistent results and has not proved helpful in ITP in determining which patients will benefit from splenectomy.[111] In is a more promising label for the quantitative analysis of platelet kinetics;[16,17,23] it is possible, with this isotope, to distinguish the relative importance of pooling and destruction of the platelets in the spleen in different conditions. The liver does not appear to be an important organ for platelet destruction even in patients with abnormal platelet turnover.[24]

DEMONSTRATION OF PLATELET ANTIBODIES (See also Chapter 24, p. 411)

A number of tests have been developed for detecting platelet allo- and auto-antibodies. They include platelet agglutination, complement fixation, antiglobulin consumption and immunofluorescence. None is entirely satisfactory: agglutination and complement-fixation tests fail to detect important non-agglutinating and non-complement-binding antibodies, antiglobulin-consumption tests are relatively insensitive and immunofluorescence can be non-specific. A modification of the immunofluorescent technique has been developed in which the problem of non-specific fluorescence is overcome by first stabilizing the platelets with paraformaldehyde and then examining them for surface-associated antibody.[39] Patient's platelets are used in a direct test, and normal platelets are incubated with patient's serum in an indirect test.

Immunofluorescent method

Reagents

Antiglobulin reagent. Anti-IgG and anti-IgM labelled with fluorescein isothiocyanate (FITC)*. For use, dilute in phosphate buffered saline, pH 7.4 (p. 435).

* e.g. Dakopatts, Copenhagen.

To determine the appropriate dilution, titrate a series of dilutions of an Ig antibody-containing serum and a normal AB serum, using platelets as the carrier. The optimal dilution is that which gives maximal fluorescence with the antibody-containing serum but no fluorescence with the normal serum.

Paraformaldehyde, 4% (w/v) stock solution. Dissolve 4 g in 100 ml of phosphate buffered saline, pH 7.4. Heat to 70°C to dissolve. Add 1 mol/l NaOH drop by drop until the solution becomes clear. Filter through a micropore filter (0.22 μm); store in the dark at 4°C in a bottle wrapped in aluminium foil.

Paraformaldehyde, 1% (w/v). For use, add 3 volumes of phosphate buffered saline to 1 volume of the 4% stock solution. Adjust the pH to 7.4 with 1 mol/l HCl. Store in the dark at 4°C in a bottle wrapped in foil. Discard after a week.

Buffered EDTA, pH 7.0. See p. 433.

Glycerol medium. Glycerol 3 volumes, phosphate buffered saline 1 volume.

Direct test

Collect *c* 10 ml of the patient's blood into a plastic container with EDTA as anticoagulant. Centrifuge at 800 *g* for 10 min at room temperature (18–25°C) to obtain platelet-rich plasma (PRP). Then centrifuge the PRP at *c* 3000 *g* for 20 min to obtain a platelet concentrate. Wash the platelets three times in buffered EDTA.

Resuspend the platelet pellet in 3 ml of 1% paraformaldehyde and leave at room temperature (18–25°C) for 5 min. Centrifuge and wash the platelets twice in buffered EDTA. Add 1 ml of the labelled antiglobulin reagent. Stand at room temperature for 30 min in the dark. Then centrifuge and wash the platelets three times in buffered EDTA. Resuspend in the glycerol medium. Place a drop on a glass slide, cover with a cover-glass and examine by fluorescent microscopy. A positive result is shown by a ring of fluorescence around the platelets.

Indirect test

Collect *c* 10 ml of normal group-O blood. Prepare a platelet pellet and fix with 1% paraformaldehyde, as described above. Wash the fixed platelets twice in buffered EDTA, and make a suspension of *c* 200×10^6/ml.

To 0.1 ml of the platelet suspension add 0.1 ml of patient's serum (freshly collected or used immediately after thawing serum which has been stored at −20°C). Incubate at 37°C for 30 min. Then wash the platelets three times with buffered EDTA. Add 0.1 ml of the labelled antiglobulin reagent and treat as in the direct test.

Significance

By this method it is possible to demonstrate platelet agglutinins of the IgM class and non-agglutinating platelet antibodies of the IgG class. The latter are of particular clinical importance as they can be responsible for allo-immune thrombocytopenia of the newborn, for auto-immune thrombocytopenia and for most instances of refractoriness to platelet therapy.[39] It should, however, be noted that in only 60–70% of patients with idiopathic thrombocytopenic purpura have antibodies been detected by this test.

REFERENCES

[1] Aas, K. and Gardner, F. (1958). Survival of blood platelets labelled with chromium. *Journal of Clinical Investigation*, **37**, 1257.

[2] Adelson, E., Kaufman, R. M., Berdequez, C., Lear, A. A. and Rheingold, J. J. (1965). Platelet tagging with tritium-labelled di-isopropylfluorophosphate. *Blood*, **26**, 744.

[3] Aster, R. H., Cooper, H. E. and Surger, D. L. (1964). Simplified complement fixation test for the detection of platelet antibodies in human serum. *Journal of Laboratory and Clinical Medicine*, **63**, 161.

[4] Aster, R. M. and Jandl, J. H. (1964). Platelet sequestration in man. I. Methods. *Journal of Clinical Investigation*, **43**, 843.

[5] Bloom, A. L. (1980). The von Willebrand syndrome. *Seminars in Haematology*, **27**, 215.

[6] Born, G. V. R. (1962). Aggregation of blood platelets by adenosine diphosphate and its reversal. *Nature (London)*, **194**, 927.

[7] Bowie, E. J. W. and Owen, C. A. (1973). The value of measuring platelet 'adhesiveness' in the diagnosis of bleeding disorders. *American Journal of Clinical Pathology*, **60**, 302.

[8] Bowie, E. J. W., Owen, C. A., Thompson, J. H. and Didisheim, P. (1969). Platelet adhesiveness in von Willebrand's disease. *American Journal of Clinical Pathology*, **52**, 69.

[9] CAEN, J. P., NURDEN, A. T., JEANNEAU, C., MICHEL, H., TOBELEM, G., LEVY-TOLEDANO, S., SULTAN, Y., VALENSI, F. and BERNARD, J. (1976). Bernard-Soulier syndrome: a new platelet glycoprotein abnormality. Its relationship with platelet adhesion to subendothelium and with Factor VIII/von Willebrand protein. *Journal of Laboratory and Clinical Medicine*, **87**, 586.

[10] CARVALHO, A. C. A., COLMAN, R. W. and LEES, R. S. (1974). Platelet function in hyperlipoproteinemia. *New England Journal of Medicine*, **290**, 434.

[11] CASTALDI, P. A., ROZENBERG, M. C. and STEWART, J. H. (1966). The bleeding disorder of uraemia. A qualitative platelet defect. *Lancet*, **ii**, 66.

[12] CIMO, P. L., PISCIOTTA, A. V., DESAI, R. G., PINO, J. L. and ASTER, R. H. (1977). Detection of drug dependent antibodies by ^{51}Cr platelet lysis test: documentation of immune thrombocytopenia induced by diphenylhydantoin, diazepam, and sulfisoxazole. *American Journal of Hematology*, **2**, 65.

[13] HARDISTY, R. M. (1977). Disorders of platelet function. *British Medical Bulletin*, **33**, 207.

[14] HARDISTY, R. M. and HUTTON, R. A. (1965). The kaolin clotting time of platelet-rich plasma: a test of platelet factor 3 availability. *British Journal of Haematology*, **11**, 258.

[15] HARDISTY, R. M., MILLS, D. C. B. and KETSA-ARD, K. (1972). The platelet defect associated with albinism. *British Journal of Haematology*, **23**, 679.

[16] HEATON, W. A., DAVIS, H. H., WELCH, M. J., MATHIAS, C. J., JOIST, J. H., SHARMAN, L. A. and SIEGEL, B. A. (1979). Indium-111: a new radionuclide label for studying human platelet kinetics. *British Journal of Haematology*, **42**, 613.

[17] HEYNS, A. DuP., LOTTER, M. G., BADENHORST, P. W., VAN REENEN, O. R., PIETERS, H., MINNAAR, P. C. and RETIEF, F. P. (1980). Kinetics, distribution and sites of destruction of ^{111}indium-labelled human platelets. *British Journal of Haematology*, **44**, 269.

[18] HOLMSEN, H. and WEISS, H. J. (1970). Hereditary defect in the platelet release reaction caused by a deficiency in the storage pool of platelet adenine nucleotides. *British Journal of Haematology*, **19**, 643.

[19] INCEMAN, S. and TANGÜN, Y. (1972). Platelet defects in the myeloproliferative disorders. *Annals of the New York Academy of Sciences*, **201**, 251.

[20] INGERMAN, C. M., SMITH, J. B., SHAPIRO, S., SEDAR, A. and SILVER, M. J. (1978). Hereditary abnormality of platelet aggregation attributable to nucleotide storage pool deficiency. *Blood*, **52**, 332.

[21] International committee for standardization in hematology (1977). Recommended methods for radioisotope survival studies. *Blood*, **50**, 1137.

[22] KARPATKIN, S., STRICK, J. and KARPATKIN, M. B. (1972). Cumulative experience in the detection of antiplatelet antibody in 234 patients with idiopathic thrombocytopenic purpura, systemic lupus erythematosus and other clinical disorders. *American Journal of Medicine*, **52**, 776.

[23] KLONIZAKIS, I., PETERS, A. M., FITZPATRICK, M. L., KENSETT, M. J., LEWIS, S. M. and LAVENDER, J. P. (1980). Radionuclide distribution following injection of ^{111}indium-labelled platelets. *British Journal of Haematology*, **46**, 595.

[24] KLONIZAKIS, I., PETERS, A. M., FITZPATRICK, M. L., KENSETT, M. J., LEWIS, S. M. and LAVENDER, J. P. (1981). Spleen function and platelet kinetics. *Journal of Clinical Pathology*, **34**, 377.

[25] LAGARDE, M., BYRON, P. A., VARGAFTIG, B. B. and

DECHAVANNE, M. (1978). Impairment of platelet thromboxane A_2 generation and of the platelet release reaction in two patients with congenital deficiency of platelet cyclo-oxygenase. *British Journal of Haematology*, **38**, 251.

[26] LEEKSMA, C. H. W. and COHEN, J. A. (1956). Determination of the life span of human blood platelets using labelled diisopropylfluorophosphate. *Journal of Clinical Investigation*, **35**, 964.

[27] MACFARLANE, D. E. (1976). A method for assaying von Willebrand factor: erratum. *Thrombosis and Haemostasis*, **36**, 282.

[28] MACFARLANE, D. E., STIBBE, J., KIRBY, E. P., ZUCKER, M. B., GRANT, R. A. and McPHERSON, J. (1975). A method for assaying von Willebrand factor (ristocetin cofactor). *Thrombosis et Diathesis Haemorrhagica*, **34**, 306.

[29] MUSTARD, J. F. and PACKHAM, M. A. (1977). Platelets and diabetes mellitus. *New England Journal of Medicine*, **297**, 1345.

[30] O'BRIEN, J. R. (1962). Platelet aggregation. II. Some results from a new method of study. *Journal of Clinical Pathology*, **15**, 452.

[31] OLSON, J. D., FASS, D. N., BOWIE, E. J. W. and MANN, K. G. (1973). Ristocetin-induced aggregation of gel filtered platelets: a study of von Willebrand's disease and the effect of aspirin. *Thrombosis Research*, **3**, 501.

[32] RABINER, S. F. and HRODEK, O. (1968). Platelet factor 3 in normal subjects and patients with renal failure. *Journal of Clinical Investigation*, **47**, 901.

[33] SHOA'I, I., LAVERGNE, J. M., ARDAILLOU, N., OBERT, B., ALA, F. and MEYER, D. (1977). Heterogeneity of von Willebrand's disease: study of 40 Iranian cases. *British Journal of Haematology*, **37**, 67.

[34] SILVER, M. J., SMITH, J. B., INGERMAN, C. and KOCSIS, J. J. (1973). Arachidonic acid-induced human platelet aggregation and prostaglandin production. *Prostaglandins*, **4**, 863.

[35] SMITH, J. B. and WILLIS, A. L. (1971). Aspirin selectively inhibits prostaglandin production in human platelets. *Nature (New Biology)*, **231**, 235.

[36] TEN CATE, J. W., VOS, J., OOSTERHUIS, H., PRENGER, D. and JENKINS, C. S. P. (1978). Spontaneous platelet aggregation in cerebrovascular disease. *Thrombosis and Haemostasis*, **39**, 223.

[37] THACKER, M. L., COLEMAN, R. E. and WELCH, M. J. (1977). Indium-111 labelled leukocytes for the localisation of abscesses: preparation, analysis, tissue distribution and comparison with gallium-67 citrate in dogs. *Journal of Laboratory and Clinical Medicine*, **89**, 217.

[38] TSCHOPP, T. B., WEISS, H. J. and BAUMGARTNER, H. R. (1974). Decreased adhesion of platelets to subendothelium in von Willebrand's disease. *Journal of Laboratory and Clinical Medicine*, **83**, 296.

[39] VON DEM BORNE, A. E. G. K., VERHEUGT, F. W. A., OOSTERHOF, F., VON RIECZ, E., BRUTEL DE LA RIVIÉRE, A. and ENGELFRIET, C. P. (1978). A simple immunofluorescence test for the detection of platelet antibodies. *British Journal of Haematology*, **39**, 195.

[40] WEISS, H. J. (1975). Platelet physiology and abnormalities of platelet function. *New England Journal of Medicine*, **293**, 580.

[41] WEISS, H. J. and LAGES, B. A. (1977). Possible congenital defect in platelet thromboxane synthetase. *Lancet*, **i**, 760.

[42] ZAHAVI, J. (1977). The role of platelets in myocardial infarction, ischemic heart disease, cerebrovascular disease, thromboembolic disorders and acute idiopathic pericarditis. *Thrombosis and Haemostasis*, **38**, 1073.

16

Laboratory control of anticoagulant and thrombolytic therapy

(*Written in collaboration with W. R. Pitney and M. Brozovic*)

Anticoagulant therapy may prevent the occurrence of thrombosis or the further propagation of an existing thrombus. Anticoagulant drugs have little, if any, effect upon an already existing thrombus; thrombus dissolution can be achieved, however, by thrombolytic agents. There are three main classes of anticoagulant drugs:

1. The oral anticoagulants, coumarins and indanediones, which act by interfering with the synthesis by the liver of the vitamin K-dependent coagulation factors (factors II, VII, IX and X).

2. Heparin and heparinoids which have a complex action on blood clotting, the main effects being interference with the thrombin-mediated conversion of fibrinogen to fibrin and enhanced inactivation of factor Xa.

3. Defibrinating agents such as ancrod (Arvin) and Reptilase which induce hypocoagulability by the removal of fibrinogen from the blood.

Heparin and ancrod are useful in the short-term initial management of patients with deep venous thrombosis and pulmonary embolism, whereas the oral anticoagulants are reserved for thrombosis prophylaxis, usually on a long-term basis. Heparin may be indicated also in the treatment of patients with disseminated intravascular coagulation, microangiopathic haemolytic anaemia, some types of renal failure and impending renal homograft rejection as well as during haemodialysis, cardiac catheterization and cardio-pulmonary by-pass surgery.

Control of oral anticoagulant therapy

It is not possible to produce a therapeutic derangement of haemostasis without accepting some risk of haemorrhage. The purpose of laboratory control is to maintain a level of hypocoagulability which is effective in preventing thrombosis but not so low that the risk of spontaneous bleeding becomes appreciable. Three methods in current use are:

1. The one-stage prothrombin time of Quick (p. 216).

2. The prothrombin/proconvertin (P and P) method of Owren and Aas.[17]

3. The Thrombotest of Owren.[16]

Of these, the one-stage prothrombin-time test is the most popular in the United Kingdom, one or other modifications being used in about 80% of laboratories. The most important variable is in the type of thromboplastin used in the test. The original thromboplastin prepared by Quick was an acetone-dried rabbit-brain preparation, but thromboplastins from other animal sources and from human brains have been used also. Rabbit-brain preparations are relatively insensitive to the plasma defect induced by oral anticoagulants. In addition, not all rabbit- or human-brain preparations have similar sensitivities and there may also be considerable batch-to-batch variability in potency with either rabbit or human preparations. For these reasons, a laboratory using a standard technique may record quite different prothrombin times on a plasma sample from a patient on oral anticoagulants when more than one thromboplastin is used.

ONE-STAGE PROTHROMBIN TIME TEST

Recording the results

The simplest method is to record the result with the test plasma in seconds together with the result obtained from a pool of normal plasma samples, e.g. test plasma 24 s, normal control 12 s. It is a simple exercise to record the result of the test plasma as a ratio of the control value and this method of reporting was recommended by the *British Committee for Standards in Haematology**.[20] Using the above example, the ratio would be 2.0. Some laboratories record the result with the test plasma as a percentage of normal clotting activity. This percentage figure is derived from the prothrombin time by reference to a graph prepared by plotting the prothrombin times of a range of dilutions of pooled normal plasma in a diluent such as saline or adsorbed plasma. There are objections to this procedure since a diluted normal plasma is not comparable to an undiluted test plasma. Even if the fibrinogen and factor V concentrations are kept relatively constant by diluting the normal plasma with adsorbed plasma, the samples are still not comparable since plasma from patients on oral anticoagulants contains inhibitors known as PIVKA†.[8] Furthermore, reporting results as a percentage of normal clotting activity implies a degree of accuracy which is not justified from the nature of the test employed. A further method of reporting results, which is used in a few laboratories, is the prothrombin index, which is the reciprocal of the ratio, reported as a percentage. The index of the sample quoted above would be 50%. The prothrombin index has little to recommend it and it is easily confused with percentage clotting activity.

STANDARDIZATION OF THE PROTHROMBIN-TIME TEST

There are a number of commercial rabbit-brain thromboplastins available, some containing added calcium. Human-brain thromboplastins are usually home-made and may be prepared by suspending acetone-dried material in 9 g/l NaCl (saline) immediately prior to use or by suspending an emulsion of brain in saline and storing at −20°C (see Appendix, p. 433). These various thromboplastins give different ratios with the same test plasma, and

it is not possible to define the therapeutic range unless the thromboplastin used is also specified.[2] For instance, a ratio of 2.5 may represent good therapeutic control if the result was obtained with a human-brain preparation, but the same ratio would indicate excessive anticoagulation if the result was obtained with rabbit brain. However, the reactivity of two thromboplastins may be compared by the method recommended by the *WHO Expert Committee on Biological Standardization*.[23] If a number of plasma samples from patients on oral anticoagulants and normal subjects are tested with both reagents, a straight-line relationship is found to exist between the prothrombin times obtained.[5]

By means of such a correlation, it is possible to use a reference thromboplastin to assess the sensitivities of the thromboplastins (commercial or home-made) used in individual laboratories. Furthermore, the results obtained in individual laboratories may be corrected for any difference in sensitivity between the local thromboplastin and the reference reagent. Reference preparations are available which can be used for this purpose.[10,14] These include International Reference Materials of human, rabbit and bovine thromboplastins from WHO* and similar materials from the European Community Bureau of Reference.†

Standardization procedure

All the reference preparations referred to above have been calibrated in terms of a primary WHO human brain thromboplastin (67/40) which was established with a nominal value of 1.0. The relative potency of each is defined by an *international sensitivity index (ISI)*‡.

The standardization procedure described below is intended for an inter-species comparison of a working preparation with the appropriate reference preparation by an individual laboratory. The prothrombin times (PTs) obtained with the two preparations on a set of samples of normal plasma

---

* Now the British Committee for Standardization in Haematology.
† PIVKA: proteins induced by vitamin K absence or antagonists.

* From the National Institute for Biological Standards and Control, Holly Hill, Hampstead, London NW3.
† From European Community Bureau of Reference (BCR), Rue de la Loi 200, B-1049, Brussels.
‡ This term has been introduced by WHO to replace the term international calibration constant which has been used to defined the relationship obtained by comparison with prothrombin time *ratios*.

and of plasma from patients on oral anticoagulants are plotted on double-log graph paper. From the slope of the correlation line obtained, the sensitivity index of the working preparation can be defined.

Method

Collect plasma from four normal healthy adults and from 12 patients who have been stabilized on oral anticoagulant treatment for at least 6 weeks. Warm the thromboplastins and 0.025 mol/l $CaCl_2$ to 37°C in a water-bath. Carry out prothrombin time tests as described on p. 217. Allow the plasma and thromboplastin mixtures to warm for at least 2 min before adding the calcium. Test each plasma in duplicate with each of the two thromboplastins in the following order with the minimum delay between tests:

	Reference reagent	Local reagent
Plasma 1	Test 1	Test 2
	Test 4	Test 3
Plasma 2	Test 5	Test 6
	Test 8	Test 7 etc.

Record the mean time for each plasma. If there is a discrepancy of more than 10% in the clotting times between duplicates, repeat the tests on that plasma. Plot the times on double-log graph paper, with PTs for the reference preparation (y) on the vertical axis and PTs for the working preparation (x) on the horizontal axis. Obtain the best fit of a straight line (Fig. 16.1). The relationship between the two preparations is determined by the slope of the line (b). Estimate the slope from the formula: $b = (y - a) \div x$, where x and y represent linked measurements on the two axes of the graph and (a) is the intercept of x on y. For a more precise estimation calculate the regression line of the slope from the formula:

$$b = m + \sqrt{m^2 + 1}, \text{ where}$$

$$m = \frac{\sum(y - \bar{y})^2 - \sum(x - \bar{x})^2}{2\sum(y - \bar{y})(x - \bar{x})}, \text{ and where}$$

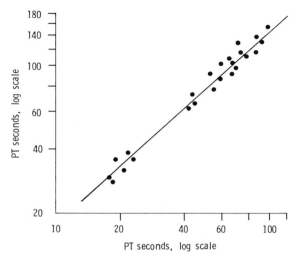

Fig. 16.1 Standardization of thromboplastin. Plot of prothrombin times for determining the sensitivity index of a thromboplastin reagent.

y and x are the logarithms of the individual PTs and $\bar{y}$ and $\bar{x}$ are their means, using the reference preparation and the working preparation, respectively.

Estimate the sensitivity index of the working preparation as follows:

SI of working preparation = ISI of reference preparation × b.

Standardization of commercial thromboplastins

A more complex procedure has been recommended for the standardization of commercial thromboplastins.[5] A total of 20 normal plasma samples and 40 specimens from patients stabilized on oral anticoagulant therapy should be tested in batches over a 10-day period. A statistical analysis is applied, taking account of the SD of the measurements. An orthogonal* regression line is calculated, and from this, the ISI can be derived.

The *European Community Bureau of Reference (BCR)* preparations are provided with certified values of the slope (b) and intercept (a) of the calibration line. The relationship of the logarithms of any prothrombin time obtained with these reference materials to the corresponding logarithm of the prothrombin time with the WHO primary

---

* This is a statistical procedure which is used to take into account differences in the SDs of the measurements obtained with the two thromboplastins (5).

reference preparation (67/40) is described by the formula:

$$y = a + bx.$$

To convert the actual measured prothrombin time to the equivalent on the international scale, carry out the following procedures:

1. Find the log to base 10 of the measured PT (=x).
2. Calculate $y = a + bx$.

The antilog to base 10 of y is then the measurement which would have been obtained on that plasma with the WHO (67/40) reference preparation. A commercial thromboplastin which has been standardized against one of the BCR reference preparations will thus be directly related to the WHO Reference Preparation.

Therapeutic range

In the anticoagulant clinic the measured PT is converted to a prothrombin ratio by dividing the patient's PT by the averaged values of the PT of a series of normal samples (p. 226).

If the sensitivity index of the thromboplastin is known, each patient's ratio can be converted into an international normalized ratio (INR).[12] This is calculated as follows:

$$INR = x^c$$

where x = the patient's measured prothrombin ratio and c = the sensitivity index of the thromboplastin. x^c can be obtained by means of logarithmic tables: it is the antilog of $(\log x \times c)$.

The British Committee for Standardization in Haematology recommended that the values obtained with the British Comparative Thromboplastin be adjusted to prothrombin-time ratios between 2.0 and 4.0 for various clinical conditions.[1,3] This has proved to be a safe range. The optimal therapeutic range for the INR is, in general, also 2.0–4.0[14] This is valid for all thromboplastins which have been standardized by the procedure described above.

Other standardization procedures

Lyophilized plasma standards may be used to check the sensitivity of thromboplastin reagents. Such standards are prepared from normal plasma artificially depleted of coagulation factors II, VII, IX and X. The standards span the therapeutic range and appear to be stable and to give reproducible results. Lyophilized plasma from patients on oral anticoagulant therapy are preferable to artificially depleted standards, since such standards will demonstrate the PIVKA effect.

Estimation of prothrombin time by the P and P (Prothrombin and Proconvertin) method of Owren and Aas[17]

Principle. The plasma sample is diluted and mixed with a source of factor V and fibrinogen before testing. The effect of dilution makes the test more sensitive to small fluctuations in the activity of factors II, VII and X. It is insensitive to deficiency of factors V and IX.

Reagents

Test and control plasma. Citrated plasma is used, as in the one-stage prothrombin-time test. Before use, dilute the plasma samples 1 in 10 in barbitone buffer, pH 7.4, diluted in citrate-saline (Solution B, see below).

Diluting solutions.
   A. 32 g/l trisodium citrate 240 ml, water 760 ml.
   B. Barbitone buffer, pH 7.4 (see p. 435) 200 ml, solution A 200 ml, 9 g/l NaCl (saline) 600 ml.
   C. 32 g/l trisodium citrate 100 ml, saline 600 ml.

Prothrombin-free ox plasma. Adsorb oxalated plasma with barium sulphate in the proportion of 50 mg of barium sulphate per ml of plasma. Centrifuge the adsorbed plasma after 10–15 min at 37°C.

Thromboplastin. Saline extract of human brain. The method of preparation is described in the Appendix (p. 433).

Calcium chloride. The optimal concentration giving minimum clotting times has to be determined for each batch of ox plasma. A 0.03 mol/l solution is usually satisfactory.

Method

Mix 0.1 ml of prothrombin-free ox plasma in a 75 × 12 mm glass tube with 0.1 ml of diluted test (or control) plasma and 0.1 ml of brain-thromboplastin suspension. After allowing 1–2 min for the mixture to warm in the 37°C water-bath, add 0.1 ml of calcium chloride, and measure the clotting time of the mixture by means of a stop-watch. Repeat the test at least once and record the mean time. Include normal plasma control samples in each batch tested.

Normal range of prothrombin time. (P and P method): 30–40 s. It must be emphasized that a normal range has to be established for each particular laboratory and set of reagents.

Recording results of the P and P method

The clotting time of the patient's plasma can be converted into 'Percent P and P activity' from a graph. Pool about six samples of normal plasma and dilute the pool 1 in 2, 1 in 4, 1 in 8 and 1 in 16 with diluting solution C. Then dilute the undiluted plasma and these diluted samples 1 in 10 to 1 in 160. Record the clotting times obtained with each dilution. Plot the observed times against plasma dilutions on double-log paper when a straight line should result. Read the dilution off the graph and hence percent activity corresponding with the observed time for the patient's plasma.

Comment on the P and P method

The P and P method is suitable for the control of anticoagulant therapy on specimens submitted through the post. Contact activation does not affect the results and loss of factor V activity is not a problem since factor V is added in the test. The usually accepted therapeutic range using the P and P method is 10–25%, ideally about 15%.

This method has not achieved much popularity and is seldom used in the United Kingdom for the control of oral anticoagulant therapy. It is more sensitive than the one-stage prothrombin time, particularly when the prothrombin activity is relatively high, as measurements are made on diluted plasma. The concentrations of factor V and fibri-

nogen are optimal in the clotting mixtures and independent of the concentrations of the factors in the test plasma. The test is relatively insensitive to the presence of heparin in the test plasma, since the inhibiting effect is diluted out. However, the extra reagents required and the rather elaborate testing procedure are obstacles to the more widespread use of the test in place of the one-stage prothrombin time.

Thrombotest[16]

The Thrombotest reagent* is a commercial preparation containing adsorbed bovine plasma, bovine thromboplastin and cephalin. The material in lyophilized and dispensed under vacuum in sealed ampoules. Batches of reagents are subjected to rigid quality control and there is little batch-to-batch variability. The reagent can be used to test capillary blood, in which case the reagent is dissolved in water, or citrated venous blood, when the reagent is used dissolved in a solution of 3.2 mol/l calcium chloride provided with the thrombotest reagent. Sealed ampoules of the material in lyophilized and dispensed under and the reconstituted reagent (see below) may be stored at −20°C for up to 2 months without appreciable loss of activity.

Thrombotest measures overall clotting activity and the result is influenced by deficiencies of factors II, VII, IX and X as well as by the PIVKA effect. Bovine thromboplastin appears to be as sensitive as human thromboplastin to factor VII deficiency.

The actual technique of the test is different according to whether capillary or venous blood is used. The most practical for the control of oral anticoagulant therapy is the venous-blood technique, and this will be described.

Preparation of reagent

The ampoule containing the freeze-dried reagent is vacuum-sealed and care must be taken in opening the ampoule that the sudden in-rush of air does not disperse the powder.

* Nyegaard and Co., Oslo.

Dissolve the powder in the calcium chloride solution previously warmed to 37°C. Use 2.2 ml of the solution to dissolve the contents of a small ampoule and 11 ml for a large ampoule. It is convenient to pipette out the whole content of the ampoule in 0.25 ml volumes into 75 × 12 mm glass tubes. Cap those not required for immediate use and store frozen at −20°C. They can be kept for up to 2 months.

Method

Blood collection. Collect venous blood in a plastic or siliconized syringe and mix with a one-ninth volume of 32 g/l sodium citrate in a plastic or siliconized tube. The blood should be tested within 1 h of collection, although it is stated that the test gives satisfactory results if carried out within 6 h.

Procedure. Place 0.25 ml of the reagent in a 75 × 12 mm glass tube and allow it to warm up in a water-bath at 37°C. Then add 50 μl of whole citrated blood and record the clotting time in the usual way. The mixture may be left undisturbed for *c* 30 s for normal blood and for *c* 50 s for the blood from patients receiving anticoagulants before being tilted to inspect for coagulation.

Calculation

Read the percentage activity from a correlation curve supplied with the reagent. Correction for abnormal PCV is rarely necessary as patients receiving oral anticoagulants are not usually anaemic. However, a correction may be made from a graph supplied with the reagent.

Therapeutic range

The usually accepted therapeutic range for anticoagulant therapy using the Thrombotest method is 6–11%.

Comment on thrombotest

The Thrombotest is a very satisfactory method for anticoagulant clinics. The use of capillary blood or uncentrifuged venous blood enables the test to be performed while the patient is waiting and there is minimal delay in obtaining the result. The ISI of the Thrombotest is about 1.0 and the recommended therapeutic range of 6–11% corresponds roughly to a range of 2.5–4.0 expressed as an international normalized ratio.[13] The Thrombotest is used in a number of centres known for their special interest in the prevention and management of thromboembolism.

CONTROL OF HEPARIN THERAPY

Intravenous heparin therapy

Heparin is usually administered intravenously for the treatment of venous thrombosis or pulmonary embolism; it is also given subcutaneously in low dosage for thrombosis prophylaxis in patients at high risk, e.g. following surgical operations or myocardial infarction. Intravenous heparin may be given by intermittent injections every 4 h or by constant infusion, preferably with a constant-infusion pump. Constant infusion produces a reasonably steady concentration of heparin in the plasma, whereas the concentration fluctuates widely with intermittent injections.

In patients who receive *intermittent* intravenous injections, blood should be withdrawn for the control of dosage 30 min before the next injection is due. If the blood is not collected at the correct time, the result cannot be interpreted and is of no use for regulating the dosage of heparin. If heparin is given by *constant* infusion, the blood sample may be obtained at any convenient time. With either form of therapy, blood should be tested every 24 h and the dosage altered, if necessary, in the light of the results obtained. Heparin is a powerful anticoagulant and the incidence of bleeding complications, despite laboratory control, is appreciable.[11] Bleeding is not always associated with laboratory results indicating overdosage.[18,19] Nevertheless, it appears reasonable to use some method of laboratory control to identify those patients with a plasma-heparin concentration outside the accepted therapeutic range. Tests available include the partial thromboplastin time with kaolin, thrombin time, chromogenic assays for heparin, and protamine neutralization assay.

The whole-blood coagulation time (as described in the 5th edition) was widely used in the past as a method for the control of heparin therapy. It has the major disadvantage that it is relatively insensitive to heparin. Moreover, the test must be performed at the bedside; a portable water-bath is essential and the test is time-consuming, especially when clotting times are unduly prolonged.

PARTIAL THROMBOPLASTIN TIME WITH KAOLIN (PTTK) (p. 219)

This test is performed in the laboratory on samples of citrated plasma, and is, at present, one of the most commonly used tests for monitoring heparin therapy.[11] The test is very sensitive to heparin but has a number of disadvantages that should be kept in mind. The first is that different phospholipids have different sensitivities to heparin, and some do not show a linear relationship between clotting times and heparin concentration in the therapeutic range. Such reagents are not suitable for the control of heparin therapy.

If a phospholipid reagent carries no manufacturer's information on its sensitivity to heparin, or is home-made, it is necessary to establish whether it is a reliable guide to plasma-heparin concentration. The testing is carried out by adding known concentrations of heparin to a normal plasma pool and performing a PTTK test on each concentration as shown on Table 16.1. The relationship between clotting times and heparin concentration is in this case linear, and the reagent satisfactory.

Table 16.1 Testing a phospholipid reagent for heparin sensitivity

Heparin concentration of normal plasma (iu/ml)	Partial thromboplastin time with kaolin (s)
0	34
0.1	34
0.2	38
0.3	49
0.4	62
0.5	76
0.8	98
1.0	128

The second disadvantage of the PTTK test is that it is affected by a number of variables not related to heparin. The most important of these is the high concentration of factor VIII:C commonly found in acute phase reaction. High factor VIII:C causes a marked shortening of the clotting time and in such patients the PTTK test may remain nearly normal despite an adequate concentration of heparin in the plasma. If this effect of factor VIII:C is suspected, another test, such as protamine neutralization or a chromogenic assay for heparin, or thrombin time, should be carried out.

A range of clotting times covering heparin concentrations between 0.3 and 0.8 iu/ml of plasma is considered to represent effective heparin therapy. This is usually between 1.5 and 2.5 times the control value.[11,22] With the reagent shown in Table 16.1, the therapeutic range would be 50–100 s. Oxalated plasma should never be used for this test, since sensitivity to heparin in the presence of oxalate is much less than when citrate is present.[21]

THROMBIN-CLOTTING TIME OF PLASMA (p. 218)

This test is simple and popular, since it can be performed rapidly on batches of plasma processed in the laboratory. A range of thrombin times between 25 and 100 s (normal control 10–15 s) is considered to represent effective heparin therapy.[15]

CHROMOGENIC SUBSTRATE ASSAY FOR HEPARIN[4]

Chromogenic assay kits are available from different commercial firms*. Thrombin or Xa specific substrates are used. The values are read off a standard heparin curve determined at the time of the test.

Plasma heparin assay

The assay is an extension of the thrombin-clotting time test, various amounts of pro-

* (Coatest Heparin Kit, Kabi Vitrum; Heparin Kit BCL, Coagulation Diagnostica, Lewes, Sussex; Heparin Kit, Boehringer, Mannheim).

tamine sulphate being added to the plasma before the addition of thrombin. When all the heparin present in the plasma has been neutralized, the clotting time should become normal. From the amount of protamine sulphate required to produce this effect, the concentration of heparin in the plasma can be calculated. Heparin assays are used mainly to calculate the dose of protamine sulphate used to neutralize circulating heparin after cardiopulmonary surgery and haemodialysis, but they have also been used to control therapy.

Reagents

Protamine sulphate. Prepare dilutions made in barbitone buffer, pH 7.4, from 0 to 50 mg/dl.

Dilute 5 ml of protamine sulphate (10 g/l) 1 in 20 with buffer to give 1 dl of a stock solution containing 50 mg/dl. Then make working solutions to cover the range 0–50 mg/dl in 5 mg steps from the stock solution by dilution with buffer. The solutions keep indefinitely at 4°C.

Thrombin. Dilute thrombin in barbitone buffer to a concentration of about 20 NIH units per ml. Adjust the concentration so that 0.1 ml of thrombin will clot 0.2 ml of normal plasma at 37°C in 10 ± 1 s. Keep the thrombin in a plastic tube in melting ice during the assay.

Plasma. Citrated platelet-poor plasma from the patient.

Method

Place 0.2 ml of test plasma and 20 μl of barbitone buffer in a 75 × 12 mm glass tube kept at 37°C. Allow the mixture to warm to 37°C and then blow in 0.1 ml of thrombin. Record the clotting time. If this is 10 ± 1 s, there is no demonstrable heparin in the plasma. If the thrombin clotting time is prolonged, repeat the test using 20 μl of protamine sulphate, 50 mg/dl, instead of buffer. Repeat the test, if necessary, until a concentration of protamine is found which gives a clotting time of 10 ± 1 s.

Calculation

If 20 μl of protamine sulphate of concentration 15 mg/dl produce a normal thrombin clotting time (whereas the clotting time is prolonged when a concentration of 10 mg/dl is used), then 15 μg of protamine is clearly sufficient to neutralize the heparin in 1 ml of plasma. Assuming weight-for-weight neutralization, the patient's plasma contains 15 μg of heparin per ml, i.e. 1.5 iu/ml, assuming that 1 mg of heparin is equivalent to 100 iu. This figure can be converted to concentration of heparin per ml of whole blood by multiplying by 1 − PCV.

In the above example, for the in vivo neutralization of heparin by protamine sulphate, assuming a total blood volume of 75 ml/kg, the dose of protamine required would be:

$$\frac{15 \times \text{total blood volume (l)}}{1/(1 - PCV)} \text{ mg}$$

$$= \frac{15 \times 75 \times \text{weight (kg)} \times (1 - PCV)}{1000} \text{ mg.}$$

Comment

It is apparent from the number of tests available that the control of heparin therapy is not entirely satisfactory. Each test measures a different aspect of heparin action on the coagulation cascade, and the correlation between the results of different tests is not good. Furthermore, clinically significant bleeding may occur even when the plasma concentration of heparin is within the accepted therapeutic range (0.3–0.8 iu/ml).

Subcutaneous heparin therapy

Heparin is often administered subcutaneously in an attempt to prevent the development of venous thrombosis following major surgery or during the course of some medical illnesses. It is also used prophylactically to prevent the recurrence of venous thrombosis in situations where warfarin therapy may be contraindicated, e.g. pregnancy. The usual dose is 5000 iu administered at 8 or 12 h intervals and the plasma concentrations achieved are too low to be measured by the methods used to control intravenous heparin therapy. However, these low concentrations are sufficient to increase the activity of antithrombin III, thus neutralizing the thrombin and factor Xa generated during incipient thrombosis. There is an increased, although slight, risk of post-operative bleeding with subcutaneous heparin and some patients still develop thrombosis even with this therapy. It has been suggested that the frequency of bleeding or thrombosis might be reduced if subcutaneous heparin therapy was monitored with estimations of the plasma-heparin concentration. The peak plasma value usually occurs between 2 and 4 h after each dose and an estimation performed at this time could indicate the probable effectiveness of therapy.

The PTTK test can be used to assess whether the concentration of heparin is unacceptably high. The result should be within 8 s of the control time; if longer, the plasma-heparin concentration is probably in excess of 0.2 iu/ml and the patient is likely to bleed, especially if undergoing surgery. The PTTK test gives only a rough estimate of excessively high concentrations. In contrast, heparin assay by factor Xa inhibition measures accurately the very low concentrations of heparin in plasma (0.05–0.2 iu/ml) usually found during subcutaneous therapy.

Plasma heparin assay by factor Xa inhibition[6]

Principle. The plasma is heated at 56°C to inactivate clotting factor inhibitors other than anti-Xa (antithrombin III) and then incubated with a standard amount of factor Xa for a fixed period. The residual factor Xa in the mixture is measured by recording the clotting time after the addition of factor X-free substrate plasma, calcium and phospholipid. In the presence of heparin, the action of anti-Xa is potentiated and more factor Xa is destroyed in the incubation mixture, resulting in a longer clotting time.

Reagents

Pooled normal plasma. Collect citrated blood from 6 to 10 normal subjects and sepa-

rate the plasma by centrifugation. The pooled plasma may be stored in 1–2 ml volumes at −20°C.

Citrated test plasma. See p. 215.

Calcium chloride. Use a 0.05 mol/l solution.

Citrate-albumin-glyoxaline buffer. Prepare glyoxaline buffer, pH 7.4, by dissolving 0.68 g of imidazole and 1.17 g of sodium chloride in c 100 ml of water. Add 37.2 ml of 0.1 mol/l HCl and make up the volume to 200 ml with water. Then add to 150 ml of glyoxaline buffer, 30 ml of 32 g/l trisodium citrate and 1 ml of 20% bovine albumin. Add sodium azide at a final concentration of 0.04%.

Phospholipid. Purified phospholipid is obtainable from Diagnostic Reagents Ltd., Thame, Oxon. Add 5.0 ml of distilled water to the content of the vial.

Factor X-deficient substrate plasma. This is obtainable from Diagnostic Reagents Ltd., Thame, Oxon. Add 3.0 ml of water to the contents of the vial.

Activated bovine factor X (factor Xa). This is obtainable from Diagnostic Reagents Ltd., Thame, Oxon. Add 0.5 ml of water to the contents of the vial. Then dilute the solution 1 in 100 with citrate-albumin-glyoxaline buffer.

Substrate plasma-phospholipid mixture. Mix equal volumes of factor X-deficient substrate plasma and phospholipid. The mixture may be kept at room temperature (18–25°C) for up to 3 h.

Heparin for standard curve. Heparin is a mixture of different molecular species with varying molecular weights and activities and different brands show variable activity per unit weight. For preparation of the standard curve use, if possible, the same batch of heparin as that used for therapy.

Method

Make a series of dilutions of heparin in the pooled normal plasma to give concentrations of 0.02, 0.04, 0.06, 0.08, 0.10, 0.15 and 0.20 iu/ml. A convenient way to do this is to take a vial containing heparin 5000 iu/ml and add 0.4 ml to 500 ml of 9 g/l NaCl (saline) to give a heparin concentration of 4 iu/ml. Add

Table 16.2 Heparin dilutions for plasma-heparin assay

Diluted heparin (ml)	Plasma (ml)	Final heparin concentration (u/ml)
0.1	1.9	0.2
0.075	1.925	0.15
0.05	1.95	0.10
0.04	1.96	0.08
0.03	1.97	0.06
0.02	1.98	0.04
0.01	1.99	0.02

the diluted heparin to plasma as shown in Table 16.2.

Into 75 × 12 mm glass tubes place, respectively, 1 ml volumes of normal plasma, the heparinized normal plasma samples and the test plasma. Stand the tubes in a 56°C waterbath for 15 min, then cool and centrifuge at 1200–1500 *g* for 10 min. Transfer the clear supernatants into clean dry glass tubes. Into each of a series of 60 × 8 mm plastic tubes, place 0.3 ml of diluted factor Xa. Place one of the tubes in the water-bath at 37°C and add to it 0.1 ml of heated normal plasma—this provides the incubation mixture. Start a stop-watch, stopper the tube, invert twice and then discard the stopper. Place two 75 × 12 mm glass tubes in the water-bath and add 0.1 ml of calcium chloride solution to each. At 4 min 45 s, transfer duplicate 0.1 ml volumes from the incubation mixture into the tubes containing calcium chloride. At 5 min, pipette 0.2 ml of the substrate plasma-phospholipid mixture into each of these tubes and record the clotting times with separate stop-watches. Average the duplicate clotting times. Repeat the procedure with 0.1 ml volumes of the heparinized normal plasma samples and then with the test samples.

Calculation

Plot the clotting time of the standard heparin dilutions, ranging from zero to 0.2 units/ml, against concentrations of heparin on log/ linear paper. This should give a straight line. Read the heparin concentrations in the test samples directly off the graph. If the test

plasma contains more than 0.2 units of heparin per ml, dilute it appropriately in heated pooled normal plasma and repeat the procedure.

For the same batches of factor Xa and factor X-free substrate plasma, a single calibration graph may be used; and on different days it is only necessary to check the zero heparin and 0.1 iu/ml heparin samples. If these samples give clotting times a second or so different from the standard line, but the line joining them is parallel to the standard line, use the new line for interpolation of the test results.

Thrombolytic therapy

Two thrombolytic agents are currently in use: streptokinase and urokinase.

Streptokinase, a purified fraction of the filtrate from cultures of haemolytic streptococci, will cause lysis of plasma clots in vitro and may produce lysis of thrombi when injected intravenously. The chief indications for streptokinase therapy are massive pulmonary embolism and ilio-femoral vein thrombosis. Streptokinase therapy produces a complex derangement of haemostasis. The concentration of circulating plasminogen activator is greatly increased, plasma plasminogen values fall to low levels and fibrinogen/fibrin degradation products (FDPs) appear in the blood. The concentration of plasma fibrinogen falls and there may be a reduction in the concentration of other clotting factors, especially factors V and VIII. Platelet function may be impaired at high plasma concentrations of FDP and the plasma concentration of α_2-macroglobulin (which contains antiplasmin) falls.

The blood of most people contains antistreptococcal antibodies which neutralize the action of streptokinase. The agent must therefore be administered intravenously in a loading dose sufficiently large to overcome the effect of these antibodies in order to set up an intense systemic fibrinolysis. The size of the loading dose may be calculated by an in vitro test (see below). However, it has been shown that the initial dose required would not be more than 250 000 iu in 88% of patients, not more than 400 000 iu in 94% and not more than 600 000 in

98%.[9] The practice in many hospitals is to dispense with the titrating procedure and administer a standard loading dose of 600 000 iu to all adult patients. Maintenance therapy is usually 100 000 iu each hour.

Urokinase is a β-globulin produced by the kidney and present in urine. Unlike streptokinase it is not antigenic in man. Urokinase directly converts plasminogen into plasmin; the effects on haemostasis are similar to those described for streptokinase. It is usually administered in a dose of 4000 CTA* units per kg body weight per hour for 12–72 h, and there is no need for an initial loading dose.

Titration of the initial dose of streptokinase[7]

Principle. Different amounts of streptokinase are added to 1 ml volumes of the patient's plasma and the samples are clotted with thrombin. The smallest amount of streptokinase which causes clot lysis to occur in less than 10 min is multiplied by the presumed plasma volume.

Reagents

Test plasma. Prepare citrated platelet-poor plasma from venous blood in the usual way (p. 215).

Streptokinase. Vials containing 5000 iu (Behring) or 10 000 iu (Kabi) of freeze-dried material are suitable. Open the vial carefully and add sufficient 9 g/ NaCl to make a solution containing 2000 iu/ml. From this initial solution, make further dilutions containing 1500, 1000 and 500 iu/ml.

Thrombin. A solution containing *c* 50 NIH units per ml of 9 g/l NaCl is suitable.

Method

Place four 75 × 12 mm glass tubes in the water-bath at 37°C. Pipette 1 ml of plasma into each tube followed by 0.1 ml of one of the

---

* This is an arbitrary unit which was established by the Committee on Thrombolytic Agents; another arbitrary unit is the Ploug unit. 1 iu = 0.67 Ploug units or 0.96 CTA units.

four streptokinase dilutions and 0.1 ml of thrombin. Mix the contents of the tubes by inversion and start a stop-watch when clotting has taken place. Observe the tubes for clot lysis. Lysis will commence first in the tube with the highest concentration of streptokinase. Note the tube containing the smallest amount of streptokinase which will cause clot lysis in 10 min.

Calculation

Suppose that clot lysis occurred in less than 10 min in the three tubes containing 0.1 ml volumes of streptokinase of strength 1000 iu, 1500 iu and 2000 iu/ml. The least amount of streptokinase able to induce lysis in 1 ml of plasma was 100 iu. If the patient was an adult with a presumed plasma volume of 3000 ml, the necessary initial dose of streptokinase would be 100 × 3000 = 300 000 iu.

Laboratory control of thrombolytic therapy

A number of laboratory tests are abnormal during streptokinase therapy. The level of circulating plasminogen activator will be high and the plasma-plasminogen concentration will be greatly reduced. Unfortunately, neither of these can be measured quickly and accurately. The simplest method of measuring plasminogen activator activity is by the euglobulin clot-lysis time (p. 242), but in its unmodified form this test is sensitive to deficiencies of plasminogen and fibrinogen and may give fallacious results in streptokinase therapy. The ability of the euglobulin fraction to produce lysis of untreated fibrin plates is a more accurate method for assessing plasminogen activator, but is too time-consuming for routine use. Measurement of plasma plasminogen is also a complex, lengthy procedure.

The concentration of fibrinogen/fibrin degradation products can be assessed roughly by the degree of prolongation of the thrombin clotting time of plasma, and this test is used in many laboratories as an index of effective therapy.

The thrombin clotting time is also sensitive to the plasma-fibrinogen concentration and it is therefore not a specific test of fibrinolytic activity. A few hours after the commencement of therapy, the thrombin clotting time may be prolonged to 40 s or more (normal 10 ± 1 s), but then it usually settles down in the range 20–30 s. Very prolonged thrombin clotting times during therapy indicate high levels of FDP or low levels of plasma fibrinogen, both the result of hyperplasminaemia.

Hyperplasminaemia can only occur when there is plasminogen available in the plasma for conversion to plasmin, and it has been suggested that, in such an event, the dose-rate of streptokinase should be increased so as to reduce the plasma-plasminogen concentration further. This is a controversial recommendation and it is not clear at present what action should be taken in the event of a very prolonged thrombin clotting time. In view of the difficulties of laboratory control and the uncertainty in interpreting laboratory data, there is some justification for using a standard dosage scheme for streptokinase[9] and urokinase without laboratory control.

Therapeutic defibrination

Therapeutic defibrination with Ancrod is now used infrequently. For details of monitoring see the 5th edition of this book.

REFERENCES

[1] BARKHAN, P. (1976). Therapeutic range with BCTR. *Thrombosis and Haemostasis*, **36**, 485.

[2] BIGGS, R. and DENSON, K. W. E. (1967). Standardization of the one-stage prothrombin time for the control of anticoagulant therapy. *British Medical Journal*, i, 84.

[3] BLACKBURN, E. K. (1976). Long term anticoagulant therapy. *Prescriber's Journal*, **16**, 73.

[4] BLOMBACK, M. (1981). Chromogenic substrates in the laboratory diagnosis of clotting disorders. In *Haemostasis and Thrombosis*, eds. A. L. Bloom and D. P. Thomas, p. 809. Churchill Livingstone, Edinburgh.

[5] Commission of European Communities (1982). BCR Information: certification of three reference materials for thromboplastins. EEC, Brussels.

[6] DENSON, K. W. E. and BONNAR, J. (1973). The measurement of heparin. A method based on the potentiation of anti-Factor Xa. *Thrombosis et Diathesis Haemorrhagica*, **30**, 471.

[7] HAWKEY, C. and HOWELL, M. (1964). The laboratory control of thrombolytic therapy. *Journal of Clinical Pathology*, **17**, 287.

[8] HEMKER, H. C., VELTKAMP, J. J. and LOELIGER, E. A. (1968). Kinetic aspects of the interaction of blood clotting enzymes. III. Demonstration of the existence of an inhibitor of prothrombin conversion in vitamin K deficiency. *Thrombosis et Diathesis Haemorrhagica*, **19**, 346.

[9] HIRSH, J., O'SULLIVAN, E. F. and MARTIN, M. (1970). Evaluation of a standard dosage schedule with streptokinase. *Blood*, **35**, 341.

[10] International Committee on Thrombosis and Haemostasis/International Committee for Standardization in Haematology. (1979). Prothrombin time standardization: report of the Expert Panel on anticoagulant control. *Thrombosis and Haemostasis*, **42**, 1073.

[11] KELTON, J. G. and HIRSH, J. (1980). Bleeding associated with antithrombotic therapy. *Seminars in Hematology*, **27**, 259.

[12] KIRKWOOD, T. B. L. (1983). Calibration of reference thromboplastins and standardization of the prothrombin ratio. *Thrombosis and Haemostasis*, **49**, 238.

[13] LOELIGER, E. A. (1972). Progress in the control of oral anticoagulants. *Thrombosis et Diathesis Haemorrhagica*, **28**, 109.

[14] LOELIGER, E. A. and LEWIS, S. M. (1982). Progress in laboratory control of oral anticoagulants. *Lancet*, ii, 318.

[15] O'SHEA, M. J., FLUTE, P. T. and PANNELL, G. M. (1971). Laboratory control of heparin therapy. *Journal of Clinical Pathology*, **24**, 542.

[16] OWREN, P. A. (1959). Thrombotest: a new method for controlling anticoagulant therapy. *Lancet*, ii, 754.

[17] OWREN, P. A. and AAS, K. (1951). The control of dicumarol therapy and the quantitative determination of prothrombin and proconvertin. *Scandinavian Journal of Clinical and Laboratory Investigation*, **3**, 201.

[18] PITNEY, W. R. (1972). *Clinical Aspects of Thromboembolism*, p. 124. Churchill Livingstone, Edinburgh.

[19] PITNEY, W. R., PETTIT, J. E. and ARMSTRONG, L. (1970). Control of heparin therapy. *British Medical Journal*, iv, 129.

[20] POLLER, L. (1970). The British comparative thromboplastin: the use of the national thromboplastin reagent for uniformity of laboratory control of oral anticoagulants and expression of results. *Association of Clinical Pathologists Broadsheet* No. 71.

[21] SOLOWAY, H. B., COX, S. P. and DONAHOO, J. V. (1973). Sensitivity of the activated partial thromboplastin time to heparin: effect of anticoagulant used for sample collection. *American Journal of Clinical Pathology*, **59**, 760.

[22] SPECTOR, I. and CORN, M. (1967). Control of heparin therapy with activated partial thromboplastin times. *Journal of the American Medical Association*, **201**, 157.

[23] WHO Expert Committee on Biological Standardization. 31st Report, Annex 7: requirements for thromboplastins and plasma used to control oral anticoagulant therapy. *World Health Organization Technical Report Series 1981* No. 658, p. 185.

17

Use of radionuclides in haematology

In this chapter a brief general account will be given of the methods of using radionuclides in medical diagnosis. For a more complete account of the theory and practice of nuclear medicine techniques the reader is referred to textbooks by Sorenson and Phelps[9] and Bowring,[1] and the issue of *Clinics in Haematology* which was devoted to the use of radioisotopes in haematology.[7] The main properties of the radionuclides useful in diagnostic haematology are summarized in Tables 17.1 and 17.2. Specific instructions for their use are given in Chapters 15, 18, 19 and 20.

FORMS OF RADIATION

Radioactivity results from the spontaneous decay of unstable atomic nuclei; this is accompanied by the emission of charged particles (α, $\beta+$ and $\beta-$) or photons (γ rays). Isotopes* which emit γ rays are particularly useful as they have the advantage that these are 'hard' rays with good powers of penetration so that they can be detected at the surface of the body when they have originated within organs. The radiation from α and β ray emitters has little penetration; these are less useful for certain clinical purposes and are potentially more harmful than γ-ray emitters. The different types of radiation can be detected and distinguished by their ionization effect, by chemical and photochemical effects and by the production of scintillations in certain materials. The systems used for measuring radioactivity are described on p. 274.

RADIATION DOSAGE

When using radionuclides, account must be taken of their potential risk both for the recipient and the

Table 17.1 Radionuclides used in haematological diagnosis

Element	Physical half-life	Principal radiations	Energies (MeV)	Availability
^{57}Co	270d	γ	0.122, 0.136	†
^{58}Co	71.3d	$\beta+$ γ	0.48 0.811, 0.511	†
^{51}Cr	27.8d	γ X-rays	0.320	†
^{52}Fe*	8.2h	$\beta+$ γ	0.804 0.511, 0.165	Cyclotron
^{55}Fe	2.6yr	X-rays		†‡
^{59}Fe	45d	$\beta-$ γ	0.475, 0.273 1.09, 1.29	†
^{3}H	12.3yr	$\beta-$	0.0186	†
^{125}I	60d	γ	0.035	†
^{131}I	8.05d	$\beta-$ γ	0.606, 0.33 0.364, 0.637	†
^{111}In	2.81d	γ	0.247, 0.173	†
^{113m}In	1.67h	γ	0.393	^{113}Sn generator
^{32}P	14.3d	$\beta-$	1.71	
^{99m}Tc	6h	γ	0.140	^{99}Mo generator

* Decays to ^{52}Mn ($T_{1/2}$ 21 min).
† Radiochemical Centre, Amersham, Bucks.
‡ A small amount occurs as contaminant in ^{52}Fe production.

---

* Isotopes occur in radioactive and non-radioactive forms. For convenience, in this and in subsequent chapters the term 'isotope' will be used when referring to radioactive chemicals (i.e. radionuclides).

Table 17.2 Application of radionuclides in haematological diagnosis

Element	Radiopharmaceutical	Application	Usual dose (μCi)*
^{57}Co ^{58}Co	Vitamin B$_{12}$	Investigation of megaloblastic anaemias	0.5–1 0.5–1
^{51}Cr	Sodium chromate Sodium chromate Sodium chromate Sodium chromate Sodium chromate Sodium chromate Sodium chromate	Red-cell volume Red-cell life-span Sites of red-cell destruction Measurement of gastro-intestinal bleeding Platelet life-span Spleen scan Spleen pool	10–20 30–50 100 100 25–50 100–150 250
^{52}Fe	Ferric chloride or citrate	Ferrokinetics	100
^{59}Fe	Ferric chloride or citrate	Absorption of iron Ferrokinetics and erythropoiesis	5–20 5–10
^{3}H	Folic acid DFP	Folic acid metabolism Red-cell life-span	20–40 500
^{125}I ^{131}I	Iodinated human serum albumin	Plasma volume	2–5 2–5
^{111}In	Indium chloride ($\rightarrow$ oxine or acetyl acetone)	Platelet life-span Red-cell volume Spleen scan	200 25–50 200
^{113m}In	Indium chloride ($\rightarrow$ oxine or acetyl acetone)	Red-cell volume Spleen scan Spleen pool	50–100 250 500
^{32}P	DFP	Red-cell life-span Platelet life-span	50–70 50–70
^{99m}Tc	Pertechnetate	Red-cell volume Spleen scan Spleen pool	50–100 1000 2000

* 1 μCi = 3.7 $\times$ 10^4 Bq.

laboratory worker. The extent of radiation hazard in relation to the small amount of isotope employed in diagnostic work depends on a number of factors: e.g. whether the isotope is widely distributed in the body or becomes localized in specific organs; the physical half-life of the isotope and its biological half-time in the body, and compounded from these, the effective half-life from which the amount of radiation to which the person is exposed can be calculated. As far as possible, the isotope should have as short a half-life as is compatible with the duration of the test. An isotope with a very short half-life can be administered in much higher amounts than isotopes which are likely to remain active in the body for a considerably longer time.

Doses of radioactivity for diagnostic tests are generally in microcurie (μCi) amounts; but some short-lived isotopes may be administered in millicurie (mCi) amounts*.

The effect of radiation depends, essentially, on the amount of energy deposited in the body. This is expressed in grays (Gy). 1 Gy is the amount of radiation which deposits 1 joule of energy per kg of

* The basic unit of radioactivity has been the curie (Ci) which is the amount of isotope undergoing 3.7 $\times$ 10^{10} nuclear disintegrations per second. In SI, the basic unit is the bequerel (Bq), 1 Bq corresponding to one disintegration per second, so that 1 Ci = 3.7 $\times$ 10^{10} Bq. 1 millicurie (mCi) = 10^{-3} Ci = 3.7 $\times$ 10^7 Bq or 37 MBq, and 1 microcurie (μCi) = 10^{-6} Ci = 3.7 $\times$ 10^4 Bq or 0.037 MBq.

tissue. This has in the past been expressed in rads (1 rad = 0.01 Gy). The reaction of the body to the radiation is also affected by the type of the particular ionizing ray, and the biological effect of the radiation is calculated from the amount in Gy (or rad) multiplied by an ionization quality factor; this factor varies with the type of ray and is 20 times more for α rays than for β and γ rays. The unit for describing the biological effect is the sievert (SV) or the rem (1 rem = 0.01 SV). This important quantity determines the total amount of isotopes which can be administered (the maximum permissible dose), which for an adult must not exceed 0.05 SV (5 rem) per year. Isotopes should not be given to pregnant women, especially during the early weeks and, because of possible genetic effects, only minimal doses should be given to persons of reproductive age.

RADIATION PROTECTION

Before using radionuclides, workers should familiarize themselves with the problem of radiation protection for themselves, their fellow workers and patients. In Britain there is a code of practice which describes the procedures which must be followed in medical and dental practice.[2,3] An important recommendation is that radioactive isotopes should only be handled in designated laboratories. The DHSS regulations under the Medicines Act[4] also require that they be used under the direction of an authorized person and that the doses administered must not exceed the limits laid down by the International Committee on Radiological Protection.[5]

The safe handling of radionuclides by laboratory workers requires knowledge and skill. The possibility of hazard due to radiation from a well-contained external source is negligible in view of the small amounts of isotope used, and the greatest danger is from direct contact, while contamination of apparatus and working area will affect the validity of tests. Working with radionuclides requires the same order of technical competence, experience, discipline and precautions as are used in handling infective materials. To monitor radiation, each designated radiation worker must wear a personal monitor which records the radiation dose it receives. This is usually in the form of a photographic film badge or a thermo-luminescent dosemeter (TLD) badge.* The laboratory should be equipped with a monitoring device to detect contamination in the working area, including sinks and drains. In general, the radioactive waste from isotopes used in haematological diagnostic procedures may be poured down a single designated laboratory sink. It should be washed down with a large quantity of running water. If the waste material exceeds the amount allowed for disposal in this way, it should be stored in a suitable place until its radioactivity has decayed sufficiently for it to be disposed of via the refuse system. All working and storage areas and disposal sinks should be clearly labelled with the internationally recognised trefoil symbol.

Decontamination of working surfaces, walls and floors can usually be achieved by washing with a detergent such as Decon 90 (Decon Laboratories Ltd.). Glassware can be decontaminated by soaking in Decon 90 and plastic laboratory ware by washing in dilute (e.g. 1%) nitric acid. Protective gloves must always be worn when handling isotopes; any activity which does get on to the hands can usually be removed by washing with soap and water, or if that fails, with detergent solution. For each laboratory handling isotopes, a radiological safety officer should be nominated to supervise protection procedures.

SOURCES OF RADIONUCLIDES

The long-lived isotopes which are used for haematological investigations are generally available from commercial suppliers (e.g. Radiochemical Centre, Amersham). Short-lived isotopes with a half life of hours or at most 1–2 days can be produced by a cyclotron, but these expensive units are established in only a few centres. Another way of obtaining certain short-lived isotopes is by means of a radionuclide generator, in which a moderately long-lived parent isotope decays to produce the required short-lived isotope. The parent isotope is

* The National Radiological Protection Board, Harwell, Didcot, provide a film badge service; the TLD system is available from Pitman Instruments, Weybridge, Surrey.

adsorbed on to a support material such as an ion exchange resin, surrounded by an aqueous buffer. The daughter nuclide dissolves in the buffer as it forms, and may be obtained by elution of the generator column. In this way ^{99m}Tc ($T_{1/2}$ 6 h) can be derived from ^{99}Mo ($T_{1/2}$ 66 h); ^{113m}In ($T_{1/2}$ 100 min) from ^{113}Sn ($T_{1/2}$ 120 days).

Radioactive elements are often mixed with a proportion of a non-radioactive but chemically identical element which is known as 'carrier'. The specific activity is a measure of the radioactivity per unit mass of total material. A compound which is carrier-free offers the highest attainable specific activity (sp act). As the isotope decays, its sp act decreases. The dose of isotope which is administered is chosen in order to have sufficient radioactivity for the subsequent sample measurements; it is important to ensure that the concentration of the chemical element is not so great as to be non-physiological or even toxic.

APPARATUS FOR MEASUREMENT OF RADIOACTIVITY

Geiger-Müller counters (GM tubes)

If the electrical field between electrodes is high enough, an electron may be accelerated sufficiently between collisions with gas molecules to acquire enough energy to produce further pairs of ions, and each electron so freed repeats the process. Increasing the voltage intensifies the gas-multiplication process as well as the size of the current pulse. A stage is reached when all the pulses are of the same size, and the output signal is independent of the nature of the energy of the radiation which triggers it. While the avalanche of electrons is close to the anode, the ions which approach the cathode cause the electrical field to be screened and the discharge ceases, or is 'quenched'. The quenching is aided by the addition of an alcohol or formate to the gas (organically-quenched tubes) or by means of a trace of chlorine or bromine (halogen-quenched tubes).

GM counters are used mostly in survey meters for radiation protection. The detector is of an end-window type. The window is a thin layer of mica which is sufficiently thin to permit the passage of α and β particles into the counter. If intended for detecting γ rays the window will be thicker, and made of aluminium or stainless steel, and the inner walls will be coated with lead to induce secondary emission of electrons.

Ionization chambers

A known volume of air or other gas is subjected to irradiation by a radioactive material. Ions produced in the gas are collected on a pair of electrodes and this collection of ions results in the flow of a very small current in an external circuit. This current, which is proportional to the intensity of radiation passing through the chamber, is measured by an electrometer. This type of apparatus is adequate for the measurement of comparatively large quantities of radioactivity (>1 mCi); its main use is for the measurement of the activity of a stock isotope.

Semi-conductor detectors

These are essentially solid state analogs of gas-filled ionization chambers. Germanium and silicon are the usual materials used, sometimes in combination with lithium and, as these are many times more dense than gases, they have much better stopping power and are much more efficient detectors of γ rays. Their main use is for analytic studies on mixtures of different isotopes, as they have narrow spectrum resolution which permits unequivocal identification of each isotope. The system is, however, expensive and germanium detectors require liquid nitrogen cooling.

Scintillation detectors

These are widely used for the detection and measurement of γ radiation. Detection is based on the fact that certain crystals (phosphors) have the property of emitting a flash of light (a scintillation) when energetic photons enter them. The light is detected by the photocathode of a photomultiplier tube which produces a response to this light. The electrons are accelerated towards a series of metal grids ('dynode') each held at a higher positive voltage than the previous dynode. For each electron striking this dynode several electrons are emitted. The number of electrons is progressively increased at each dynode; they accumulate at the

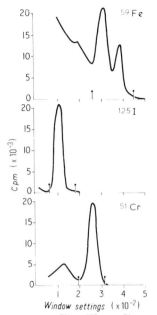

Fig. 17.1 Spectragrams of ^{59}Fe, ^{125}I and ^{51}Cr obtained on a scintillation spectrometer. The gain settings were 6%, 100% and 20%, respectively. These were chosen as they yielded the maximum count-rate at the mid-window settings. These isotopes should be counted with the window set at the limits indicated by the vertical lines.

anode where they constitute a small pulse, the size of which is proportional to the total energy absorbed by the crystal. The pulses are amplified and are counted in a scaler or ratemeter (see below).

The magnitude of the pulses from the scintillation detector is proportional to the energy of the γ rays which give rise to the scintillations. In a gamma-ray spectrometer the pulses are analysed by an analyser with respect to their height (Fig. 17.1). The number of pulses within a selected channel are counted. By selecting a part of the spectrum in which energies produced by other isotopes are either not counted or are minimized, a selected isotope can be counted when present in a mixture. Pulse selection also enables background noise to be minimized in instruments set to count with a high degree of sensitivity. Care must be taken in in vivo counting to exclude components of a spectrum which result from scattered activity arising from activity not within the required field of view.

The most commonly used phosphor for γ ray measurements is a thallium-activated sodium

iodide crystal. They are available in various shapes and sizes. A 'well-type' crystal contains a cavity into which is inserted a small container or test tube holding up to 5 ml of fluid. Another form is a solid circular cylinder, 2.5–10 cm in diameter. In this form it is used for in vivo measurements on patients and occasionally for the measurement of bulky samples, e.g. 24 h urine specimens.

The geometric efficiency of a well-counter depends on the position of the sample in relation to the crystal; thus, it is important to use the same volume for each sample in a series.

Liquid scintillation counters

Low-energy β-emitters can be counted with high efficiency in a liquid scintillator in which the radioactive material is mixed with an organic scintillator in a solvent, and the scintillation activity is then measured between a pair of photomultiplier tubes. The apparatus is usually operated in a refrigerated unit at 4°C to reduce spurious electrical signals. Liquid scintillation solutions have three components:

1. A solvent (e.g. xylene or toluene).
2. A primary solute such as p-terphenyl, 1-phenyl, 4-phenyloxazole (PPO), and various conjugated phenyls.
3. A secondary solute such as 1,4-di-(2-5-phenyloxazole) benzene ('POPOP') which traps the excitation energy from the primary solute, emitting photons of a longer wavelength which are measured more efficiently.

A problem of liquid scintillation which is particularly pertinent to haematological work is that a quenching effect with a decrease in counting efficiency is caused by material which is coloured or contains proteins or insoluble substances. To count such material accurately requires careful preparation and adoption of special procedures to correct for the quenching effect.

Gas-flow counters

The sample is dried on to a planchette which when inserted into the instrument is separated from the detector chamber by a thin membrane. A gas (e.g. helium) flows into the chamber and radiation from the sample is measured by the ionization produced within the gas-filled chamber. This technique is suitable for β-ray emitters (^{3}H, ^{14}C, ^{32}P etc.) and is particularly useful for measuring low activities in preparations which are not suitable for liquid scintillation counting. Unfortunately, these useful counters are being phased out of production.

Measurement of radioactivity in bulky material

By using two end-on crystals in a single counting system, it is possible to measure, with relative precision, the radioactivity in a sample of faeces or an organ without the necessity for homogenization. Similarly, the radioactivity in a large volume of urine or other fluid can be measured without the necessity of concentrating to a smaller volume. The sample is contained in a 450 ml waxed cardboard carton with a screw-top lid, and positioned between two counters, placed above and below it, respectively. It is separated from the lower counter by a plastic ring to ensure that the specimen in the carton is approximately equidistant from both crystals. The counting system is surrounded by lead and the responses of both crystals are counted together. If a single detector system is used it is essential to homogenize the samples.

Another large-volume counting system which is available commercially consists of a counting chamber surrounded by a scintillation fluid and linked to a series of photomultiplier tubes.

Scalers, timers and ratemeters

These instruments record the output signals from radiation detection after pulse height analysis of the signals. A device that only counts pulses is called a *scaler*. An auxiliary device that controls the scaler counting time is called a *timer* and an instrument that incorporates both functions in a single unit is called a *scaler-timer*. Ratemeters record the mean rate of arrival of pulses from the analyzer where extraneous pulses are excluded. A recorder may be fitted in place of the meter, with an inked pointer, tracing a line on to a moving paper chart on which is a calibrated scale. This instrument is useful for observing changes in count rates over periods of time.

Associated with the scaler or ratemeter is a high voltage unit. Its function is to supply the high voltage necessary to operate the radiation detector. In addition, each counter has a pulse amplifier, the function of which is to increase the voltage of the pulse produced to a size suitable for operating the scaler or ratemeter.

Dead-time

After each pulse there is a short period during which the apparatus cannot respond to a further stimulus. This is the 'dead-time', during which any ray entering the counter will not be registered. Dead-time losses also occur in pulse-height analysers and scalers. In modern instruments the dead-time is short (less than 1 μs) and correction is unnecessary in clinical investigations unless the count is more than about $1–3 \times 10^5$/min.

IN VIVO MEASUREMENT OF RADIOACTIVITY

Surface counting

This depends on shielding the crystals by means of a lead collimator to exclude as far as possible the radiation from outside a well defined area of the body.[6] It is thus possible to measure the radioactivity in individual organs. Positioning of the counter in relation to the patient is critical, and if the collimation is sufficiently narrow, it is possible by counting over individual organs to detect sites of concentration of radioactivity. For most purposes a crystal with a diameter of 5–7 cm is suitable, and increased sensitivity, as well as more reliable positioning, can be achieved by using a dual counting system, with two counters positioned in apposition above and below the patient.

Imaging

Radionuclide imaging has become an important application of radioactivity in clinical medicine. Its purpose is to obtain a picture of the distribution of a labelled substance within the body after it has been administered. This requires an isotope which yields γ rays, the energies of which are sufficiently penetrating in body tissues to be detected from deep lying organs. The most efficient method for imaging is by the gamma camera. This consists of a large diameter (25–40 cm) thallium-activated sodium iodide detector crystal, an array of photo-multiplier tubes, standard pulse-height analysers a collimator (usually with multiple parallel holes), a cathode ray tube for image display and a polaroid film recording system.

Scanning camera

The gamma camera will normally visualize a cir-cumscribed area of the body. To obtain a whole-body image on a single sheet of film a modification of the gamma camera, called the scanning camera, is used. The detector passes linearly head to foot over the patient's body, recording and displaying the image on the cathode ray tube. The image moves on the display in synchrony with the move-ment of the detector head, so that the whole-body image is built-up and recorded on one film.

An alternative scanning procedure is the recti-linear scanner. This uses a detector crystal 7.5–12 cm in diameter in a collimated scintillation counter which moves relative to the patient's body. The count distribution is displayed as dots either in black with varied density or as colours determined individually by the count rate, or as an image on X-ray film.

The gamma camera or rectilinear camera can be used not only to obtain the image but also to measure the quantity of the isotope in various parts of the body. This requires calibration of the scan-ner by means of a calibration factor which relates the intensity of the image or the number of dots in the scan of the area to the activity obtained from a phantom containing a known amount of the isotope.[8]

Whole-body counting

It is possible by means of a whole-body counter to measure the fraction of an administered isotope still present in the body with the passing of time. The technique is particularly useful in studying reten-tion and turnover, as it overcomes the problems of collecting and measuring excreta. As the distribu-tion of an isotope in the patient's body may vary during the course of an investigation, it is necessary to use several large crystals encompassing the entire body area and to apply careful calibration proce-dures. Extensive shielding around the detector ('shadow shield') is required to reduce background counts, or if very long-term studies are envisaged, a shielded low background room. Alternatively, a gamma camera can be used as a whole-body counter.[8]

Method of using a scintillation counter

Standardization of working conditions

Three controls require adjustment:

1. High voltage applied to the photomultiplier.
2. Amplifier gain applied to the incoming pulses before they reach the pulse-height analyser.
3. Analyser threshold and window.

The pulse-height analyser threshold and window are arbitrary settings and for simp-lification it is convenient to make the analy-ser setting correspond to the energy of the γ rays. Thus, a threshold scale of 0–100 can be made to correspond to a range of 0–1000 KeV.*

The procedure is as follows: a radionuclide of known γ emission, preferably one with a single energy such as ^{99m}Tc (0.140 MeV) or ^{51}Cr (0.320 MeV) is placed in front of the detector. The high voltage is fixed at a conve-nient level (e.g. 1000 V). The threshold scale is then set to correspond to the photo-peak of the isotope (i.e. the energy at which the max-imum number of pulses in the pulse-height spectrum are emitted) and the window is set at about 10% of the threshold reading. The amplifier gain is varied until the spectro-meter's ratemeter shows a definite peak. It should be established that the peak corre-sponds to the photopeak of the isotope and is not a scattered peak by starting with a high analyzer setting and then gradually reducing it. The settings may be checked by means of another isotope of different energy when the

* eV = electron volt; 1 MeV = 10^3 KeV.

analyser threshold should yield a maximum ratemeter deflection at a scale reading corresponding to the new energy. Examples of spectra and selected settings are illustrated in Fig. 17.1.

The setting of the apparatus, once determined, should remain constant for many months. The sensitivity of the equipment should be checked from time to time using a known standard. Ideally, this should be a sample of the isotope that is being measured; with a short-lived isotope this is not practical, and, instead, an isotope with a low decay rate and comparable emission, e.g. ^{60}Co (5.3 yr half-life), can be used. A further standard of sensitivity is the background itself, as this tends to vary little from day to day.

Counting technique

Standardization of counter

As described above, the counter is set at optimal working conditions for the particular radionuclide to be measured.

Measurement of radioactivity

Measurements are usually carried out for a fixed period of time, the results being recorded as counts per s (cps) or counts per min (cpm). Radioactivity is subject to random but statistically predictable variation. The accuracy of the count depends upon the total number of counts recorded. The SD of a radioactive count $= \sqrt{total count}$ and the CV is is given by

$$\frac{SD}{count} \times 100\%.$$

Thus, on a count of 2500, the CV is 2%; it is 1% on a count of 10 000. Any measured activity represents the difference between the sample count and the background count, in which the errors of both counts are cumulative. Other errors include those related to the calibration of the apparatus and those related to techniques, so that in vivo radioactive measure-

ments rarely have a CV <5% unless the count rate is very high or the counting time unusually prolonged. In practice, a net count of 2500 is adequate for the accuracy required in in vivo clinical studies.

Background counts should be measured alongside that of the radioactive material. If the count rate of the sample is not much above background, then the background should be counted for as long a time as the sample. If the sample count rate is less than the background accurate measurement requires extremely long counting times.

Correction for physical decay

As physical decay is a continuous process which proceeds at an exponential rate and is specific for each particular radionuclide it is possible to correct for the loss of radioactivity with time and so convert any measurement back to that on Day 0. This is necessary when successive observations made at different times after the administration of an isotope to a patient are compared. An alternative method is to prepare a standard from an accurately measured sample of the originally administered material and to compare the measurements at any time with the measurements of the standard at the same time; the loss of radioactivity due to physical decay can then be ignored as both are decaying at identical rates.

Correction for dead-time

With a scintillation counter the dead-time is usually that of the scaler (p. 276). It varies between instruments but is constant for any one instrument and should be provided by the manufacturer. If the count rate is so high that the interval between counts is shorter than the dead-time, some counts will not be recorded. In this case the solution being counted should be diluted or allowed to decay until the count rate decreases to a level where loss due to dead-time becomes negligible.

DOUBLE ISOTOPE MEASUREMENTS

If more than one isotope is present in a sample, it is possible to measure the radioactivity of each isotope separately by one of several techniques:

Mechanical separation

When plasma is labelled with ^{131}I and red cells with ^{51}Cr, the separation of the two components is simple. For example:

(a) counts per ml whole blood
   = activity of ^{131}I + ^{51}Cr per ml of blood;
(b) counts per ml plasma $\times$ (1 − PCV)
   = activity of ^{131}I per ml of blood;
   (a) − (b) = activity of ^{51}Cr per ml of blood.

Differential decay

This is of value especially when one of the isotopes has a very short half-life (e.g. ^{99m}Tc, half-life 6 h). The method is to count the activity in the mixture twice, with the time interval between the counts chosen to allow for the decay of three or more half-lives of the short-lived isotope.

Physical separation

When the two isotopes produce γ rays of widely different energies they can be counted separately at different settings in a γ ray spectrometer, as determined by pulse-height analysis. If there is interference of one isotope by the other because of overlap of the spectra a correction can be applied by establishing a ratio of counts from a standard of the particular isotope measured at the setting for that isotope and at the setting for the other isotope. For example, to separate ^{99m}Tc and ^{51}Cr in a mixture, a ^{51}Cr source is counted in window 1 (optimal for Tc) and window 2 (optimal for Cr). The ^{51}Cr ratio (R) is calculated as counts of ^{51}Cr source in window 1 divided by counts of ^{51}Cr source in window 2. Then, when the mixture is measured, the counts due to ^{51}Cr interference in window 1 (N_1) = R $\times$ ^{51}Cr counts in window 2, and the true ^{99m}Tc count in window 1 = total count in window 1 − N_1 ^{51}Cr.

REFERENCES

[1] Bowring, C. S. (1981). *Radionuclide Tracer Techniques in Haematology*. Butterworth, London.

[2] *Code of Practice for the Protection of Persons exposed to Ionising Radiations in Research and Teaching* (1968). HMSO, London.

[3] *Code of Practice for the Protection of Persons against Ionising Radiations arising from Medical and Dental Use* (1975). HMSO, London.

[4] Department of health and social security (1979). Health Service Management: Administration of Radioactive Substances to Persons HC(79)17. DHSS, London.

[5] International commission on radiological protection (1977). Recommendations of the ICRP. A Summary (Publication No. 26). Pergamon, Oxford.

[6] International committee for standardization in haematology (1975). Recommended methods for surface counting to determine sites of red-cell destruction. *British Journal of Haematology*, **30**, 249.

[7] Lewis S. M. (ed.) (1977). Radioisotopes in Haematology. *Clinics in Haematology*, **6**, 541.

[8] Short, M. D., Richards, A. R. and Glass, H. I. (1972). The use of a gamma camera as a whole-body counter. *British Journal of Radiology*, **45**, 289.

[9] Sorenson, J. A. and Phelps, M. E. (1980). *Physics in Nuclear Medicine*. Grune and Stratton, New York.

18

Blood volume

The Hb content, total red-cell count and PCV do not invariably reflect the total red-cell volume. Whilst in most cases there is a good correlation between peripheral-blood values and (total) red-cell volume,[2] there will be a discrepancy if the plasma volume is reduced or increased disproportionately. Some of the causes and the variations are given in Table 18.1.

It may therefore be necessary in some instances to measure separately the component parts of the

Table 18.1 Clinical effect of variable relationship between red-cell volume and plasma volume

Red-cell volume	Plasma volume	Cause	Effect
Normal* (or low)	High	Pregnancy Cirrhosis Nephritis Congestive cardiac failure Myelomatosis Macroglobulinaemia	Pseudo-anaemia or anaemia less severe than indicated by red-cell count
Normal	Low	Stress Peripheral circulatory failure Essential hypertension Diuretic drugs Dehydration Oedema Prolonged bed rest High altitude (1st 2 weeks)	Pseudo-polycythaemia
Low	Normal	Anaemia	Accurate reflection of degree of anaemia
Low	High	Anaemia	Anaemia less severe than indicated by red-cell count
Low	Low	Haemorrhage Severe anaemia (when PCV below 0.2)	Anaemia more severe than indicated by red-cell count
High	Normal to low	Polycythaemia	Accurate reflection of polycythaemia or polycythaemia less severe than apparent
High	High	Polycythaemia	Polycythaemia more severe than apparent
Normal (or even high)	High	Marked splenomegaly	Pseudo-anaemia

* Some of the conditions listed may also cause true anaemia.

total blood volume, i.e. the red-cell volume and plasma volume. This is particularly important (a) in polycythaemia, when the demonstration of an absolute increase in red-cell volume is necessary for the diagnosis to be made and for the assessment of severity, and (b) in the elucidation of obscure anaemias when the possibility of an increase in plasma volume cannot be excluded.

METHODS OF MEASUREMENT OF BLOOD VOLUME

Principle. A small volume of a readily identifiable material is injected intravenously and its dilution is measured after time has been allowed for the injected material to become thoroughly mixed in the circulation, but before significant quantities have left the circulation. Formerly, Evans blue dye was commonly used as the marker. It is still used occasionally and the method is described in detail by Mollison.[19b] However, the most practical method now available is to use a small volume of the patient's red cellls labelled with radioactive chromium (^{51}Cr), technetium (pertechnetate) (^{99m}Tc) or indium ([113m]In). The labelled red cells are diluted in the whole blood of the patient and from their dilution the total blood volume and the red-cell volume can be calculated from knowledge of the PCV. The plasma volume can be measured directly by injecting human albumin labelled with radioactive iodine (^{125}I or ^{131}I): the albumin is diluted in the plasma compartment only and thus gives values for plasma volume only.

In contrast to measurement of red-cell volume, plasma-volume measurements are often only approximations as the plasma volume is capable of rapid fluctuation. The labelled albumin, too, not only undergoes continuous slow interchange between the plasma and extracellular fluids, but part of it also probably exchanges with a small rapidly exchanging pool, even during the mixing period. For these reasons it is undesirable to attempt to calculate red-cell volume from plasma volume, on the basis of the observed PCV. The reverse calculation of total blood volume from red-cell volume is more reliable, provided that the difference between whole body and venous PCV is appreciated and allowed for (see p. 285). Measurement of red-cell and plasma volumes by direct methods gives the most reliable calculation of total blood volume.

The subject of blood volume and its measurement has a large literature. Much information is to be found in the reviews of Mollison,[19a] Mayerson[17] and Najean and Cacchione[23] and in the recommendations on standard techniques of the International Committee for Standardization in Haematology.[14]

DETERMINATION OF RED-CELL VOLUME

Radioactive chromium method

Add approximately 10 ml of blood to 1.5 ml of sterile NIH-A acid-citrate dextrose (ACD) solution (see p. 432), in a 30 ml bottle with a screw cap. Centrifuge at 1200–1500 *g* for 5 min. Discard the supernatant plasma and buffy coat and slowly add to the cells, with continuous mixing, 0.1–0.2 μCi of $Na_2{}^{51}CrO_4$* per kg of body weight. The sodium chromate should be in a volume of at least 0.2 ml, being diluted in 9 g/l NaCl (saline). Allow the blood to stand for 15 min at 37°C for labelling to take place. Wash the red cells twice in 4–5 volumes of sterile saline[†]. Finally, resuspend the cells in a volume of sterile saline sufficient for an injection of about 10 ml and the preparation of a standard. Take up the appropriate volume to the mark in a precalibrated syringe or into a syringe which is weighed before and after the injection. In the latter case the volume

* Available in concentration of 1 mCi/ml, specific activity 100–350 μCi/μg Cr (Radiochemical Centre, Amersham).
[†] 12 g/l NaCl should be used when red-cell osmotic fragility is greatly increased, e.g. in cases of hereditary spherocytosis.

injected is calculated from the following formula:

volume injected (ml)

$$= \frac{\text{weight of suspension injected (g)}}{\text{density of suspension (g/ml)}}$$

where density of suspension =

$$1.000 + \frac{\text{Hb conc. of suspension (g/l)} \times 0.097}{340}$$

(This assumes that packed red cells have a MCHC of 340 g/l and a density of 1.097.)

The accurate and aseptic filling of the syringe and exclusion of air bubbles are facilitated by drawing up the solution beyond the required volume and then returning the excess to the original bottle by means of a U-shaped needle or a length of plastic tubing attached to the nozzle of the syringe.

Inject the suspension intravenously without delay and note the time. 10 and 20 min later, collect 5–10 ml of the patient's blood and add it to the appropriate amount of a solid anticoagulant (e.g. EDTA). This blood should preferably be withdrawn from a vein other than that used for the injection. However, it is often convenient to insert a self-retaining (e.g. butterfly) needle; in this case care must be taken to ensure that the isotope is well dispersed into the blood stream when injected by flushing through with 10 ml of sterile saline. When the mixing time is likely to be prolonged as in splenomegaly,[33] cardiac failure[28] or shock,[24] another sample should be taken 60 min after the injection.

Measure the PCV of each sample and lyse the remainder with saponin. Deliver known volumes (2 or 3 ml) into counting tubes and measure their radioactivity in a scintillation counter. Then dilute the residue of the original suspension which was not injected 1 in 100 in 0.4 g/l ammonia (for use as a standard) and determine the radioactivity of a 2 or 3 ml volume. Then red-cell volume (RCV) (ml) =

$$\frac{\begin{array}{c}\text{radioactivity of standard (cpm/ml)}\\ \times \text{diln. of standard}\\ \times \text{volume injected (ml)}\end{array}}{\begin{array}{c}\text{radioactivity of post-injection}\\ \text{sample (cpm/ml)}\end{array}} \times \text{PCV*.}$$

The total blood volume (BV) can be calculated by multiplying the value for RCV by 1/(whole-body PCV) (see p. 285). Plasma volume can be calculated by subtracting RCV from BV.

If a sample has been taken at 60 min in cases where delayed mixing is suspected and there is a significant difference between the measurements at 10–20 and 60 min, the 60 min measurement should be used for calculating the red-cell volume.

Technetium method[15]

Deliver approximately 10 ml of blood into a sterile container to which has been added 200 iu of liquid heparin. Place 20 ml of 9 g/l NaCl (saline) into another container and add to it exactly 5 ml of this blood. Centrifuge and remove as much of the supernatant as possible.

In advance of the test weigh out 2 mg of stannous chloride ($SnCl_2.2H_2O$). Dissolve in 20 ml of saline. Pass this solution through a micropore filter (0.22 μm) into a sterile container. With a 1 ml (tuberculin-type) syringe, transfer 0.2 ml into 100 ml of sterile saline. With a 1 ml syringe withdraw 0.3 ml and add this to the packed red cells ($\equiv 10 \pm 5$ μg stannous ions per ml red cells). The time between dissolving the stannous chloride and adding it to the blood must not exceed 10 min. Allow to stand for 5 min at room temperature. Then add 50 μCi of freshly generated ^{99m}Tc in approximately 0.2 ml of saline. Allow to stand at room temperature for 5 min. Centrifuge; wash once in cold sterile saline and resuspend in a sufficient volume of cold sterile

---

* As measured by an electronic counting system or corrected for trapped plasma (see p. 34).

saline for an injection of 10 ml and preparation of a standard. Reinject and carry out subsequent procedures as for the chromium method. Because of the short half-life of ^{99m}Tc, radioactivity must be measured on the day of the test. Because up to 5% of the radioactivity is eluted from the red cells within 1 h, the method is less suitable than the chromium method when there is splenomegaly or another cause of delayed mixing is suspected. If technetium is used in such cases, specimens should be collected at 10 and 30 min. If there is a significant difference between these measurements, the 30 min measurement is likely to be more reliable, and this should be used for calculating the red-cell volume.

An alternative method of labelling red cells with technetium is to give the patient a preliminary intravenous injection of 'Pyrolite'*, a mixture of sodium pyrophosphate, sodium trimetaphosphate and stannous chloride. Dissolve a vial of Pyrolite in 8 ml of sterile saline and inject 3.7 ml intravenously. After 15 min, collect 10 ml of blood and centrifuge to remove the plasma. Add 50 μCi of freshly generated ^{99m}Tc to the packed cells and roller mix for 5 min. Then wash the cells once in cold sterile saline, resuspend in c 12 ml of cold sterile saline and reinject. Carry out subsequent procedures, as described above.

Indium method

Indium is available as ^{111}In chloride or it can be produced as ^{113m}In in a generator by elution of ^{113}Sn with HCl. For labelling blood cells, the indium is complexed with oxine[38] or acetylacetone.[30] The latter complex is easier to prepare.

1. Preparation of oxine complex

Dissolve 50 μg of 8-hydroxyquinolone in 50 μl of ethanol and add to approximately 1 mCi of ^{111}In chloride in 0.05 mol/l HCl. After 1 min

* Available in a sterile kit from New England Nuclear.

add 200 μl of sodium acetate buffer, pH 5.0. Add 2 ml of chloroform. Mix briefly in a vortex mixer. Evaporate to dryness on a hot plate. Then dissolve the residue in 100 μl of ethanol. Again evaporate to dryness to remove traces of chloroform and redissolve in 50 μl of ethanol. Immediately before use, dilute with 100 μl of 9 g/l NaCl (saline). Take approximately 5 ml of blood into a sterile container containing 100 iu of heparin. Wash once with sterile saline and add the In-oxine to the packed cells. Allow to stand for 5 min; then wash with saline. Resuspend in a sufficient volume of saline for an injection of 10 ml and preparation of a standard.

2. Preparation of acetylacetone complex

Take approximately 5 ml of blood into a sterile container containing 100 iu of liquid heparin. Wash once in sterile saline. To the packed cells, add 10 ml of 1.9 g/l acetylacetone (Sigma or E. Merck) in HEPES or tris buffer, pH 7.6 (p. 436). The acetylacetone should be stored at 4°C but brought to room temperature before use. Mix gently for 1 min, then add 50–100 μCi of freshly generated ^{113m}In. Mix on a roller mixer for 5 min, then wash once in saline. Resuspend in a sufficient volume of saline for an injection of 10 ml and preparation of a standard.

Repeated blood-volume measurements

When repeated blood-volume measurements are required, the ^{51}Cr method can be used if the residual radioactivity is measured in the blood immediately before each test. However, the residual radioactivity increases the counting error and it may be necessary to increase the amount of tracer injected. The short-lived isotopes (^{99m}Tc, ^{111}In) have the advantage that they can be used for repeated tests without this problem and also that the patient will be subjected to lower doses of radioactivity. The isotopes are slowly eluted in vivo and in vitro. With ^{99m}Tc elution is slight within the first 10–20 minutes; it gives results which compare closely with those of ^{51}Cr but the method is less satisfactory when delayed mixing necessitates sampling at 60 min post-injection.

The labelling procedure using indium is much simpler than with technetium and, as elution is less than with ^{99m}Tc during the first hour, it is particularly suitable for delayed sampling.[27]

Determination of plasma volume

^{125}I- or ^{131}I-human serum albumin (HSA) method[14]

Human albumin labelled with ^{125}I or ^{131}I is available commercially*. The albumin concentration should not be less than 20 g/l. To guard against the risk of serum hepatitis, the user must be reassured that only Australia-antigen-negative donors are used as the source of the albumin. ^{125}I has the advantage that it is readily distinguished from ^{51}Cr, ^{99m}Tc and ^{113m}In, and this makes possible the simultaneous direct determination of red-cell volume and plasma volume (see below).

Take up c 20 ml of blood into a syringe containing a few drops of sterile heparin solution and transfer to a 30 ml sterile bottle with a screw cap. After centrifuging at 1200–1500 g for 5–10 min, transfer c 7 ml of plasma to a second sterile bottle and add 0.05 μCi of the isotope-labelled HSA per kg body weight. Inject a measured amount (e.g. 5 ml) and retain the residue for preparation of a standard.

^{125}I-HSA is also available commercially, pre-packed in 1 ml volumes containing 3–5 μCi. The contents of an ampoule can be injected intravenously and a similar ampoule should then be used to prepare a standard. After 10, 20, and 30 min, withdraw blood samples from a vein other than that used for the original injection (or after flushing through with 10 ml of sterile 9 g/l NaCl (saline) if a butterfly needle has been used) and deliver into bottles containing EDTA or heparin.

Measure the PCV, centrifuge the sample and separate the plasma. Prepare a standard

by diluting part of the residue of the uninjected HSA 1 in 100 in saline.

Measure the radioactivity of the plasma samples in a scintillation counter, and by extrapolation on semilogarithmic graph paper calculate the radioactivity of the plasma at zero time. If only a single sample is collected 10 min after the injection, the radioactivity at zero time may be obtained approximately by multiplying by 1.015. Reliance on a single 10 min sample will lead to error if the mixing of the albumin in the plasma is delayed. After measuring the radioactivity of the standard, the plasma volume (ml) is calculated as follows:

$$\frac{\begin{array}{c}\text{radioactivity of standard (cpm/ml)}\\ \times \text{ diln. of standard}\\ \times \text{ volume injected (ml)}\end{array}}{\begin{array}{c}\text{radioactivity of post-injection sample}\\ \text{(cpm/ml, adjusted to zero time).}\end{array}}$$

Other isotope methods for determination of plasma volume

Trivalent ^{51}CrCl$_3$ has been used[8,31] but this does not appear to offer any advantage over ^{125}I- or ^{131}I-HSA. ^{132}I has the very short half-life of 2.26 h and, like ^{131}I and ^{125}I, it can be combined with human serum albumin[35], but the advantage of the isotope—its short half-life—is outweighed by the necessity of labelling the albumin shortly before it is used. ^{99m}Tc has also been used in combination with human serum albumin[4] and ^{113m}In with transferrin.[37]

DETERMINATION OF TOTAL BLOOD VOLUME

As has already been indicated, the total blood volume is frequently calculated from the red-cell volume and PCV. But before this can be done the observed PCV has to be corrected for the difference between the whole-body and venous PCV. The reason for this difference is described below.

* ^{125}I-HSA at 50 μCi/ml, sp activity 2.5 μCi/mg albumin; ^{131}I-HSA at 0.4–1.5 mCi/ml, sp activity 20–80 μCi/mg (Radiochemical Centre, Amersham).

Whole-body and venous PCV ratio

It is well known that the PCV measured on venous blood is not identical with the average PCV of all the blood in the body. This is mainly because the red-cell:plasma ratio is less in small blood vessels (capillaries, arterioles and venules) than in large vessels. The ratio between the whole-body PCV and venous-blood PCV is normally about 0.9,[14] and it is thus necessary in the calculation of total blood volume from measurements of red-cell volume to multiply the observed PCV by 0.9. Thus total blood volume is given by:

$$\text{red cell volume} \times \frac{1}{\text{PCV} \times 0.9}.$$

Unfortunately, the ratio varies from 0.85 to 0.95 in normal subjects[3] and may fall outside this range in some pathological states. Thus, the ratio is often notably raised in splenomegaly[9,11] because of the increased volume of splenic blood of relatively high PCV, while in oedema or cardiac failure it may be lower than normal.[9,19c] The ratio is increased in pregnancy[5] and at high altitudes.[18] In such cases it is better to estimate red-cell volume and plasma volume by separate measurements rather than to attempt to calculate one of these from an estimate of the other. Nevertheless, in many diseases the ratio is not far from 0.9 and total blood volumes can be calculated from red-cell volume measurements with reasonable accuracy.

Simultaneous measurement of red-cell volume and plasma volume

Add c 14 ml of blood to 2 ml of ACD. Centrifuge at 1200–1500 **g** for 5 min. Discard the plasma and buffy coat. Label the red cells with ^{51}Cr, ^{99m}Tc or ^{113}In (see p. 281), wash twice in 9 g/l NaCl (saline) and resuspend to a volume of approximately 12 ml. Add ^{125}I-HSA (see p. 284) and mix it with the red-cell suspension. Inject an accurately measured amount and dilute the remainder 1 in 100 in 0.4 g/l ammonia for use as a standard. Collect three blood samples at 10, 20 and 30 min, respectively, after the administration of the labelled blood and estimate the radioactivity of a measured volume of each sample and a similar volume of the standard.

When ^{99m}Tc or ^{113m}In has been used, count on the same day; then leave for 2 days to allow that isotope to decay and count again for the ^{125}I activity. Subtract the ^{125}I counts (corrected for decay) from the original counts to obtain a measurement of the counts due to the ^{99m}Tc or ^{113m}In.

When ^{51}Cr has been used in combination with ^{125}I, and a multi-channel counter is available, measure the radioactivity due to the ^{51}Cr and ^{125}I at the appropriate settings for ^{51}Cr and ^{125}I. Whereas the ^{51}Cr counts are obtained free from ^{125}I counts, some ^{51}Cr radioactivity will be counted in the ^{125}I channel. A correction factor for this can be calculated by measuring a standard of ^{51}Cr in the ^{125}I channel.

Calculate the radioactivity due to ^{51}Cr, ^{99m}Tc or ^{113m}In in the blood from the mean of the three samples; obtain that due to ^{125}I from the value extrapolated to zero time. Calculate red-cell volume as described on p. 282.

Plasma volume is calculated from the formula:

$$\frac{\begin{array}{c}\text{radioactivity of standard (cpm/ml)} \\ \times \text{ dilution of standard} \\ \times \text{ volume* injected (ml)}\end{array}}{\begin{array}{c}\text{radioactivity of post-injection} \\ \text{sample (cpm/ml, corrected} \\ \text{to zero time)}\end{array}} \times (1 - \text{PCV}).$$

Total blood volume = red-cell volume
+ plasma volume.

EXPRESSION OF RESULTS OF BLOOD-VOLUME ESTIMATIONS

Red-cell volume, plasma volume and total blood volume are usually expressed in ml/kg of body weight. Because fat is relatively avascular, low values are obtained in obese subjects and the

* See p. 282.

relation between blood volume and body weight varies according to body composition. Blood volume is more closely correlated with lean body mass[13,21] but the determination of lean body mass is not practical as a routine procedure.

An alternative is to discount excess fat by using an estimate of so-called 'ideal weight' from a formula, i.e. weight in kg = height in cm − 100, or to refer to standard tables which are based on height, age, build and sex.[6] These methods are somewhat arbitrary and tend to overcorrect for the avascularity of fat.

More complicated formulae have been proposed for predicting the normal blood volume.[12,22,29,36] These are slightly more reliable than those based on weight alone. The table given by Hurley[12] which relates both red-cell and plasma volume to surface area is derived from a relatively large series of measurements; even so, the 95% confidence limits for the volumes at different surface areas include a range of at least ±10% of the mean values given.

Range in health

Red-cell volume: men, 30 ml/kg (2SD 5 ml); women, 25 ml/kg (2SD 5 ml).
Plasma volume: men and women, 40–50 ml/kg.
Total blood volume: men and women, 60–80 ml/kg.

In newborn infants, at comparable levels of PCV, the red-cell volume and plasma volume are the same, relative to body weight, as in adults.[20] The total blood volume is thus *c* 250–350 ml at birth. After infancy the volume increases gradually until adult life. As a rule, the blood volume remains remarkably constant in an individual and rapid adjustments take place within a few hours after blood transfusion or intravenous infusion.

In pregnancy both the plasma volume and total blood volume increases. The plasma volume increases especially in the first trimester, the total volume later,[16] and by full term the plasma volume has increased by *c* 40% and total volume by 32% or more. The blood volume returns to normal within a week post partum.

Bed rest causes a reduction in plasma volume[32], and muscular exercise and changes in posture cause transient fluctuations. In practice, the patient should always be allowed to rest in a recumbent position for 15 min prior to measuring the blood volume.

SPLENIC RED-CELL VOLUME

The red-cell content of the normal spleen is less than 5% of the total red-cell volume (i.e. <70 ml in an adult). In splenomegaly the red-cell 'pool' is increased, e.g. by as much as 5–10 times in myelofibrosis, polycythaemia, hairy cell leukaemia and lympho-proliferative disorders.[25] Increase in the volume of the splenic red-cell pool may by itself be a cause of anaemia; measurement of the pool is thus useful in the investigation of the anaemia which occurs in these conditions. It is also useful in determining the cause of erythrocytosis, as the increased pool in polycythaemia vera contrasts with secondary polycythaemia in which it is normal.[1]

An approximate estimate of the splenic red-cell volume can be obtained from the difference between the apparent red-cell volume, as measured immediately after the injection of isotope-labelled cells, and that measured after mixing has been completed, i.e. after a delay of *c* 20 min,[26] or from the difference in surface counts over the spleen before and after mixing has been completed.[34] The splenic red-cell volume can be estimated more accurately by quantitative scanning, after injecting viable red cells labelled with ^{99m}Tc or ^{113m}In[10] (p. 276). The blood volume is measured in the usual way using 2–4 mCi of ^{99m}Tc or 1 mCi of ^{113m}I. The splenic area is scanned 20 min after the injection. To delineate the spleen more precisely, it may be necessary to carry out a second scan after an injection of heat-damaged labelled red cells (see p. 308). From the radioactivity in the spleen, relative to that in a standard, and knowledge of the total red-cell volume, the proportion of the total red-cell volume contained in the spleen can be calculated.

REFERENCES

[1] BATEMAN, S., LEWIS, S. M., NICHOLAS, A. and ZAAFRAN, A. (1978). Splenic red cell pooling: a diagnostic feature in polycythaemia. *British Journal of Haematology*, **40**, 389.
[2] BENTLEY, S. A. and LEWIS, S. M. (1976). The relationship between total red cell volume, plasma volume and venous haematocrit. *British Journal of Haematology*, **33**, 301.
[3] BROZOVIC, B., KORUBIN, V., LEWIS, S. M. and SZUR, L. (1966). Simultaneous red cell and plasma volume

determinations by a differential absorption method. *Journal of Laboratory and Clinical Medicine*, **68**, 142.

4 CALLAHAN, R. J., MCKUSICK, K. A., LAMSON, M., CASTRONOVO, F. P. and POTSAID, M. S. (1976). Technetium-99m-human serum albumin: evaluation of a commercially produced kit. *Journal of Nuclear Medicine*, **17**, 47.

5 CATION, W. L., ROBY, C. C., REID, D. E., CASEWELL, R., MALETSKOS, C. J., FLUMARTY, R. G. and GIBSON, J. G. (1951). The circulating red cell volume and body hematocrit in normal pregnancy and the puerperium by direct measurement using radioactive red cells. *American Journal of Obstetrics and Gynecology*, **61**, 1207.

6 Documenta Geigy (1970). *Scientific Tables* 7th edn., p. 712. J. R. Geigy, Basel.

7 FERRANT, A., LEWIS, S. M. and SZUR, L. (1974). The elution of ^{99m}Tc from red cells and its effect on red cell volume measurement. *Journal of Clinical Pathology*, **27**, 983.

8 FRANK, H. and GRAY, S. J. (1953). The determination of plasma volume in man with radioactive chromic chloride. *Journal of Clinical Investigation*, **32**, 991.

9 FUDENBERG, H., BALDINI, M., MAHONEY, J. P. and DAMESHEK, W. (1961). The body hematocrit/venous hematocrit ratio and the 'splenic reservoir'. *Blood*, **17**, 71.

10 HEGDE, U. M., WILLIAMS, E. D., LEWIS, S. M., SZUR, L., GLASS, H. I. and PETTIT, J. E. (1973). Measurement of splenic red cell volume and visualization of the spleen with ^{99m}Tc. *Journal of Nuclear Medicine*, **14**, 769.

11 HUBER, H., LEWIS, S. M. and SZUR, L. (1964). The influence of anaemia, polycythaemia and splenomegaly on the relationship between venous haematocrit and red-cell volume. *British Journal of Haematology*, **10**, 567.

12 HURLEY, P. J. (1975). Red cell and plasma volumes in normal adults. *Journal of Nuclear Medicine*, **16**, 46.

13 HUFF, R. L. and FELLER, D. D. (1956). Relation of circulating red cell volume to body density and obesity. *Journal of Clinical Investigation*, **35**, 1.

14 International committee for standardization in haematology (1980). Recommended methods for measurement of red-cell and plasma volume. *Journal of Nuclear Medicine*, **21**, 793.

15 JONES, J. and MOLLISON, P. L. (1978). Simple and efficient method of labelling red cells with ^{99m}Tc for determination of red cell volume. *British Journal of Haematology*, **38**, 141.

16 LUND, C. J. and SISSON, T. R. C. (1958). Blood volume and anemia of mother and baby. *American Journal of Obstetrics and Gynecology*, **76**, 1013.

17 MAYERSON, H. S. (1965). Blood volume and its regulation. *Annual Review of Physiology*, **27**, 307.

18 METZ, J., LEVIN, N. W. and HART, D. (1962). Effect of altitude on the body/venous haematocrit ratio. *Nature (London)*, **194**, 483.

19 MOLLISON, P. L. (1979). *Blood Transfusion in Clinical Medicine*, 6th edn., (a) p. 114, (b) p. 121, (c) p. 134. Blackwell Scientific Publications, Oxford.

20 MOLLISON, P. L., VEALL, N. and CUTBUSH, M. (1950). Red cell and plasma volume in newborn infants. *Archives of Disease in Childhood*, **25**, 242.

21 MULDOWNEY, F. P. (1957). The relationship of total red cell mass to lean body mass in man. *Clinical Science*, **16**, 163.

22 NADLER, S. B., HIDALGO, J. U. and BLOCH, T. (1962).

Prediction of blood volume in normal human adults. *Surgery*, **51**, 224.

23 NAJEAN, Y. and CACCHIONE, R. (1977). Blood volume in health and disease. *Clinics in Haematology*, **6**, 543.

24 NOBLE, R. P. and GREGERSEN, M. I. (1946). Blood volume in clinical shock. I. Mixing time and disappearance rate of T-1824 in normal subjects and in patients in shock; determination of plasma volume in man from 10-minute sample. *Journal of Clinical Investigation*, **25**, 158.

25 PETTIT, J. (1977). Spleen function. *Clinics in Haematology*, **6**, 639.

26 PRYOR, D. S. (1967). The mechanism of anaemia in tropical splenomegaly. *Quarterly Journal of Medicine*, **36**, 337.

27 RADIA, R., PETERS, A. M., DEENMAMODE, M., FITZPATRICK, M. L. and LEWIS, S. M. (1981). Measurement of red cell volume and splenic red cell pool using ^{113m}Indium. *British Journal of Haematology*, **49**, 587.

28 REILLY, W. A., FRENCH, R. M., LAU, F. Y. K., SCOTT, K. G. and WHITE, W. E. (1954). Whole blood volume determined by radiochromium-tagged red cells: comparative studies on normal and congestive heart failure patients. *Circulation*, **9**, 571.

29 RETZLAFF, J. A., TAUXE, W. N., KIELEY, J. M. and STROEBEL, C. F. (1969). Erythrocyte volume, plasma volume and lean body mass in adult men and women. *Blood*, **33**, 649.

30 SINN, H. and SILVESTER, D. J. (1979). Simplified cell labelling with indium-111-acetylacetone. *British Journal of Radiology*, **52**, 758.

31 SMALL, W. J., and VERLOOP, M. C. (1956). Determination of the blood volume using radioactive ^{51}Cr: modifications of the original technique. *Journal of Laboratory and Clinical Medicine*, **47**, 255.

32 TAYLOR, H. L., ERICKSON, L., HENSCHEL, A. and KEYS, A. (1945). The effect of bed rest on the blood volume of normal young men. *American Journal of Physiology*, **144**, 227.

33 TIZIANELLO, A. and PANNACCIULLI, I. (1959). The effect of splenomegaly on dilution curves of tagged erythrocytes and red blood cell volume. *Acta Haematologica (Basel)*, **21**, 346.

34 TOGHILL, P. J. (1964). Red-cell pooling in enlarged spleens. *British Journal of Haematology*, **10**, 347.

35 VEALL, N., PEARSON, J. D. and HANLEY, T. (1955). The preparation of ^{132}I and ^{131}I labelled human serum albumin for clinical tracer studies. *British Journal of Radiology*, **28**, 633.

36 WENNESLAND, R., BROWN, E., HOPPER, J. Jnr, HODGES, J. L. Jnr, GUTTENTAG, O. E., SCOTT, K. G., TUCKER, I. N. and BRADLEY, B. (1959). Red cell, plasma and blood volume in healthy men measured by radiochromium (^{51}Cr) cell tagging and hematocrit: influence of age, somatotype and habits of physical activity on the variance after regression of volumes to height and weight combined. *Journal of Clinical Investigation*, **38**, 1065.

37 WOCHNER, R. D., ADATEPE, M., van AMBURG, A. and POTCHEN, E. J. (1970). New method for estimation of plasma volume with the use of the distribution space of transferrin-113m indium. *Journal of Laboratory and Clinical Medicine*, **75**, 711.

38 WISTOW, B. W., GROSSMAN, Z. D., McAFEE, J. G., SUBRAMANIAN, G., HENDERSON, R. W. and ROSKOPF, M. L. (1978). Labelling of platelets with oxine complexes of Tc-99m and In-111. Part 1. In vitro studies and survival in the rabbit. *Journal of Nuclear Medicine*, **19**, 483.

19

Erythrokinetics

Although much can be learnt about the rate and efficiency of erythropoiesis from the red-cell count, blood film and bone marrow, radioactive isotopes* of iron may sometimes provide useful additional data. In much the same way, whereas increased haemolysis can be suspected from the peripheral-blood film and bone marrow, techniques are available which permit the measurement of red-cell life-span with a considerable degree of accuracy. An indirect assessment can be obtained from measurements of Hb catabolism: namely from the bilirubin turnover, the daily faecal urobilinogen (a rough estimate); from the excretion of carbon monoxide; [8,22,43] or (experimentally) using ^{15}N-glycine to label haem. More directly, red-cell life-span can be estimated by the differential-agglutination method of Ashby (now seldom used) or by tagging the red cells with radioactive sodium chromate (^{51}Cr) or radioactive di-*iso*propyl phosphofluoridate (DF^{32}P). The ^{51}Cr method is a practical technique of wide application.

The measurement of products of Hb catabolism includes those derived from erythroblasts which are destroyed in the bone marrow. Thus, major discrepancies are found between the results obtained from ^{51}Cr red-cell life-span estimations and catabolism estimations when there is marked ineffective erythropoiesis.

USE OF RADIOACTIVE IRON

^{59}Fe

This isotope has a moderately short half-life, 45 days, and labels Hb after ingestion or injection. If injected intravenously, it labels, too, the plasma iron pool and this allows measurement of iron clearance and the calculation of plasma-iron turnover. Its subsequent appearance in Hb permits the assessment of the rate of Hb synthesis and of the completeness of the utilization of iron. Being a γ-ray emitter, radioactivity can be measured in vivo by surface counting, and the sites of distribution of the administered iron and the probable sites of erythropoiesis can thus be determined.

^{52}Fe

This isotope has a very short half-life, 8.2 h, and this has advantages as well as disadvantages. Because of its very short half-life, it cannot be kept in stock, and has to be freshly prepared for each individual patient. On the other hand, it can be administered successively, if required, at short intervals, and, because of its physical characteristics and the fact that it can be given in a relatively large dose, it can be used for identifying the sites and rate of the absorption of iron in the intestine[25] and for tracing the extent of active marrow in the bones and elsewhere,[28,54] neither of which can be satisfactorily accomplished using ^{59}Fe in permissible dosages. However, its very short half-life prevents it from being used to study the utilization of iron by red cells (see below).

^{55}Fe

The long half-life (2.6 yr) of this isotope makes it unsuitable for use in studies in man because of the radiation hazard. It has, nevertheless, been used in double-isotope investigations, e.g. for measuring iron absorption.[12c] It occurs in a small amount as a contaminant in the production of ^{52}Fe. This can be

* or 'radionuclides' see p. 271.

turned to an advantage as it can be used to study the utilization of iron by red cells after the administration of ^{52}Fe.[48] However, specialized equipment and complex preparation of the samples are required.

ESTIMATION OF IRON ABSORPTION

Principle. A small amount of labelled inorganic iron is administered by mouth and the amount of radioactivity eliminated in the faeces subsequently is measured. The difference between the radioactivity administered and that excreted is taken as the amount absorbed. Alternatively, the absorption of iron can be estimated by measuring whole-body radioactivity before and after ingestion of the iron and its elimination in the faeces, using a whole-body counter.[12c]

Method using inorganic iron

Prepare the test dose no longer than 30 min prior to administration. To 15 mg of iron sulphate ($FeSO_4.7H_2O$) add 18 mg of ascorbic acid in a beaker containing 10 ml of 0.001 mol/l HCl. Add 2 μCi of ^{59}Fe in the form of ferric chloride in 0.01 mol/l HCl (sp activity 2 μCi/μg). Make up the solution to c 25 ml with water. Keep 1 ml as a standard. Measure an exact volume of the remainder. The patient takes this by mouth, in the early morning after an overnight fast, and is not allowed to eat for a further 3 h. The faeces passed during the following 5–7 days (see below) are collected in plastic or cardboard cartons.

Count each sample in a large-volume scintillation counter against the standard (1 ml) after diluting it in approximately 100 ml of water in a similar carton.

Calculation

% excreted

$$= \frac{\text{cpm/ml of sample}}{\text{cpm/ml of standard} \times \text{volume administered (ml)}} \times 100.$$

Stool collections are continued until <1% of the administered dose is excreted in a 24 h collection. If a whole-body counter is used, measurements should be continued for about 1 week. Then:

$$\% \text{ excreted} = \frac{\text{cpm after 7–10 days}}{\text{original cpm after dose}} \times 100.$$

$$\% \text{ absorbed} = 100 - \text{total } \% \text{ excreted}.$$

Interpretation of results

Iron absorption is a complex process (for reviews see Bothwell et al,[12a] Cook and Lipschitz[18]) and a test based on the absorption of a small dose of a soluble iron salt is not a reliable indicator of the ability of the lumen of the gastro-intestinal tract to absorb less available forms of iron from different foods. The situation is further complicated by the role of ascorbic acid and chelators in the diet, the presence or absence of achlorhydria, dietary food interactions and the fact that iron may be absorbed but retained in the epithelial cells of the intestine and lost subsequently by the normal process of desquamation.

In normal subjects the absorption averages about 15–30% of a test dose of a soluble iron salt, but it varies enormously; in iron-deficiency anaemia absorption depends on the degree of iron deficiency and transferrin saturation, but it is usually in the range 50–80%. Absorption is decreased in the malabsorption syndromes (e.g. in sprue and 'idiopathic' steatorrhea).

Because of the variation in normal subjects it is difficult to conclude from a single test dose that absorption is impaired. The test is of more use in demonstrating normal absorption (i.e. >10% of the test dose absorbed) in a patient suspected of having an absorption defect. However, the validity of the result depends on the completeness of the faecal collection. In doubtful cases help can be obtained by demonstrating a corresponding degree of radioactivity in the patient's blood 10–14 days later, provided that there has been no increased haemolysis or haemorrhage.

In iron deficiency, in which the absorption of iron from a test dose is generally greater than normal, almost all of the administered radioactivity may be expected to appear in the peripheral blood if the patient is absorbing iron normally. Blood radioactivity figures can thus be used in such cases as a simple test of iron absorption obviating the necessity of stool collection. In other cases, by using $^{131}BaSO_4$ as a marker of the passage of the dose of ^{59}Fe through the intestinal tract, it is possible to identify the extent to which the initially absorbed iron is retained. This has some value in distinguishing between primary and secondary iron overload.[11]

PLASMA-IRON CLEARANCE, IRON TURNOVER AND UTILIZATION

Principle. Iron for incorporation into erythroblasts is transported to the bone marrow as a transferrin-bound complex. At the surface of the erythroblasts the complex releases its iron which enters the cell to be incorporated into haem, leaving the transferrin free for recycling. Iron not bound to transferrin finds its way to the liver and to other organs rather than to the bone marrow, whilst colloidal particles of iron are rapidly removed by phagocytic cells.

The ferrokinetic studies with ^{59}Fe which provide information on erythropoiesis include the rate of clearance of the radioiron from the plasma, plasma-iron turnover, iron incorporation into circulating red cells (iron utilization) and surface counting to measure the uptake and turnover of iron by organs. These are relatively simple procedures which provide clinically useful information. They do not, however, take account of the recirculation of iron which is refluxed into the plasma or iron turnover resulting from dyserythropoiesis or haemolysis. To take account of these factors requires much more detailed compartmental analysis with multiple sampling over an extended period.[14,15,55] These more complex and time-consuming procedures are essential for quantitative measurement of effective and ineffective erythropoiesis. Even so, they are based on models which do not necessarily correspond to the biological mechanism.

In ferrokinetic studies it is important to ensure that any iron administered is bound to transferrin. As a rule, normal (or patient's) plasma has an adequate amount of transferrin. The unsaturated iron-binding capacity (UIBC) or transferrin concentration of the patient's plasma should be measured before the test is carried out and, if the UIBC is less than 1 mg/l (20 μmol/l) or the transferrin concentration is less than 0.6 g/l, normal donor plasma (hepatitis antigen (HB_s)-negative) should be used instead of that of the patient for the subsequent labelling procedure. Some workers recommend passing the labelled plasma through an exchange resin to ensure removal of non-transferrin-bound iron prior to injection.[13]

The subject of ferrokinetics in health and disease was extensively reviewed in an early monograph by Finch et al[27] and has been more recently dealt with by Bothwell et al.[12b]

Method

Under sterile conditions, obtain 5–10 ml of plasma from freshly collected heparinized blood. Add 7–10 μCi of ^{59}Fe ferric citrate (sp activity >5 μCi/μg). Incubate at 37°C for 30 min. Fill a syringe with all but 1 ml of the mixture. Weigh the syringe to the nearest 10 mg. Inject its contents intravenously into the patient, starting a stop-watch at the mid-point of the injection. Re-weigh the empty syringe and calculate the volume injected:

$$\text{volume of plasma (ml)} = \text{wt of plasma (g)} \times \frac{1}{1.015}.$$

Dilute the residual portion of the dose (1 ml) 1 in 100 in 0.1 mol/l HCl, and use as a measuré of the total amount of radioactivity and as a standard in subsequent measurements.

Plasma-iron clearance

Commencing 10 min after injection, take four or five blood samples over a period of 1–2 h, collecting them into heparin or EDTA. Retain a portion of one sample for measurement of plasma iron. Measure the radioactivity in unit volumes of plasma from the samples and plot the values obtained on log-linear graph paper. A straight line will usually be obtained for the initial slope. The radioactivity at the moment of injection is inferred by extrapolation back to zero time and the time taken for the plasma radioactivity to decrease to half the initial value ($T_{1/2}$-plasma clearance) is read off the graph.

Range of $T_{1/2}$-plasma clearance in health. 60–140 min.

The clearance rate is influenced by the intensity of erythropoiesis and also by the activity of the macrophages of the reticulo-endothelial system, especially in the liver, spleen and bone marrow, where the iron is retained as storage iron. Also, to a lesser extent, circulating reticulocytes may take up some of the iron. A rapid clearance indicates hyperactivity of one or more of these mechanisms, as for instance, in iron-deficiency anaemias, haemorrhagic anaemias, haemolytic anaemias and polycythaemia vera. The clearance rate is decreased in aplastic anaemia. In leukaemia and in myelosclerosis the results are variable, depending upon the amount of erythropoietic marrow and the extent of extramedullary erythropoiesis; in myelosclerosis, however, rapid clearance is by far the more common finding. In dyserythropoiesis the clearance may be normal or accelerated.

Plasma-iron turnover (PIT)

When the plasma-iron clearance is related to the iron content of the plasma, a value can be obtained for plasma-iron turnover in mg/l or μmol/l of blood per day.

PIT (mg/l/day) is calculated from the formula:

$$\frac{\text{plasma iron (mg/l)}^\star \times 0.693^\dagger \times (60 \times 24)}{T_{1/2} \text{ (min)}} \times (1 - \text{PCV}).$$

This may be simplified to:

$$\frac{\text{plasma iron (mg/l)} \times 10^3}{T_{1/2} \text{ (min)}} \times (1 - \text{PCV}).$$

or PIT (μmol/l/day) =

$$\frac{\text{plasma iron } (\mu\text{mol/l}) \times 10^3}{T_{1/2} \text{ (min)}} \times (1 - \text{PCV}),$$

* Because of marked diurnal variation, the plasma iron should be measured on a sample of blood collected during the plasma clearance study.
† Natural log of 2.

The range in normal subjects is 4–8 mg/l/day; 70–140 μmol/l/day.

The PIT is increased in iron-deficiency anaemia, haemolytic anaemias and myelosclerosis. It is increased also in ineffective erythropoiesis, particularly so in thalassaemia. In aplastic anaemia the PIT is normal or decreased, but when the plasma iron is raised, the PIT may be above normal. The calculation of PIT assumes a constant rate of iron transport and, while it is an indicator of total erythropoiesis, it does not distinguish between effective and ineffective erythropoiesis. For the reasons discussed earlier and because the findings in health and disease overlap, measurement of the PIT has only limited clinical usefulness.

Iron utilization

Collect blood samples at intervals for a period of about 2 weeks after the administration of the ^{59}Fe. Measure the radioactivity per ml of whole blood and calculate the percentage utilization from the formula:

$$\frac{\text{cpm/ml of day 14 whole-blood sample}}{\text{cpm/ml whole-blood sample at zero time}} \times 100\% \times f,$$

where f is a PCV correction factor, i.e.

$$\frac{0.9 \text{ PCV}}{1 - 0.9 \text{ PCV}}.$$

When there is reason to suspect that the body: venous PCV ratio is not 0.9 (see p. 285), measure the red-cell volume and calculate percentage utilization from the formula:

$$\frac{{}^\star\text{red-cell volume (ml)} \times \text{cpm/ml red cells} \times 100}{\text{total radioactivity injected (cpm)}^\dagger}.$$

* It is preferable to measure the red-cell volume by a direct method (p. 281). Calculation of plasma volume from extrapolation of the ^{59}Fe disappearance curve is often unreliable and the figure for plasma volume should not be used as the basis for the calculation of red-cell volume.
† The radioactivity is adjusted for physical decay up to the day of measurement.

The calculation gives a measure of effective erythropoiesis. In normal subjects red-cell radioactivity rises steadily from 24 h, and reaches a maximum of 70–80% utilization on the 10–14th day.

A rapid plasma clearance is usually associated with early and relatively complete utilization and the converse also applies. The results are inconsistent in megaloblastic anaemias and in haemoglobinopathies in which there is ineffective erythropoiesis; and also in myelosclerosis and polycythaemia vera, depending on the extent of extramedullary erythropoiesis and whether the red-cell life-span is reduced. If there is rapid haemolysis, the utilization curve will be distorted by destruction of some of the labelled red cells; this may be recognized if frequent (daily) samples are measured. In aplastic anaemia the utilization is usually 10–15%; in ineffective erythropoiesis it is as a rule 30–50%.

If the iron utilization is known, it is possible to determine the red-cell iron turnover expressed as mg/l blood per day (PIT × % maximum utilization). This provides a measure of effective erythropoiesis. In normal subjects it is about 5 mg/l, but it gives an underestimate if there is increased haemolysis. In normal subjects the ratio of plasma-iron turnover to red-cell iron turnover is 1.2–1.3 : 1.0.[27]

Marrow transit time

This can be determined from the red-cell utilization data and is the time taken to reach one-half the maximum. It is normally about 3.5 days. It is thought to be a fairly reliable reflection of marrow stimulation by erythropoietin.[39]

Surface counting of [59]Fe

The technique of surface counting is similar to that for ^{51}Cr; as described on p. 304. In addition to measurements over the heart, liver and spleen, the ^{59}Fe activity in the marrow can be measured by placing a collimated counter over the upper portion of the sacrum with the patient lying prone. In order to obtain a pattern of the distribution of the radioactive iron, count the sites mentioned as soon as possible after the administration of the isotope; again after 5, 20, 40 and 60 min, and hourly for 6–10 h. Then make measurements daily or on alternate days for the next 10 days or so. In order to compare the pattern in different patients express the initial counts at each site as 100% and convert subsequent counts proportionately after correction for the physical decay of the isotope. The results obtained in a normal subject are illustrated in Fig. 19.1.

Surface counting after the administration of ^{59}Fe is laborious, but the technique has a place in the investigation of patients thought to be suffering from aplastic anaemia, myelosclerosis or 'refractory' anaemia. It may be helpful to know the sites and extent of extramedullary erythropoiesis, especially if splenectomy is contemplated. The patterns of surface counts in disease are illustrated in Figs. 19.1–19.3.

WHOLE-BODY SCANNING

When [52]Fe is available it can be used to visualize iron distribution and erythropoiesis. The isotope is prepared and administered in the same way as [59]Fe.

Obtain blood samples for measurement of plasma clearance. At 3 h after administration, and again at about 20 h, scan the skeleton by a gamma camera. The extent of skeletal erythropoiesis and the presence of splenic erythropoiesis can be readily identified (Fig. 19.4).

In aplastic anaemia, characteristically, the radioiron accumulates in the liver. [52]Fe disintegrates to [52m]Mn, which also accumulates in the liver. This isotope decays rapidly (half-life 21 min) and should not cause interference, especially in the scan at 20 h.[42] As ^{111}In chloride also binds to transferrin it has been suggested as a convenient and more readily available substitute for [52]Fe. However, results with this isotope are inconsistent and its distribution in the body does not always parallel that of iron.[16]

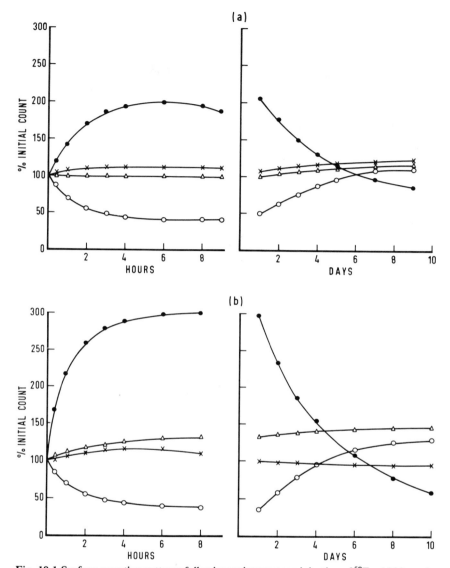

Fig. 19.1 Surface-counting patterns following an intravenous injection of ^{59}Fe. (a) Normal subject and (b) a subject suffering from iron-deficiency anaemia. Radioactivity was measured over the heart ($\bigcirc$), sacrum ($\bullet$), spleen ($\triangle$) and liver (X). The patient with the iron-deficiency anaemia showed an excessive uptake of ^{59}Fe by the bone marrow.

MEASUREMENT OF BLOOD LOSS FROM THE GASTRO-INTESTINAL TRACT USING ^{51}Cr

The ^{51}Cr method of red-cell labelling can be used to measure quantitatively haemorrhage into the gastro-intestinal tract, as ^{51}Cr is neither excreted nor more than minimally reabsorbed.[57] Accordingly, when the blood contains ^{51}Cr-labelled red cells faecal radioactivity is at a very low level unless bleeding has taken place somewhere within the gastro-intestinal tract. Measurement of the faecal radioactivity then gives a reliable indication of the extent of the blood loss.

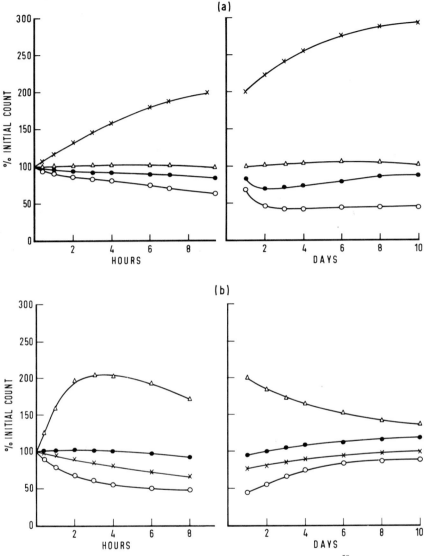

Fig. 19.2 Surface-counting patterns following an intravenous injection of ^{59}Fe. (a) Aplastic anaemia and (b) myelosclerosis. Radioactivity was measured over the heart ($\bigcirc$), sacrum ($\bullet$), spleen ($\triangle$) and liver (**X**). In aplastic anaemia the rate of clearance of the ^{59}Fe from the blood (heart counts) is unusually slow and the bulk of the ^{59}Fe is taken up by the liver. In myelosclerosis there is little or no uptake of ^{59}Fe by the bone marrow but a clear excess uptake by the spleen. The subsequent decrease in radioactivity over the spleen is an indication that the iron is being used for erythropoiesis and is not merely being stored in the organ (cf. the liver in aplastic anaemia).

Method

Label the patient's own blood with approximately 100–150 μCi of ^{51}Cr, as described on p. 281. On each day of the test the faeces are collected in plastic or waxed cardboard cartons. Prepare a standard by adding a measured volume (3–5 ml) of the patient's blood, collected on the same day, to approximately 100 ml of water in a similar carton. Compare the radioactivity of the faecal samples and the standard in a large-volume counting system

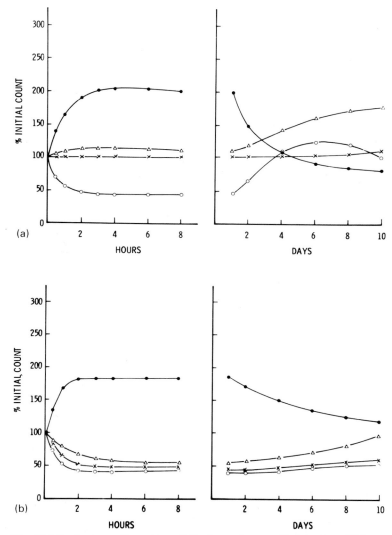

Fig. 19.3 Surface-counting patterns following an intravenous injection of ^{59}Fe.
(a) Haemolytic anaemia and (b) dyserythropoiesis. Radioactivity was measured over
the heart (○), sacrum (●), spleen (△) and liver (X). In the haemolytic anaemia there
is a delayed excess uptake of ^{59}Fe by the spleen which was the main site of red-cell
sequestration. In dyserythropoiesis there is active uptake of ^{59}Fe by the bone marrow.
The subsequent retention of most of the radioactivity in the marrow is an indication of
ineffective erythropoiesis.

(see p. 276). Then, volume of blood in faeces
(in ml) =

$$\frac{cpm/24 \text{ h faeces collection}}{cpm/ml \text{ standard}}.$$

Blood loss from any other source, e.g. surgical operation or menstruation, can be measured in a similar way by counting swabs,
dressings etc., placed in a carton. It is not,
however, possible to measure blood or
haemoglobin loss in the urine (haematuria or
haemoglobinuria) by this method as free ^{51}Cr
is normally excreted in the urine.

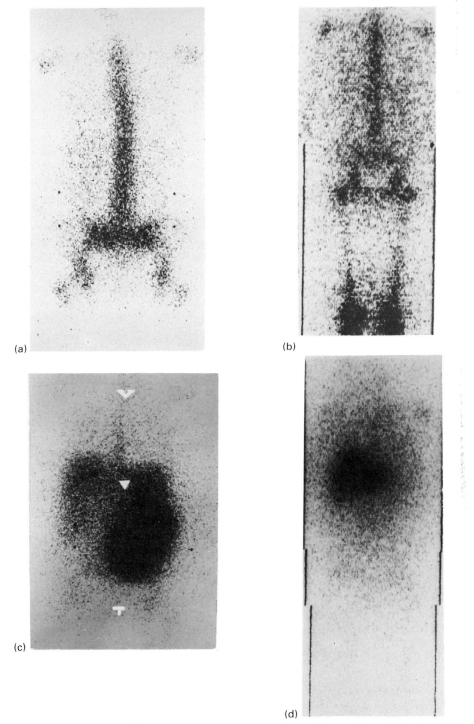

Fig. 19.4 Scans showing distribution of ^{52}Fe. (a) Normal subject, (b) polycythaemia vera, (c) myelofibrosis and (d) aplastic anaemia. In myelofibrosis there is extramedullary erythropoiesis in the liver and spleen; in aplastic anaemia the iron accumulates slowly in the liver.

ESTIMATION OF THE LIFE-SPAN OF RED CELLS IN VIVO

The differential agglutination method of Ashby

The recipient is transfused with red cells of a different but compatible blood group; the resulting mixture of cells is separated in vitro by means of a potent agglutinating serum which agglutinates the recipient's red cells but not those of the donor, and the unagglutinated cells are counted by a standard method of red-cell counting.

It is essential to use a highly avid agglutinating serum, and this often restricts the method to tracing the survival of group-O red cells given to a group-A or -B, or -AB recipient, using an anti-A or anti-B serum. In practice, too, it is necessary to transfuse a major amount of blood, e.g. in an adult the red cells from 1 l of blood in order to obtain a substantial number of donor cells to count. Moreover, it is impossible to measure the life-span of a patient's red cells in his own circulation. Accordingly, with the advent of ^{51}Cr, this method has become outmoded; it is still sometimes used, however, when it is necessary to study the behaviour of donor cells alongside that of the patient's own cells (labelled by ^{51}Cr) or when it is undesirable to expose the patient to a radioactive isotope. The technique is essentially that described by Dacie and Mollison[45b] with the exception that now an electronic cell counter can be used to count the unagglutinated cells.[30,31] More recently, too, a technique has been described in which agglutination is enhanced with bromelin or polyvinylpyrrolidone (PVP).[59]

ISOTOPIC METHODS

There are two ways in which red cells can be labelled by isotopes:

1. Cohort labelling in which red cells produced over a restricted period of time are labelled.
2. Random labelling in which a population of circulating red cells, of all ages, are labelled.

In cohort labelling the isotope (^{15}N, ^{14}C or ^{59}Fe) is incorporated into haemoglobin during its synthesis by erythroblasts or reticulocytes. For random labelling either radioactive chromium (^{51}Cr) or radioactive phosphorus (^{32}P) can be used. ^{51}Cr is used as a label for anionic hexavalent sodium chromate ($Na_2\,^{51}CrO_4$) and ^{32}P as a label for di-*iso*propyl phosphofluoridate (DF^{32}P). While ^{51}Cr can only be used as an in-vitro label, DF^{32}P is normally used as an in vivo label. DF^{32}P inhibits cholinesterase, to which it becomes irreversibly bound, and it thus labels red-cell membranes. However, in the amount required for labelling it does not damage the red cells. Neither ^{51}Cr nor DF^{32}P is reutilised or transferred to other cells in the circulation.

Cohort labelling

Cohort labelling has the potential advantage that it provides information about the relative importance of random destruction and red-cell senescence. The isotope is introduced into the red cells at the time of their formation, and the labelled cells appear in the circulation as a cohort of cells of closely similar age. The total radioactivity of the blood increases steeply and eventually reaches a plateau which is maintained until the cell population reaches the end of its life-span, provided that there is no intervening random destruction. Average life-span is determined by the time which elapses between corresponding points on the rising and falling parts of the curve. The exact form of the curve varies according to the technique used, the rate of incorporation of the label and the extent of its reutilization. The mathematical interpretation of the data is complex.[10]

The most satisfactory label is [^{14}C] glycine which labels both the haem and globin components of Hb.[9] However, measurement of radioactivity requires the use of a liquid scintillation counter and the preparation of the blood samples for counting is laborious. Red cell life-span can also be calculated from measurements of red-cell iron turnover obtained with ^{59}Fe.[56] But the results have to be interpreted with caution because of the major reutilization for haem synthesis of iron derived from effete red cells.

Random labelling

Random labelling is a much more practical method than is cohort labelling. Whether to use ^{51}Cr or

DF^{32}P depends on a number of circumstances. ^{51}Cr is a γ-ray emitter and its radioactivity can be counted externally over the liver and spleen, and it is also practicable to combine a study of red-cell survival with measurement of blood volume. The main disadvantage of ^{51}Cr is that it elutes from circulating red cells; also, there may be an increased early loss over the first 1–3 days, and this may make it impossible to estimate red-cell life-span accurately.

DF^{32}P has the advantage over ^{51}Cr in that elution of the isotope from red cells is less. Whilst there is some early loss of radioactivity this can be minimized and confined to the first 24 h or so by the use of high-specific-activity material. The radioactivity curves are thus relatively easy to interpret. A disadvantage of DF^{32}P is that surface counting is not possible because the label (^{32}P) is a β-emitter.

THE RADIOACTIVE CHROMIUM METHOD

^{51}Cr has a half-life of 27.8 days. After passing through the surface membrane of the red cells, the labelled sodium chromate is reduced to the trivalent form which binds to protein, preferentially to the β-polypeptide chains of haemoglobin.[50] Chromium is toxic to red cells, probably by its oxidizing action; it inhibits glycolysis when present at a concentration of 10 μg/ml of red cells or more [35] and blocks glutathione reductase activity at a concentration exceeding 5 μg/ml.[36,37] Blood should thus not be exposed to more than 2 μg of chromium per ml of packed red cells.

Na$_2$^{51}CrO$_4$ is available commercially at a specific activity of 50–150 μCi/μg; it is usually dissolved in 9 g/l NaCl (saline) in 1–2 mCi amounts. It is convenient to dilute this stock in saline and to dispense 50–150 μCi amounts in ampoules which can then be sterilized by autoclaving. ACD must not be used as a diluent as this reduces the chromate to the cationic chromic form.

Care must be taken to avoid lysis when the red cells are washed; and it may be necessary, especially if the blood contains spherocytes, to use a slightly hypertonic solution, e.g. 12 g/l NaCl. This should certainly be used if an osmotic-fragility test has demonstrated lysis in 9 g/l NaCl. In patients whose plasma contains high-titre, high-thermal-amplitude cold agglutinins the blood must be collected in a warmed syringe, delivered into ACD solution previously warmed to 37°C and the labelling and washing in saline carried out in a 'warm room' at 37°C.

Method

The technique of labelling red cells is the same as for blood-volume measurement (see p. 281). To ensure as little damage to red cells as possible, with subsequent minimal early loss and later elution, it is important to maintain the blood at optimal pH. This can be achieved by adding 10 volumes of blood to 1.5 volumes of the recommended (NIH-A) ACD solution[33] (see p. 432)*.

For a red-cell survival study 0.5 μCi of Na$_2$^{51}CrO$_4$ per kg body weight is recommended. But if surface counting is to be carried out also, a higher dose (e.g. 1 μCi/kg) should be used, bearing in mind that <2 μg of chromium should be added per ml of packed red cells.

After injection, allow the labelled cells to circulate in the recipient for 10 min (or for 60 min in patients with cardiac failure or splenomegaly in whom mixing may be delayed). Then collect a sample of blood from a vein other than that used for the injection (or after washing the needle through with saline if a butterfly needle is used) and mix with EDTA anticoagulant. The radioactivity in this sample provides a base line for subsequent observations. Retain part of the labelled cell suspension which was not injected into the patient to serve as a standard. This enables the blood volume to be calculated if required.

Take further 4–5 ml blood samples from the patient 24 h later (Day 1) and subsequently at intervals, the frequency of the samples depending on the rate of red-cell destruction. The recommended procedure is to take three specimens between Day 2 and Day 7, and

* or CPD solution (see p. 432).

then two specimens per week for the duration of the study.[33] Measurements should be continued until at least half the radioactivity has disappeared from the circulation.

Measure the Hb or PCV in a part of each sample; then lyse the samples with saponin, mix well and deliver a measured volume (1–2 ml) into counting tubes, if possible in duplicate.

Measurement of radioactivity

Estimate the percentage survival (of ^{51}Cr) on any Day(t) by comparing the radioactivity of the sample taken on that day with that of the Day 0 sample, i.e. the sample withdrawn 10 (or 60) min after the injection of the labelled cells. Thus, ^{51}Cr survival on Day t (%) =

$$\frac{\text{cpm/ml of blood on Day t}}{\text{cpm/ml of blood on Day 0}} \times 100.$$

No adjustment is necessary for the physical decay of the isotope, provided that the standard is counted within a few minutes of the Day t sample.

Carry out the measurements in any high-quality scintillation counter, at least 2500 counts being recorded in order to achieve an accuracy of ±2%.

INTERPRETATION OF RADIOACTIVITY MEASUREMENTS

Before the data can be analysed and interpreted, factors, other than physical decay, which are involved in the disappearance of radioactivity from the circulation have to be considered. There are two processes; ^{51}Cr-labelled red cells are lost from the circulation by lysis, phagocytosis or haemorrhage and, in addition, ^{51}Cr is eluted from intact red cells.

Elution is random, the rate differing to a small extent from one individual to another. It is thought to vary to a greater extent in some diseases,[17] especially when the red-cell life-span is considerably reduced. However, in such cases elution and variation in the rate of elution become relatively unim-

portant. The rate of elution is also influenced by technique, especially by the anticoagulant solution into which the blood is collected prior to labelling. With the NIH-A ACD solution the rate of elution is c 1% per day.[33]

Sometimes, in addition to the elution which occurs continuously and at a constant rate, up to 10% of the ^{51}Cr may be lost within the first 24 h. The cause of the early loss is obscure and several components may be involved. If the early loss does not continue beyond the first two days, it is often looked upon as an artefact, in the sense that it does not denote an increased rate of lysis in vivo, and it is usually ignored by replotting the figures as described on p. 301. This procedure is acceptable, at least for clinical studies, but it does not take into account the possibility that a small proportion of red cells are present which are unusually prone to lysis and that the rate of elimination of the rest of the labelled cells is not representative of the entire cell population. Even when the ^{51}Cr data are corrected for elution the survival curve may not be strictly comparable with an Ashby survival curve. This is, however, not of great importance provided the findings are compared with normal ^{51}Cr survival curves, obtained by an identical technique (see Table 19.1 and Fig. 19.5). It is common practice to calculate the T_{50}Cr*, i.e. the time taken for the concentration of ^{51}Cr in the blood to fall to 50% of its initial value, after correcting the data for physical decay but not for elution. The chief objection to the use of T_{50}Cr is that it may be misleading without additional information on the pattern of the survival curve; moreover, the mean red-cell life-span cannot be calculated from it. With the technique described above, the mean value of T_{50} in normal subjects is c 30 days, range 25–33 days.

Correction for elution

When haemolysis is marked, elution is of minor importance and can be ignored. When haemolysis is not greatly increased, it is essential to correct for elution. This can be done using the factors given in Table 19.1.[33]

---

* T_{50} is used rather than $T_{1/2}$ when the fractional elimination does not have a constant gradient.

Table 19.1 Normal range for ^{51}Cr survival curves

Day	% ^{51}Cr (corrected for decay; *not* corrected for elution)	Elution correction factors[33]
1	93–98	1.03
2	89–97	1.05
3	86–95	1.06
4	83–93	1.07
5	80–92	1.08
6	78–90	1.10
7	77–88	1.11
8	76–86	1.12
9	74–84	1.13
10	72–83	1.14
11	70–81	1.16
12	68–79	1.17
13	67–78	1.18
14	65–77	1.19
15	64–75	1.20
16	62–74	1.22
17	59–73	1.23
18	58–71	1.25
19	57–69	1.26
20	56–67	1.27
21	55–66	1.29
22	53–65	1.31
23	52–63	1.32
24	51–60	1.34
25	50–59	1.36
30	44–52	1.47
35	39–47	1.53
40	34–42	1.60

Drawing survival curves and deriving the mean red-cell life-span[7,10,20,33]

Plot the % radioactivity figures or count rates per ml of whole blood (corrected for physical decay and for elution) on arithmetical and semi-logarithmic graph paper and attempt to fit straight lines to the data. Then:

1. If a straight line *can* be fitted to the arithmetical plot, the mean red-cell life-span is given by the point in time at which the line or its extension cuts the abscissa (Fig. 19.6).

2. If a straight line *can* be fitted to the semi-logarithmic plot, the mean cell life-span can be read as the time when 37% of the cells are still surviving (Fig. 19.7) or calculated by multiplying the half-time of the fitted line by 1.44.

3. If a straight line *cannot* be fitted satisfactorily as in (1) or (2), the mean cell life-span can be deduced approximately by extrapolation to the abscissa of a tangent drawn to the initial slope of the data plotted on arithmetical paper (Fig. 19.8).

The mean cell life-span can also be deduced from mathematical formulae with the aid of a computer programme.[33]

INTERPRETATION OF SURVIVAL CURVES

In the auto-immune haemolytic anaemias, the slope of elimination is usually markedly curvilinear when the data are plotted on arithmetical graph paper. Red-cell destruction is typically random and the curve of elimination is thus exponential and produces a straight line on semi-logarithmic graph paper.

In some cases of haemolytic anaemia (? only when there are intra-corpuscular defects) the survival curve appears to consist of two components, an initial steep slope being followed by a much less steeply falling slope. This suggests the presence of cells of widely varying life-span. This type of 'double population' curve is seen in paroxysmal nocturnal haemoglobinuria and in sickle-cell anaemia, and in some cases of hereditary enzyme-deficiency haemolytic anaemias, and when the labelled cells consist of a mixture of transfused normal cells and patient's cells. The mean cell life-span of the entire cell population can be deduced by extrapolation of the initial steep slope to the abscissa. The proportion of cells belonging to the longer-lived population can be estimated by extrapolating the less steep slope, if linear, to the ordinate, and the life-span of this population can be estimated by extending the same slope to the abscissa (Fig. 19.8). The life-span of the short-lived cells can be deduced from the formula:

$$MCL_S = \frac{\%S}{\dfrac{100}{MCL_T} - \dfrac{\%L}{MCL_L}},$$

where S = short-lived population, L = longer-lived population, T = entire cell population and MCL = mean cell life.

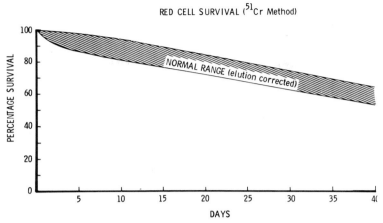

Fig. 19.5 ⁵¹Cr red-cell survival. The hatched area shows the normal range.

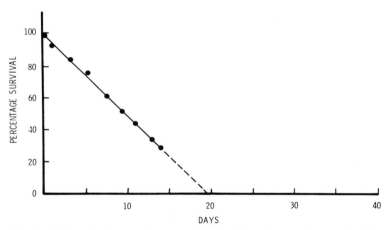

Fig. 19.6 ⁵¹Cr red-cell survival curves. Patient with hereditary spherocytosis. The results give a straight line when plotted on arithmetic graph paper. The mean cell life-span is indicated by the point at which its extension cuts the abscissa (20 days).

Correction for early loss

The simplest method is to ignore the early loss by taking as 100% the radioactivity still present at the end of 24–48 h. Alternatively, the following more laborious method can be employed; it has the advantage that the slope of the survival curve is not altered. The data are plotted on arithmetical graph paper, the line of the slope beyond the initial steep part is extrapolated back to the ordinate and the point of intersection is taken as 100% and the ordinate scale recalibrated accordingly.

Blood-volume changes

There is no need to correct the measurements of radioactivity per ml of whole blood for alterations in PCV provided that the total blood volume remains constant throughout the study. However, when it is suspected that the blood volume may be changing, e.g. in patients with renal disease or during red-cell regeneration, if serial determinations of blood volume are carried out, the observed radioactivity should be multiplied by the observed blood volume and divided by the initial blood volume. In practice, if a patient receives a blood

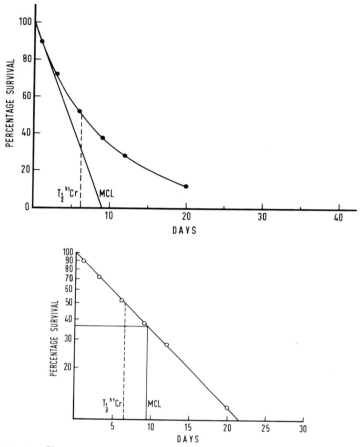

Fig. 19.7 ^{51}Cr **red-cell survival curves.** Patient with auto-immune haemolytic anaemia. In the upper chart the results have been plotted on arithmetic graph paper and the mean cell life-span was deduced by extrapolation of a tangent at the initial slope to the abscissa (9 days). In the lower chart the results have been plotted on semilogarithmic graph paper and the mean cell life-span was read as the time when 37% of the cells were still surviving (9–10 days). The T_{50}Cr was 6–7 days. MCL = mean cell life-span.

tranfusion during a survival study, it can, as a general rule, be assumed that the blood volume will have returned to its pre-transfusion level within 24–48 h.

Correction of survival data for blood loss

When there is a relatively constant loss of blood during a red-cell survival study, the true mean red-cell life-span can be obtained by the following equation:

$$\text{true MCL} = Ta \times \frac{\text{RCV}}{\text{RCV} - (Ta \times L)},$$

where Ta = apparent MCL (days), RCV = red-cell volume (ml), and L = mean rate of loss of red cells (ml/day).

STUDIES WITH NORMAL BLOOD IN NORMAL RECIPIENTS

In about one-third of studies involving the injection of small volumes of apparently compatible ^{51}Cr-labelled normal red cells into a normal recipient (or into recipients who have intrinsic red-cell defects), a sudden collapse of the curve may follow after a period of 1–2 weeks of apparently normal

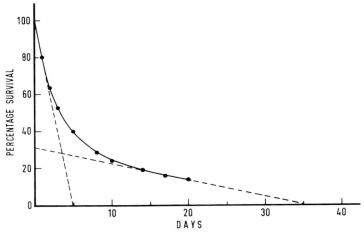

Fig. 19.8 ^{51}Cr red-cell survival curve showing a 'double population'. The mean cell life-span (MCL) of the entire cell population was deduced by extrapolation of a tangent at the initial slope to the abscissa (5 days). By extrapolation of the less steep slope to the ordinate it was deduced that approximately 30% of the red cells belonged to one population, and by extrapolation of the same slope to the abscissa the MCL of this population was deduced as 35 days. The life-span of the remaining 70% of cells was calculated to be 3.6 days (see formula below). The T_{50}Cr was 3–4 days.

survival.[2,45a] The likely cause of this is latent incompatibility, but it has not always been possible to demonstrate the responsible antibody by in vitro tests.

Compatibility test

The behaviour of [51]Cr-(or [113m]In-) labelled donor cells in a recipient will provide important information on the compatibility or otherwise of a donor blood:

1. When serological tests suggest that all normal donors are incompatible.
2. When in the presence of an allo-antibody no non-reacting donor can be found.
3. When the recipient has had an unexplained haemolytic transfusion reaction.

Method[33]

Remove 1–2 ml of blood from the donor bag using a sterile technique. Label 0.5 ml of the red cells with 20 μCi of ^{51}Cr in the standard way (p. 281) and administer to the recipient. Collect 5–10 ml of blood into EDTA or heparin at 3, 10, and 60 min from a vein other than that

used for the injection. Prepare 1–2 ml samples in counting vials. Centrifuge the remainder of the specimens and pipette 1–2 ml of the plasma into counting vials. Measure the radioactivity in the usual way. Calculate the activity in the blood and plasma samples as a percentage of the 3 min blood sample.

Interpretation

With compatible blood the activity in the 60 min sample is, on average, 99% of that of the 3 min sample, but this may vary between 94% and 104%. If survival at 60 min is not less than 70% and the plasma activity is not more than 3%, the donor cells may be transfused with minimal hazard.[33]

DF[32]P method[32]

Labelling with DF[32]P in vivo is carried out by the intravenous injection of DF[32]P or ^{3}H-DFP in propylene glycol. Dilute a stock solution (The Radiochemical Centre, Amersham), if necessary, in sterile 9 g/l NaCl (saline) immediately before injection so as to obtain an amount of DFP not greater than 0.02 mg/kg body weight, with radioactivity not exceeding 0.7 μCi/kg body weight for DF^{32}P, or 7 μCi/kg body weight for ^{3}H-DFP. Inject the solution slowly (over a period of 10–15 min) through a butterfly needle inserted into one of the patient's veins.

Collect the first blood sample 60 min after the injection, and a second sample at 24 h; collect three further samples between Day 2 and Day 7 and take thereafter at least three further samples each week for the duration of the study. Estimate the PCV of each sample and pipette a measured volume of the blood into a tube marked at 10 ml. Centrifuge the blood, remove the plasma carefully and wash the red cells three times with saline. Care must be taken that no red cells are lost during this procedure. Then lyse the cells by a small amount of saponin; add saline to the 10 ml mark and measure the radioactivity of the lysate in a liquid scintillation or gas-flow counting system after appropriate treatment of the samples (see p. 275).

Plotting the radioactivity data

Express the radioactivity per ml of whole blood and plot the figures on graph paper as for ^{51}Cr. Do not use the 60 min sample as 100%, but obtain a value for 100% by extrapolating a line fitted to the data back to the ordinate.

Normal red-cell life-span. The mean red-cell life-span in health is usually taken as 120 days, and the SD 15 days.[33]

Determination of sites of red-cell destruction using ^{51}Cr

The sites of destruction of red cells, with special reference to the spleen and liver, can be determined by in vivo surface counting using a shielded scintillation counter placed, respectively, over the heart, spleen and liver.

A collimated scintillation detector with a crystal of not less than 7.5 cm diameter and not less than 3.75 cm thickness is required.

The collimator should exclude radiation from extraneous sources and should be capable of surveying an adequate area of the organ being studied. A cylindrical-hole collimator about 7 cm deep, 5 cm internal hole diameter and 10 cm external diameter is suitable. However, more reliable results are probably obtained by using two counters, 25–30 cm apart, positioned above and below the counting couch. It is essential when counting on successive days to make the measurements over the chosen points under standardized conditions. Thus, the patient should always be supine in the same position.

Mark the following selected points with marking ink and cover by a layer of transparent dressing:

Heart: third interspace at left sternal border.

Liver: halfway between mid-clavicular and anterior axillary lines on the right side of the body, 3–4 cm above the costal margin.

Spleen: select the site of maximum activity on the first occasion by means of a preliminary count for a few seconds over each of several adjacent sites; then mark this position as the point for subsequent counting.

Some workers recommend that the spleen should first be visualized by injecting ^{99m}Tc-labelled heat-damaged red cells (see p. 308); this will not interfere with the surface counting if 24 h are allowed to elapse.

If a single detector is used, this should be placed vertically over the liver and heart counting points and horizontally over the splenic point, just touching the skin. Dual counters, if used, should be placed above and below the selected point in the same vertical axis, and at a fixed distance from each other.

In haemolytic anaemias the first measurements are normally made 30–60 min after injection of the ^{51}Cr-labelled red cells and they are usually made thereafter daily or on alternate days depending on the rate of haemolysis. At least 2500 counts should be recorded at each site, and it is convenient to

Table 19.2 Example of method for calculation of surface counting data

Day	0	1	2	5	8	10	12	14
Heart	1000	850	780	720	670	600	500	370
Liver								
Actual counts	670	670	660	560	640	630	550	530
Expected counts		570	522	482	449	402	335	248
Excess		100	138	78	191	228	215	282
Spleen								
Actual counts	970	1265	1490	1800	2130	2370	2210	2020
Expected counts		825	756	698	650	582	485	359
Excess		440	734	1102	1480	1788	1725	1661
Spleen: Liver ratio								
Actual*	1.45	1.89	2.26	3.21	3.33	3.76	4.02	3.81
Adjusted	1.00	1.30	1.56	2.21	2.30	2.59	2.77	2.62

The actual count rate over the heart on Day 0 was 7500 counts per min. This was recorded as 1000 and all other counts were adjusted proportionately.
* Obtained from the actual counts of the organs. The ratio obtained on Day 0 was recorded as 1.00 and the results on subsequent days were adjusted proportionately.

count at each site for two periods of 1 min and to average the counts. The measurements should be repeated if there is a difference of more than 2% between the counts. After Day 0, the counts have to be corrected for physical decay of the isotope by reference to a standard counted on each occasion under conditions of constant geometry.

In order to compare the results in different patients irrespective of the amount of isotope administered, the initial count over the heart is taken as the base-line. This is recorded as '1000 counts', irrespective of the actual number of counts recorded, and all the other counts at every site are adjusted ('normalized') proportionately. The fall in heart counts parallels the loss of the labelled red cells from the circulation, although the actual counts usually fall off more slowly than the radioactivity of the blood measured in vitro, probably because ^{51}Cr is deposited in all tissues before it is excreted. Alternatively, the changes in blood radioactivity can be used to normalize the observed count-rate over liver and spleen. This may at times give more consistent results. Theoretically, the counts over the spleen and the liver should fall at the same rate as the heart and blood counts unless lysis or sequestration of red cells is taking place within the organ(s) or unless ^{51}Cr eluted from red cells in the blood stream accumulates in the organ(s). When the counts over the liver or spleen exceed the calculated amount (based on the fall in heart or blood count), the excess radioactivity is recorded by subtracting the expected counts from the counts actually obtained. The counts recorded in a patient suffering from haemolytic anaemia are illustrated in Table 19.2.

It is useful to calculate an index, the Spleen : Liver Ratio, which reflects the relative accumulation of ^{51}Cr in the spleen and liver. The ratio between the counts on Day 0 is recorded as 1.00 and all subsequent ratios are related to this.

Normal surface-counting patterns are illustrated in Fig. 19.9. The interrupted lines indicate the limits of accumulation observed in normal subjects. In haemolytic anaemias the results differ from case to case. Four patterns can be distinguished[41] (Fig. 19.10):

1. Excess accumulation in the spleen, as in hereditary spherocytosis and hereditary elliptocytosis and some cases of auto-immune haemolytic anaemia (AIHA).

2. Excess accumulation chiefly in the liver; seen only in sickle-cell anaemia, especially in older patients.

3. Little or no excess accumulation in either spleen or liver, as in some hereditary enzyme-

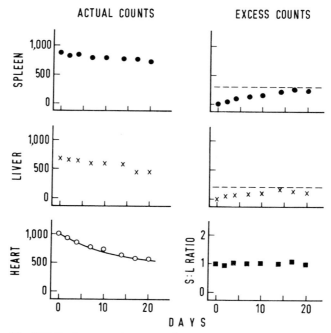

Fig. 19.9 Surface-counting pattern in a normal subject following labelling of his red cells with ⁵¹Cr. The interrupted lines indicate the limits of accumulation in normal subjects.

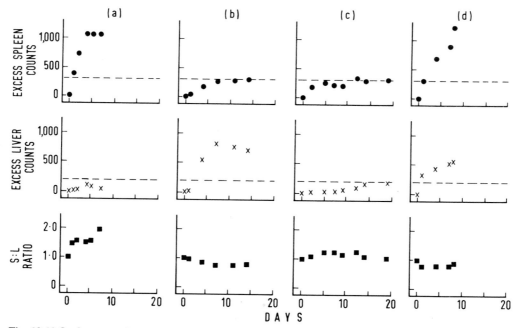

Fig. 19.10 Surface-counting patterns following labelling of patients' red cells with ⁵¹Cr in various haemolytic anaemias. The interrupted lines indicate the limits of accumulation in normal subjects. Only excess counts and the spleen:liver ratio are shown. (a) Hereditary spherocytosis; (b) sickle-cell disease; (c) pyruvate-kinase deficiency; (d) auto-immune haemolytic anaemia. See text.

deficiency haemolytic anaemias and in paroxysmal nocturnal haemoglobinuria.

4. Excess accumulation in both liver and spleen, as in some cases of auto-immune haemolytic anaemia.

Clinical experience has shown that splenectomy usually benefits patients showing the pattern (1) and to a more limited degree, in parallel with the Spleen:Liver Ratio, patients showing the pattern (4). The degree of improvement is not, however, closely correlated with the magnitude of the ^{51}Cr accumulation in the spleen.[3]

Surface-counting studies have their limitations. Even minor alterations in the conditions of counting and positioning of the patient may produce significant changes. Isolated readings may, therefore, be misleading. Amongst the variables which affect the count-rate are the volume of the organ counted in relation to its total volume, the distance of the organ from the surface of the body, the absorption of radiation by the overlying tissues and the rate of loss of deposited ^{51}Cr from the organ. Nevertheless, despite these difficulties, surface counting has proved to be of value in the management of patients with some types of haemolytic anaemia when used in conjunction with other clinical and laboratory investigations.

Methods have been developed by which the counts over the spleen can be related quantitatively to red-cell destruction within the spleen.[61] After the usual surface-counting study, the spleen is scanned; heat-damaged ^{51}Cr-labelled cells are then injected and the scan is repeated together with a surface count. The increase in surface count due to the damaged cells which enter the spleen is recorded. By counting the dots in the scan produced by these cells (a quantitative measurement of the radioactivity of a known volume of cells) the surface counter can be calibrated; the radioactivity due to the splenic destruction or sequestration of the not-heat-damaged cells can then be calculated and expressed as a fraction of the radioactivity which has disappeared from the circulation during the period of study. In hereditary spherocytosis up to 95% or more of the loss of the labelled cells from the circulation has, in some cases, been accounted for in the spleen;[61] in other haemolytic anaemias it has varied, depending on the mechanism of haemolysis. Thus, it has been 1–2% in hexokinase deficiency, 15–50% in auto-immune haemolytic anaemias and up to 80% in thalassaemia.[26,61] However, the measurements are of more theoretical interest than of clinical value.

Simultaneous measurements of ^{51}Cr and ^{59}Fe

It is possible to study simultaneously the rate and sites of both erythropoiesis and haemolysis. This has been carried out using ^{59}Fe and ^{51}Cr and the separate measurement of the radioactivity due to each isotope in blood and plasma is relatively simple (see p. 279). However, in practice the reliability of the ^{51}Cr measurement may be invalidated by the presence of ^{59}Fe and if possible the procedures should not be performed together.

VISUALIZATION OF THE SPLEEN BY SCINTILLATION SCANNING

This procedure is a development and extension of the techniques of surface counting described above. It has been used:

1. To demonstrate enlargement or abnormal position of the spleen or accessory splenic tissue.
2. To identify the nature of a mass in the left hypochondrium.
3. To demonstrate the presence of space-occupying lesions within the spleen.
4. To assess splenic function.

It is especially useful for demonstrating splenic atrophy in conditions such as thrombocythaemia and idiopathic steatorrhea. Mention has been made of the value of delineating the spleen for surface counting (p. 304) and for estimation of the splenic blood pool (p. 286).

Methods which have been used to alter red cells in vitro to ensure that after re-injection they are selectively removed from the circulation by the spleen include heat-damage, antibody sensitization and exposure to chemicals such as N-ethyl maleimide (NEM), mercuri-hydroxypropane (MHP) and paramercuribenzoate (PMB) (for review of the literature, see Pettit.[53])

By appropriate isotope labelling of these altered cells the accumulation of radioactivity within the organ provides a means of demonstrating its size and position. The heat-damage method is recommended using ^{51}Cr, ^{99m}Tc or ^{113m}In as the label. Scintillation scanning is usually started about 1 h after the injection of the damaged cells, but it can be performed up to 3–4 h later; satisfactory scans can also be obtained with ^{51}Cr and ^{113m}In up to 24 h after the injection.

Methods using heat damage

With ^{51}Cr as the label[44]

Deliver approximately 10 ml of blood into 1.5 ml of sterile ACD solution. Centrifuge the sample at 1200–1500 **g** for 5–10 min. Keep the plasma in a sterile container. Label the red cells with Na$_2$ ^{51}CrO$_4$ using 1.5–2.0 μCi per kg body weight. Wash the labelled cells three times in sterile 9 g/l NaCl (saline). Place approximately 6 ml of the packed cells in a sterile 30 ml glass bottle with a screw cap. Heat the bottle in a water-bath at a constant temperature of 49.5–50°C for exactly 20 min with occasional gentle mixing. Resuspend the cells in their own plasma and inject intravenously as soon as possible. Follow a standardized technique meticulously.

With ^{99m}Tc as the label

Deliver 5–10 ml of blood into a sterile bottle containing 100 iu of heparin. Centrifuge the sample at 1200–1500 **g** for 5–10 min and discard the plasma. Transfer 2 ml of the packed red cells to a 30 ml glass bottle with a screw cap; heat the bottle in a water-bath at a constant temperature of 49.5–50°C for exactly 20 min with occasional gentle mixing. Wash the cells twice in saline and discard the supernatant. Add 0.3 ml of stannous chloride and label with 1 mCi of ^{99m}Tc or label with 1 mCi of ^{99m}Tc by the alternative method as described on p. 282. After standing for 5 min, wash once in 12 g/l NaCl. Resuspend in about 10 ml of 12 g/l NaCl and inject as soon as possible.

With ^{111}In or ^{113}In as the label

Prepare 2 ml of heat-damaged red cells as for the ^{99m}Tc method. Wash twice in 12 g/l NaCl.

Add 250 μCi of ^{111}In or ^{113}In, as described on p. 283. Then wash once in 12 g/l NaCl. Resuspend in about 10 ml of 12 g/l NaCl and inject as soon as possible.

RATE OF CLEARANCE OF DAMAGED RED CELLS

Information on splenic activity may be obtained by measuring the rate of clearance of heat-damaged labelled red cells from the circulation. A blood sample is taken exactly 3 min after the mid-point of the injection and further samples are collected at 5 min intervals for 30 min and a final sample at 60 min. The radioactivity in each sample is measured and expressed as a percentage of the radioactivity in the 3 min sample. The results are plotted on semi-logarithmic graph paper, the 3 min sample being taken as 100% radioactivity.

In normal subjects the half-time of disappearance (T_{50}) is 5–15 min.[53] The time is considerably longer in thrombocythaemia and in conditions associated with splenic atrophy such as sickle-cell anaemia, coeliac disease, dermatitis herpetiformis.

Peters and colleagues[51,52a,52b] have demonstrated that the disappearance curve is a complex one (Fig. 19.11); its first phase (8–10 min) is influenced by the rapid uptake of some of the labelled material by the liver, followed by a phase in which the damaged cells pass through the spleen where they are held up transiently in the sinusoids and some of them are phagocytosed by reticulo-endothelial cells. Within 30 min the cells in the splenic pool will have equilibrated with those still in circulation, but subsequently more cells are taken up irreversibly by the spleen and this is the main factor in the later part of the curve. Thus, the middle phase of the curve (Fig. 19.11) best reflects the two main components of splenic function, i.e. blood flow and phagocytosis. This is expressed as the fraction of radioactivity disappearing from circulation between 8 and 28 min.[51] Thus, fractional clearance (20 min) =

$$\frac{\% \text{ of 3 min count at 8 min} - \% \text{ of 3 min count at 28 min}}{\% \text{ of 3 min count at 8 min}}.$$

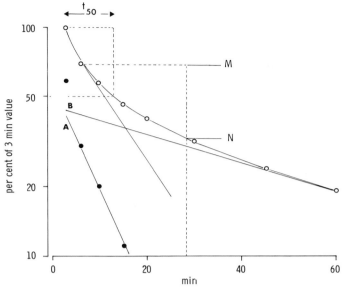

Fig. 19.11 Curve of disappearance from circulation of labelled heat-damaged red cells. The half-time of disappearance (T_{50}) was 10 min. The fractional disappearance between 8 min (M = 56%) and 28 min (N = 34.5%), i.e. (M − N/M was 38% (1.9% per min). Extrapolation of the early component (A) reflects liver clearance and extrapolation of the late component (B) represents the irreversible trapping of cells in the spleen.

When the spleen is functioning normally this is in the range of 30–60% or 1.5–3.0% per min.

For consistent results a carefully standardized technique is necessary. The extent of red-cell damage should be checked by a plot of cell size distribution as measured by a Channelyzer (p. 38) (Fig. 19.12). It is also advisable to check for plasma radioactivity in the blood samples; if present, the measurements of radioactivity in the whole-blood samples will be misleading.

ASSAY OF ERYTHROPOIETIN

Erythropoietin is a glycoprotein hormone which regulates red-cell production. Only a small quantity is demonstrable in normal human plasma or urine. Increased amounts are found in various anaemias. Considerable amounts of erythropoietin are found in the blood and urine of patients with secondary polycythaemia (erythrocytosis) occurring in respiratory and cardiac diseases, in abnormal Hbs with high oxygen affinity, in association with hypernephroma and other renal lesions, and with erythropoietin-secreting tumours such as hepatoma, uterine fibroma, ovarian carcinoma and some other rare tumours. In contrast, in polycythaemia vera, the levels appear to be normal or lower than normal.[5,24,38] A sex difference and diurnal variation have been reported.[1,4]

The original method for measurement of erythropoietin was by an in vivo biological assay, based on the measurement of the ^{59}Fe uptake by laboratory animals (usually rats) following the injection of test plasma or extract.[23,38] Variations in the techniques include differences in the methods of preparation of the test plasma or extract and the modification of the test animals for the purpose by hypoxia-induced polycythaemia, hypertransfusion or starvation, all of which manoeuvres result in a decrease in normal erythropoiesis so that any detectable ^{59}Fe uptake can be attributed to stimulation by the administered plasma or extract. More recently, in vitro methods have been developed using a fetal mouse liver-cell culture,[21,46,49,60] haemagglutination inhibition[40] or radio-immune assay.[29,58]   The   haemagglutination-inhibition

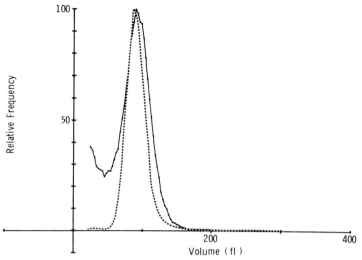

Fig. 19.12 Effect of heat-damage on red cells. This is an example of a satisfactory end-result. The morphological features are paralleled by alteration in the Channelyzer plot of cell size distribution. (- - - pre-damage; — post-damage).

method does not appear to be consistently reliable and has shown poor correlation with bioassay methods.[49] The radio-immune assay is based on pure human erythropoietin as the labelled antigen and also as the primary standard; this seems a promising method for routine use. It may be especially useful for distinguishing polycythaemia vera from secondary polycythaemia in which there is a small but significant overproduction of erythropoietin. The in vivo bioassay method is not sufficiently sensitive for this level of discrimination unless the erythropoietin content of plasma or urine is first concentrated by a fairly laborious procedure.[24] It is thus not practical for routine clinical purposes but it reflects the physiological effects of erythropoietin and should remain as a reference method.[47]

An international (WHO) reference preparation is available. The international unit was originally defined as the activity contained in 1.48 mg of the first international reference preparation. This has been replaced by a second international reference preparation with a potency of 10 iu per ampoule.[6,19] In the published series referred to in the previous paragraph, the normal level in plasma has been reported to be 5–10 iu/l and the urinary excretion about 0.5–5.0 iu per day. The reported normal ranges, however, have varied considerably according to the method of assay.

REFERENCES

[1] ADAMSON, J. W., ALEXANIAN, R., MARTINEZ, C. and FINCH, C. A. (1966). Erythropoietin excretion in normal man. *Blood*, **28**, 354.

[2] ADNER, P. L., FOCONI, S. and SJÖLIN, S. (1963). Immunization after intravenous injection of small amounts of ^{51}Cr-labelled red cells. *British Journal of Haematology*, **9**, 288.

[3] AHUJA, S., LEWIS, S. M. and SZUR, L. (1972). Value of surface counting in predicting response to splenectomy in haemolytic anaemia. *Journal of Clinical Pathology*, **25**, 467.

[4] ALEXANIAN, R. (1966). Urinary excretion of erythropoietin in normal men and women. *Blood*, **28**, 344.

[5] ALEXANIAN, R. (1977). Increased erythropoietin production in man. In *Kidney Hormones, Vol II: Erythropoietin* (ed. J. W. Fisher), p.531. Academic Press, London.

[6] ANNABLE, L., COTES, P. M. and MUSSETT, M. V. (1972). The second international reference preparation of erythropoietin, human, urinary, for bioassay. *Bulletin of World Health Organization*, **47**, 99.

[7] BENTLEY, S. A. (1977). Red cell survival studies reinterpreted. *Clinics in Haematology*, **6**, 601.

[8] BERK, P. D., RODKEY, F. L., BLASCHKE, T. F., COLLISON, H. A. and WAGGONER, J. G. (1974). Comparison of plasma bilirubin turnover and carbon monoxide production in man. *Journal of Laboratory and Clinical Medicine*, **83**, 29.

[9] BERLIN, N. I., LAWRENCE, J. H. and LEE, H. C. (1954). The pathogenesis of the anaemia of chronic leukemia: measurement of the life-span of the red blood cell with glycine-2-^{14}C. *Journal of Laboratory and Clinical Medicine*, **44**, 860.

[10] BERLIN, N. I., WALDMANN, T. A. and WEISSMAN, S. M. (1959). Life span of red blood cell. *Physiological Reviews*, **39**, 577.

[11] BOENDER, C. A. and VERLOOP, M. C. (1969). Iron absorption, iron loss and iron retention in man: studies after oral administration of a tracer dose of $^{59}FeSO_4$ and $^{131}BaSO_4$. *British Journal of Haematology*, **17**, 45.

[12] BOTHWELL, T. H., CHARLTON, R. W., COOK, J. D. and FINCH, C. A. (1979). *Iron Metabolism in Man*, (a) Ch. 12, (b) Ch. 20, (c). Ch. 21. Blackwell Scientific Publications, Oxford.

[13] CAVILL, I. (1971). The preparation of ^{59}Fe-labelled transferrin for ferrokinetic studies. *Journal of Clinical Pathology*, **24**, 472.

[14] CAVILL, I., RICKETTS, C. and JACOBS, A. (1977). Radioiron and erythropoiesis: methods, interpretation and clinical application. *Clinics in Haematology*, **6**, 583.

[15] CAZZOLA, M., BAROSI, G. ORLANDI, E. and STEFANELLI, M. (1980). The plasma ^{59}Fe clearance curve in man: an evaluation of methods of measurement and analysis. *Blut*, **40**, 325.

[16] CHIPPING, P., KLONIZAKIS, I. and LEWIS, S. M. (1980). Indium chloride scanning: a comparison with iron as a tracer for erythropoiesis. *Clinical and Laboratory Haematology*, **2**, 255.

[17] CLINE, M. J. and BERLIN, N. I. (1963). The red cell chromium elution rate in patients with some hematologic diseases. *Blood*, **21**, 63.

[18] COOK, J. D. and LIPSCHITZ, D. A. (1977). Clinical measurement of iron absorption. *Clinics in Haematology*, **6**, 567.

[19] COTES, P. M. and BANGHAM, D. R. (1966). The international reference preparation of erythropoietin. *Bulletin of the World Health Organization*, **35**, 751.

[20] DORNHORST, A. C. (1951). The interpretation of red cell survival curves. *Blood*, **6**, 1284.

[21] DUNN, C. D. R., JARVIS, J. H. and GREENMAN, J. M. (1975). A quantitative bioassay for erythropoietin using mouse fetal liver cells. *Experimental Haematology*, **3**, 362.

[22] ENGEL, R., BERK, P. D., RODKEY, F. L., HOWE, R. B. and BERLIN, N. I. (1969). Estimation of heme turnover (HT) and erythrocyte red cell survival (RBCLS) in man from clearance of bilirubin (BR)-^{14}C and from carbon monoxide production (COP). *Clinical Research*, **17**, 325.

[23] ERSLEV, A. J. (1977). Erythropoietin assay. In *Haematology* (ed. W. J. Williams, E. Beutler, A. J. Erslev and R. W. Rundles), 2nd edn., p. 1616. McGraw Hill, New York.

[24] ERSLEV, A. J., CARO, J., KANSU, E., MILLER, O. and COBBS, E. (1979). Plasma erythropoietin in polycythemia. *American Journal of Medicine*, **66**, 243.

[25] FAWWAZ, R. A., WINCHELL, H. S., POLLYCOVE, M., SARGENT, T., ANGER, H. and LAWRENCE, J. H. (1966). Intestinal iron absorption studies using iron-52 and Anger positron camera. *Journal of Nuclear Medicine*, **7**, 569.

[26] FERRANT, A., CAUWE, J. L., MICHAUX. C., BECKERS, C., VERWILGHEN, R. and SOKAL, G. (1982). Assessment of the sites of red-cell destruction using quantitative measurement of splenic and hepatic red-cell destruction. *British Journal of Haematology*, **50**, 591.

[27] FINCH, C. A., DEUBELBEISS, K., COOK, J. D., ESCHBACH, J. W., HARKER, L. A., FUNK, D. D., MARSAGLIA, G., HILLMAN, R. S., SLICHTER, S., ADAMSON, J. W., GANZONI, A. and GIBLETT, E. R. (1970). Ferrokinetics in man. *Medicine*, **49**, 17.

[28] FRANCOIS, P. E. and SZUR, L. (1958). Use of iron-52 as a radioactive tracer. *Nature (London)*, **182**, 1665.

[29] GARCIA, J. F. (1977). Assays for erythropoietin. In *Kidney Hormones*, Vol II: Erythropoietin, ed. J. W. Fisher, p. 7. Academic Press, London.

[30] GREENDYKE, R. M., BOWDLER, A. J. and SWISHER, S. N. (1969). Studies of differential red cell agglutination utilising an electronic particle counter. I. Quantitative analysis of red cell mixtures prepared in vitro. *American Journal of Clinical Pathology*, **51**, 24.

[31] GREENDYKE, R. M., KNOLL, P. J. and SWISHER, S. N. (1969). Studies of differential agglutination utilising an electron particle counter. II. Simultaneous determination of red cell survival by ^{51}Cr tagging and differential agglutination. *American Journal of Clinical Pathology*, **51**, 30.

[32] International committee for standardization in haematology (1971). Recommended methods for radioisotope red-cell survival studies. *British Journal of Haematology*, **21**, 241.

[33] International committee for standardization in haematology (1980). Recommended method for radioisotope red-cell survival studies. *British Journal of Haematology*, **45**, 659.

[34] International committee for standardization in haematology (1975). Recommended methods for surface counting to determine sites of red-cell destruction. *British Journal of Haematology*, **30**, 249.

[35] JANDL, J. H., GREENBERG, M. S., YONEMOTO, R. H. and CASTLE, W. B. (1956). Clinical determination of the sites of red cell sequestration in hemolytic anaemias. *Journal of Clinical Investigation*, **35**, 842.

[36] KOUTRAS, G. A., HATTORI, M., SCHNEIDER, A. S., EBAUGH, F. G. and VALENTINE, W. N. (1964). Studies of chromated erythrocytes. Effect of sodium chromate on erythrocyte glutathione reductase. *Journal of Clinical Investigation*, **43**, 323.

[37] KOUTRAS, G. A., SCHNEIDER, A. S., HATTORI, M. and VALENTINE, W. N. (1965). Studies on chromated erythrocytes. Mechanisms of chromate inhibition of glutathione reductase. *British Journal of Haematology*, **11**, 360.

[38] KRANTZ, S. B. and JACOBSON, L. O. (1970). *Erythropoietin and the Regulation of Erythropoiesis*. University of Chicago Press, Chicago.

[39] LABARDINI, J., PAPAYANNOPOULOU, T., COOK, J. D., ADAMSON, J. W., WOODSON, R. D., ESCHBACH, J. W., HILLMAN, R. S. and FINCH, C. A. (1973). Marrow radioiron kinetics. *Haematologia*, **7**, 301.

[40] LANGE, R. D., McDONALD, T. P. and JORDAN, T. (1969). Antisera to erythropoietin: partial characterization of two different antibodies. *Journal of Laboratory and Clinical Medicine*, **73**, 78.

[41] LEWIS, S. M., SZUR, L. and DACIE, J. V. (1960). The pattern of erythrocyte destruction in haemolytic anaemia, as studied with radioactive chromium. *British Journal of Haematology*, **6**, 122.

[42] LILLICRAP, S. C., STEERE, H. and CLINK, H. M. (1976). Distribution and dosimetry of ^{52}Fe and ^{59}Fe in bone marrow and other organs. *Radioaktive Isotope in Klinik und Forschung*, **12**, 79.

[43] LUNDH, B., CAVALLIN-STAHL, E. and MERCKE, C. (1975). Heme catabolism, carbon monoxide production and red cell survival in anaemia. *Acta Medica Scandinavica*, **197**, 161.

[44] MARSH, G. W., LEWIS, S. M. and SZUR, L. (1966). The use of ^{51}Cr-labelled heat-damaged red cells to study splenic

function. I. Evaluation of method. *British Journal of Haematology*, **12**, 161.

45 MOLLISON, P. L. (1979). *Blood Transfusion in Clinical Medicine*, 5th edn., (a) p. 537, (b) p. 727. Blackwell Scientific Publications, Oxford.

46 NAPIER, J. A. F., and EVANS, J. (1980). Erythropoietin assay using fetal mouse liver cultures: a modified technique using semi-automatic harvesting of ^{125}I deoxyuridine labelled erythroblasts. *Clinical and Laboratory Haematology*, **2**, 13.

47 National committee for clinical laboratory standards (1979). Standard assay for the determination of erythropoietin activity in body fluids. NCCLS, Villanova, Pa, USA.

48 O'CONNELL, M. E. A., HOWS, J. and LEWIS, S. M. (1977). The combined use of iron-52 and its contaminant iron-55 in studies of the bone marrow. *British Journal of Radiology*, **50**, 419.

49 OMRAN, N. and NEUMANN, E. (1979). A haemagglutination inhibition test kit for routine analysis of erythropoietin. *Blut*, **39**, 225.

50 PEARSON, H. A. (1963). The binding of ^{51}Cr to hemoglobin. I. In vitro studies. *Blood*, **22**, 218.

51 PETERS, A. M., RYAN, P. F. J., KLONIZAKIS, I., ELKON, K. B., LEWIS, S. M. and HUGHES, G. R. V. (1981). Analysis of heat-damaged erythrocyte clearance curves. *British Journal of Haematology*, **49**, 581.

52a PETERS, A. M., RYAN, P. F. J., KLONIZAKIS, I., ELKON, K. B., LEWIS, S. M. and HUGHES, G. R. V. (1981). Measurement of splenic function in humans using heat damaged autologous red blood cells. *Scandinavian Journal of Haematology*, **27**, 374.

52b PETERS, A. M., RYAN, P. F. J., KLONIZAKIS, I., ELKON, K. B., LEWIS, S. M., HUGHES, G. R. V. and LAVENDER, J. P.

(1982). Kinetics of heat damaged autologous red blood cells. *Scandinavian Journal of Haematology*, **28**, 5.

53 PETTIT, J. E. (1977). Spleen function. *Clinics in Haematology*, **6**, 639.

54 PETTIT, J. E., LEWIS, S. M., WILLIAMS, E. D., GRAFTON, C. A., BOWRING, C. S. and GLASS, H. I. (1976). Quantitative studies of splenic erythropoiesis in polycythaemia vera and myelofibrosis. *British Journal of Haematology*, **34**, 465.

55 RICKETTS, C., JACOBS, A. and CAVILL, I. (1975). Ferrokinetics and erythropoiesis in man: the measurement of effective erythropoiesis, ineffective erythropoiesis, and red cell lifespan using ^{59}Fe. *British Journal of Haematology*, **31**, 65.

56 RICKETTS, C., CAVILL, I. and NAPIER, J. A. F. (1977). The measurement of red cell lifespan using ^{59}Fe. *British Journal of Haematology*, **37**, 403.

57 ROCHE, M. and PÉREZ-GIMÉNEZ, M. E. (1959). Intestinal loss and reabsorption of iron in hookworm infection. *Journal of Laboratory and Clinical Medicine*, **54**, 49.

58 SHERWOOD, J. B. and GOLDWASSER, E. (1979). A radioimmunoassay for erythropoietin. *Blood*, **54**, 885.

59 SZYMMANSKI, I. O., VALERI, C. R., ALMOND, D. V., EMERSON, C. P. and ROSENFELD, R. E. (1967). Automated differential agglutination for measurement of red-cell survival. *British Journal of Haematology*, **13**, Suppl, 50.

60 WARDLE, D. F. H., BAKER, I., MALPAS, J.S. and WRIGLEY, P. F. M. (1973). Bioassay of erythropoietin using foetal mouse liver cells. *British Journal of Haematology*, **24**, 49.

61 WILLIAMS, E. D., SZUR, L., GLASS, H. I., LEWIS, S. M., PETTIT, J. E. and AHUJA, S. (1974). Measurement of red cell destruction in the spleen. *Journal of Laboratory and Clinical Medicine*, **84**, 134.

20

Investigation of megaloblastic and iron-deficiency anaemias
(*Written in collaboration with A. V. Hoffbrand**)

MEGALOBLASTIC ANAEMIA

Megaloblastic anaemia can be suspected from the presence in a blood film of macrocytes, oval red cells, pear-shaped poikilocytes and polymorphonuclear neutrophils with hypersegmented nuclei (see Chapter 5). The first indication in many cases is the finding of a raised MCV, especially when the blood count is performed in an electronic counter, and this may occur in non-anaemic cases. The diagnosis is confirmed by finding megaloblasts and giant metamyelocytes in the marrow. Assay of serum vitamin B_{12} (B_{12}) and folate can provide the additional evidence for a firm diagnosis to be made. Serum B_{12} assay is particularly important in the diagnosis of B_{12} neuropathy, as this is often associated with only slight haematological abnormality.

Vitamin B_{12} deficiency can be detected by estimating the serum B_{12} or the urinary excretion of methylmalonic acid. However, since the assay of methylmalonic acid excretion is no longer in general use the methods of estimation will not be described here. The reader is referred to the previous edition of this book or to Chanarin[20] for details of appropriate methods. Estimation of the serum and red-cell folate concentrations will demonstrate folate deficiency. The deoxyuridine suppression test can also be used to diagnose B_{12} or folate deficiency. Measurement of formiminoglutamic acid (Figlu) excretion after a histidine load was used formerly for assessing folate status but is now obsolete.

The elucidation of the cause of deficiency of B_{12} or folate depends both on the clinical diagnosis and on laboratory tests. The latter include measurement of the absorption of B_{12} or folate, demonstration of serum antibodies to intrinsic factor or gastric parietal cells, and measurement of gastric secretion of intrinsic factor. The measurement of serum B_{12}-binding capacity and transcobalamins are useful ancillary tests.

MICROBIOLOGICAL ASSAY OF VITAMIN B_{12} IN SERUM

Two methods are available, using *Euglena gracilis* and *Lactobacillus leichmannii,* respectively. The former method requires a specially designed water-bath and an incubation period of 4 days; it is, on the other hand, probably the more sensitive and accurate of the two and it is especially suitable for the assay of a large number of specimens. The *L. leichmannii* method requires the use of routine apparatus only and the incubation period is shorter. It is probably the method of choice when small batches are to be assayed.

Descriptions of both methods are given below. A few points of general importance common to both methods will be made first.

Glassware. Carry out the assays in Pyrex glass test-tubes*. Clean all glassware before use by washing in a detergent, thoroughly

* Professor Hoffbrand wishes to thank Martine Laulicht and Beverley Jackson for technical help, Mrs M. Evans and Miss J Allaway for secretarial assistance.

* 150 × 16 mm tubes are recommended for the *Euglena* assay and 150 × 19 mm tubes for the *L. leichmannii* assay.

rinsing in running tap-water and then with glass-distilled water.* Finally, autoclave twice in order to remove inhibiting or stimulating contaminants. Plug test-tubes, bottles and pipettes with non-absorbent cotton wool and sterilize in a hot-air oven at 160°C for $1\frac{1}{2}$ h.

Collection of samples. Collect 7–10 ml of blood; separate the serum and store at −20°C until assayed. Sera can be kept frozen for a year or longer. The sera must be separated by an aseptic technique as it is most important that they should be free from bacterial contamination. Ascorbic acid, added to sera to protect serum folate, should not be added to the serum for B_{12} assay since it destroys B_{12}.

If possible, two samples of serum should be provided from each patient and ideally each sample should be assayed on two separate occasions.

The *Lactobacillus leichmannii* method[60,81]

Media

Inoculum broth. Dissolve Bacto-B_{12} Inoculum Broth USP (Difco 0542),32 g/l and Bacto-B_{12} Culture Agar USP (Difco 0541), 47 g/l in water; dispense in 10 ml volumes in 30 ml screw-capped bottles and autoclave for 15 min at 121°C.

Double-strength medium. Dissolve Bacto-B_{12} Assay Medium USP (Difco 0457), 85 g/l in water.

Single-strength medium. Prepare this as required by dilution with water; autoclave for 3 min at 121°C.

Maintenance of organism and preparation of inoculum

Lactobacillus leichmannii (National Collection of Industrial Bacteria 8117[†]) is maintained as a stab in the culture agar and subcultured fortnightly. The sub-culture is

---

* Throughout this chapter, glass-distilled water is implied when water is referred to.
† Torrey Research Station, Aberdeen, Scotland, AB9 9DG.

incubated at 37°C for 24 h and then stored at 4°C. For the preparation of the inoculum, sub-culture the organism into Inoculum Broth and incubate at 37°C for 24 h; then again sub-culture into Inoculum Broth for 18–24 h. On the morning of the assay, sub-culture into another tube of Inoculum Broth for 6–8 h. Then centrifuge the suspension, wash twice in sterile Single Strength Medium, with vigorous shaking to ensure resuspension. Finally, re-suspend in 10 ml of this medium and mix well. Use this suspension for the subsequent inoculations.

Reagents

Sodium cyanide. 1 g/l.

Acetate buffer. 0.4 mol/l, pH 4.6. Dissolve 54.5 g of sodium acetate trihydrate in 900 ml of water; adjust the pH to 4.5 with glacial acetic acid and make up the volume to 1 l with water.

Potassium phosphate. 0.2 mol/l. 34.84 g/l $K_2HPO_4 . 2H_2O$.

Standard solutions. Dilute a solution of pure crystalline vitamin B_{12}, e.g. Cytamen (Glaxo), containing 1 mg/ml, 1 in 10,000 (i.e. 1 in 100 × 1 in 100) in the acetate buffer. Store this stock (containing 100 μg/l B_{12}) under toluene at 4°C; it should be made up freshly at monthly intervals. Immediately before setting up an assay, prepare a Working Standard ($\equiv$100 ng/l B_{12}) by diluting 1 ml of the stock in 1 l of water. Into a series of assay tubes (in triplicate) place increasing volumes of the Working Standard as shown in Table 20.1. Make up the volume in each tube to 5 ml with water and perform the assay as shown in Table 20.1.

Assay procedure

Place 1 ml of serum, 0.5 ml of acetate buffer, 0.05 ml of cyanide solution and 6.95 ml of water in a 30 ml screw-capped bottle and autoclave for 10 min at 115°C. After cooling, add 1.5 ml of the potassium phosphate solution; shake the solution well and filter. (The

Table 20.1 *L. leichmannii* method for vitamin B_{12} assay—standard solutions

Tube No.	1	2	3	4	5	6	7	8	9	10	11
Working standard (ml)	0	0.05	0.1	0.2	0.4	0.6	0.8	1.0	1.2	1.5	0
Water (ml)	5	4.95	4.9	4.8	4.6	4.4	4.2	4.0	3.8	3.5	5
Final B_{12} concentration (ng/l)	0	0.5	1.0	2.0	4.0	6.0	8.0	10.0	12.0	15.0	0 (blank)

serum dilution is now 1 in 10). For the assay, place 0.5, 1.0 and 2.0 ml volumes of the diluted filtrate in assay tubes and make up the volume to 5 ml with water. These represent dilutions of 1 in 200, 1 in 100 and 1 in 50, respectively. If the serum B_{12} concentration is expected to be unusually low or high, use alternative appropriate volumes.

Add 5 ml of Double-Strength Medium to each of the assay tubes; close with aluminium caps and autoclave for 10 min at 115°C. Then inoculate with 1 drop of inoculum, delivered from a 50-dropper Pasteur pipette. Incubate the tubes at 37°C for 20–24 h.

Measure the turbidity against a water blank in a spectrophotometer at 700 nm in 1 cm cuvettes or in a photoelectric colorimeter using a red (e.g. Ilford 204) filter. Subtract the reading of the blank tube, in which growth should be very slight, from the readings given by the test sera and standards. Plot the mean of the three standards at each concentration against their B_{12} content and draw a standard curve on arithmetical graph paper. From this, read the B_{12} content of the test serum extracts and multiply by the original dilution of the serum.

For quality control, sera of known B_{12} content must be included in each assay. It is usual to use samples of low, intermediate and normal values from stock pooled sera from which volumes have been unfrozen for each assay. Recovery experiments with the addition of crystalline B_{12} (e.g. 100 or 200 pg/ml) to known sera are useful additional controls. Assay of some sera in successive assay batches also helps to guarantee reproducibility of the assay.

Normal values.[60] 120–1150 ng/l; 95% range, 170–970 ng/l.

The *Euglena gracilis* method (Anderson's modification of the method of Hutner, Bach and Ross)[3,43]

In this method whole serum is assayed, so no previous extraction of the serum proteins is required. Although serum has an inhibitory effect on the growth of the Euglena, within limits inhibition does not depend on the amount of serum added. In practice, similar conditions for growth can be obtained both in the standards and the test solution by adding trace amounts (0.01 ml) of B_{12}-deficient serum, containing less than 30 ng/l of B_{12}, to the standards.[3]

Water-bath

A suitable design has been described by Anderson.[3] This consists of a specially designed Perspex tank with Perspex racks for holding the assay tubes. It is illuminated from beneath by fluorescent strip lighting. As the Euglena is extremely sensitive to alterations in light intensity, standard and optimal conditions must be aimed at. A light intensity of 50 foot-candles, measured by a Weston Master III Universal Exposure Meter held 17.5 cm above the bottom of the Perspex racks is suitable. The bath is maintained at an optimal temperature of 28.5°C by means of a thermostatically-controlled fan and a constant mixing stirrer. The lighting unit provides the heat.

Preparation of basal (double-strength) medium[43]

Grind the following chemicals together in a mortar:

$FeSO_4(NH_4)_2SO_4 \cdot 6H_2O$, 14.0 g; $ZnSO_4 \cdot 7H_2O$, 4.4 g; $MnSO_4 \cdot H_2O$, 1.55 g; $CuSO_4 \cdot 5H_2O$, 0.31 g; $CoSO_4 \cdot 7H_2O$, 0.48 g; H_3BO_3, 0.57 g; $(NH_4)_6Mo_7O_{24} \cdot 4H_2O$*, 0.64 g; $Na_3VO_4 \cdot 16H_2O$[†], 0.093 g.

After mixing, add 0.22 g of the mixture to the following ingredients:

KH_2PO_4, 3.0 g; $MgSO_4 \cdot 7H_2O$, 4.0 g; L-glutamic acid, 30.0 g; $CaCO_3$, 0.8 g; sucrose, 150.0 g; DL-aspartic acid, 20.0 g; DL-malic acid, 10.0 g; glycine, 25.0 g; ammonium succinate, 6.0 g; thiamine hydrochloride, 0.006 g; p-aminobenzoic acid, 0.0125 g.

Dissolve the ingredients in water; adjust the pH if necessary to 3.6 with NaOH or H_2SO_4 and make the volume up to 5 l with water. Autoclave the medium for 10 min at 115°C and store at 4°C. Prepare Single-Strength Basal Medium from this by adding an equal volume of water.

Culture medium

Place the following substances in a Pyrex test-tube (150 × 16 mm), cover with an aluminium cap and heat at 100°C for 15 min:

Vitamin B_{12} (1 in 100 dilution of stock solution, see below) 0.25 ml ($\equiv$ 1000 pg).
0.4% tryptone   4.75 ml.
Basal (double-strength) Medium   5.0 ml.

Stock culture

Euglena gracilis var. *z* (Culture Collection of Algae, Cambridge University Botany School, Downing Street, Cambridge).

The culture is maintained by weekly subculturing into tubes containing the culture

* Ammonium molybdate.
[†] Sodium vanadate.

medium and incubating in the special water-bath for 5–7 days. The culture should be examined for motility and purity by microscopic observation and plating on a Sabaroud plate. For use, centrifuge a 7-day-old culture at 2000 rpm (600 *g*) and discard the supernatant; wash the deposit twice in sterile Single-Strength Basal Medium and resuspend in 20 ml of the same medium. Shake gently to obtain a homogeneous suspension. This is now ready for use as an inoculum.

B_{12} standards

Dilute 1 ml of pure crystalline B_{12} (Cytamen [Glaxo]), 1 mg/ml, 1 in 250 in water. Add 10 ml of this solution to 90 ml of water ($\equiv$ 400 μg/l B_{12}). Make up a fresh stock solution each month. To obtain a Working Solution ($\equiv$ 40 ng/l), dilute the stock solution 1 in 10 000 (i.e. 1 in 100 × 1 in 100) on the day of the assay.

Preparation of standard B_{12} curve

Set up a series of tubes, as shown in Table 20.2, with 4–6 tubes at each concentration.

Test Sera

Set up the sera in duplicate using a dilution (1 in 20 to 1 in 400) appropriate for the serum (Table 20.3). Normally, sera are set up initially at a 1 in 80 dilution. Quality control sera should be included in each assay batch, as described for the *L. leichmannii* assay (p. 315).

Steam all the tubes (test, controls and standard) for 15 min at 100°C. When cooled to c 20°C, inoculate each tube with 1 drop of the inoculum (see above). Incubate the tubes in the special water-bath for 3–4 days.

Reading of results

At the end of 3–4 days' incubation, shake the tubes. Read the turbidity against a water blank in a 1 cm cuvette in a colorimeter or spectrophotometer at 620 nm. Very occasionally, the supernatant may be turbid due to slight

Table 20.2 Preparation of standard B_{12} curve for the *E. gracilis* assay

Tube No.	1	2	3	4	5	6	7	8	9
B_{12} Working solution (ml)	0	0.05	0.1	0.2	0.4	0.6	0.8	1.0	1.2
B_{12}-deficient serum (diluted 1 in 10) (ml)	0.1	0.1	0.1	0.1	0.1	0.1	0.1	0.1	0.1
Water (ml)	1.9	1.85	1.8	1.7	1.5	1.3	1.1	0.9	0.7
Basal Medium (ml)	2.0	2.0	2.0	2.0	2.0	2.0	2.0	2.0	2.0
Final B_{12} concentration (ng/l)	0	0.5	1.0	2.0	4.0	6.0	8.0	10.0	12.0

Table 20.3 Preparation of test sera for the *E. gracilis* assay

Serum (ml)	0.20	0.10	0.05	0.20 (1 in 10)	0.10 (1 in 10)
Water (ml)	1.80	1.90	1.95	1.80	1.90
Basal Medium (ml)	2.0	2.0	2.0	2.0	2.0
Final concentration of serum	1 in 20	1 in 40	1 in 80	1 in 200	1 in 400

precipitation of protein. If this occurs, measure the turbidity of the supernatant after centrifugation and subtract this figure from the total turbidity to correct for the turbidity of the original fluid.

Plot a standard curve for B_{12} concentration on arithmetic graph paper; interpolate the readings of the serum under test and multiply by the original dilution.

Normal values. 160–925 ng/l; mean 472 ng/l.[3] Using standards to which no B_{12}-deficient serum has been added, the normal mean is a little lower, i.e. 360 ng/l, range 140–980 ng/l.[64]

Effect of drugs on microbiological serum B_{12} assays

Antibiotics in general do not inhibit the growth of *E. gracilis*. Sulphonamides are inhibitory but this can be prevented by adding *p*-aminobenzoic acid to the growth medium. Chlorpromazine was reported to be inhibitory but this has not been confirmed.

On the other hand, *L. leichmannii* is inhibited by penicillins, erythromycin, cotrimoxazole, pyrimethamine, methotrexate, lincomycin, chloramphenicol, cephalothin, tetracycline and rifampicin. Drugs which do not appear to inhibit growth include methicillin, streptomycin, trimethoprim, sulphadimidine and cytotoxics, e.g. chlorambucil, busulphan, 6-mercaptopurine and vincristine.

However, not all studies have given the same findings and inhibition is obviously dose-dependent. For a more complete review of the effects of drugs on the assays, see Chanarin.[20c]

MEASUREMENT OF SERUM VITAMIN B_{12} BY RADIOASSAY

Principle. A known amount of radioactive B_{12} is diluted with non-radioactive B_{12} derived from the patient's serum, the patient's serum having been first heated and acid and cyanide added to give optimum release of B_{12}. An aliquot of the mixture of 'hot' and 'cold' B_{12} is bound to a binding protein and the excess (free) B_{12} is separated from the protein-bound B_{12}, for example, by means of albumin-coated charcoal. The radioactivity in the aliquot attached to the binding protein is measured. This count will be inversely proportional to the patient's initial serum-B_{12} concentration, as the higher the serum-B_{12} level the greater will be the dilution of the radioactive B_{12}, and thus less radioactivity will be attached to the binding protein. Conversely, the lower the patient's serum-B_{12} level, the less the dilution of the radioactive B_{12} and the greater the radioactivity remaining attached to the binding protein. By comparison with measurements of standards of known B_{12} content, the B_{12} content of the serum can be calculated.

Various techniques have been proposed:

1. The binding protein may be intrinsic factor,[53,72] normal human serum,[16,91] human unsaturated transcobalamin 1[74] or chicken serum.[39]

2. The separation of free and bound B_{12} may be brought about by albumin-coated charcoal,[53,71] haemoglobin-coated charcoal,[55] Sephadex gel,[95] DEAE-cellulose[35,88,91] or a solid-phase medium. Recently the need for either pure intrinsic factor or a non-intrinsic factor binder in which binding sites for B_{12} analogues have been blocked has been recognized (see below).

In some two-phase techniques, the patient's serum B_{12} is freed from protein and then completely bound to an excess of the binding protein *before* the addition of excess radioactive B_{12} which saturates the binding protein completely and leaves a proportion of the radioactive B_{12} free.

In general, isotope assays have the advantage over microbiological assays in that they are simpler and because the results can be obtained more rapidly and are unaffected by antibiotics, chemotherapeutic agents and other drugs which may inhibit the living organisms.[84] Some isotope assays, however, tend to give higher results than microbiological assays[64,71] with the sera of certain patients, for example, following partial gastrectomy, in pregnancy, in folate deficiency and when the serum B_{12} values are borderline for other reasons.[71]

In some cases, vitamin-B_{12} deficiency may be missed because of a false normal result.[24] Kolhouse et al suggested that the discrepancy might be caused by the presence in human serum of analogues of B_{12} which bind to proteins other than the pure intrinsic factor (IF) used in the radioassays but which are not microbiologically or physiologically active.[51] Such proteins or 'R' binders (R = rapid electrophoretic mobility) include serum transcobalamin 1 and an R binder in gastric juice and saliva.[18] The presence of these proteins will lead to falsely high serum B_{12} values, depending on the amount of analogue in the serum. B_{12} analogues differ from the cobalamins either by having no nucleotide portion ('cobinamide') or an altered nucleotide portion (e.g. 'cobamides'). Pure IF is thought to bind true B_{12} only and not to bind the analogues. Although some studies have not confirmed the presence of B_{12} analogues in serum[10,80] most recent evidence[22] does support Kolhouse's findings.

On the basis of this suggestion, radioassays for serum B_{12} have been designed either employing pure IF as the binding agent or, alternatively, adding an excess of B_{12} analogues (e.g. cobinamide) to the binding protein in order to block those sites which bind analogues. Pure IF is difficult to prepare and in several kits IF is undoubtedly contaminated by R binder.

Tests have shown, nevertheless, that the use of a blocked binder, or pure IF, results in lower radioassay figures which are more closely correlated with those obtained microbiologically.[7,52] However, in some hands, an increased number of false or low results are being encountered using assays with 'blocked' binders.[54,85] It is recommended, therefore, that if a radioassay is used, it should be one that gives results both in normal subjects and in untreated pernicious anaemia patients similar to those given by microbiological assays. Analysis of the results obtained with commercial kits for serum B_{12} assay have been published.[29,30,66]

DEOXYURIDINE SUPPRESSION TEST

Principle. Pre-incubation of normal bone marrow with an appropriate concentration of deoxyuridine (dU) suppresses the subsequent incorporation of tritiated thymidine (^{3}H-TdR) into DNA. This suppression is less in patients with B_{12} or folate deficiency.[36,50,61] The addition of B_{12} corrects the dU suppression in B_{12} deficiency, The addition of methyl tetrahydrofolate (CH_3 THF) corrects the suppression in folate deficiency, while folinic acid (formyl tetrahydrofolate) corrects the suppression whether there is deficiency of either B_{12} or folate. The test gives a normal result when the cause of megaloblastic anaemia is neither B_{12} nor folate deficiency, nor due to any other defect in thymidylate synthesis.

Materials

Bone marrow. $10-50 \times 10^6$ nucleated cells or 0.5–2.0 ml aspirated marrow, in EDTA. It is preferable to test the marrow freshly but it can be left overnight at 18–25°C without affecting the results significantly. The test may also be performed on phytohaemagglutinin-stimulated lymphocytes.[27]

Blood. 10 ml of heparinized blood.

Reagents

Hanks balanced salt solution (GIBCO Cat. No. 041–4020) ready for use.

KCl, 0.6 mol/l. 4.473 g in 100 ml water.

Phosphate buffered saline, pH 7.4. Add 90 ml of 0.15 mol/l $NaH_2PO_4 . 2H_2O$ (23.4 g/l) and 410 ml of 0.15 mol/l Na_2HO_4 (21.3 g/l) to 500 ml of saline.

Perchloric acid, 0.5 mol/l. Make up 20.8 ml of concentrated perchloric acid to 500 ml with water.

Hydroxocobalamin (Glaxo), 1000 μg/ml.

Folinic acid (calcium leucovorin) (Lederle). 3 mg/ml.

DL 5-methyltetrahydrofolic acid (Sigma), 1 mg. Reconstitute with 0.33 μl saline immediately before use.

Tritiated thymidine TRA 120 (Amersham), 5.0 Ci/mmol. Dilute 0.1 ml in 10 ml of saline (1 μCi/0.2 μmol/100 μl).

Deoxyuridine (Sigma), 100 mmol. Prepare a working solution of 11.4 mg in 0.5 ml of saline. This is stable at 4°C.

Scintillation fluid. e.g. Packard emulsifier scintillator 299™ Cat. No. 6013079.

Method

Whenever possible, except where stated, carry out all procedures at 4°C.

Wash marrow once in buffered Hanks solution, centrifuging at 4°C at 1000 *g* for 5 min.

Lyse the red cells by adding 3 ml of cold water; mix for 30 s; add 1.0 ml of 0.6 mol/l KCl; add 1–2 ml of buffered Hanks solution to maintain the pH, and then centrifuge at 4°C at 1000 *g* for 5 min.

Wash the deposit with buffered Hanks solution, centrifuging at 1000 *g* for 5 min. Discard the supernatant. Repeat the lysing process if a visible button of red cells remains.

Suspend the pellet in 1 ml of Hanks solution, checking that there are no clumps in the final suspension. If necessary, pass the suspension through a 19-gauge needle attached to a 1 ml syringe.

Count the number of cells present and express the results as $\times 10^6$/ml.

Add 1 volume of autologous plasma to 4 volumes of Hanks solution and dilute the cells with this solution to obtain $1-3 \times 10^6$ cells/ml.

Set up the 10-ml plastic centrifuge tubes as shown in Table 20.4.

Transfer the tubes into an ice-bath.

Centrifuge at 1000 *g* for 5 min and discard the supernatant.

Vortex-mix and wash the pellets once with 2.0 ml of cold phosphate buffered saline. Discard the supernatant.

Mix and add 2 ml of the perchloric acid to each pellet.

Mix and stand in the ice-bath for 10 min. Centrifuge and discard the supernatant. If necessary the pellet can be left overnight at this stage.

Mix, add 0.5 ml of the perchloric acid, mix and place the tubes in a water-bath at 80°C for 20 min.

Centrifuge at 18–25°C at 1000 *g* for 5 min.

Transfer 100 μl of the supernatant into counting vials. Add 10 ml of scintillation fluid,

---

Table 20.4 Preparation of assay tubes for the deoxyuridine suppression test

Tubes	Saline	Vitamin B_{12}	Folinic acid	5-methyl-THF	Cells		dU		^{3}H-TdR	
1 & 2	100 μl	—	—	—	1 ml		—		100 μl	
3 & 4	100 μl	—	—	—	1 ml	Mix—incubate	10 μl	Mix—incubate	100 μl	Mix—incubate
5 & 6	—	100 μl	—	—	1 ml	at	10 μl	at	100 μl	at
7 & 8	90 μl	—	10 μl	—	1 ml	37°C 15 min	10 μl	37°C 15 min	100 μl	37°C 1 hour
9 & 10	90 μl	—	—	10 μl	1 ml	with shaking	10 μl	with shaking	100 μl	with shaking
11 & 12	90 μl	—	—	—	1 ml		10 μl		100 μl	

allow to equilibrate for 30 min and count for 200 s.

Calculate % counts per min (cpm) using the counts of ^{3}H-TdR alone (tubes 1 and 2) as 100%.

Results

Deoxyuridine suppression in normal marrow <8%.

Deoxyuridine suppression in megaloblastic marrow >8%.

Correction with added B$_{12}$, in B$_{12}$ deficiency.

Correction with added folinic acid to <5%, in both B$_{12}$ and folate deficiencies.

Correction with added 5 methyl-tetra-hydrofolic acid, in folate deficiency.

There is a partial correction with both B$_{12}$ and 5 methyl-tetrahydrofolic acid in a mixed B$_{12}$ and folate deficiency. In megaloblastic anaemias refractory to B$_{12}$ or folate, e.g. in erythroleukaemia, or drug-induced following 6-mercaptopurine therapy, the result is normal.[93]

INVESTIGATION OF THE ABSORPTION OF VITAMIN B$_{12}$

An important step in the study of a patient suffering from B$_{12}$ deficiency is to establish whether or not he or she has the capacity to absorb the vitamin normally. This is best accomplished with the aid of B$_{12}$ labelled by a radioactive isotope of cobalt. Originally, ^{60}Co was employed but the shorter-lived isotopes, ^{58}Co (half-life 71 days) and ^{57}Co (half-life 270 days), are more suitable. ^{57}Co emits one gamma ray and no particulate energy; it can be used in larger tracer doses than ^{58}Co and is the isotope of choice when a well-type scintillation counter is used. ^{58}Co can be used with all counting methods, but its counting efficiency is low and relatively large amounts must be given to obtain adequate count-rates, especially for measuring blood radioactivity. Labelled cyanocobalamin (B$_{12}$) is used routinely.

Method

Give an oral dose of 1 μg (1 μCi) of ^{57}Co or ^{58}Co-B$_{12}$ in c 100 ml of water to a subject who has fasted overnight; he or she takes no further food for a further 2 h. Prepare a standard form a similar dose of radioactive B$_{12}$ suitably diluted in water.

One (or more) of the procedures outlined below is then adopted to assess the absorption of the test dose. The urinary-excretion test has been recommended by ICSH as being the most convenient and reliable in practice.[46]

If absorption is found to be subnormal, the test is repeated with the simultaneous administration of a source of intrinsic factor, such as 100 mg of a concentrate of hog stomach of known potency. Intrinsic Factor Concentrate capsules are available* in a dose of 10 mg blended with lactose.

Urinary-excretion (Schilling) test[77].

Give 1.0 μg of radioactive B$_{12}$ (^{57}Co or ^{58}Co) by mouth, and at the same time give 1000 μg of non-radioactive hydroxycobalamin intramuscularly (a 'flushing' dose). Collect urine over a 24 h period. Measure the radioactivity of this urine and of a standard. Calculate the percentage dose excreted in the urine as follows:

$$\frac{\text{total cpm in 24 h urine sample}}{\text{cpm in standard } (\equiv \text{test dose})} \times 100.$$

A dual isotope ('Dicopac') kit of free ^{58}Co-B$_{12}$ bound to intrinsic factor is available.[9,69] In this technique 0.25 μg (0.8 μCi) of ^{58}Co-B$_{12}$ is given alone and 0.25 μg (0.5 μCi) of ^{57}Co-B$_{12}$ is given bound to human gastric juice. Standards are provided. The dual isotope test can be used with whole body counting.[11]

Interpretation of results

The normal urinary excretion is >10% of the test dose in the first 24 h; in patients with pernicious anaemia or with B$_{12}$ deficiency associated with

* Radiochemical Centre, Amersham, Bucks.

intestinal malabsorption, the excretion is <5%. This can be increased in pernicious anaemia by the simultaneous administration of a source of intrinsic factor, whereas absorption remains subnormal if the malabsorption is due to an intestinal defect. The second test dose, with intrinsic factor, can be given 48 h after the first, provided that an additional flushing-out injection of 1000 μg is given 24 h after the first oral dose and flushing-out injection. Low results may be found in patients with renal disease, when excretion may be delayed. In such cases urine should be collected for 48 h.

The method is generally reliable (except in renal disease); the results are clear-cut and the technique is simple. The need for large flushing out doses of B_{12} is a disadvantage in that they may interfere with other studies, and the tests depend on a *complete* collection of urine.

With the Dicopac test the results differ from those of separately performed tests, partly because of the difference in size of oral doses and partly because some exchange of isotopes occurs in the combined test.

In normal subjects the quoted figures are: [58]Co (dose alone) 11–28%, [57]Co (dose with intrinsic factor) 12–30%; in pernicious anaemia: [58]Co 0.5–5.5% and [57]Co 14–15%. A ratio of % [57]Co excreted/% [58]Co excreted may be calculated and this may be of value even if the urine collection is incomplete. Normal subjects and patients with intestinal malabsorption give a ratio of 0.7–1.5, whereas patients with pernicious anaemia give ratios >1.8.[9,20,69]

Faecal-excretion method[65]

Give 1 μg of radioactive B_{12} by mouth as described above. Collect all faeces passed in 450 ml waxed cardboard cartons and measure their radioactivity in a GM ring counter, or other large-sample counting system. Continue the collection until less than 2% of the dose appears in a 24 h sample (usually 4–6 days). Calculate the percentage of the dose which has been absorbed as follows:

$$\frac{\text{cpm standard} \ (\equiv \text{test dose}) - \text{cpm faeces}}{\text{cpm standard}} \times 100.$$

Interpretation of results

Normal subjects absorb >0.45 μg of a 1 μg dose. Patients with pernicious anaemia or with B_{12} deficiency associated with intestinal malabsorption absorb <0.30 μg, usually <0.2 μg.[65] As in the Schilling test, these causes of B_{12} deficiency can be distinguished from each other if the test is repeated, adding intrinsic factor to the test dose. Under these conditions patients with pernicious anaemia absorb normal amounts of the test dose, whereas absorption remains subnormal if the malabsorption is due to an intestinal defect.

The test has the advantage that it is one in which the absorption of B_{12} is measured directly; it has the disadvantage that it entails collection of faeces and that incomplete collection may lead to erroneous conclusions. Moreover, the test takes some days to complete. It is less practical as a routine diagnostic procedure than the Schilling test.

Plasma radioactivity[12,32,34,57]

In normal subjects the plasma radioactivity due to absorbed labelled B_{12} increases 3 h after an oral dose and subsequently reaches a peak between 8 h and 12 h when about 2% of the dose will be detected in the plasma of patients with pernicious anaemia unless a source of intrinsic factor has been given with the labelled B_{12}. As the amount of radioactivity in the plasma will be small, it is essential to use B_{12} labelled with [57]Co.

Measurement of plasma radioactivity is suitable as a rapid screening test for the detection of absorption but it is not possible to measure absorption quantitatively with any degree of accuracy, and discrepancies have been reported between the results of this test and the Schilling test in patients with malabsorption.[25,57] Both methods can be combined in a single test with advantage.[57,59]

Method

Give an oral dose of labelled B_{12} (without and subsequently with intrinsic factor) in the morning after an overnight (10 h) fast; give no food or fluid for a further 2 h. Instruct the patient to empty the bladder 6 h after the dose and discard the urine. Then give a flushing injection of 1000 μg of non-radioactive B_{12} and collect all the urine passed during the following 24 h for a Schilling test. Collect 15–20 ml of blood 8 hours after the oral dose for measurement of plasma radioactivity.[25]

Liver and whole-body counting

As most of the B_{12} which is absorbed goes to the liver, it is possible to measure liver radioactivity by a directional scintillation counter placed over the organ after a 1 μg dose of labelled B_{12} has been given by mouth.[37]

The liver counting (hepatic-uptake) method is time-consuming, and low results are of doubtful significance in the presence of liver disease. It is also affected by the positioning of the probe. A whole-body counting method overcomes these disadvantages and can give reliable results, but this requires specialized equipment and, normally, a low-background room.[1,11,67] Initial counting (100% value) is performed 1 h after swallowing the dose. Repeat counting is performed after 7 days to establish how much has been retained. A system has been described which can be used in the absence of a low-background room and fairly accurate measurements of ^{58}Co absorption have been reported.[19]

^{57}Co labelled B_{12} can also be used[86] and a double isotope test has been described.[11,15]

Estimation of intrinsic factor (IF) in gastric juice[6,38]

Direct measurement of the IF content of gastric juice is useful in the diagnosis of pernicious anaemia, particularly when there is associated small intestinal disease which complicates interpretation of B_{12}-absorption studies.

Reagents

Activated albumin-coated charcoal (100 g/l). This is prepared fresh for each as-

say. Heat 2.5 g of charcoal (Norit A)* at 110°C overnight. Suspend in 50 ml of water. Add 6.8 ml of bovine albumin (Stayne) in 50 ml of water, and mix well for 10 s. Activated charcoal is stable for several months.

Vitamin B_{12}. Dilute ^{57}Co-B_{12} (10–20 μCi/μg) with water to a final concentration of 200 μg/l. A solution of non-radioactive cyanocobalamin, e.g. 200 μg/l, can also be used for this dilution in order to conserve radioactive B_{12}.

Collection of gastric juice. This is collected into an ice-cooled container after pentagastrin or maximum histamine stimulation. Add sufficient 5 mol/l NaOH to the gastric juice to obtain a pH of 11.0, stand for 20 min at c 20°C to inactivate peptidases and then neutralize to pH 7.0 with 1 mol/l HCl; measure the volume. It may then be stored at −20°C for some weeks without loss of IF activity.

Method

Set up controls and samples as shown in Table 20.5. Shake the tubes well and incubate at c 20°C for 10 min. Add 0.5 ml of ^{57}Co-B_{12} ($\equiv$100 ng of B_{12}) to each tube. After mixing, again incubate the tubes at c 20°C for 20 min. Add 1 ml of coated-charcoal suspension (100 g/l) to each tube *except* A. Mix well for 10 min; centrifuge the tubes and pipette 3 ml of each supernatant into a counting vial. Measure the radioactivity and correct for background activity.

Calculation

Counts equivalent to 100 ng of B_{12} = A − B. Total B_{12}-binding concentration (u/ml) =

$$\frac{E - C}{A - B} \times 100 \times 2.$$

Specific IF concentration (u/ml)[†] =

$$\frac{(E - B)}{(A - B)} - \frac{(F - D)}{(A - B)} \times 100 \times 2.$$

* Sigma.
† By definition, 1 unit of IF binds 1 ng of B_{12}.

Table 20.5 Preparation of control and sample tubes for estimation of intrinsic factor in gastric juice

Tube	Saline (9 g/l NaCl) (ml)	Gastric Juice (ml)	IFAP-PA* (ml)	Normal serum (ml)
A Control	7.0	0	0	0
B Control	6.0	0	0	0
C Control	5.5	0	0	0.5
D Control	5.5	0	0.5	0
E Sample	5.0	0.5	0	0
F Sample	5.0	0.5	0.5	0

* IFAP-PA = intrinsic-factor-antibody-positive serum from a patient with PA, which should contain 80–100 u of IFA/ml of serum. A = control for counts per 100 ng of B_{12}; B = control for efficiency of absorption by charcoal; C = control for serum effect; D = control for serum containing intrinsic-factor antibody.

* Radiochemical Centre, Amersham, Bucks.

Interpretation

The normal range varies widely from 15 to 115 u/ml with a total secretion per hour of 500 to several thousand units.[20b] In females the concentration is the same as in males, but because of a smaller volume of gastric juice there is only half the total secretion, and never more than 250 u in 1 h. The concentration in pernicious anaemia is usually zero and never more than 10 u/ml.

INTRINSIC-FACTOR ANTIBODIES[20f]

Two types of antibody to intrinsic factor (IF) have been detected in the sera of patients with PA. Type 1 (blocking antibody) prevents the attachment of B_{12} to IF, while Type 11 (precipitating or co-precipitating antibody) prevents the attachment of IF or the IF-B_{12} complex to ileal receptors. Type 1 antibody is present in the serum of 50–60% of cases of PA, Type 11 in about 30%. Only those with Type-1 antibody have Type-11 antibody, so about 40–50% of PA patients have neither antibody in serum. The antibodies occur only with extreme rarity in conditions other than PA; e.g. they have been described in a few patients with thyroid disorders or diabetes mellitus. The gastric juice in PA may also contain IF antibodies, but tests for these are not carried out routinely and will not be described here.

Parietal-cell antibody

This is present in the sera of about 90% of patients with PA but also occurs in other conditions. It is usually detected by an immunofluorescent technique, using human or rat stomach.[73]

Estimation of Type-1 (Blocking) intrinsic-factor antibody

Reagents

Normal gastric juice.
1. Measure the IF content of the gastric juice (see p. 322) and then store the juice in 10–15 ml volumes at −20°C.
2. Determine the B_{12}-binding capacity with ^{57}Co-B_{12} in various dilutions of gastric juice, from undiluted to 1 in 20, using albumin-coated charcoal to remove excess ^{57}Co-B_{12}.
3. Dilute the gastric juice in 9 g/l NaCl (saline) to make up a solution which binds 10–15 ng of ^{57}Co-B_{12} per ml; i.e. a binding capacity of 10–15 u/ml.
Albumin-coated charcoal. 25 g/l (p. 322).
^{57}Co-B_{12}. 15 ng/ml.

Method

Arrange a series of 10-ml conical centrifuge tubes, as shown in Table 20.6, and set up controls and tests. Mix the contents of each

Table 20.6 Preparation of control and sample tubes for estimation of Type 1 intrinsic-factor antibody

Tube	Saline (9 g/l NaCl) (ml)	Serum (ml)	Gastric juice (ml)
A Radioactive control	4.5	0	0
B Supernatant control	2.5	0	0
C Gastric juice control	1.5	0	1.0
D Normal serum control	2.4	0.1	0
E Positive serum control	1.4	0.1	1.0
F Negative serum control	1.4	0.1	1.0
G Test serum	1.4	0.1	1.0

tube. Incubate at c 20°C for 10 min. Add 1 ml of ^{57}Co-B$_{12}$ solution to each tube. Mix well and incubate at c 20°C for 30 min with intermittent mixing at 10-min intervals. Add 2.0 ml of charcoal suspension to each tube *except* A. Mix again and then leave the tubes to stand for 10 min with intermittent mixing. Centrifuge at 1500 *g* for 15 min. Remove 3 ml of the supernatant from each (including A), transfer to counting vials, and measure the radioactivity.

Calculation

Serum IF antibody titre (u/ml) =

$$\frac{(C - B) - (G - D)}{A} \times 15 \times 10.$$

It is important to ensure that the patient has not been given B$_{12}$ (e.g. in a Schilling test) in the week prior to the test, as this will give a false positive result unless the serum is previously absorbed with albumin-coated charcoal to remove free B$_{12}$.

Estimation of Type-11 (precipitating or co-precipitating) intrinsic-factor antibody

Reagents

Barbitone buffer, pH 8.3. 0.04 mol/l sodium diethyl barbitone 100 ml; 0.2 mol/l HCl 6.21 ml. Make up the solution freshly every 4 weeks, and keep at 4°C.

Anhydrous sodium sulphate. 300 g/l and 150 g/l.

Albumin-coated charcoal. See p. 322.

Gastric intrinsic factor/^{57}Co-B$_{12}$ complex. For every 1 ml of normal gastric juice add an excess of ^{57}Co-B$_{12}$, e.g. 200 ng. Leave at c 20°C for 30 min, and then remove excess (free) B$_{12}$ by adding 1 ml of charcoal suspension. After a further 10 min at c 20°C, centrifuge the suspension for 15 min at 1500 *g*; dispense the supernatant in 2-ml volumes and store at 20°C.

Method

Place 0.3 ml of serum, including negative and positive control sera, in 10 ml centrifuge tubes. Add 0.5 ml of barbitone buffer and 1.0 ml of IF/^{57}Co-B$_{12}$ complex, diluted 1 to 5 with saline. Incubate at 37°C for 30 min. Add 2 ml of 300 g/l sodium sulphate, warmed to 37°C. After mixing, incubate for a further 10 min, and then centrifuge the suspensions at 1500 *g* for 15–20 min. Discard the supernatant and add 1 ml of 150 g/l sodium sulphate and centrifuge twice. After discarding the supernatant, add 3.5 ml of saline to each tube to dissolve the precipitate. Place 3-ml volumes from each tube in counting vials and count the radioactivity. A radioactive control containing 1.0 ml of the diluted IF/^{57}Co-B$_{12}$ complex and 2.0 ml of water is also set up and counted.

Interpretation

Precipitating antibodies are indicated by a high count in the precipitate, usually ten times higher than that of the negative controls.

Plasma vitamin-B$_{12}$ binding capacity[20a,38]

The total B$_{12}$ binding capacity (TBBC) of plasma comprises the sum total of the serum B$_{12}$ concentration and the plasma unsaturated binding capacity (UBBC). Estimation of the binding capacities of the individual transcobalamins (TC) 1, 11 and 111 requires column chromatography or other separation techniques, and a number of simple assays have recently been described.[47,79].

Estimation of the UBBC is simple and useful. Because of variable release of TC 1 and TC 111 into serum in vitro by granulocytes, blood should be collected into an anticoagulant mixture of 1 mg of EDTA and 2 mg of sodium fluoride per ml of blood*.[78] If serum is used, this should be separated within 2 h of blood collection.

Materials

^{57}Co-B$_{12}$. Dilute the contents of a vial containing 10 μCi/ml of ^{57}Co (with a specific activity of 15 μCi/μg of B$_{12} \equiv c$ 0.66 μg/ml[†]) in 100 ml of water to give a stock solution of approximtely 6.6 μg/l. On the day of assay, dilute it further to provide a working standard of 2000 ng/l.

Albumin-coated charcoal. See p. 322.

Method

Set up a series of 10 ml conical centrifuge tubes containing plasma or 9 g/l NaCl (saline) as shown in Table 20.7. Add 1 ml of ^{57}Co-B$_{12}$ to each tube. After mixing and incubating at c

Table 20.7 Preparation of tubes for estimation of plasma vitamin-B$_{12}$ binding capacity

Tube	Saline (ml)	Plasma (ml)
A Standard	2.5	0
B Supernatant control	0.5	0
C Test	0	0.5

* Available commercially, e.g. Vacutainer 3200XF42.
† Radiochemical Centre, Amersham, Bucks.

20°C for 30 min, add 2 ml of charcoal suspension to each tube *except* A. After standing for 10 min, centrifuge the tubes at 1500 **g** for 10 min. Pipette 3-ml volumes of the supernatant into counting vials. Measure the radioactivity and correct for background counts.

Calculation

UBBC (ng/l) =

$$\frac{C - B}{A} \times \text{ng/l } ^{57}\text{Co-B}_{12} \times \text{plasma dilution.}$$

If the UBBC is equal to or greater than the amount of ^{57}Co-B$_{12}$ added, the test should be repeated after appropriately diluting the plasma with saline.

Normal range. The normal range for serum UBBC is 670–1200 ng/l; that of plasma collected into EDTA-sodium fluoride is 505–1208 ng/l.[78]

Raised levels are found when the blood granulocyte pool is increased, particularly in chronic granulocytic leukaemia and other myeloproliferative disorders. The TBBC may also be increased in benign conditions associated with an increase in blood granulocyte pool and in patients with liver disease.

ASSAY OF SERUM AND RED-CELL FOLATE

The folate activity of serum is due mainly to the presence of a folic acid co-enzyme, 5-methyltetrahydrofolic acid. Because this compound is a growth requirement for *Lactobacillus casei*, this organism is used for the assay of naturally-occurring folates in serum and in red cells.

The material necessary for the growth of *L. casei* is extremely labile, but it can be protected during assay with ascorbic acid.[26,92] When this precaution is taken, the serum folate (*L. casei*) levels of patients with megaloblastic anaemia due to folate deficiency are lower than in normal subjects and patients with pernicious anaemia.[20d,92]

Serum to which 5 mg/ml of ascorbic acid has been added can be stored at −20°C for up to 2 months. For assay of red-cell folate, whole blood anticoagulated with EDTA can be stored for up to 1 week at 4°C. A lysate is prepared by adding 0.2 ml of whole blood (of known PCV) to 1.8 ml of 10 g/l aqueous ascorbic acid. The lysate can then be stored for up to 5 months at −20°C.[42]

Previously, an extraction procedure[42,92] was recommended, but most laboratories using microbiological methods, including our own, use a whole-serum technique and a chloramphenicol-resistant strain of *L. casei* as assay organism. This method is therefore described in detail.

Chloramphenicol-resistant L. casei method[28,63]

This modified whole-serum assay obviates the need for a strict aseptic technique and facilitates automation; it is easier to carry out and requires less serum than the original extraction method.[41]

Reagents and materials

Glassware. This is prepared as for B_{12} assays.

Water. Use glass-distilled water throughout.

Organism. Chloramphenicol-resistant *Lactobacillus casei* NC1B 10463 (National Collection of Industrial Bacteria*).

Maintain the organism in dried gelatin discs by the method of Stamp.[83] Store in a desiccator over phosphorus pentoxide at 18–25°C. Use a fresh disc for each assay.

Chloramphenicol solutions.

1. 1 mg/ml. Dissolve 100 mg of chloramphenicol base B.P. in 1 ml of absolute ethanol and make up the volume to 100 ml with water.

2. 3 mg/ml. Dissolve 300 mg of chloramphenicol base B.P. in 1 ml of absolute ethanol and make up the volume to 100 ml with water.

Maintenance medium. Bacto Lactobacillus Broth AOAC (Difco 0901–15–3). Suspend 19 g of dehydrated medium in 450 ml of water and boil for 2 min, protected from light. To 180 ml

of broth add 20 ml of 3 mg/ml chloramphenicol solution (300 µg/l). To 270 ml of broth add 30 ml of 1 mg/ml chloramphenicol solution (100 µg/l). Distribute 10-ml volumes into 30 ml screw-capped glass bottles, and autoclave at 121°C for 15 min. Store at 4°C protected from light. Use the broth containing 300 µg chloramphenicol per ml for the stock culture, and subculture the organism for assay in the broth containing 100 µg chloramphenicol per ml.

Propagation of organism

Transfer a disc of dried culture to 10 ml of maintenance medium containing 300 µg/ml chloramphenicol and incubate at 37°C for 48 h. Store the stock culture at 4°C in liquid culture. Subculture every 10–15 days by transferring 1 ml of the stock culture into 10 ml of maintenance medium containing 300 µg chloramphenicol per ml; incubate at 37°C for 48 h.

Assay medium

Prepare Folic Acid Casei Medium Difco 0822 or Dano (Ferrosan of Denmark, marketed by Hopkin & Williams) according to instructions. Protect it from light during heating and use, to avoid destruction of riboflavin and impaired growth of *L. casei*.[5] Dilute the medium to *single strength* (1:1) with water. Add 10 ml of 1 mg/ml chloramphenicol solution and 250 mg of ascorbic acid to each litre of single-strength medium and adjust the pH to 6.4 with 3 mol/l KOH if Dano Medium is used.

Preparation of standards

Dry pteroylglutamic acid (folic acid) powder at 100°C for 2 h.

Stock solution (A) Prepare an aqueous folic acid solution (1 g/l) by bringing the folic acid into solution with a few drops of 0.2 mol/l NaOH. Store this solution at − 20°C.

Solution (B) Dilute the stock solution A l in 100 in 20% ethanol to give a solution of 10 mg/l. Store in a dark bottle at 4°C

Table 20.8 Preparation of standard solutions for the *L. casei* method for assay of serum and red-cell folate

* Folic acid solution C 100 μg/l (ml)	0	0.1	0.2	0.4	0.6	0.8	1.0	1.2	1.4
Water (ml)	5	4.9	4.8	4.6	4.4	4.2	4.0	3.8	3.6
Concentration of standard (μg/l)	0	2.0	4.0	8.0	12.0	16.0	20.0	24.0	28.0

* Store at -20°C; use a fresh set for each assay.

Solution (C) Dilute Solution B l in 100 with water to give a solution of 100 μg/l.

Standard curve. Dilute solution C in water according to Table 20.8.

Controls

Serum folate controls. Store pooled, previously assayed sera with values of approximately 4 and 6 μg/l in *c* 1 ml volumes at -20°C.

Haemolysate with a previously assayed value of approximately 10 μg/l. Store in *c* 1 ml volumes at -20°C.

Recoveries. These are used in some laboratories routinely. Add an equal volume of 12 μg/l standard to the serum control. Add an equal volume of 12 μg/l standard to the red-cell folate control (haemolysate).

Inoculum

On the day before setting up the assay, subculture 1 ml of the stock culture into a bottle of maintenance medium (10 ml) containing 100 μg/ml chloramphenicol and incubate at 37°C for 24 h. On the morning of the assay centrifuge the culture at 1200 **g** for 5 min, discard the supernatant and wash the organism with 20 ml of single-strength medium. Repeat this washing. Centrifuge again, discard the supernatant and reconstitute the culture with 2 ml of single-strength medium. Store this inoculum in liquid nitrogen. For each assay, thaw an ampoule of the culture.

Method

Set up 0.05 ml volumes of the sera or lysates in duplicate and the standards in triplicate,

using 150 $\times$ 16 mm glass tubes. Include one blank for the standards, one for the sera and one for each lysate. Add 0.25 ml of inoculum to 1 l of the assay medium and stir continuously. Add 4.95 ml of inoculated assay medium to each tube. Incubate all the tubes at 37°C for 20–22 h.

Reading the assay

Remove the tubes from the incubator and cool at 4°C for 30 min. Mix in a vortex mixer and read the turbidity at 620 nm in a spectrophotometer, preferably with a flow-through cell and recorder, using the appropriate uninoculated blanks.

Calculation

Plot the absorbance against the folic-acid concentration in μg/l to prepare a standard curve on arithmetic graph paper. Read the serum folate directly from the curve. Calculate the red-cell folate from the readings of serum folate and whole-blood folate (multiplied by the dilution factor of 10) according to the following formula:

$$\text{red-cell folate } (\mu\text{g}/\text{l}) = \frac{\left(\begin{array}{c}\text{whole blood folate} \\ -\text{serum folate}\end{array}\right) \times (1 - \text{PCV})}{\text{PCV}}.$$

Normal range

Serum folate. 3–20 μg/l; mean 10 μg/l.
Red-cell folate. 160–640 μg/l; mean 316 μg/l.

In the series reported by Waters and Mollin,[92] patients with megaloblastic anaemia due to folate deficiency had serum folate levels of <4.0 μg/l and patients with pernicious anaemia had levels of 4.0–17.0 μg/l (mean 16.6 ± 1.1 μg/l).

Other workers have found slightly different normal ranges, e.g. 2.1–28 μg/l; mean 7.8 μg/l),[82] with correspondingly lower levels in megaloblastic anaemia due to folate deficiency. For a full summary of normal ranges see Chanarin.[20d]

Red-cell folate levels correlate well with the severity of folate deficiency as assessed by the degree of anaemia and by blood and bone-marrow morphology. The results are low in B$_{12}$ deficiency and high if the reticulocyte count is raised.[42]

Effect of drugs on the serum folate (L. casei) assay[20d]

The growth of *L. casei* is inhibited by antibiotics that inhibit the growth of *L. leichmannii*. These include penicillin, ampicillin, chloramphenicol, tetracycline, leucomycin, erythromycin, streptomycin, carbenicillin, methicillin, rifampicin and trimethoprim-sulphamethoxazole. Methotrexate and pyrimethamine also inhibit the assay. Alkylating agents do not usually inhibit the assay at conventional doses whereas some antimetabolites do. Drug inhibition will depend on the doses of drugs given as well as on the nature of the drug. Serious inhibition is evident if the growth of the organism is less in the test serum than in the blank (zero folic acid) tube of the standard curve and inhibition can also be detected by assay of a mixture of the patient's serum and a normal serum.

RADIOASSAYS FOR SERUM AND RED CELL FOLATE

The principle of these assays is similar to that of the radioassay for serum B$_{12}$. As for the serum B$_{12}$ assay, a variety of binding proteins (milk protein, lactoglobulin or pig serum) and separation techniques have been used. Moreover, a number of different isotopically labelled folate compounds have been used, including [^{3}H] folic acid, [^{14}C] folic acid, [^{14}C]methyl-THF and [^{75}Se]selenofolate.[48,49,75]

Methyl-THF is not recommended since it is unstable; and binding of folic acid and methyl-THF, the form of folate in serum, is similar at alkaline pH (e.g. pH 9.3). A bewildering variety of kits are available and some of these have recently been evaluated.[30] The results have emphasized the need for each laboratory using one of these kits to establish its own normal range. They also showed in general a lack of precision, the coefficient of variation both within a batch and between batches being greater than 10% and at low levels of folate, often greater than 30%. In general, the kits that perform best for serum folate also perform best for red-cell folate, but red-cell folate seems to be more difficult to estimate by radioassay than serum folate.[68]

TESTS OF FOLIC-ACID ABSORPTION

Folic-acid absorption may be measured following an oral dose of folic acid. The test can be carried out:

1. With non-radioactive folic acid and the subsequent measurement of the folic-acid level in serum by microbiological assay using *Streptococcus faecalis*.[21]

2. With [^{3}H] folic acid,[4] the absorption of which is measured by a procedure analogous to that for radioactive B$_{12}$.

For the latter test the patient is given a 'flushing' dose of 15–30 mg of non-radioactive folic acid by intramuscular injection, followed immediately by an oral dose of 15 μg/l of [^{3}H] folic acid (specific activity 100 μCi/mg). The percentage excreted in the urine in 24 h is estimated by measuring the radioactivity of the urine and of a standard in a liquid scintillation counting system. Tests using natural folate compounds rather than folic acid have been used in some centres but are not widely available.

Therapeutic trials

Deficiency of B$_{12}$ or folate can be distinguished in a patient with megaloblastic anaemia by administering daily physiological doses of one or other vitamin and observing whether there is an appropriate haematological response. To do this trial successfully, the following precautions must be taken:

1. The patient must be in a clinically satisfactory state and anaemia must be fairly severe with the haemoglobin between 60 and 100 g/l. With lower haemoglobin concentrations, the risk of clinical deterioration if there is failure to respond is increased, while with an initial haemoglobin over 100 g/l, the reticulocyte response is difficult to assess.

2. A preliminary period of observation, e.g. 3–4 days, should be allowed to ensure that the patient is not responding to a previously administered haematinic.

3. The megaloblastic anaemia must be uncomplicated, e.g. by iron deficiency, infection, malignancy or any other cause of anaemia.

4. A diet low in B_{12} and folate must be given. In practice, this entails omitting liver and large quantities of fresh vegetables or yeast from the diet.

5. A dose of 1 μg of B_{12} or of 200 μg of folic acid is given daily parenterally. Orally administered vitamins may also produce a satisfactory response if the deficiency is due to nutritional lack of the appropriate vitamin.

6. The trial should be continued for 10 days with one vitamin and daily red-cell and reticulocyte counts carried out. A response is indicated by a clinical improvement and a peak reticulocyte count on the 6th or 7th day.

ESTIMATION OF SERUM IRON

The method to be described for the estimation of serum iron is that recommended by the International Committee for Standardization in Haematology (ICSH).[44] It is an adaptation of the method of Peters et al,[70] and is based on the development of a coloured complex when ferrous iron is treated with bathophenanthroline(4:7-diphenyl-1:10-phenanthroline).

Reagents and materials

Protein precipitant. 100 g/l trichloracetic acid and 30 ml/l thioglycollic acid in 2 mol/l HCl. This solution should be stored in a dark brown bottle; it is stable for 2–3 months.

Chromagen solution. 2 mol/l sodium acetate, containing 250 mg of sulphonated 4:7-diphenyl-1:10-phenanthroline (bathophenanthroline sulphonate; BDH or Sigma).

Iron standard; stock. Dissolve 100 mg of freshly cleaned pure iron wire in 4 ml of 7 mol/l HCl and make up the volume to 1 l with water.

Iron standard; working. Dilute 2 ml of the stock iron standard in 100 ml with water ($\equiv$ 2 mg/l).

Preparation of glassware. It is essential to avoid contamination by iron. Wash all glassware, including reagent bottles, in a detergent solution; soak in 2 mol/l HCl for 24 h and finally rinse in iron-free water.

Iron-free water. Use de-ionized, double distilled water for the preparation of all solutions and for rinsing glassware.

Method

Place 2 ml of serum (free of haemolysis), 2 ml of working iron standard and 2 ml of iron-free water (as a blank), respectively, in three separate iron-free glass test tubes. Add 2 ml of protein precipitant to each. Mix the contents vigorously, e.g. with a vortex mixer, and allow to stand for 5 min. Centrifuge the tube containing the serum to obtain an optically clear supernatant. To 2 ml of this supernatant, and to 2 ml of each of the other mixtures, add 2 ml of the chromagen solution with thorough mixing. After standing for 5 min, measure the absorbance in a spectrophotometer against water at 535 nm.

Calculation

Serum iron (mg/l) =

$$\frac{A^{535} \text{ test} - A^{535} \text{ blank}}{A^{535} \text{ standard} - A^{535} \text{ blank}} \times 2.$$

To convert to μmol/l, multiply the result in mg/l by 18 (i.e. 1000/55.8).

The same procedure can be used in a micromethod.[17] Only 0.1 ml of serum is required when measurement is carried out in an AutoAnalyzer.

Normal range of serum iron. 13–32 μmol/l (0.7–1.8 mg/l).

The serum iron is slightly lower in women than in men. Diurnal variation of up to 30%, with the level lower at night than during the day, has been described.[13a] Characteristically, the serum iron is very low in iron-deficiency anaemia and in infections; it is high in haemochromatosis and following multiple transfusions, and usually high in pernicious anaemia.

IRON-BINDING CAPACITY

In the plasma, iron is bound to a β-globulin (transferrin) and the total iron-binding capacity depends on the concentration of this globulin. The transferrin to which iron is not actually bound is known as the 'unsaturated iron-binding capacity'. The serum-iron concentration plus the unsaturated iron-binding capacity together give the total iron-binding capacity.

Iron-binding capacity is usually measured by adding an excess of iron and measuring the iron retained after the action of a suitable reagent such as light magnesium carbonate, an ion-exchange resin, Hb-coated charcoal or Sephadex G-25. All methods are empirical, and none is completely satisfactory.[33] That described below is fairly reliable.

Estimation of total iron-binding capacity[33,45]

Principle. Excess iron, as ferric chloride, is added to serum. Any iron which does not bind to transferrin is adsorbed on to magnesium carbonate and removed. An iron estimation is then carried out on the iron-saturated serum.

Method

To 2 ml of serum add 4 ml of ferric chloride solution (containing 5 μg of Fe per ml in 5 mmol/l HCl). After standing for 5 min, add 400 mg of light magnesium carbonate, shake well and allow to stand for 30 min. Centrifuge the mixture for at least 15 min at 1500 **g**. Remove 2 ml of the supernatant and treat as serum for an iron estimation, as described above. Multiply the final result by a factor of 3.

Estimation of unsaturated iron-binding capacity

This may be deduced from the total iron-binding capacity and serum iron concentration or measured directly by an isotope method. In the latter method the amount of radioactive iron required to saturate the serum (i.e. the unsaturated iron-binding capacity) is measured directly. In the original method of Bothwell et al[14] ^{59}Fe-ammonium citrate was used and adsorption was carried out on Amberlite resin. The following modification makes use of the same reagents as are used for the estimation of total iron-binding capacity.

Method

Add approximately 5 μCi of ^{59}ferric chloride to 5 ml of a stock solution of stable ferric chloride containing 100 μg of Fe per ml in 0.1 mol/l HCl. Dilute the mixture to 100 ml in water and measure the exact iron content by a chemical method. Add 1 ml of this working solution to 0.05 ml of serum in one tube and to 0.5 ml of water in another tube (standard). After standing for 5 min, add approximately 125 mg of light magnesium carbonate to each tube. Shake the tubes vigorously from time to time over a period of about 2 min, and then centrifuge for at least 15 min at 1500 **g**. Remove 1 ml of the supernatant from each tube for counting the radioactivity.

Calculation

Unsaturated iron-binding capacity (mg/l) =

$$\frac{\text{cpm in test}}{\text{cpm in standard}} \times 2$$

$$\times \text{ Fe concentration (mg/l) in working solution.}$$

Estimation of serum transferrin by immunological methods

In addition to the iron-binding capacity method described above, transferrin in serum may be estimated by direct measurement of the specific protein, using immunoelectrophoresis or immunodiffusion.[33,89,90] These methods have the advantages of sensitivity and specificity. Standard sera and antisera are now available commercially.*

Normal range of transferrin and total iron-binding capacity

In health the serum transferrin is 1.2–2.0 g/l, and 1 mg of transferrin binds 1.4 μg of iron. The normal serum total iron-binding capacity is 45–70 μmol/l (2.5–4.0 mg/l), with about 33% saturation.

The iron-binding capacity is raised in iron-deficiency anaemia, when saturation may be as low as 5% and in pregnancy; it is lower than normal in infections. In haemochromatosis the iron-binding capacity of the serum is typically completely saturated with iron. In hypoproteinaemia both serum iron and iron-binding capacity may be proportionately reduced.

ASSAY OF SERUM FERRITIN

With the recognition that the small quantity of ferritin in human serum (normally 15–350 μg/l) reflects body iron stores, measurement of serum ferritin has been widely adopted as a test for iron deficiency and overload. A number of different assay techniques are described and a variety of commercial kits are available.

The first reliable method to be described was the immunoradiometric (IRMA) assay of Addison et al.[2] The principle of this method is to react radiolabelled antibody with serum ferritin and then to remove excess free antibody with an immunoad-

* Behringwerke (Hoechst).

sorbent. The bound labelled antibody is counted and the counts related to those of standards. This assay is sensitive and does not suffer from the high dose 'hook' effect (see p. 333) of other assays.[58] It requires high quality reagents (immunoabsorbent and ^{125}I-labelled antibody) and is rather tedious since two incubations are necessary and long counting times are needed.

The two-site IRMA assay of Miles et al[62] is easier to perform and is less dependent on reagent quality. In this assay, tubes are first coated with unlabelled antibody to ferritin, the diluted serum to be tested is then added, and finally labelled antibody to ferritin is added in excess; the excess is then removed and the tubes counted. Because of the high dose hook effect (p. 333), sera are assayed in two dilutions. The concentration of serum is also critical and standards are buffered to give a pH and protein concentration similar to that in the serum samples. This assay is particularly sensitive at low serum ferritin concentrations; it uses ^{125}I-labelled antibody.[40,62] Alternative procedures have been described with enzyme labelling of antibody.[87,98]

A further technique for assay of serum ferritin, and that employed in most commercial kits, e.g. those of The Radiochemical Centre, Amersham, Becton and Dickinson, Clinical Assays (Travenol), is the radioimmunoassay. This depends on competition for binding sites on limited amounts of a ferritin-specific antibody between ^{125}I-labelled ferritin and the ferritin in the serum to be assayed. The antibody-bound ferritin can be precipitated by a second antibody to immunoglobulin (e.g. goat anti-rabbit immunoglobulin). The radioimmunoassays are simpler to perform than the IRMA of Addison et al,[2] but are not simpler than the two-site IRMA. They are probably slightly less sensitive than are the IRMAs. Excellent critical reviews of the various assays for serum ferritin have been published.[23,96,97] ICSH is at present developing lyophilized liver ferritin standards. Ferritin prepared from either liver or spleen is suitable as a secondary standard.

Immunoradiometric assay

The method which is recommended is that of Worwood.[98]

Reagents and materials

Ferritin (human spleen).
Immunoadsorbent.
Ferritin antibody (antihuman spleen).
[125]I-ferritin antibody.

The preparation of these reagents requires complicated techniques.[13b,98] They will not be described and it is suggested that training in the preparative techniques be acquired by visiting a laboratory already carrying them out. The method for the assay is described below.

Bicarbonate buffer, pH 9.6. Dissolve 1.72 g Na_2CO_3 and 2.8 g $NaHCO_3$ in 1 l of distilled water.

Protein wash solution. Dissolve 9 g NaCl, 0.1 g thiomersal ($C_2H_5HgS \cdot C_6H_4$-COONa) and 5 g of bovine serum albumin (BSA) in 1 l of distilled water.

Barbitone BSA buffer. See p. 435.

Buffered rabbit serum. Dilute normal rabbit serum (Wellcome Reagents Ltd., rabbit serum inactivated, TC 69) 1 in 20 in barbitone-BSA buffer.

Preparing a control serum

Collect 20 ml of venous blood from 10–12 normal subjects (an equal number of men and women) and separate the serum. Discard any haemolyzed samples. Pool the sera and mix thoroughly. Dispense 0.5 ml volumes in small plastic tubes. These can be stored for up to 2 years at −20°C. For use thaw a vial and dilute 1 in 20 in buffered rabbit serum.

Preparation and storage of a standard ferritin solution

Dilute a sample of human ferritin to approximately 200 μg/l in distilled water. Measure the protein concentration, e.g. by the method of Lowry. This should be 20–50 μg/ml. Then dilute the ferritin solution in barbitone-BSA buffer to obtain a concentration of 10 μg/ml. Deliver 300 μl volumes into polyethylene miniature centrifuge tubes*. Cap tightly and

* Beckman type EET 23 or Walter Sarstedt type 46/6.

store at 4°C. The solution will be stable for about 1 yr. For use, dilute in buffered rabbit serum to 1 μg/ml. Then prepare a range of standard solutions between 0.2 and 100 μg/l.

Preparation of coated tubes

Thaw a vial of ferritin antibody. This solution will remain stable for 1 month at 4°C. Dilute 10 μl in 100 ml of bicarbonate buffer, pH 9.6. This may be kept for 2 weeks at 4°C. Place 200 μl of the diluted solution into each of a batch of miniature centrifuge tubes*. Make sure that any bubbles disappear by tapping the tubes. Place the tubes in the refrigerator, cover with a sheet of paper or plastic film, and leave for 6–24 h. Decant or aspirate and refill with saline three times so as to wash the interior of the tubes. Finally wash once with the protein wash solution, and decant or aspirate through a vacuum pump. Then drain the tubes over absorbent paper for 30 min. The tubes may be stored dry, for up to 2 weeks at 4°C.

Preparation of test sera

Collect venous blood and separate the serum in the usual way. Samples may be stored for a week at 4°C or for 2 yr at −20°C. Plasma obtained from heparinized blood is also suitable.

For assay, dilute 20 μl 1 in 20 in barbitone-BSA buffer and then further dilute part of the solution 1 in 10 in buffered rabbit serum.

Method

Pipette into the coated tubes 200 μl of each of the series of standard solutions, the controls, and the test sera (diluted 1 in 20 and 1 in 200). Dispense the standard solutions and the serum controls in quadruplicate with duplicates at the beginning and end of the batch of tubes, and dispense the sera in duplicate. Also include four tubes with buffered rabbit serum and four tubes without any reagents. Incubate the racks of tubes in the water-bath for 3 h at 37°C. Wash twice with barbitone-BSA buffer, aspirating as described above. Dilute the ^{125}I-antibody in barbitone-BSA buffer so as to give c 5×10^4 cpm/ml. Then add 200 μl of the ^{125}I-antibody to each tube. Leave overnight at 4°C. On the following day wash the tubes twice with barbitone-BSA buffer and measure the radioactivity left in the tubes in a gamma counter.

Calculation

Calculate the mean radioactivity of the set of four tubes for each dilution of the standard and plot against the ferritin concentration on four-cycle semilogarithmic paper. Read concentrations for the serum samples at the two dilutions from the curves. It is essential to assay at two dilutions because of the so-called 'high-dose hook'. This is the *fall* in count rate which occurs at high concentrations of ferritin, as the concentration increases. Check that the count rate for the 1 in 200 diluted serum sample is less than that for the 1 in 20 diluted sample; if this is not the case, the serum should be reassayed at dilutions 1 in 200 and 1 in 2000. The working range of the assay is 0.1–10 μg/l, and if the above condition is satisfied, and if the ferritin concentration in one or both samples falls within this range, calculate the absolute serum ferritin concentration by multiplying by the appropriate dilution.

Rapid assay procedure

Saab et al[76] have described a modification of the assay which makes it possible to complete the process, from tube coating to calculation of results, within one working day.

RADIOIMMUNOASSAY FOR THE MEASUREMENT OF SERUM FERRITIN CONCENTRATION

Most laboratories using RIAs will employ commercial kits. For a laboratory wishing to set up its own RIA, suitable methods include those described in detail by Worwood,[98] Barnett et al,[8] Luxton et al,[56] Wide and Birgegård,[94] Deppe et al,[31] all of which give satisfactory results. In general, these procedures have the advantage of labelling ferritin rather than antibody, but they are tedious to perform and are probably insensitive at low levels.

Interpretation of results

Normal subjects. The serum concentrations probably reflect the amount of iron stored in the tissues and, in general, correlate well with the amount of bone marrow stainable iron. The normal range differs in different countries and at different ages and in males and females. In Britain, the normal male adult range is 39–340 μg/l and in females and children it is 15–140 μg/l. The level is low in iron deficiency (<14 μg/l). It is high in patients with iron overload, whether primary haemochromatosis or secondary, e.g. to blood transfusions for refractory anaemia, with levels up to 20 000 μg/l or more. In primary haemochromatosis, however, 'falsely' normal levels may occur. Raised levels of serum ferritin may also occur in liver diseases, in malignant diseases and in infections and other inflammatory diseases in the absence of iron overload, and when these conditions complicate genuine iron deficiency, a result above 15 μg/l may be found.

A proportion of serum ferritin is glycosylated and this may vary according to the origin of the ferritin, whether derived from reticulo-endothelial or parenchymal cells.

Serum ferritin is composed of a mixture of acidic and basic isoferritins, which may be separated by isoelectric focussing. Its heterogeneity is, however, caused by the presence or absence of sialic acid residues. Serum ferritin is immunologically similar to liver or spleen ferritin in normal subjects and in patients with iron overload. The occurrence of high concentrations of acidic isoferritins has been reported in patients with cancer, but this has not been confirmed; for a review of these aspects see Worwood.[97]

REFERENCES

[1] ADAMS, J. F., CLOW, D. J., ROSS, S. K., BODDY, K., KING, P. and MAHAFFY, M. A. (1972). Factors affecting the absorption of vitamin B$_{12}$. *Clinical Science*, **43**, 233.
[2] ADDISON, G. M., BEAMISH, M. R., HALES, C. N., HODGKINS, M., JACOBS, A. and LLEWELLIN, P. (1972). An

immunoradiometric assay for ferritin in the serum of normal subjects and patients with iron deficiency and iron overload. *Journal of Clinical Pathology*, **25**, 326.

[3] ANDERSON, B. (1964). Investigations into the Euglena method for the assay of vitamin B_{12} in serum. *Journal of Clinical Pathology*, **17**, 14.

[4] ANDERSON, B., BELCHER, E. H., CHANARIN, I. and MOLLIN, D. L. (1960). The urinary and faecal excretion of radioactivity after oral doses of ^{3}H-folic acid. *British Journal of Haematology*, **6**, 439.

[5] ANDERSON, B. B. and COWAN, J. D. (1968). Effect of light on the *Lactobacillus casei* microbiological assay. *Journal of Clinical Pathology*, **21**, 85.

[6] ARDEMAN, S. and CHANARIN, I. (1963). Method for assay of human gastric intrinsic factor and for detection and titration of antibodies against intrinsic factor. *Lancet*, **ii**, 1350.

[7] BAIN, B., BROOM, G. W., WOODSIDE, J., LITWINCZUK, R. A. and WICKRAMASINGHE, S. N. (1982). An assessment of a radioisotopic assay for vitamin B_{12} using an intrinsic factor preparation with R proteins blocked by cobinamide. *Journal of Clinical Pathology*, **35**, 1110.

[8] BARNETT, M. D., GORDON, Y. B., AMESS, J. A. L. and MOLLIN, D. L. (1978). The measurement of ferritin in serum by radioimmunoassay. *Journal of Clinical Pathology*, **31**, 742.

[9] BAYLY, R. J., BELL, T. K. and WATERS, A. (1971). A dual isotope modification of the Schilling test. In *Ergebnisse der klinischem Nuklearmedizin*, p. 911. Schattauer Verlag, Stuttgart.

[10] BEGLEY, J. A. and HALL, C. A. (1981). Forms of vitamin B_{12} in radioisotope dilution assays. *Journal of Clinical Pathology*, **34**, 630.

[11] BODDY, K., MAHAFFY, M. E. and WILL, G. (1972). A double-tracer test of the oral absorption of ^{57}Co- and ^{58}Co-vitamin B_{12} using a whole-body monitor: clinical experience and technical factors. *American Journal of Clinical Nutrition*, **25**, 703.

[12] BOOTH, C. C. and MOLLIN, D. L. (1956). Plasma, tissue and urinary radioactivity after oral administration of ^{56}Co-labelled vitamin B_{12}. *British Journal of Haematology*, **2**, 223.

[13] BOTHWELL, T. H., CHARLTON, R. W., COOK, J. D. and FINCH, C. A. (1979). *Iron Metabolism in Man*. (a) p. 196; (b) p. 376. Blackwell Scientific Publications, Oxford.

[14] BOTHWELL, T.H., JACOBS, P. and KAMENER, R. (1959). The determination of the unsaturated iron-binding capacity of serum using radioactive iron. *South African Journal of Medical Sciences*, **24**, 93.

[15] BRIEDIS, D., McINTYRE, P. A., JUDISCH, J. and WAGNER, H. N. (1973). An evaluation of a dual-isotope method for the measurement of vitamin B_{12} absorption. *Journal of Nuclear Medicine*, **14**, 135.

[16] BRITT, R. P., BOLTON, F. G., CULL, A. C. and SPRAY, G. H. (1969). Experience with a simplified method of radio-isotopic assay of serum vitamin B_{12}. *British Journal of Haematology*, **16**, 457.

[17] BROZOVIĆ, B. and PURCELL, Y (1974). An automated micromethod for measuring iron concentration in serum using thioglycollic acid and bathophenantroline sulphonate. *Journal of Clinical Pathology*, **27**, 222.

[18] BURGER, R. L., MEHLMAN, C. S. and ALLEN, R. H. (1975). Human plasma R-type vitamin B_{12} binding proteins. *Journal of Biological Chemistry*, **250**, 7700.

[19] CALLENDER, S. T., WITTS, L. J., WARNER, G. T. and OLIVER, R. (1966). The use of a simple whole-body counter for haematological investigations. *British Journal of Haematology*, **12**, 276.

[20] CHANARIN, I. (1979). *The Megaloblastic Anaemias*, 2nd edn. (a) p. 59; (b) p. 87; (c) p. 131; (d) p. 190; (e) p. 230; (f) p. 362. Blackwell Scientific Publications, Oxford.

[21] CHANARIN, I., ANDERSON, B. B. and MOLLIN, D. L. (1958). The absorption of folic acid. *British Journal of Haematology*, **4**, 156.

[22] CHANARIN, I. and MUIR, M. (1982). Demonstration of vitamin B_{12} analogues in human sera not detected by microbiological assay. *British Journal of Haematology*, **51**, 171.

[23] COOK, J. D. (1980). Iron methodology: an overview. In *Methods in Hematology. Vol 1: Iron*. Ed. J. D. Cook, p. 1. Churchill Livingstone, Edinburgh.

[24] COOPER, B. A. and WHITEHEAD, V. M. (1978). Evidence that some patients with pernicious anaemia are not recognized by radiodilution assay for cobalamin in serum. *New England Journal of Medicine*, **299**, 816.

[25] COTTRALL, M. F., WELLS, D. G., TROTT, N. G. and RICHARDSON, N. E. G. (1971). Radioactive vitamin B_{12} absorption studies: comparison of the whole-body retention, urinary excretion and eight-hour plasma levels of radioactive vitamin B_{12}. *Blood*, **38**, 604.

[26] COWAN, J. D., HOFFBRAND, A. V. and MOLLIN, D. L. (1966). Effect of serum factors other than folate on the Lactobacillus casei assay. *Lancet*, **i**, 11.

[27] DAS, K. C. and HOFFBRAND, A. V. (1970). Lymphocyte transformation in megaloblastic anaemia: morphology and DNA synthesis. *British Journal of Haematology*, **19**, 459.

[28] DAVIS, R. E., NICOL, D. J. and KELLY, A. (1970). An automated method for the measurement of folate activity. *Journal of Clinical Pathology*, **23**, 47.

[29] DAWSON, D. W., FISH, D. I., FREW, I. D. O., ORTON, B. and ROOME, T. (1981). Vitamin B_{12} quality control trials. *Clinical and Laboratory Haematology*, **3**, 323.

[30] DAWSON, D. W., DELAMORE, I. W., FISH, D. I., FLAHERTY, T. A., GOWENLOCK, A. H., PUNT, L. P., HYDE, K., MACIVER, J. E., THORNTON, J. A. and WATERS, H. M. (1980). An evaluation of commercial radioisotope methods for the determination of folate and vitamin B_{12}. *Journal of Clinical Pathology*, **33**, 234.

[31] DEPPE, W. M., JOUBERT, S. M. and NAIDOO, P. (1978). Radioimmunoassay of serum ferritin. *Journal of Clinical Pathology*, **31**, 872.

[32] DOSCHERHOLMEN, A. and HAGEN, P. S. (1956). Radioactive vitamin B_{12} absorption studies: results of direct measurement of radioactivity in the blood. *Journal of Clinical Investigation*, **35**, 699.

[33] FIELDING, J. (1980). Serum iron binding capacity. In *Methods in Hematology Vol 1: Iron*. Ed. J. D. Cook, p. 25. Churchill Livingstone, Edinburgh.

[34] FINNEY, R. D. and PAYNE, R. W. (1972). Plasma radioactivity following simultaneous oral administration of intrinsic factor-bound and free radioactive vitamin B_{12}. *Acta Haematologica*, **48**, 137.

[35] FRENKEL, E. P., WHITE, J. D., REISCH, J. S. and SHEENAN, R. G. (1973). Comparison of two methods for radioassay of vitamin B_{12} in serum. *Clinical Chemistry*, **19**, 1327.

[36] GANESHAGURU, K. and HOFFBRAND, A. V. (1978). The effect of deoxyuridine, vitamin B_{12}, folate and alcohol on the uptake of thymidine and on the deoxynucleoside triphosphate concentrations in normal and megaloblastic cells. *British Journal of Haematology*, **40**, 29.

[37] GLASS, G. B. J., BOYD, L. J., GELLIN, G. A. and STEPHANSON, L. (1954). Uptake of radioactive vitamin B_{12} by the liver in humans: test for measurement of intestinal

absorption of vitamin B_{12} and intrinsic factor activity. *Archives of Biochemistry and Biophysics*, **51**, 251.

[38] GOTTLIEB, C., LAU, K.-S., WASSERMAN, L. R. and HERBERT, V. (1965). Rapid charcoal assays for intrinsic factor (IF), gastric juice, unsaturated B_{12} binding capacity, antibody to IF and serum unsaturated B_{12} binding capacity. *Blood*, **25**, 6.

[39] GREEN, R., NEWMARK, P. A., MUSSO, A. M. and MOLLIN, D. L. (1974). The use of chicken serum for measurement of serum vitamin B_{12} concentration by radioisotope dilution. Description of method and comparison with microbiological assay results. *British Journal of Haematology*, **27**, 507.

[40] HALLIDAY, J. W., GERA, K. and POWELL, L. W. (1975). Solid phase radioimmunoassay for serum ferritin. *Clinica Chimica Acta*, **58**, 207.

[41] HERBERT, V. (1966). Aseptic addition method for *Lactobacillus casei* assay of folate activity in human serum. *Journal of Clinical Pathology*, **19**, 12.

[42] HOFFBRAND, A. V., NEWCOMBE, B. F. A. and MOLLIN, D. L. (1966). Method of assay of red cell folate activity and the value of the assay as a test for folate deficiency. *Journal of Clinical Pathology*, **19**, 17.

[43] HUTNER, S. H., BACH, M. K. and ROSS, G. I. M. (1956). A sugar-containing basal medium for vitamin B_{12} assay with Euglena; application to body fluids. *Journal of Protozoology*, **3**, 101.

[44] International committee for standardization in haematology (1978). Recommendation for measurement of serum iron in human blood. *British Journal of Haematology*, **38**, 291.

[45] International committee for standardization in haematology (1978). The measurement of total and unsaturated iron-binding capacity in serum. *British Journal of Haematology*, **38**, 281.

[46] International committee for standardization in haematology. (1981). Recommended method for the measurement of vitamin B_{12} absorption. *Journal of Nuclear Medicine*, **22**, 1091.

[47] JACOB, E., WONG, K. T. J. and HERBERT, V. (1977). A simple method for the separate measurement of transcobalamins I, II and III: Normal ranges in serum and plasma in men and women. *Journal of Laboratory and Clinical Medicine*, **89**, 1145.

[48] JALALUDDIN, M., CAMPBELL, J. B., SANHUEZA, J. and SESLER, A. (1977). Observations on the determination of serum and red-cell folate levels by a radiometric assay method. *Clinical Biochemistry*, **10**, 38.

[49] JOHNSON, I., GUILDFORD, H. and ROSE, M. (1977). Measurement of serum folate: experience with ^{75}Se-selenofolate radioassay. *Journal of Clinical Pathology*, **30**, 645.

[50] KILLMANN, S.-A. (1964). Effect of deoxyuridine on incorporation of tritiated thymidine: difference between normoblasts and megaloblasts. *Acta Medica Scandinavica*, **175**, 483.

[51] KOLHOUSE, J. F., KONDO, H., ALLEN, N. C., PODELL, E. and ALLEN, R. H. (1978). Cobalamin analogues are present in human plasma and can mask cobalamin deficiency because current radioisotope dilution assays are not specific for true cobalamin. *New England Journal of Medicine*, **299**, 785.

[52] KUBASIK, N. P., RICOTTA, M. and SINE, H. E. (1980). Commercially supplied binders for plasma cobalamin (vitamin B_{12}), analysis— 'purified' intrinsic factor, 'cobinamide'-blocked R-protein binder, and non-purified intrinsic factor-R protein binder—compared to microbiological assay. *Clinical Chemistry*, **26**, 598.

[53] LAU, K.-S., GOTTLIEB, C., WASSERMAN, L. R. and HERBERT, V. (1963). Measurement of serum vitamin B_{12} level using radioisotope dilution and coated charcoal. *Blood*, **26**, 202.

[54] LEFEBVRE, R. J., VIRJI, A. S. and MERTENS, B. F. (1980). Erroneously low results due to high non-specific binding encountered with a radioassay kit that measures 'true' serum vitamin B_{12}. *American Journal of Clinical Pathology*, **74**, 209.

[55] LIU, Y. K. and SULLIVAN, L. W. (1972). An improved radioisotope dilution assay for serum vitamin B_{12} using hemoglobin-coated charcoal. *Blood*, **39**, 426.

[56] LUXTON, A. N., WALKER, W. H. C., GAULDIE, J., ALI, M. A. M. and PELLETIER, C. (1977). A radioimmunoassay for serum ferritin. *Clinical Chemistry*, **23**, 683.

[57] McINTYRE, P. A. and WAGNER, H. N. (1966). Comparison of the urinary excretion and 8 hour plasma tests for vitamin B_{12} absorption. *Journal of Laboratory and Clinical Medicine*, **68**, 966.

[58] MARCUS, D. M. and ZINBERG, N. (1975). Measurement of serum ferritin by radioimmunoassay: results in normal individuals and patients with breast cancer. *Journal of the National Cancer Institute*, **55**, 791.

[59] MATHAN, V. I., SWARNABAI, S. and BAKER, S. J. (1973). Intestinal absorption of radioactive vitamin B_{12}: a comparison of plasma, faecal and urinary tests. *Indian Journal of Medical Research*, **61**, 714.

[60] MATTHEWS, D. M. (1962). Observations on the estimation of serum vitamin B_{12} using Lactobacillus leichmannii. *Clinical Science*, **22**, 101.

[61] METZ, J., KELLY A., SWETT, V. C., WAXMAN, S. and HERBERT, V. (1968). Deranged DNA synthesis by bone marrow from vitamin B_{12}-deficient humans. *British Journal of Haematology*, **14**, 575.

[62] MILES, L. E. M., LIPSCHITZ, D. A., BIEBER, C. P. and COOK, J. D. (1974). Measurement of serum ferritin by a 2-site immunoradiometric assay. *Analytical Biochemistry*, **61**, 209.

[63] MILLBANK, L., DAVIS, R. E., RAWLINS, M. and WATERS, A. H. (1970). Automation of the assay of folate in serum and whole blood. *Journal of Clinical Pathology*, **23**, 54.

[64] MOLLIN, D. L. (1959). The Megaloblastic Anaemias. In: *Lectures on the Scientific Basis of Medicine 1957–58*, vol. 7, p. 94, Athlone Press, London.

[65] MOLLIN, D. L., BOOTH, C. C. and BAKER, S. H. (1957). The absorption of vitamin B_{12} in control subjects, in Addisonian pernicious anaemia and in the malabsorption syndrome. *British Journal of Haematology*, **3**, 412.

[66] MOLLIN, D. L., HOFFBRAND, A. V., WARD, P. G. and LEWIS, S. M. (1979). Interlaboratory comparisons of serum vitamin B_{12} assays. *Journal of Clinical Pathology*, **33**, 243.

[67] MOLLIN, D. L. and WATERS, A. H. (1968). The study of vitamin B_{12} absorption using labelled cobalamins. Medical Monograph 6. The Radiochemical Centre, Amersham, England.

[68] MORTENSON, E. (1976). Determination of erythrocyte folate by competitive protein binding assay preceded by extraction. *Clinical Chemistry*, **22**, 982.

[69] PAYNE, R. W. and FINNEY, R. D. (1972). An evaluation of the double isotope test in the diagnosis of pernicious anaemia. *Scottish Medical Journal*, **17**, 359.

[70] PETERS, T., GIOVANNIELLO, T. J., APT, L. and ROSS, J. F. (1956). A new method for the determination of serum iron-binding capacity. I. *Journal of Laboratory and Clinical Medicine*, **48**, 274.

[71] RAVEN, J. L., ROBSON, M. B., MORGAN, J. O. and HOFFBRAND, A. V. (1972). Comparison of three methods for measuring vitamin B$_{12}$ in serum: radioisotopic, *Euglena gracilis* and *Lactobacillus leichmannii*. *British Journal of Haematology*, **22**, 21.

[72] RAVEN, J. L., ROBSON, M. B., WALKER, P. L. and BARKHAN, P. (1969). Improved method for measuring vitamin B$_{12}$ in serum using intrinsic factor, ^{57}Co B$_{12}$ and coated charcoal. *Journal of Clinical Pathology*, **22**, 205.

[73] ROITT, I. M. and DONIACH, D. (1972). *W.H.O. Manual of Immunological Techniques*. World Health Organization, Geneva.

[74] ROTHENBERG, S. P. (1968). A radioassay for serum B$_{12}$ using unsaturated transcobalamin I as the B$_{12}$ binding protein. *Blood*, **31**, 44.

[75] RUDZKI, Z., NAZARUK, M. and KIMBER, R. J. (1976). The clinical value of the radioassay of serum folate. *Journal of Laboratory and Clinical Medicine*, **87**, 859.

[76] SAAB, G. A., GREEN, R. and CROSBY, W. H. (1978). Rapid assay for the measurement of serum ferritin. *American Journal of Clinical Pathology*, **70**, 275.

[77] SCHILLING, R. F. (1953). Intrinsic factor studies. II. The effect of gastric juice on the urinary excretion of radioactivity after the oral administration of radioactive vitamin B$_{12}$. *Journal of Laboratory and Clinical Medicine*, **42**, 860.

[78] SCOTT, J. M., BLOOMFIELD, F. J., STEBBINS, R. and HERBERT, V. (1974). Studies on derivation of transcobalamin III from granulocytes. Enhancement by lithium and elimination by fluoride of *in vitro* increments in vitamin B$_{12}$-binding capacity. *Journal of Clinical Investigation*, **53**, 228.

[79] SELHUB, J., RACHMILEWITZ, B. and GROSSWICZ, N. (1976). Fractionation of serum transcobalamins on charged cellulose filters. *Proceedings of the Society of Experimental Biology and Medicine*, **152**, 204.

[80] SOURIAL, N. A. (1981). Use of an improved *E. coli* method for the measurement of cobalamin in serum: comparison with the *E. gracilis* assay results. *Journal of Clinical Pathology*, **34**, 351.

[81] SPRAY, G. H. (1955). An improved method for the rapid estimation of vitamin B$_{12}$ in serum. *Clinical Science*, **14**, 661.

[82] SPRAY, G. H. (1964). Microbiological assay of folic acid activity in human serum. *Journal of Clinical Pathology*, **17**, 660.

[83] STAMP, LORD (1947). The preservation of bacteria by drying. *Journal of General Microbiology*, **1**, 251.

[84] STREETER, A. M., SHUM, H. Y. and O'NEILL, B. J. (1970). The effect of drugs on the microbiological assay of serum folic acid and vitamin B$_{12}$ levels. *Medical Journal of Australia*, **i**, 900.

[85] STURGEON, M. F. (1981). Erroneously low results due to high non-specific binding encountered with a radioassay kit that measures 'true' serum vitamin B$_{12}$. *American Journal of Clinical Pathology*, **75**, 767.

[86] TAIT, C. E. and HESP, R. (1976). Measurement of ^{57}Co-vitamin B$_{12}$ uptake using a static whole-body counter. *British Journal of Radiology*, **49**, 948.

[87] THERIAULT, L. and PAGE, M. (1977). A solid-phase enzyme immunoassay for serum ferritin. *Clinical Chemistry*, **23**, 2142.

[88] TIBBLING, G. (1969). A method for determination of vitamin B$_{12}$ in serum by radioassay. *Clinica Chimica Acta*, **23**, 209.

[89] TSUNG, S. H., ROSENTHAL, W. A. and MILELUSKA, K. A. (1975). Immunological measurement of transferrin compared with chemical measurement of total iron-binding capacity. *Clinical Chemistry*, **21**, 1063.

[90] VON SCHMIDT, H., EBELING, H. and KRAFT, D. (1975) Vergleiche konventionelle Methoden zur Albumin, Transferrin und Coeruloplasmin. Bestimmung in Serum mit immunologishen Referenmethoden. *Zeitschrift fur klinische Chemie und klinische Biochemie*, **13**, 117.

[91] WAGSTAFF, M. and BROUGHTON, A. (1971). A simple routine radioisotopic method for the estimation of serum vitamin B$_{12}$ using DEAE cellulose and human serum binding agent. *British Journal of Haematology*, **21**, 581.

[92] WATERS, A. H. and MOLLIN, D. L. (1961). Studies on the folic acid activity of human serum. *Journal of Clinical Pathology*, **14**, 335.

[93] WICKRAMASINGHE, S. N. and LONGLAND, J. E. (1974). Assessment of deoxyuridine suppression test in diagnosis of vitamin B$_{12}$ or folate deficiency. *British Medical Journal*, **ii**, 148.

[94] WIDE, L. and BIRGEGÄRD, G. A. (1977). A solid phase radioimmunoassay of serum ferritin. *Uppsala Journal of Medical Science*, **82**, 15.

[95] WIDE, L. and KILLANDER, A. (1971). A radiosorbent technique for the assay of serum vitamin B$_{12}$. *Scandinavian Journal of Clinical and Laboratory Investigation*, **27**, 151.

[96] WORWOOD, M. (1979). Serum ferritin. *CRC Critical Reviews in Clinical and Laboratory Sciences*, **10**, 171.

[97] WORWOOD, M. (1980). Serum ferritin. In *Iron and Biochemistry in Medicine II*, Eds. A. Jacobs and M. Worwood. Academic Press, London and New York.

[98] WORWOOD, M. (1981). Serum ferritin. In *Methods in Hematology Vol 1: Iron*. Ed. J. D. Cook, p. 59. Churchill Livingstone, Edinburgh.

21

The human red-cell blood groups and the identification of the blood-group antigens and antibodies
(*Written in collaboration with P. Chipping and E. Lloyd*)

In one short chapter it is impossible to give a detailed survey of the human blood groups. Facts basic to an understanding of blood-group serology will be described here and selected practical techniques will be found in the next chapter. For a more detailed exposition the reader is referred to the monograph of Race and Sanger.[21]

THE HUMAN BLOOD GROUPS

Since Landsteiner's discovery in 1901 that human blood groups existed, a vast body of serological, genetical and more recently biochemical data on red-cell blood-group antigens has been accumulated. At least 100 antigens can be recognized with specific antisera, and 15 well-defined systems of antigens have so far been demonstrated in people of European ancestry. In order of discovery these are ABO, MNSs, P, Rh, Lutheran, Kell, Lewis, Duffy, Kidd, Diego, Yt, Ii, Xg, Dombrock and Colton. Some antigens that are rare in Europeans occur with appreciable frequency in certain racial groups, e.g. Diego (Di^a) in South American Indians, Japanese and Chinese and Sutter (Js^a) in blacks. In addition there are antigens of very high incidence such as Vel, Ge and En^a, as well as 'private' antigens of very low incidence (see p. 345).

Fortunately, for most practical purposes, it is only the ABO and Rh red-cell systems which are of major clinical importance. Others are of less importance because the antigens are weak and/or because the corresponding antibodies are not normally present or occur only following multiple transfusions, or, because when present, they usually react only at low temperatures.

In recent years platelet and leucocyte antigen systems have been identified. These are referred to in Chapter 24. The present chapter deals exclusively with red-cell antigens and their corresponding antibodies. For all practical purposes antibodies against red-cell antigens are immunoglobulins of the IgM or IgG class. IgA antibodies do exist, but they normally occur only in association with IgM or IgG antibodies of the same specificity.

NATURALLY-OCCURRING ANTIBODIES

Some antibodies are found in human sera without there having been any obvious exposure to the corresponding human red-cell antigens. The commonest of these, anti-A and/or anti-B, are found in almost all normal individuals over the age of 6 months, who lack the appropriate A and/or B antigens. Amongst other common naturally-occurring blood-group antibodies are anti-A$_1$, anti-H, anti-P$_1$, anti-Lewis and anti-I. Anti-M and anti-N are common in some parts of Africa, as is anti-i in some parts of New Guinea and South America. Anti-E occurs occasionally.

Substances with chemical groups similar to the A and B antigens are widely distributed in nature, and it is postulated that the naturally-occurring anti-A and anti-B are produced in response to these substances, i.e. they are hetero(xeno)- rather than allo-antibodies. However, it is difficult to accept this explanation for all naturally-occurring antibodies, for some react with antigens which seem to occur only on the red-cell surface, e.g. antigens in the Rh and MN systems. Thus, no satisfactory explanation of naturally-occurring anti-E has yet been provided.

Naturally-occuring antibodies are usually of high mol wt (900 000 daltons) and are IgM in type. Characteristically, they react as 'cold' antibodies, i.e. they react with the appropriate red-cell antigens more strongly at lower temperatures than at 37°C, and may not react at all at 37°C. IgM antibodies usually cause red cells to agglutinate in saline media and have in the past been referred to as 'complete' antibodies. They do not pass through the placental barrier and they cannot, therefore, cause haemolytic disease of the newborn.

IMMUNE ANTIBODIES

Immune antibodies are produced as a direct result of the parenteral introduction of red-cell allo-antigens not possessed by the individual. They can be produced not only by blood transfusion but also by the intramuscular or even intradermal injection of blood and the passage of fetal cells into the mother's circulation during pregnancy.

Immune antibodies are 'warm' in type, i.e. they combine with the appropriate red-cell antigens as readily at 37°C as at lower temperatures. Most Rh antibodies (except for some forms of anti-E) and most Kell, Duffy and Kidd antibodies are immune in origin. When first developed, they may be IgM in type; if so, the IgM molecules are usually rapidly replaced by the IgG type. The latter are smaller (mol wt, 140 000 daltons) than IgM molecules and often do not agglutinate red cells when suspended in saline media. Because of this IgG antibodies used to be called 'incomplete'.

The red-cell surface is normally negatively charged (mainly due to sialic acid residues) and the force of this charge keeps individual cells apart. It is thought that agglutination is brought about by the linkage of red cells by antibodies connecting the antigen sites on one cell to the antigen sites on another. If this is so, the distance between the antigen binding sites on a single antibody molecule will be important. For IgG this seems to be about 12.5–25 nm and in saline media this is insufficient to link the red cells. IgM molecules are larger and the distance between antigen binding sites (30–50 nm) is greater; the antibodies are thus able to link red cells and bring about agglutination in saline. IgG antibodies, nevertheless, often bring

about the agglutination of cells in albumin and other media of high dielectric constant, which, it is thought, dissipate the charge between red cells and thereby allow closer contact. These antibodies also readily cause agglutination of red cells which have been treated with enzymes such as trypsin, bromelin, papain or ficin. These enzymes are thought to remove neuraminic (sialic) acid and part of the protein to which it is attached from the surface of the red cells and in this way to lower the charge between them. Some red-cell antigens, however, are destroyed by treatment with enzymes (e.g. M, N, and Fy^a) and this, in practice, limits their usefulness.

The suspension of red cells in a medium of low ionic strength increases the rate of association of antibody with erythrocyte antigen. This fact is exploited in antibody detection using a low ionic strength medium (LISS) which allows an increase in sensitivity while reducing the necessary incubation period in the indirect antiglobulin test (IAT).[17]

IgG antibodies pass freely through the placenta and can thus cause haemolytic disease of the newborn. IgG levels in the neonate are very similar to those of its mother; the levels of IgM and IgA, on the other hand, will be very low since the infant has to synthesize these for itself.

Complement fixation by anti-red-cell antibodies

Complement (C) is a term used to cover a complex mixture of proteins, the complement components, which are present in all fresh normal sera. These components can be activated in at least two ways:

1. By the so-called classical pathway as the result of antigen–antibody reaction.

2. By the so-called alternative (Pillemer) pathway without antibody being necessarily involved at all.

When antigen–antibody reactions occur on the red cells, the activated complement components are bound to the cell membranes in an ordered sequence, and if the process is completed 'holes' about 9 nm in diameter are produced in the membrane, which lead to the passage of water into the cell and its eventual rupture with the liberation of haemoglobin (lysis). In fact, the process does not always go to completion: nevertheless, in these circumstances the adsorption of complement components can be detected by means of the antiglobulin test, which thus can provide a convenient measure of the lytic potential of an antibody.

Most IgM antibodies bind complement components in the presence of the appropriate red-cell antigens and excess fresh normal human serum, and they sometimes produce lysis in vitro. IgG antibodies bind complement less readily and the lytic potential of this type of antibody, if present at all, can, as a rule, only be demonstrated by the IAT using anti-complement (anti-C) sera. Rh and MN antibodies are the most important of the blood-group antibodies which do not bind detectable amounts of complement; their failure to do so may be related to a peculiarity of the antigen sites, for it applies to both IgM and IgG antisera of these specificities. IgA blood-group antibodies do not as a class seem to bind complement.

The usefulness of using antisera against complement for detecting sub-lytic and sub-agglutinating amounts of IgM and IgG antibodies has been the subject of much discussion, and the ICSH working party on the standardization of antiglobulin reagents recommended that anti-complement as well as anti-IgG components should be present in antiglobulin sera used in routine cross-matching techniques.[11]

THE ABO BLOOD-GROUP SYSTEM

The antigens

There are four main groups, i.e. AB, A, B, and O, based on the presence or absence of two antigens A and B. These antigens are under the control of the A and B genes, which, with a third allelomorphic gene, O, are inherited as simple dominants. (The O gene is thought to be an amorph, and to exert no effect on the basic antigenic structure.) The A and B substances on the red cell are glycosphingolipids. The basic carbohydrate substance is called the H antigen and its formation is controlled by another gene which is separate from the A and B genes. The H antigen is present in virtually all red cells but the amount formed is influenced by the A and B genes. The presence of the A and B genes results in the addition of sugars to the H antigen to produce the A and B antigens: N-acetyl-D-galactosamine in the case of the A gene and D-

galactose in the case of the B gene. The incidence of ABO phenotypes varies in different populations. In the British Caucasian population the frequency of ABO groups is O 46%, A 42%, B 9% and AB 3%.[21]

There are two common sub-groups of the A blood group; slightly more than 20% of group 'A' and group 'AB' subjects belong to group A_2 and group A_2B, respectively, and the remainder belong to group A_1, and group A_1B. The distinction is most conveniently made using the lectin *Dolichos biflorus*. The A_2 gene seems able to convert less H antigen to A than does the A_1 gene. When human red cells are exposed to anti-H they react in the following order of strength: $O > A_2 > A_2B > B > A_1 > A_1B$. Forms weaker than A_2 are occasionally found (called A_3, Ax, Am etc.). Very rarely an individual's red cells are not agglutinated by either anti-A, anti-B or anti-H. These 'Bombay' red cells are thought to be the consequence of homozygosity of the gene *h*, allelomorphic to *H*. These individuals cannot form basic H antigen and thus the A and B antigens cannot be expressed even if the A and B genes are present. Anti-A, anti-B and anti-H, all active at 37°C, are present in their sera.

Secretors and non-secretors

In a white population *c* 80% are secretors. Figures vary from series to series. They have H substance present in the saliva together with A and/or B substances if of the appropriate blood group; *c* 20% are 'non-secretors'. The ability to secrete A, B and H substances is governed by a dominant secretor gene called *Se* (allele *se*) (Table 21.1). A and/or B substances are also present in the serum of group-A, -AB, or -B subjects and in most human tissues as well as in red cells.

The A, B and H antigens are detectable early in fetal life but the antigens are not fully developed on the red cells at birth. Antigens reach 'adult' strength by the age of 1 yr and remain at the same strength throughout life until old age when a slight weakening occurs. Certain pathological conditions affect their strength—thus, in acute leukaemia, a weakening of the A antigen has been described. Rarely, lesions of the large intestine lead to a 'pseudo-B' antigen appearing on the group-A red cells.

Table 21.1 Secretor status

	Genes	Blood group of red cells	ABH antigens present in saliva	Incidence
Secretors (soluble ABH antigens secreted)	*SeSe*	A B	A + H B + H	
	Sese	AB O	A + B + H H	80%
Non-secretors (soluble ABH antigens not secreted)	*sese*	A, B, AB or O	None	20%

Table 21.2 The ABO antigens and antibodies

Blood group	Antigens	Antibodies normally present in serum	Antibodies occasionally present in serum
A_1B	$A + A_1 + B$	None	Anti-H
A_2B	A + B	None	Anti-A (25–30% of sera)
A_1	$A + A_1$	Anti-B	Anti-H
A_2	A	Anti-B	Anti-A_1 (1–2% of sera)
B	B	Anti-A + Anti-A_1	Anti-H
O	None	Anti-A + Anti-A_1 + Anti-B	None

The antibodies

The serum of a group-O person normally contains anti-A and anti-B; that of a group-A person anti-B; that of a group-B person anti-A, and that of a group-AB person neither anti-A nor anti-B (Table 21.2). Anti-A and anti-B are always, to some extent, naturally-occurring and IgM in type. Although they are cold antibodies they still react at 37°C, and potentially dangerous haemolytic reactions result if transfusions are given without regard to ABO groups. IgM and IgG anti-A and anti-B of immune type do occur and are discussed below.

An antibody reacting only with A_1 and A_1B cells, called anti-A_1, is occasionally found in the serum of group-A_2 subjects and not uncommonly in the serum of group-A_2B subjects. An antibody reacting most strongly with O and A_2 cells, probably best referred to as anti-H, is sometimes found in the serum of group-A_1 or -A_1B, or -B subjects (Table 21.2). These two antibodies normally act as cold agglutinins and rarely react with the appropriate red-cell antigens at temperatures over 30°C. They

seldom cause haemolytic reactions in vivo, but they may be a source of confusion in compatibility testing.

In most instances immune anti-A and anti-B develop in response to transfusion of the corresponding red-cell antigens or to pregnancy, but immune anti-A may also be formed following the injection of tetanus toxoid and some vaccines (including pneumococcal vaccines)—recently described as stimulating IgG anti-A.[2] This appears to be due to the use of material bearing antigens similar to human ABO antigens in the production of the vaccines. Immune anti-A and anti-B antibodies, whether IgM or IgG, readily lyse A and B cells, respectively: the naturally-occurring antibodies, on the other hand, cause lysis much less easily. This is of practical importance in selecting group-O donors, as powerfully lytic (i.e. immune) anti-A and anti-B may cause transfusion reactions when whole blood is transfused to group-A, -B or -AB recipients. Group-O donors should therefore always be tested for lytic antibodies, and, if their serum causes marked lysis, the blood should be reserved for group-O recipients only. It is not practical to give a lysis titre which will indicate a 'dangerous universal donor' because the extent to which lysis can be demonstrated depends so much on technique. Immune anti-A and anti-B may be responsible for causing ABO haemolytic disease of the newborn.

THE RHESUS BLOOD-GROUP SYSTEM

The Rhesus (Rh) system was so named because the original antibody was raised by injecting red cells of rhesus monkeys into rabbits and guinea-pigs and testing the resulting sera against human red cells; it has proved to be a system of considerable complexity. The clinical importance of the system is a consequence of the fact that Rh-negative individuals are relatively easily stimulated to form Rh antibodies if transfused with Rh-positive blood or, in the case of pregnant women, if exposed to Rh-positive cells which have leaked through the placenta into the maternal circulation.

The antigens

For most clinical purposes it is sufficient to determine whether a subject is Rh-positive or Rh-negative. This division is made by testing the red cells with the commonest type of Rh antibody, known in the Fisher nomenclature as anti-D. For routine hospital work at least two different anti-D sera should be used. In transfusion centres the red cells of Rh-negative donors are further tested for the presence of the C and E antigens and only those giving negative results, i.e. those which are cde/cde, are called Rh-negative.

Fisher suggested that the Rh antigens were determined by three pairs of allelomorphic genes situated close together on the same chromosome. In his nomenclature the alternative antigens were C or c, D or d, and E or e. Subsequently, less common antigens such as C^w, D^u and e^s have been described. (The C^w and D^u antigens give some but not all the reactions expected of the C and D antigens, respectively.) Most authors, however, now agree with Wiener that the genes determining C, D and E are not separable.

Table 21.3 The Rh genes in order of frequency (Fisher nomenclature) and the corresponding short notations

Fisher	Short notations	Approximate frequency (%)
CDe	R^1	41
cde	r	39
cDE	R^2	14
cDe	R^0	3
C^wDe	R^{1w}	1
cdE	r"	1
Cde	r'	1
CDE	R^z	rare
CdE	r^y	rare

There are racial differences in the distribution of Rh antigens, D^u being commoner in blacks than in Caucasians and e^s being frequent in blacks and rare in Caucasians. The antigens C, c and C^w, D and d, E and e can be combined in twelve ways. These are in order of their frequency: CDe, cde, cDE, cDe, C^wDe, cdE, Cde, CDE, C^wde, CdE, C^wDE and C^wde. In pairs these give rise to 78 combinations (genotypes). The frequencies of the most common genotypes are as follows: CDe/cde (31.7%), CDe/CDe (16.6%), cde/cde (15.1%), CDe/cDE (11.5%), cDE/cde (11.0%), cDe/cde (2.0%) and cDE/cDE (2.0%)—these figures were based on the results of testing 2000 English blood samples.[20] The most commonly used short symbols corresponding with these genotypes are given in Table 21.3.

The antigens seem only to be present on the red cells. They are well developed before birth and can be demonstrated on the red cells of very early fetuses. There is substantial evidence that the Rh antigen is a protein.

Like the ABO blood-group system, the final antigens seem to be influenced by at least two pairs of gene complexes which are inherited independently. One pair is the CDE complex already mentioned and the other is the LW complex. The LW gene, which is seldom absent, produces the antigen LW which reacts with true anti-Rhesus serum, i.e. the serum of guinea pigs immunized against monkey red cells.[12] Although it is now known that this antigen is not the same as that which reacts with human anti-D sera, the products of these two pairs of genes are obviously closely related. Since it is too late to change the name of the whole system, the 'true' anti-Rhesus antigen is called LW in honour of Landsteiner and Wiener.

The antibodies

Fisher's nomenclature is convenient when applied to Rh antibodies, and antibodies acting against all the Rh antigens except d, have been described. These are called anti-D, anti-C, anti-E etc.

The importance of the system lies in the fact that D-negative individuals (d/d) are relatively easily stimulated to form immune anti-D antibodies. In men these antibodies are only harmful if D-positive blood is transfused, but in women, since the antibodies are often IgG in type, they can also cause haemolytic disease of the newborn (HDN). Except for some forms of anti-E, naturally-occurring anti-Rh antibodies are seldom found.

An immune Rh antibody (whether IgM or IgG) is often only demonstrable at first by the use of enzyme-treated red cells. However, the IAT provides a more useful way of predicting the development of HDN, because this technique demonstrates most sensitively the all-important IgG antibodies. Rhesus HDN is most commonly the result of the destruction of an infant's D-positive red cells by IgG anti-D antibodies. This is discussed more fully on p. 373.

THE MNSs BLOOD-GROUP SYSTEM

In England c 28% of people are group M, 50% group MN and 22% group N; 55% are S-positive and 45% S-negative. In this country, human anti-M and anti-N sera are rarely met with but they are not unknown. Most seem to be naturally occurring and act as cold antibodies; however, immune antibodies may be formed. Both types of antibodies show marked dosage effects, e.g. anti-M may react strongly with homozygous MM cells but fail to react with heterozygous MN cells. Anti-S is also a rarity, but when formed it is usually immune in type and appears in the sera of patients who have had many blood transfusions; even so, it is often best detected by the IAT at temperatures below 37°C. Very rarely anti-S may cause HDN. Anti-s is extremely rare.

Anti-M, anti-N and anti-S are quite common in some parts of Africa. In Ibadan, Nigeria, for instance, they were found, active at temperatures over 22°C, in 1.9% of all serum samples received[22]: the antibodies mainly had anti-N specificity and

although they appeared to be naturally-occurring, they occasionally reacted up to 37°C.

Rarely, red cells from blacks fail to be agglutinated by anti-S or anti-s sera. Of these, approximately four out of five also lack the U antigen, their genotype being designated S^uS^u.

MN antigens are on the major sialoglycoprotein (glycophorin A or PAS-1) of the red cell membrane;[1] S, s and N activity are expressed on a minor sialoglycoprotein (glycophorin B; PAS-3). The M and N antigens are destroyed by proteolytic enzymes.

THE P BLOOD-GROUP SYSTEM

The antigens and antibodies of the P system are summarized in Table 21.4.

In P_1 subjects there is considerable variation in the strength of the P_1 antigen. People of genotype pp (phenotype p) appear to represent the 'Bombay' type of the P system. Anti-P is found in the serum of most P_2 subjects; it is, however, a cold antibody which usually has a low thermal amplitude and seldom reacts at temperatures over 30°C, thus rarely leading to transfusion reactions. The relationship between the Donath-Landsteiner autoantibody and the P blood-group system is well known and is discussed in Chapter 23.

THE LUTHERAN BLOOD-GROUP SYSTEM

About 8% of English blood samples are Lutheran-positive (Lu^a+) and 92% are Lutheran-negative (Lu^a−). Anti-Lu^a is not infrequently formed after the transfusion of Lu^a + blood to Lu^a− persons but it is often an extremely transient antibody. It usually reacts best as an in-saline agglutinin at 20°C

Table 21.4 The P blood-group system

Phenotype	Incidence	Antigens on red cells	Antibodies in serum
P_1	75–80%	P_1P	None
P_2	20–25%	P	Anti-P_1
P_1^k	Very rare	P_1P^k	Anti-P
P_2^k	Very rare	P^k	Anti-P
p	Very rare	None	Anti-P, Anti-P_1 and Anti-P^k (Anti-Tj^a)

Table 21.5 The Lewis blood-group system

Genes	Blood-group substances in saliva			Blood-group substances in serum		Red cells	Frequency %
	Le^a	Le^b	ABH	Le^a	Le^b		
Se Le	+	+	+	Trace	+	Le(a − b +)	73%
se Le	+	−	−	+	−	Le(a + b −)	22%
Se le	−	−	+	−	−	Le(a − b −)	4%
se le	−	−	−	−	−	Le(a − b −)	1%

and the antigen may be destroyed by enzyme treatment. Anti-Lu^a gives a distinct type of agglutination in which many of the cells remain free. Anti-Lu^b is rare and is thought to be mainly IgA in type.

THE KELL BLOOD-GROUP SYSTEM

About 9% of the population in Southern England are Kell-positive (genotype *Kk or KK*) the remainder being Kell-negative (*kk*). An antibody (anti-Cellano) against the alternate allele (*k*) agglutinates all Kell-negative and most Kell-positive blood samples.

The Kell antigen is a powerfully immunogenic antigen, and anti-K has been quite frequently identified as an immune antibody formed as a result of pregnancies or transfusions. Most reported examples are IgG and have often been complement-binding; they are best detected by the IAT. Anti-K may cause severe transfusion reactions and HDN.

The Kell system has by now been greatly expanded; it includes the antigen Js^a which is racially distinctive, being found in 20% of blacks but not in Caucasians.

THE LEWIS BLOOD-GROUP

The Lewis system is best thought of as a system of tissue antigens, the expression of the group on the red cells being only secondary to antigens in the plasma. Lewis, secretor and ABH genes act closely together although they are not genetically linked. If the Lewis groups are determined by testing saliva for the ABH and the Le^a and Le^b antigens, four different combinations are found:

1. All three antigens (Le^a, Le^b and ABH) are present.

2. Only the Le^a antigen is present.
3. Only the ABH antigens are present.
4. None of the antigens is present.

The first group (1) have trace amounts of Le^a antigen and large amouns of Le^b antigen in their plasma and their red cells group as Le(a − b+)— they are secretors of ABH substances. The second group (2) have large amounts of Le^a antigen in their plasma and the red cells group as Le(a+ b−)—they are all non-secretors of ABH substances. Groups (3) and (4) have no Lewis antigens in their plasma and their red cells group as Le (a− b−) (Table 21.5).

Anti-Lewis antibodies are naturally-occurring and IgM. They can be found in about 1% of unselected serum samples from Caucasians. Subjects who make these antibodies usually have red cells which group as Le(a− b−) and in countries where this group is frequent Lewis antibodies may be very common indeed. In Nigeria, for example, about 40% of the population are Le(a− b−) and Lewis antibodies, reacting at 22°C or over, are found in 10% of unselected serum samples.

Lewis antibodies are potentially lytic and often lyse enzyme-treated cells. They are cold antibodies but many have a high thermal amplitude and often bind sufficient sublytic amounts of complement at 37°C to give a positive IAT with 'broad-spectrum' antisera.

Lewis antibodies can cause severe transfusion reactions associated with intravascular haemolysis. These reactions are uncommon because much of the antibody in the recipient's plasma will be neutralized by Lewis substance contained in the donor's plasma. The deliberate neutralization of an antibody by Le^a and Le^b substances enables large volumes of potentially incompatible blood to be transfused.[16] Thus, a patient whose red cells were grouped as Le(a − b −) and who had anti-Le^a

and anti-Le^b in his plasma was given Le^a and Le^b substances to neutralize these antibodies and prepare him for open heart surgery. At operation he was given 34 bottles of Le(a−b+) blood and 13 bottles of Le(a−b−) blood without mishap. Within a few days of the operation the transfused red cells had become Le(a−b−), illustrating that the Lewis antigens on the red cells are absorbed from the plasma and are not primarily red-cell antigens.

THE DUFFY BLOOD-GROUP SYSTEM

At least two allelomorphic genes exist, Fy^a and Fy^b. In England about 66% of people are Duffy-positive, Fy(a+) (49% Fy^aFy^b and 17% Fy^aFy^a), and 34% are Duffy-negative, Fy(a−)(Fy^bFy^b). About 68% of American blacks have the phenotype Fy(a−b−), their cells reacting neither with anti-Fy^a nor with anti-Fy^b. It is of interest that the Fy(a−b−) genotype appears to confer resistance to penetration by the malaria parasite *Plasmodium vivax*.

Many examples of anti-Fy^a are known, most being found in patients who have received repeated transfusions. The antibodies are usually IgG and are thus most readily detected by the IAT. Treatment of the red cells with enzymes seems to destroy the antigen. Anti-Fy^a binds complement well and can cause severe transfusion reactions; it has often been implicated in delayed transfusion reactions. Anti-Fy^b is very rare, and the few antibodies that have been studied have been of the IgG type.

THE KIDD BLOOD-GROUP SYSTEM

Two allelomorphic genes, Jk^a and Jk^b, have been identified. In England approximately 75% of the population are Kidd-positive, Jk(a+)(Jk^aJk^a, 25%; Jk^aJk^b, 50%) and 25% Kidd-negative, Jk(a−)(Jk^bJk^b). The antibodies are always immune and while they may cause agglutination in saline, they are more reliably detected by the IAT. The reaction is enhanced by enzyme-treatment of the red cells and a stronger IAT may be obtained by using these cells. Anti-Jk^a usually binds complement very well and may show dosage effects. It has been the cause of severe transfusion reactions.

OTHER BLOOD-GROUP SYSTEMS

Diego

The antigen Di^a seems almost confined to people of the Mongoloid race; it is rare in blacks and Caucasians. Anti-Di^a is uncommon, and the antibodies studied have so far been of the immune type. Anti-Di^b has also been described.

I/i

The Ii blood group system is unusual in that the I antigen cannot be regarded as being controlled by a gene allelomorphic to that controlling the i antigen. In most adults the red cells are agglutinated strongly by anti-I and only weakly by anti-i. The red cells from cord blood samples give the opposite results with the two antisera— such red cells are known as 'cord i'. As the child matures there is an increasing agglutinability with anti-I and decreasing agglutinability with anti-i, so that by about 18 months of age, they give the expected reactions of adult cells (Fig. 21.1).

Unlike the blood-group antibodies so far described, antibodies to the I/i antigens are typically cold auto-antibodies. Almost all normal adults have a low titre, low thermal amplitude anti-I in their serum (titre <32 at 4°C; upper limit of activity

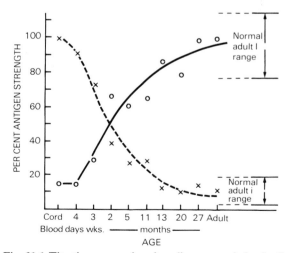

Fig. 21.1 Titration scores given by saline-suspended red cells of infants of selected ages calculated as a percentage of the scores of normal adult (I) and normal cord (i) blood. I titration scores = ○; i titration scores = X. (From W. L. Marsh [1961], British Journal of Haematology, 7, 200. By kind permission of the authors and the publishers).

15°C). High titre anti-I is found in patients suffering from chronic cold haemagglutinin disease and may develop transiently following infection with *Mycoplasma pneumoniae* (see Chapter 23).

'Private' blood groups

There are antigens of very low frequency which have been for the most part demonstrated in single families only. Usually they have been discovered as the result of finding an unusual antibody in the sera of recipients of blood transfusion or of pregnant women, which, while reacting with antigens on the red cells of the donor (or husband) and their immediate relatives, fails to react with many hundreds of other blood samples chosen at random. These 'private' blood groups have, in most cases, been named after the family involved, e.g. By (Batty), Bx (Box), Levay, Sw (Swann), Wb (Webb) and Wr (Wright).

From the practical point of view, 'private' antibodies are unimportant in blood transfusion practice as it is easy to find compatible blood for patients who have formed antibodies against rare antigens. On the other hand, although a rare event, the possibility of any antibody being a 'private' one should not be overlooked and it is important, therefore, in attempting to identify an antibody always to include in the panel of test cells those of the actual blood donor(s) (or of the husband) who may have been responsible for the immunization.

General points of serological technique

Collection and storage of blood samples

Venous blood is desirable for blood-grouping purposes and 5–10 ml of blood should be taken and allowed to clot at room temperature in a sterile glass bottle. This will provide serum and cells. If serum is required urgently, the specimen may be placed in a 37°C water-bath and centrifuged as soon as the clot can be seen to have started to retract.

If necessary, the specimen, after clotting, can be stored undisturbed at 4°C overnight. If the red cells are to be kept longer than this, it is desirable to add the blood, after withdrawal, to a one-quarter volume of sterile ACD or CPD anticoagulant. If kept sterile, the red cells will be found to react well with most antibodies even after 2–3 weeks' storage. Red cells should not be washed and suspended in saline until just before use.

Red-cell suspensions

A 2% suspension of washed red cells in phosphate buffered saline, pH 7.0, is generally suitable for agglutination tests in tubes. Unless otherwise specified, throughout this text 'saline' or 'buffered saline' refers to 9 g/l NaCl buffered to pH 7.0 (see Appendix, p. 436).

Preservation of red cells in glycerol

Red cells can be stored at −20°C for up to 2 yr if glycerol at a final concentration of 3.0 mol/l is added.

Add 4 volumes of glycerol (e.g. BDH 'Analar') to 6 volumes of 50 g/l trisodium citrate. Centrifuge ACD or CPD blood at 1200–1500 **g** for 10 min. Remove the supernatant plasma and add, drop by drop with continuous mixing, the glycerol-citrate solution in a volume equal to that of the packed red cells. Then freeze the mixture at −20°C in small (e.g. 0.5 ml) volumes. For use, warm a vial of glycerol-frozen red cells in a 37°C water-bath and wash the cells successively with 16%, 12%, 8% and 2% glycerol in 50 g/l trisodium citrate or dialyse them at room temperature for 1 h in a beaker containing at least 500 ml of saline. Then wash the cells recovered by either method in saline until the supernatant contains no visible haemoglobin. Such cells appear to react in serological tests almost as well as fresh red cells.

Preservation of red cells in liquid nitrogen

The antigens of red cells stored in liquid nitrogen at −196°C appear to be well preserved over a period of years. The storage method of Huntsman et al[10] is satisfactory for the preservation of small volumes of cells for laboratory use.

To 2 volumes of EDTA blood add 1 volume of 400 g/l sucrose and deliver the mixture, drop by drop, into a vacuum flask containing liquid nitrogen. Adjust the drop-rate until each drop of blood freezes separately. Collect the individual frozen drops from the bottom of the flask with a pre-cooled long-handled spoon, transfer to a pre-cooled pillbox and store in the liquid nitrogen or in the vapour. To thaw the red cells place about eight individual drops in 5 ml of 10 g/l NaCl pre-warmed to 45°C and shake vigorously. 7–10% of the cells lyse, the percentage lysing being approximately the same with cells stored for up to 2 yr. For use, centrifuge the red cells and then wash them at least twice in saline.

Panels of red cells

A panel of red cells of known genotype is essential for the identification of allo-antibodies. A panel of group-O cells, the red-cell antigens of which differ considerably, such that they give clearly negative or positive reactions with almost all the important antibodies, may be purchased from commercial sources or may be supplied in the United Kingdom by a Blood Transfusion Centre. It is, however, convenient to group and genotype as far as is practical all members of the laboratory staff and to select six to eight group-O subjects whose red-cell antigens fulfil the above criteria.

For screening purposes it is useful to use a mixture of two or three group-O subjects whose red cells so differ from each other that all the common antigens are represented. Samples taken into ACD or CPD will keep 2–3 weeks at 4°C. Care must be taken to avoid too much dilution of any antigen, i.e. the pool used as a screening mixture must be a small one.

Storage of sera

Grouping and other sera are best stored frozen at −20°C in 1–2 ml volumes in separate glass or plastic vials. Repeated thawing of a sample is harmful. If the sera are stored at −20°C, no precautions as to sterility are necessary. At 4°C sterility is essential; if this can be maintained, it will be found that the sera will retain their potency for months.

Complement deteriorates quickly on storage, but sera separated from blood as quickly as possible and stored at −20°C retain most of their complement activity for 1–2 weeks. For compatibility tests, samples of serum should be separated from the red cells as soon as possible and stored at −20°C until used, as the content of complement may be important for the detection of some antibodies.

Use of enzyme-treated cells

Enzyme-treated red cells have proved to be valuable reagents in the detection and investigation of auto- and allo-antibodies. Papain, trypsin, ficin and bromelin have all been used in antibody investigation. Enzyme treatment is known to increase the avidity of both IgM and IgG antibodies. The receptors of some blood-group antigens, however, may be inactivated by enzyme-treatment, e.g. M, N, Fy^a and Pr.

Löw's method for the preparation and use of papain solutions[13]

A 1% solution of activated papain is made as follows:

Grind 2 g of papain (Merck) in a mortar in 100 ml of Sörensen's phosphate buffer, pH 5.4 (p. 436). Centrifuge for 10 min and add 10ml of 0.5 mol/l cysteine hydrochloride to the supernatant to activate the enzyme. Dilute the solution to 200 ml with the phosphate buffer and incubate for 1 h at 37°C. Dispense the enzyme in small volumes (e.g. 0.1–0.2 ml); it will keep satisfactorily for many months at −20°C, but once a tube is unfrozen, any of the solution not immediately used should be discarded.

Addition of papain to the serum. Add equal volumes of the papain solution to the serum immediately before the addition of the cells.

This method has the advantage of speed as no pre-treatment of the red cells is required; it has the disadvantage of being relatively insensitive compared with methods in which the red cells are pre-treated with the enzyme before being added to the serum. If papain, prepared by this technique is to be used with serum dilutions, the solution must be buffered to pH 7.0 before use by the addition of a small volume of 0.2 mol/l NaOH or it will lyse the red cells.

Use of red cells pre-treated with papain[9]

Add 1 volume of 1% papain (activated as described above) to 9 volumes of Sörensen's phosphate buffer, pH 7.0 (p. 436). Incubate at 37°C equal volumes of the freshly diluted papain and packed washed red cells of appropriate group for a time which must be determined for each batch of papain and is normally 15–30 min. After incubation, wash the cells in two changes of saline, pH 7.0, then dilute as required.

Preparation of trypsin solution[18]

Crystalline trypsin (Armour) is satisfactory. Make a 1% solution by dissolving a few mg of the powder in an appropriate volume of 0.05 mol/l HCl. The solution keeps for a week or more at 4°C. Make a 0.1% solution by diluting 1 volume of the stock solution with 9 volumes of Sörensen's buffer, pH 7.8.

Trypsinization of red cells. Add 0.2 ml of packed washed red cells of appropriate group to 1 ml of the 0.1% trypsin solution. Incubate the mixture for 1 h at 37°C and wash the trypsinized cells in at least two changes of saline, pH 7.0.

Preparation of ficin solution

Dissolve 25 mg of ficin (Merck) in 2.5 ml of Sörensen's phosphate buffer, pH 7.0 (p. 436). The solution is stable for at least 2 weeks when stored at 4°C. At −20°C it retains its potency for long periods.

Ficinization of red cells. Dilute 1 volume of the stock 1% ficin with 9 volumes of buffer. Add 1 volume of the diluted ficin solution to 1 volume of washed packed red cells, mix the suspension and allow to stand for 15 min at 37°C. Re-wash the red cells in at least two changes of saline, pH 7.0. The enzyme-treated cells can be stored at 4°C for up to 12 h before use.

If the ficin-treated cells are to be used in an antiglobulin reaction, half the concentration of ficin must be used.

Preparation of bromelin solution[19]

Prepare a 0.5% solution by dissolving the bromelin powder (Light and Co. Ltd.) in a mixture of 9 volumes of saline and 1 volume of Sörensen's phosphate buffer, pH 5.4 (p. 436). Store the solution in 0.5–1.0 ml volumes at −20°C, at which temperature it will keep for months. As preservatives, add 0.1% sodium azide and 0.05% Actidione (a fungicide). Add the bromelin, as papain is added in Löw's technique, to the serum just before the addition of the red cells. There is no need to pre-treat the red cells with the enzyme.

Agglutination of red cells by antibody: the basic method

Add 1 volume of the red-cell suspension to 1 volume of serum or serum dilution in a disposable plastic tube or glass tube. Mix well and leave undisturbed for the appropriate time (see below). Alternatively, when a rapid result is required, add 1 volume of the red-cell suspension to 1 volume of serum or serum dilution previously placed on an opalescent tile. We use this method in carrying out antiglobulin tests.

Tubes. For screening agglutination tests use medium-sized (e.g. 75 × 8 mm) disposable plastic tubes. Similar tubes should be used for lysis tests when it is essential to have a relatively deep layer of serum to look through, if small amounts of lysis are to be detected. The level of the fluid must rise well above the concave bottom of the tubes.

Glass tubes of closely similar size are available and are satisfactory. They should always be used if the contents are to be heated to 50°C or higher or if organic solvents are being used. Glass tubes, however, are difficult to clean satisfactorily, particularly if of small bore, and methods such as those given in the Appendix (p. 437) should be followed in detail.

Temperature and time of exposure of red cells to antibody

In blood-grouping work tube tests are generally done at 37°C and/or room temperature. There is some advantage in using a 20°C water-bath rather than relying on 'room temperature' which in different countries and seasons may vary from 15°C (or less) to 30°C (or more).

Agglutination reactions carried out in tubes are not usually read until 1–2 h have elapsed. Strong agglutination will, however, be obvious much sooner than this. Agglutination can be read after only 5–10 min incubation if the suspension of cells in serum is centrifuged.

Reading results of agglutination tests

Agglutination may be read macroscopically, as in antiglobulin tests carried out on tiles; macroscopically in tube tests, as in reading the results of ABO grouping or an auto-antibody screening test (p. 394); or microscopically, as in all other tests.

Tile tests

Agglutination is scored in increasing strength from 0 to 5. It is useful to record the time in minutes when the first sign of agglutination appears. Agglutination which appears immediately on mixing is given a score of 5; that which appears after 1 min has passed is given a score of 4 and so on; at the end of 5 min the tile as a whole is looked at; agglutination is re-assessed and $\frac{1}{2}+$ and weak results are recorded.

A magnifying glass (reading glass) is a useful accessory.

Tube tests: microscopic reading

It is essential that a careful and standardized technique be followed. Lift the tube carefully

from its rack without disturbing the bottom of sedimented cells. Holding the tube vertically, introduce a Pasteur pipette, with its tip cut at an angle of 90°. Carefully draw up a column of supernatant about 1 cm in length and then, without introducing an air bubble, draw up a 1–2 mm column of red cells by placing the tip of the pipette in the button of deposited red cells. Gently expel the supernatant and cells on to a slide and spread over an area of about 2 × 1 cm using the end of the pipette as a spreader. It is important not to overload the suspension with cells, and the method described above achieves this.

The scheme of scoring the results, which is given in Table 21.6, was recommended by Dunsford and Bowley.[6]

Table 21.6 Scoring of results in red-cell agglutination tests

++++ or 4+ = C (complete)	One complete mass of agglutinates, easily visible on the slide before microscopic examination.
+++ or 3+ = V (visual)	Large separate masses of agglutinates, easily visible on the slide before microscopic examination. Very few unagglutinated cells.
++ or 2+ = double plus	Smaller agglutinates, still easily visible on the slide before microscopic examination.
+ or 1+ = plus	A granular appearance just visible on the slide before microscopic examination. The microscope reveals big clumps of more than 20 cells.
(+) or $\frac{1}{2}+$ = plus brackets	Smaller clumps (12–20 cells), only detectable microscopically.
gw = good weak	Clumps of 8–12 cells, only detectable microscopically.
w = weak*	Small clumps of 4–6 cells, uniformly distributed.
? = 'sticky'	Uneven distribution of cells 2 or 3 sticking together; more noticeable when the cells are 'rolling' on the slide.
− = negative	All cells free and evenly distributed.

*Weak reactions (w) are the minimum finding that should be considered definitely positive.

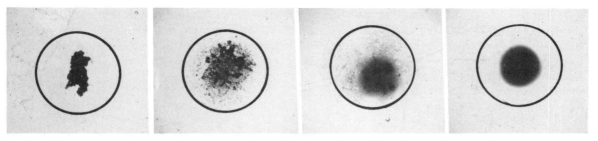

Fig. 21.2 Macroscopic appearances of agglutination in round-bottom tubes or hollow tiles. Agglutination is shown by various degrees of 'graininess'; in the absence of agglutination the sedimented red cells appear as a smooth round button, as on the extreme right.

Tube tests: macroscopic reading

It is perfectly possible to read agglutination tests macroscopically with the aid of a hand reading-glass or concave mirror, but it is then difficult to distinguish reactions weaker than + (microscopic reading) from the normal slight granular appearance of unagglutinated red cells in suspension. Macroscopic reading thus gives lower titration values than does microscopic reading. The following system of scoring can be used:

4+ is intense agglutination which results in a button of cells which remains undispersed when the tube is inverted; a (+) reaction is a distinct granularity persisting after inverting the tube compared with the control saline suspension. Intermediate degrees of agglutination visible to the naked eye are graded + (1+), ++ (2+) and +++ (3+).

A good idea of the presence or absence of agglutination can often be obtained by inspection of the deposit of sedimented cells: a perfectly smooth round button suggests no agglutination whilst agglutination is shown by varying degrees of irregularity, 'graininess' or dispersion of the deposit (Fig. 21.2). Absence of agglutination should be confirmed microscopically.

ANTIGLOBULIN REACTIONS

The antiglobulin test (Coombs test) was introduced by Coombs, Mourant and Race in 1945[5] as a method of detecting 'incomplete' Rh antibodies,, i.e. antibodies absorbed by Rh-positive red cells but incapable of causing agglutination of the same cells suspended in saline, as opposed to 'complete' antibodies which do agglutinate saline-suspended red cells. Anti-human globulin serum (Coombs serum) is prepared by immunizing animals, usually rabbits, with whole human serum or with specific fractions of human serum. Whole human serum is used for the preparation of 'broad-spectrum' sera which contain anti-IgG and anti-complement (C) components. Specific antisera can be prepared against the heavy chains of IgG, IgM and IgA and are refered to as anti-γ, anti-μ and anti-α. Specific antibodies against the complement components C4 (β_1E) and C3 (β_1C) and the breakdown product C3d can also be prepared. Suitable specific antisera are manufactured by various commercial companies; before use they require standardization and checking for specificity. (Methods for the standardization of antiglobulin sera are given on p. 355.)

Direct and indirect antiglobulin tests can be carried out. In the *direct* test (DAT) the patient's cells, after careful washing, are tested without any exposure to antibody in vitro; in the *indirect* test (IAT) normal red cells are deliberately exposed to a serum suspected of containing an antibody or antibodies and subsequently tested, after washing, to see whether they have adsorbed any antibody. The red cells can be added to the antiglobulin sera on tiles (or slides) or in tubes. The tile method has the advantage that estimates of the speed of agglutination as well as of the final strength of the reaction can be made. The tube technique is more suitable when only small volumes of red cells are available.

The IAT is applicable to the screening of sera as a means of antibody detection, in characterizing allo-antibodies when a panel of red cells is used, in typing unknown cells, and as a cross-matching procedure before a blood transfusion (see p. 369). For most purposes a single potent broad-spectrum antiglobulin serum that gives good reactions with IgG and complement components is satisfactory. However, in characterizing allo-antibodies it may be advisable to use separate anti-IgG and anti-C reagents. An anti-Lewis antibody, for example, is usually better detected by an anti-complement reagent reacting with the complement bound by the antibody rather than by an anti-IgG reacting with the antibody itself. Sometimes the presence of active complement components in the sera tested is essential for a positive test.

Direct antiglobulin test (DAT)

Tile method

Wash the patient's red cells 4 times in a large volume of saline. Prepare a 10–20% suspension of the washed cells in saline and, using a Pasteur pipette, add 1 drop to the following reagents, which have already been pipetted on to a flat opal tile*:

1. 1 drop of anti-IgG serum at optimal dilution.
2. 1 drop of anti-complement (anti-C) reagent at optimal dilution.
3. 1 drop of saline.

Rock the tile from time to time and read finally after 5 min.

Alternatively, two dilutions of a broad-spectrum antiglobulin serum can be used, one at optimal dilution for anti-IgG and one at optimal dilution for anti-C. After 5 min record the results according to strength, as previously described. If the results are negative, add 1 drop of control anti-D-sensitized cells (see p. 352) in a 10–20% suspension in saline on top of the cells being tested and rock the tile for a further 5 min. If the antiglobulin

---

* Suitable tiles are available from James Clark and Eaton, Great Suffolk St, London SE1.

---

serum is satisfactory and the patient's cells have been washed sufficiently, the suspension containing antiglobulin serum will undergo agglutination.

Tube method

Add 2 drops of a 3% suspension of red cells to 2 drops of antiglobulin serum dilution. Incubate the suspension for 1 min at 37°C and then centrifuge for 1 min at 250 *g* (rapid slow-spin technique). Read the results microscopically. The same antiglobulin reagents and control cells are used, as in the tile method.

The finding of a positive DAT will require further investigation depending on the mechanisms thought to be responsible in each particular case. This is discussed in detail in Chapter 23 where details of a quantitative DAT can also be found (p. 390).

Indirect antiglobulin test

Tile method

Add 1 volume of a 50% suspension of red cells in saline to 10 volumes of serum and incubate at 37°C (or other appropriate temperature) for 1 h. Then wash the cells four times in saline and test for adsorbed antibody and/or complement using a broad-spectrum antiglobulin serum or separate anti-IgG and anti-C reagents, as has been described.

Tube spin method

Add 2 drops of a 3% suspension of red cells to 2 drops of serum and incubate for 1 h. Following the incubation, wash the cells four times in saline and add 2 drops of an appropriately diluted antiglobulin serum to the deposited cells. Resuspend the cells and, after 1 min, centrifuge the tube slowly (150 *g*) for 1 min and assess agglutination microscopically. Check negative reactions by adding 2 drops of a 3% suspension of anti-D-sensitized cells; centrifuge after 1 min and read microscopically.

Two-stage EDTA-complement indirect antiglobulin test

Stored serum may become anticomplementary. To overcome this, a two-stage method is recommended. Antibody is taken up in the first stage and complement in the second stage.

Add 1 drop of a 20% suspension of red cells to 4 drops of EDTA-treated serum, prepared by adding 0.1 ml of neutral EDTA (i.e. 11 μmol; c 4 mg) (p. 433) per ml of serum, and incubate at 37°C for 1 h. Wash the cells three times in saline and then re-incubate with 2 drops of fresh normal serum for 15 min at 37°C. Finally wash the cells and treat them in the usual manner for the IAT.

Use of low ionic strength saline (LISS) solutions

It is known that the rate of association of antibodies with red-cell antigens is greatly enhanced by lowering the ionic strength of the medium in which the reactions take place. Nevertheless, there has been some reluctance to use low ionic strength media in routine laboratory work for two reasons: first, non-specific agglutination may occur when NaCl concentrations <2 g/l (0.03 mol/l) are used, and secondly, complement components are bound to the red cells at low ionic strengths.

A number of studies have, however, demonstrated that, provided certain precautions are observed, low ionic strength solutions (LISS) may be safely used in routine laboratory work.[14,17] The LISS solution can be made up in the laboratory (see Appendix, p. 432) or purchased commercially.[7]

The major advantage of LISS is that the incubation period in the IAT can be shortened whilst maintaining or increasing the sensitivity of the cells to the majority of red-cell antibodies. LISS can in fact be used as a substitute for saline in grouping, antibody screening and identification, and in cross-matching.

To avoid false positives, the following rules should be followed:

1. Red cells resuspended in LISS and serum should be incubated together in equal volumes.
2. The red cells should be washed in saline before suspending in LISS.
3. The red cells in LISS and the serum should be warmed to 37°C before mixing together.
4. Over spinning must be avoided, if using a spin technique.

The methods already described for red cells suspended in normal strength saline can be used for red cells suspended in LISS apart from the IAT. Using the tube technique, for the IAT reduce the incubation period from 1 h to 10–20 min. For the tile method, use 6 drops of 5% red cells in LISS; mix with the serum and incubate for 10–20 min. Wash in saline as already described; add the antiglobulin serum and read as described above.

As a short incubation time is used for the antiglobulin test, it may be convenient to read in-saline or in-albumin tests or tests using enzyme-treated cells at 20 min, if these tests are being set up at the same time. If so, a short, slow spin—as in the emergency cross-matching techniques described on p. 371—should be used prior to reading or prior to the addition of the albumin, depending on the test. With these adapations, LISS may be applied to the methods described in this chapter. But careful training of laboratory personnel is essential, and we recommended that methods employing LISS are not used by inexperienced staff.

Demonstration of lysis

Many blood-group antibodies lyse red cells under suitable conditions, i.e. in the presence of complement. This is particularly true of anti-A and anti-B, anti-P, anti-Lewis, anti-P + P_1 + P^k (anti-Tj^a) and certain auto-antibodies (see p. 338). Lysis should be looked for at the end of the incubation period before the tubes are centrifuged, if the cells have sedimented sufficiently; it may be scored roughly quantitatively after centrifuging the suspensions and comparing the colour of the supernatant with that of the control.

If the occurrence of lysis is of interest, then the final volume of the cell-serum suspension has to be greater than is required for the reading of agglutination. 75 × 8 mm tubes should be used and the level of the cell-serum suspension must rise well above the concave bottom of the tubes.

In testing for lytic activity a high concentration of complement may be required. Therefore, in contrast to tests for agglutination, it is often advantageous to add the red cells in as small a volume of saline as is possible (see p. 401).

Lysis tests are usually carried out at 37°C, but with cold antibodies a lower temperature, e.g. 20°C, 25°C or 30°C, would be appropriate, depending on the upper thermal range of activity of the antibody, or, in the case of the Donath-Landsteiner antibody, 0°C followed by 37°C (see p. 402).

Methods for titrating an antibody to demonstrate its lysis titre are described on p. 401. With certain antibodies, too, the pH of the cell-serum suspension affects the occurrence of lysis (see p. 399).

Controls

Agglutination tests

The necessity for adequate controls in all types of serological test cannot be stressed too strongly. Every reagent and manipulation must have its own control. Thus in routine grouping, red cells which will react with the grouping serum and red cells which will fail to react must be grouped at the same time as the unknown cells to provide a check on the potency of the grouping serum and its specificity. Also, when using cells of known genotype to demonstrate the corresponding alloantibodies, sera of known antibody content must be used to check the agglutinability of the test cells. Controls are particularly important when enzyme-treated cells are being used, and it must be established without question that the altered cells are reacting appropriately with known sera of known antibody content. Only in this way can the potency of the enzyme and the method of enzyme treatment be checked.

Antiglobulin tests

It is essential to demonstrate that the antiglobulin sera are potent and capable of reacting positively, when appropriately diluted, with cells coated with IgG and with cells coated with complement.

To prepare cells sensitized with IgG antibody

Incubate at 37°C, 1 volume of a 50% suspension of washed group-O, D-positive red cells with 10 volumes of an incomplete anti-D serum for 1–2 h before centrifuging and washing. It has to be determined by experiment to what extent (if any) the anti-D serum should be diluted to give (a) maximally sensitized cells (as determined in optimally diluted antiglobulin serum) and (b) weakly sensitized cells, just agglutinable by the antiglobulin serum at the end of a 5 min exposure.

To prepare cells coated with complement

Several components of complement may be demonstrated bound to red cells, and it is important, therefore, that anti-complement antiglobulin sera should react at least with the C4, C3b and C3d components of complement. Five possible sources of complement-coated cells are mentioned below:

1. *Cells sensitized in LISS.* Red cells suspended in an excess of a low ionic strength medium become coated with complement. Thus, when blood is added to 6% sucrose in 1.5 g/l NaCl, the cells become coated with C4, C3b, and C3d. If 10% sucrose in water is used instead there is a greatly increased uptake of C3. To achieve this, add 1–2 ml of group-O

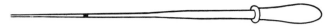

Fig. 21.3 A marked Pasteur pipette.

whole blood (fresh and without anticoagulant) to 20 ml of 100 g/l sucrose. Incubate for 15 min at 37°C and wash in four changes of saline. The treated cells can be stored at 4°C, but should be used within 3 days.

2. *Cells sensitized by fresh anti-Lewis antisera.*

3. *Cells sensitized by normal incomplete cold antibody (anti-H).*

4. *Cells sensitized by fresh anti-I antisera.*

5. *Cells from a patient with chronic cold haemagglutinin disease,* if available. Such cells are coated mainly with C3d.

Lysis tests

It is necessary to be sure that any lysis observed is not artefactual, i.e. that any present is brought about by the serum under test and not by the serum added as complement, and that the added complement is potent. A complement control (no test serum) is thus necessary and also a control using a serum known to contain a lytic antibody.

In lysis tests, great care should be taken to deliver the cell suspension directly into the serum. If the cell suspension comes into contact with the side of the tube and starts to dry up, this in itself will lead to lysis.

Titration of antibodies

Preparation of serial dilutions of patient's or other sera

When comparing the effect of different temperatures on agglutination or the different sensitivities of several types of red cells, it is important to make a set of master serial dilutions of the serum being tested and to subsample an appropriate number of small volumes from each dilution as it is made.

Doubling dilutions are usually made and can be prepared by adding an equal volume of serum to the diluent and transferring the same volume of the mixture to the next volume of diluent and so on. The dilutions may be made with a marked glass Pasteur pipette (Fig. 21.3) or by using a similar pipette to deliver drops of serum. Commercially available Pasteur pipettes are satisfactory, and provided the ends are not chipped, the pipettes, if held vertically, will deliver 30 ± 1 drops to the ml. Sometimes when the serum is in short supply it is convenient to use fine-bore '50-dropper' pipettes.

The methods of making dilutions, referred to above, suffer from 'carry over' of serum — that is to say, traces of concentrated serum remain in the pipette and tend to increase the concentration of serum in the tubes which should contain only highly diluted serum. This results in erroneously high titration figures and long drawn-out end-points. However, the titrations are easy to carry out and the results obtained have a relative value and are satisfactory for most clinical purposes. To obtain more accuracy it is necessary to use a separate accurately calibrated pipette for each dilution (Table 21.7).

Fourfold dilutions using a drop method

A method employing fourfold dilutions is economical of time and materials, and Figure 21.4 illustrates how such a titration can be carried out using a drop technique. The master dilutions can be made by the drop method or if greater accuracy is desired by using separate pipettes for each dilution.

The diluent should be buffered saline, pH 7.0, for agglutination tests; or for lysis tests undiluted ABO-compatible fresh normal human serum acidified so that the pH of the cell-serum mixture is *c* 6.8. The normal serum serves as a source of complement.

Titrations which involve reading the result by the antiglobulin method should be carried out in relatively large (e.g. 65 × 10 mm) tubes so that the red cells can be washed

Table 21.7 Comparison of titration end-points of a high-titre cold agglutinin using conventional doubling-diluting techniques with those obtained by making dilutions with separate pipettes

Final serum dilution		1 in 1024	1 in 4096	1 in 16 000	1 in 64 000	1 in 256 000	1 in 1 000 000	Control (saline)
1. Doubling dilutions using Pasteur pipette								
(a) no mixing in stem	macro	+	+	+	[+]	—	—	—
	micro	+	+	+	+	+	[+]	—
(b) with mixing in stem	macro	+	+	+	weak	—	=	—
	micro	+	+	+	+	+	[+]	—
2. Doubling dilutions using glass automatic pipette	macro	+	+	+	[+]	(?)	—	—
	micro	+	+	+	+	+	[+]	—
3. Dilutions prepared using a separate pipette for each dilution	macro	+	+	[+]	(?)	—	—	—
	micro	+	+	+	[+]	—	—	—

The titre read macroscopically was recorded as 32 000.

Only the results of readings made on the last seven alternate tubes of the titrations are recorded. The doubling dilutions were prepared commencing with undiluted serum, and the separate dilutions (Series 3) were prepared from an initial serum dilution of 1 in 256.

The titrations were carried out at room temperature (18°C) and the end-points of the titrations were determined macroscopically (macro) using a concave mirror, and also microscopically (micro). The end-points are indicated [+].

The end-points determined *macroscopically* using the conventional doubling-diluting techniques give results which closely approximate to the truth, assuming that the correct titration figure is obtained when dilutions of serum are prepared using a separate pipette for each dilution and that the result is read microscopically.

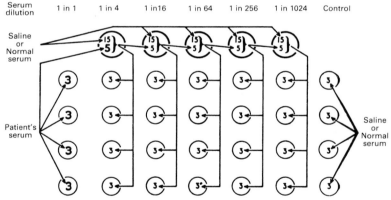

Fig. 21.4 Diagram illustrating method of preparing four sets of fourfold dilutions of a serum. The large circles at the top represent the large tubes in which the primary dilutions are made; the smaller circles the tubes in which the titrations are carried out. The figures represent drops or volumes. The patient's serum is indicated by the bold type.

thoroughly in the same tubes in relatively large volumes of saline.

The actual antiglobulin reactions can conveniently be carried out on 25 × 18 cm tiles made of flashed opal glass* on which lines have been sandblasted and painted to give five rows of eight 25 mm squares.

*See footnote p. 350.

Addition of red-cell suspensions to dilutions of serum

It is conventional to add 1 volume of red-cell suspension to 1 volume of serum or serum dilution. This means that each antibody dilution, and hence the 'final' titre, will be twice that of the original serum dilution.

Preparation and standardization of antiglobulin sera

Anti-IgG, anti-IgM, anti-IgA and anti-complement component sera, as well as 'broad-spectrum' antiglobulin sera are now so widely available from commercial firms that most hospital laboratories will find it more economical to buy the prepared reagents than to make them themselves. All the sera require careful standardization to determine their optimal dilution for use and to ensure that they contain all the wanted antibodies and do not contain unwanted antibodies.

Absorption of antiglobulin sera containing unwanted antibodies

Antiglobulin sera should be free of antibodies reacting with unsensitized red cells, but antisera prepared primarily for immunodiffusion tests may not be. It is important, therefore, to test serial dilutions of newly acquired sera with both fresh and stored washed, unsensitized A, B and O red cells. If completely negative results are not obtained with all the cells, the serum must be absorbed with the appropriate cells and retested. It is very important that the cells used for absorption should be very thoroughly washed so that all traces of human globulin are removed. At least six washes in a large volume of saline are needed and the last washing fluid should be tested subsequently with 250 g/l sulphosalicylic acid to see if it contains any protein. If the addition of a small volume of the acid results in cloudiness, further washing is necessary. The absorptions are carried out for 2 h or overnight at 4°C with an equal volume of washed packed cells.

Standardization of 'broad-spectrum' antiglobulin sera

The optimal serum dilution for the demonstration of complement components and of IgG is obtained separately.

Prepare IgG-sensitized red cells using dilutions of an 'incomplete' anti-D, so that very weakly sensitized cells are obtained as well as comparatively strongly sensitized cells. Then test the sensitized cells against doubling dilutions of the antiglobulin serum (see p. 353). It is also important, too, to test the serum with cells sensitized with IgG antibodies of specificities other than D, as the optimal dilution of the antiserum may be slightly different. In the examples given on p. 356, cells sensitized with anti-K and anti-JK^a were used, both of these sera having been treated with neutral EDTA (see p. 433) to ensure that the antibodies did not bind complement components

Methods of preparing complement-coated red cells have been outlined on p. 352. The proportions of the different complement components fixed to the red cells vary according to the method used. Several methods should, therefore, be used, e.g. cells suspended in 10% sucrose, cells from a patient with chronic cold haemagglutinin disease and cells coated with a weak IgM complement-binding antibody, for example, anti-Lewis, in the presence of fresh serum. Each type of complement-coated cell should be tested with serial dilutions of the antiglobulin serum and the dilution giving good agglutination should be noted. It is wise also at the same time to test the antiglobulin serum once more with unsensitized A, B and O cells.

The titrations illustrated in Table 21.8 show that the optimal dilution of antiglobulin serum for agglutination of IgG-sensitized cells may be very different from that required for maximal agglutination of cells coated by complement components. With a serum which reacted in the way shown in Table 21.8, it would be best always to use it at two concentrations, namely 1 in 2 and 1 in 50.

It is, however, more convenient for routine work to have a reagent which can be used at one single dilution to detect both IgG and complement components. Sometimes this can be obtained by pooling several antisera with different titres of antibodies against IgG and complement components. Usually, however, such sera have to be diluted to a more than maximal dilution for complement components in order to detect IgG satisfactorily.

Table 21.8 Chequer-board titration of an antiglobulin serum using red cells (/) sensitized with IgG and (//) coated by complement

	1 in 1	2	4	8	16	32	64	128	256
					Dilutions of antiglobulin serum				
Cells sensitized with anti-D serum diluted in saline:					*Series I*				
1 in 1	4+	4+	4+	4+	4+	4+	4+	4+	4+
1 in 2	3+	3+	3+	3+	3+	4+	4+	4+	3+
1 in 4	1+	2+	2+	3+	3+	3+	3+	3+	2+
1 in 8	—	—	1	2+	2+	2+	2+	2+	2+
1 in 16	—	—	—	1+	1+	2+	2+	2+	2+
1 in 32	—	—	—	—	$\frac{1}{2}$+	1+	1+	1+	$\frac{1}{2}$+
1 in 64	—	—	—	—	—	$\frac{1}{2}$+	1+	$\frac{1}{2}$+	—
Cells sensitized with:									
anti-K + EDTA	—	—	1+	2+	2+	2+	3+	2+	2+
anti-Jkᵃ	—	—	1+	2+	3+	3+	2+	1+	—
Cells sensitized with:					*Series II*				
Normal incomplete cold antibody (anti-H)	4+	4+	3+	3+	2+	2+	1+	$\frac{1}{2}$+	—
Anti-Leᵃ	4+	4+	4+	4+	3+	3+	2+	2+	1+
Cells from a patient with chronic cold haemagglutinin disease	4+	4+	4+	4+	3+	2+	2+	1+	$\frac{1}{2}$+
Normal (not sensitized) red cells					*Controls*				
Group A	—	—	—	—	—	—	—	—	—
Group B	—	—	—	—	—	—	—	—	—
Group O	—	—	—	—	—	—	—	—	—

Test for secretion of A or B substances

Principle. Saliva is serially diluted, then added to anti-A or anti-B serum. The sera are tested with A_2 or B cells to see whether the antibodies have been neutralized. About 20% of persons are non-secretors—they are mainly Le(a + b −) (see p. 343).

Method

Dilute an anti-A or anti-B serum so that it gives good visible agglutination with A_2 or B cells at the end of 1 h at room temperature, e.g. if the titre of the serum is 128, use it at a dilution of 1 in 16.

Collect several ml of saliva in a centrifuge tube. Place the tube in boiling water for 10 min and then centrifuge. Serially dilute the clear supernatant in saline so as to give dilutions ranging from 1 in 2 to 1 in 32. Use a tube containing saline alone as a control. Add an equal volume of the diluted anti-A (or anti-B) serum to each tube and, after shaking the rack of tubes, allow it to stand for 10–15 min at room temperature. Then add an equal volume of a 2% suspension in saline of A_2 (or B) red cells to each tube. Mix the contents, and allow to stand at room temperature for 1–2 h; then inspect for agglutination. If the saliva contains A or B substances, agglutination is usually inhibited in all the tubes except the saline-control tube. It is desirable to use saliva from a known secretor and non-secretor, respectively, as additional controls.

H substance can be demonstrated in a similar way using an extract of Ulex, eel serum or the naturally occurring 'incomplete' cold antibody as a source of anti-H.

REFERENCES

[1] ANSTEE, D. J. (1981). The blood group MNSs active sialoglycoproteins. *Seminars in Haematology*, **18**, 13.

[2] BOYER, K. M., THERAVUTHICHAI, J., VOGEL, L. C., ORLINA, A. and GOTOFF, S. P. (1981). Antibody response to group B

streptococcus type III and AB blood group antigens induced by pneumococcal vaccine. *Journal of Pediatrics*, **98**, 374.

[3] CASSELL, M., PHILLIPS, B. R. and CHAPLIN, H. JNR. (1962). Tranfusion of buffy coat-poor red cell suspensions prepared by dextran sedimentation: description of newly-designed equipment and evaluation of its use. *Transfusion (Philadelphia)*, **2**, 216.

[4] CHAPLIN, H. Jnr., BRITTINGHAM, T. E. and CASSELL, M. (1959). Methods for preparation of suspensions of buffy coat-poor red cells for transfusion. *American Journal of Clinical Pathology*, **31**, 373.

[5] COOMBS, R. R. A., MOURANT, A. E. and RACE, R. R. (1945). A new test for the detection of weak and 'incomplete' Rh agglutinins. *British Journal of Experimental Pathology*, **26**, 255.

[6] DUNSFORD, I. and BOWLEY, C. C. (1967). *Techniques in Blood Grouping*, 2nd edn., Vol. II, (a) p. 270, (b) p. 354. Oliver and Boyd, Edinburgh.

[7] DYNAM, P. K. (1981). Evaluation of commercially available low ionic strength salt (LISS) solutions. *Medical Laboratory Science*, **38**, 13.

[8] GOLDMANN, S. F. and HEISS, F. (1971). A method for preparing buffy coat-poor blood for transfusion: a modification. *Vox Sanguinis (Basel)*, **21**, 540.

[9] GOLDSMITH, K. (1955). Papain-treated red cells in the detection of incomplete antibodies. *Lancet*, **i**, 76.

[10] HUNTSMAN, R. G., HURN, B. A. L., IKIN, E. W., LEHMANN, H. and LIDDELL, J. (1963). Blood groups and enzymes of human red cells after two years' storage in liquid nitrogen. *British Medical Journal*, **ii**, 1315.

[11] International committee for standardization in haematology (1980). Working Party on Standardization of Antiglobulin Reagents of the Expert Panel on Serology. *Vox Sanguinis (Basel)*, **38**, 178.

[12] LEVINE, P., CELANO, M. J., WALLACE, J. and SANGER, R. (1963). A human 'D-like' antibody. *Nature (London)*, **198**, 596.

[13] LÖW, B. (1955) A practical method using papain and incomplete Rh-antibodies in routine Rh blood-grouping. *Vox Sanguinis (Basel)*, **5** (OS), 94.

[14] LÖW, B. and MESSETER, L. (1974). Antiglobulin test in low ionic strength salt solution for rapid antibody screening and crossmatching. *Vox Sanguinis (Basel)*, **26**, 53.

[15] LUNDSGAARD-HANSEN, P. and others. (1980). Symposium on Microfiltration of Blood and Pulmonary Function. *Vox Sanguinis (Basel)*, **39**, 46.

[16] MOLLISON, P. L., POLLEY, M. J. and CROME, P. (1963). Temporary suppression of Lewis blood-group antibodies to permit incompatible transfusions. *Lancet*, **i**, 909.

[17] MOORE, H. C. and MOLLISON, P. L. (1976). Use of low ionic-strength medium in manual tests for antibody detection. *Transfusion*, **16**, 291.

[18] MORTON, J. A. and PICKLES, M. M. (1951). The proteolytic enzyme test in the detection of incomplete antibodies. *Journal of Clinical Pathology*, **4**, 189.

[19] PIROFSKY, B. (1959). The use of bromelin in establishing a standard cross-match. *American Journal of Clinical Pathology*, **32**, 350.

[20] RACE, R. R., MOURANT, A. E., LAWLER, S. D. and SANGER, R. (1948). The Rh chromosome frequencies in England. *Blood*, **3**, 689.

[21] RACE, R. R. and SANGER, R. (1975). *Blood Groups in Man*, 6th edn. Blackwell Scientific Publications, Oxford and Edinburgh.

[22] WORLLEDGE, S. (1971). Blood transfusion. In *Tropical Surgery*, Eds. Schartz, S. I., Adesola, A. O., Elebute, E. A. and Rob, C. G., p. 28. McGraw-Hill, New York.

22

The laboratory aspects of blood transfusion
(*Written in collaboration with P. Chipping and E. Lloyd*)

This chapter will describe how knowledge of the red-cell blood groups and their corresponding antibodies, and the serological techniques used in their demonstration, can be applied to the practical problems of the provision of a hospital blood transfusion and ante-natal antibody screening service.

The investigation of transfusion reactions, haemolytic disease of the newborn and the preparation and use for transfusion of various fractions will also be briefly considered. For a detail exposition the reader is referred to Mollison's *Blood Transfusion in Clinical Medicine*.[15]

ABO GROUPING

The tube method

This is the method of choice and is particularly suitable when grouping large numbers of samples. The patient's red cells and serum are both grouped and the two results compared.

Anti-A, anti-B, and anti-A+B (group-O) sera are required for the cell grouping tests. A_1, B and O cells are required for the serum grouping tests. The anti-A+B serum acts as an additional check on blood samples which are agglutinated by anti-A or anti-B and it should also detect the rare types of A cells which may not be agglutinated by the anti-A found in group-B subjects. For ABO grouping, room temperature (18–25°C) is satisfactory.

The antisera used for red-cell grouping must be avid and cause rapid, intense and clear-cut agglutination.

Method

Small (e.g. 75 × 8 mm or 28 × 6.4 mm) glass or disposable plastic tubes can be used. Add, by means of a pasteur pipette, 1 drop of each grouping serum to 3 tubes labelled anti-A, anti-B and anti-A+B, respectively, followed by 1 drop of a 2% suspension in 9 g/l NaCl (saline) of the test cells. In addition, add 1 volume of patient's serum to 4 tubes labelled A_1 cells, B cells, O cells and 'auto-agglutination control' respectively. Then add 1 volume of 2% suspensions of the control A_1, B and O cells, and of the test red cells, to the appropriate tubes. Mix the suspensions by tapping the tubes and leave them undisturbed for $1\frac{1}{2}$–2 h. The layout for tests and controls is shown in Fig. 22.1. If avid sera have been used the results can usually be read with the naked eye. Apparent negative results should always be checked by transferring the cell–serum suspension to a glass slide and viewing it under the low power of the microscope.

It is essential to confirm the result of the red-cell grouping by examining the test subject's serum for the corresponding allo-antibodies, as described above. These tests should always be read microscopically. Any discrepancy between the results of the red-cell grouping and the serum grouping should be investigated further, except in the case of infants under 3 months of age when the corresponding allo-antibodies are usually absent.

Controls

Each grouping test (or series of tests) must be controlled by parallel tests set up exactly as described above, using cells of known group in place of the test (patient's) cells. Group-A_2 and -B cells are used to test the potency of the

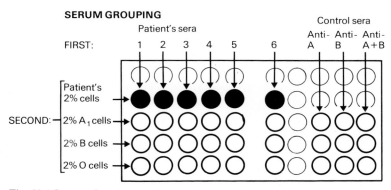

Fig. 22.1 Lay-out for tube grouping tests.

grouping sera and the use of O cells, which should not be agglutinated, guards against the possibility of false-positive reactions. In addition, the groups of the A_1, B and O cells used in the serum grouping test must be checked by setting them up against standard anti-A, anti-B and anti-A + B grouping sera.

Any agglutination of the A_1, B or O cells by the test subject's serum cannot be interpreted unless the auto-agglutination control gives a negative result. The possible causes of a positive auto-agglutination test are considered below.

The tile method

In an emergency, ABO grouping may be carried out rapidly on tiles. The method is only a little less satisfactory than the tube method in grouping a patient before transfusion: it is less satisfactory for determining the group of a blood donor.

Agglutination is rapid on flat or slightly concave surfaces, and the tile method is particularly useful when only one or two samples of blood are to be grouped. Controls must be set up with each test, and it is useful to have a perspex tile permanently ruled out and labelled as shown in Fig. 22.2, as a reminder of the controls that are necessary.

Deliver by means of a Pasteur pipette 1 drop of each grouping serum and 1 drop of the patient's serum in each of the four squares in the horizontal rows labelled anti-A and anti-B, anti- A+B and patient's serum, respectively. Add 1 drop of a 10–20% suspension of A_1 cells, B cells, O cells and the patient's cells to each of the four squares in the vertical rows under the appropriate headings. Mix the cells and serum in each square with a wooden

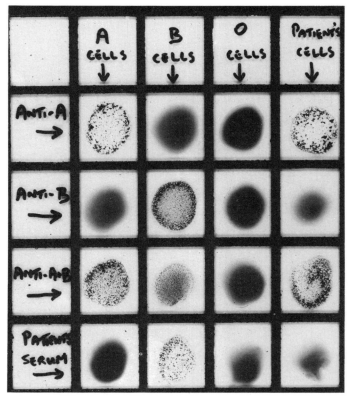

Fig. 22.2 ABO Grouping on a Perspex tile.

swab-stick, breaking off the used portion after each mixing. The results may be read within 5 min; they are usually clear-cut and indisputable (Fig. 22.2). If doubtful, the presence or absence of agglutination may be checked by viewing the suspension under the low power of a microscope.

Selection of grouping sera

Workers in hospital laboratories should not prepare their own grouping sera, but should, if possible, obtain them ready for use from a reputable source. The extensive tests necessary to ensure the specificity of such sera are beyond the resources of most hospital laboratories. Sera should be stored in the manner recommended by the manufacturer, since it is essential that they are kept free from bacterial growth, which may cause 'bacteriogenic' agglutination.[7]

CAUSES OF FALSE-POSITIVE REACTIONS IN ABO GROUPING

In addition to bacteriogenic agglutination, there are several other possible causes (see below).

Rouleaux formation

Marked rouleaux formation can simulate true agglutination. The two can be distinguished by repeating the test using serum diluted 1 in 2 or 1 in 4 in saline. Rouleaux should disappear; agglutination will hardly be affected. If rouleaux are apparent in red-cell grouping tests, the tests should be repeated after washing the red cells thoroughly.

Cold agglutinins in the patient's serum

These will cause auto-agglutination and apparent panagglutination, if active at room temperature. If this is suspected, the serum grouping test should be repeated at 37°C, at which temperature the auto-agglutination control, at least, should be negative. Any anti-A and/or anti-B present in the patient's serum will, however, still react. The patient's red cells should be washed several times in warm (37°C) saline and the cell grouping repeated. It is advisable, too, to set up an additional test of the patient's cells in group-AB serum containing no antibodies. No agglutination should result.

Warm antibodies adsorbed to the patient's red cells

When the patient's red cells are coated with anti-bodies and give a positive direct antiglobulin test (DAT), as in haemolytic anaemia caused by warm auto-antibodies, they may undergo auto-agglutination in normal serum; more often they agglutinate in albumin-containing media (see Chapter 23, p. 394).

Infected red cells

Infection of a red-cell suspension by certain bac-teria may cause the cells to become agglutinable by normal adult human sera. In vivo, this is thought to be the main cause of the rare phenomenon of polyagglutinability. Polyagglutinable red cells un-dergo agglutination in most human sera except those of young infants. Such cells might appear to be group-AB when in reality they were group O. However, the polyagglutination is less obvious or does not occur at all at 37°C and the true group can usually be determined at this temperature. Since small infants lack the normal allo-antibodies which may bring this problem to light, it is advisable to include an AB serum from a normal adult when grouping the red cells of such infants.

In view of the possibility of infection in vitro resulting in polyagglutinability, red-cell grouping should be carried out as soon as possible after the blood has been collected or, if delay is unavoidable, the blood should always be kept at 4°C. If sterility cannot be guaranteed, blood is best stored as a clot rather than as blood to which an anticoagulant has been added. Red cells should never be stored as a suspension in saline.

CAUSES OF FALSE-NEGATIVE REACTIONS IN ABO GROUPING

Failure of agglutination to take place is usually due to impotent sera. Loss of potency results if sera are carelessly left at room temperature or stored frozen in large volumes so that repeated freezings and thawings are required. In the serum grouping tests false-negative results may be recorded if lysis is not recognised as a positive result. All serum grouping tubes should be carefully inspected for lysis and its presence recorded before attempting microscopic reading of agglutination.

DIFFERENTIATION OF GROUP A_1 FROM GROUP A_2

Using lectins

Extracts from many plants, especially of their seeds, contain substances, lectins, that will agglu-tinate red cells. Some lectins have a useful blood-group specificity but most react with all red cells. A saline extract of the seeds of *Dolichus biflorus* can be diluted so that it will agglutinate A_1 and A_1B cells preferentially, and a saline extract of the seeds of *Ulex europaeus* has anti-H specificity and will agglu-tinate A_2, A_2B and O cells more strongly than A_1, A_1B and B cells. *Dolichus biflorus* extract is now used routinely in sub-typing cells carrying the A antigen.

Ulex europaeus seeds can be obtained from the plant (the common gorse bush) or from a seed merchant. *Dolichus biflorus* is not indigenous to Britain but it grows readily in India and other countries.

Using anti-A_1 sera

Group A_1 and A_2 cells can also be differentiated by absorbing group-B serum with A_2 cells. Group-B serum contains anti-A and anti-A_1, and by this method the anti-A can be removed and the anti-A_1 left behind. A satisfactorily absorbed serum should react only with A_1 cells.

Preparation of lectin solutions

The method of Dunsford and Bowley[8] is satis-factory. Soak the seeds in an excess of water for 12–18 h at room temperature. Decant off the remaining water and macerate the seeds. Add 3 volumes of saline. Leave the mixture for 1 h at room temperature, mixing constantly and then centrifuge. Filter the supernatant through Whatman No. 1 filter paper and store in 1–2 ml volumes at −20°C. The appropriate dilution of the extract has to be determined by experiment. In the case of *Dolichus biflorus* extract test serial dilutions with several examples of A_1 and A_2 cells. The dilution selected for routine use should agglutinate on a tile, within 2 min, the weakest A_1 cells and yet not agglutinate A_2 cells within the same period of time. The extract is available from commercial sources.

Rh GROUPING

Many methods have been described. Choice depends on the personal whim and experience of the serologist, the type and potency of the grouping sera available, the number of tests to be carried out and whether the result is required quickly or not. At least two different anti-D sera should be used to determine the Rh group of any one person. This is because a mistake in Rh grouping cannot usually be discovered by testing the test subject's serum. Preferably, a method using a 'saline' anti-D and one using an incomplete anti-D should be used.

Two methods will be described and some other techniques briefly referred to.

Tube method using 'saline' anti-D

Use small (e.g. 38 mm × 6.4 mm) plastic or glass tubes in order to economize with grouping sera. Place 1 small drop of grouping serum in the bottom of the tube and add 1 drop of a 2% suspension of the test red cells in saline. Mix the cells and serum and incubate for $1\frac{1}{2}$–2 h at 37°C. Read the results microscopically, as already described.

As clumps of cells agglutinated by anti-Rh sera are easily broken up, at least when using sera of low titre, care and experience are necessary for the interpretation of results. Controls of known group-O, Rh-positive and group-AB Rh-negative cells must be included with each batch of tests. As a rule, the reactions are absolutely clear-cut if a potent anti-D serum is available. A weak or doubtful reaction—when the control D-positive cells are strongly agglutinated—may be due to D^u (see p. 364).

The grouping serum

A pure anti-D serum should be used, its titre, if possible, exceeding 64. The serum may have to be absorbed with A_1 or B, D-negative cells, if anti-A and/or -B is present. If both antibodies are present, washed, packed A_1B, D-negative cells may be used for the absorption. The absorptions are best carried out at 4°C.

Because of the scarcity of complete anti-D serum, incomplete anti-D is now used by virtually all laboratories. In either case it is important to use normal human serum in place of the anti-D serum as a control in order to distinguish between genuine D-positive cells and cells which auto-agglutinate in normal serum because they have adsorbed auto-antibodies in vivo.

Tube method using incomplete anti-D

The albumin method

Set up the tests and controls exactly as with the 'saline anti-D'. After $1\frac{1}{2}$ h incubation run an additional volume (1 small drop) of 30% bovine albumin down the side of each tube so that it forms a layer above the red cells. Incubate the tubes for a further 30 min at 37°C and determine the presence of absence of agglutination microscopically.

An alternative way of grouping with albumin, favoured by some workers, is to incubate a suspension of the test red cells in the 'incomplete' anti-D serum (as described above for the tube test using saline anti-D) and at the end of $1\frac{1}{2}$ h to pipette off the supernatant serum-saline mixture and to replace this with 2 drops of 20% albumin without disturbing the button of sedimented red cells. Agglutination is read microscopically after a further 30 min incubation.

A papain method

A further alternative is to add 1 drop of Löw's activated papain solution (p. 346) to 1 drop of 'incomplete' anti-D and then add 1 drop of the test cell suspension. Read the result microscopically after 1 h at 37°C, but if required quickly the tube can be centrifuged even after a few (e.g. 5–20) minutes' incubation. Agglutination can then be read macroscopically or microscopically. It is essential to set up positive and negative controls, and controls for the absorption of the serum (i.e. using A_1B, Rh-negative cells).

Emergency Rh grouping

In an emergency, D grouping will be required in a much shorter period than the $1\frac{1}{2}$–2 h mentioned above. In this case use the saline method described above and centrifuge the tubes at 150 *g* for 1 min after a 10 min incubation. Read the results microscopically. It is essential to use potent antisera and to include positive and negative controls.

Emergency slide methods

Commercial anti-D sera are available that agglutinate Rh-positive cells within a few minutes. The manufacturer's instructions should be followed. Positive and negative and absorption controls (using A_1B, D-negative cells) must always be set up.

Rh GENOTYPING

Determination of the probable Rh genotype has often to be left to a specialist laboratory where the necessary sera are available. A brief account is given below.

The commonest reason for determining the Rh genotype is to test whether a man married to a Rh-negative woman is homozygous or heterozy-gous for the D antigen. No antisera against the 'd' antigen are available—in fact there is a growing belief that the 'd' antigen does not exist. Because of the lack of an 'anti-d' serum, the question of homo- or hetero-zygosity for the D antigen can only be guessed at from the results of tests with anti-C, anti-c, anti-E and anti-e sera, and from tables of the likelihood of the association of D or d with the other Rh antigens. These tables have been compiled for different racial groups. It is important, therefore, to tell the specialist laboratory the racial origin of the patient. This becomes essential in attempting to forecast the chances of a couple having children affected with Rh haemolytic disease of the newborn (HDN). In Nigeria, for instance, it is not worth while to attempt to determine the probable Rh genotype, for the chances of being R^0 are so high that every Rh-positive person must be assumed to be homozygous for the D antigen.

Table 22.1 gives the results of testing samples of D-positive red cells from an English population with anti-D and four other anti-Rh antisera, and the interpretation of the data in terms of homozygosity and heterozygosity for the common and not so common genotypes. The relative frequencies in the last column apply to a random population. They are applicable to D-positive husbands of D-negative women in general, but D-positive fathers of children who have had Rh HDN are a selected rather than a random population. The chances of such a father provisionally called 'heterozygous' being in reality homozygous for the D antigen becomes more likely with every child that is affected. It may be helpful to Rh group all his children or his parents.

Antisera for determining the probable Rh phenotype are available commercially. It is usually advisable to follow the manufacturers' instructions in doing the tests, but the recommended quantities of serum and cells can often be reduced. The following sera are required: anti-D, anti-C + C^w, anti-E, anti-c and anti-e. The anti-e is only necessary when the tests with anti-E are positive and anti-C + C^w are negative, i.e. to distinguish between R_2r and R_2R_2 (provided the samples are from European Caucasian donors). In this case, it is safe to assume that if the anti-E gives a negative result the anti-e would give a positive result and that a sample giving positive results with all sera is

Table 22.1 Interpretation of D-positive Rh phenotypes in terms of homozygosity (D/D) or heterozygosity (D/d) in an English population

D	C	c	E	e	Probable phenotype	% of total giving these results	Next most probable	% of total giving these results	Relative frequency of heterozygous:homozygous amongst samples giving these results
+	+	+	−		$R^1r(D/d)$	94	$R^1R^0(D/D)$	6	15:1
+	+	−	−		$R^1R^1(D/D)$	96	$R^1r'(D/d)$	4	1:21
+	+	+	+		$R^1R^2(D/D)$	88	$R^1r''(D/d)$	8	1:8
+	−	+	+	+	$R^2r(D/d)$	93	$R^2R^0(D/D)$	6	15:1
+	−	+	+	−	$R^2R^2(D/D)$	86	$R^2r''(D/d)$	14	1:6
+	−	+	−		$R^0r(D/d)$	97	$R^0R^0(D/D)$	3	30:1
+	+	−	+		$R^1R^z(D/D)$	97	$R^zr'(D/d)$	2	1:41

Table 22.2 Genotypes of the red cells to use as controls for Rh grouping sera

Antiserum	Negative control	Positive control	Absorption control
Anti-D	*Cde/cde*	*CDe/cde*	A_1B *cde/cde*
Anti-C	*cDE/cDE*	*CDe/cDE*	A_1B *cde/cde*
Anti-E	*cDe/cde*	*CDe/cDE*	A_1B *cde/cde*
Anti-c	*CDe/CDe*	*CDe/cDE*	A_1B *CDe/CDe* or A_1 + B, both *CDe/CDe*
Anti-e	*cDE/cDE*	*cDE/cde*	A_1B *cDE/cDE* or A_1 + B, both *cDE/cDE*

R_1R_2 (provided the auto-agglutination test is negative). These assumptions may not be true in people of other races.

Method

Use a fine-bore Pasteur pipette. Place 1 drop of serum at or very near to the bottom of a small (e.g. 38 mm × 6.4 mm) tube and place the 2% red-cell suspension a little higher up, taking care not to touch the bottom of the tube which has been wetted by the serum. Shake the red cells down into the serum and mix. It is convenient to set up the tubes in metal racks containing 50 holes, 8 mm in diameter, arranged in 5 rows of 10 holes. Read agglutination after $1-1\frac{1}{2}$ h incubation in a water-bath at 37°C.

If available, it is convenient to use 'saline' agglutinating sera. If sera containing 'incomplete' antibodies have to be used, 1 volume of 30% albumin must be added after $1-1\frac{1}{2}$ h incubation and a further 30 min incubation allowed. Enzyme-treated red cells or the indirect antiglobulin method may also be employed.

It is essential to use a panel of cells of known genotypes as controls. Cells that are heterozygous for the antigen under test are used as positive controls; cells that do not have the antigen under test (but would be agglutinated by the most common contaminants of the antibody) are used as negative controls. Absorption controls must also be set up. Table 22.2 lists the most readily available red cells that may be used. If there is any suggestion that the patient's red cells are be coated with antibodies, a control of patient's red cells in normal AB serum should be set up in parallel with the other tests. If albumin is used, the albumin should be added to the tube containing the patient's red cells and normal AB serum.

Detection of D^u and D variants

Occasional samples of blood may give negative results with some 'saline' anti-D sera and positive results with incomplete anti-D, at least if the antiglobulin technique is used. The donors of such samples can be thought of as having a weak D antigen which is called D^u. It is cutomary to regard D^u subjects as Rh-negative when they are recipients of transfusions and Rh-positive when they are blood donors. It is more logical, however, to regard them always as Rh-positive. It is very unusual for D^u subjects to produce anti-D antibodies after transfusions with D-positive blood but if they are $R^{1u}R^{1u}$ they are likely to produce anti-c after receiving rr blood.

Samples of blood from people who possess D variants give negative results with certain anti-D sera even by the antiglobulin method. They can be thought of as lacking part of the D antigen. Most anti-Ds are antibodies against the whole of the D complex. However, some antisera are more specific and give negative results with D variant red cells if the antibody is directed against the part of the D complex that is absent. Such people should be regarded as Rh-negative from the point of view of transfusion because the transfusion of red cells with a normal antigen can stimulate tthe production of antibodies against the absent part of the D complex.

DETECTION OF RED-CELL ANTIGENS OTHER THAN ABO AND Rh

In blood transfusion practice, although not undertaken as a routine, it is sometimes important to ascertain the patient's complete blood-group genotype as far as is practical. Particularly is this true of patients likely to need repeated transfusions, for knowledge of the patient's genotype is useful in predicting which allo-antibody he may possibly make. For this, a whole range of specific antisera are necessary, and it may be necessary to supplement a laboratory's own stock with sera purchased commercially. If so, the manufacturers' recommendations for the use of each reagent should be noted.

An additional and important use of such sera is to genotype members of the laboratory staff, so as to have fully genotyped red cells potentially available for use in the identification of unknown allo-antibodies.

The techniques used in genotyping vary according to the sera available and the antigens which they demonstrate. For example, in Kell typing the indirect antiglobulin method is appropriate while for Lewis and P antigens agglutination tests at c 20°C are best.

In order to conserve expensive antisera a tube method for the antiglobulin technique is recommended and a fine-bore pipette should be used to reduce the amount of serum required, as in Rh-genotyping. With each antiserum red cells of known genotype must be used as controls—cells known to be heterozygous for the antigen under test being used as a positive control and cells negative for the antigens tested for being used as a negative control.

BLOOD GROUPING IN BLOOD TRANSFUSIONS: SPECIAL CONSIDERATIONS

Grouping of recipients

Except in the case of identical twins or when the patient's own blood is returned to him, it is impossible to obtain blood for purposes of transfusion of *exactly* the same genotype as that of the recipient. In practice, one usually has to be content with transfusion of blood matched *only in respect of ABO and D groups*. Whilst this is usually perfectly satisfactory, allo-antibodies not infrequently develop in patients who have received many transfusions. According to Giblett's data the antibodies which are most frequently found are anti-K, anti-Le^a, anti-Le^b, anti-E and anti-c.[10] (Anti-Lewis antibodies are usually found in people who have not been transfused.) K, E and c are the antigens, in addition to A, B and D, which appear to be the most antigenic; Jk^a, C and S are amongst the antigens which appear to be less antigenic. In patients, therefore, who are destined to receive many transfusions a case can be made out for trying to avoid transfusing them with powerful antigens such as K, E and c if they themselves lack these particular antigens.

Whilst group O-blood can be given to patients of groups A, B and AB this practice is not recommended. It is inadvisable because harmful effects can follow the transfusion of large volumes of plasma containing the immune type of anti-A and anti-B—which can lead to a haemolytic transfusion reaction—and also because the practice leads to a relative shortage of group-O blood. If shortage of blood necessitates the transfusion of group-O blood to other groups then packed cells should be used.

When Rh-negative donors are in short supply and large volumes of blood are required, the problem of transfusing a Rh-negative patient with Rh-positive blood arises. This must be avoided at all costs in women in the reproductive period of life and in female children. In other cases it must be established that the recipient's serum contains no Rhesus antibodies.

Grouping of transfusion donors

In grouping prospective donors it is routine practice to carry out ABO grouping and to type the donors as D-positive or D-negative. The D-negative cells are then tested with anti-C and anti-E sera to pick up the rare combinations *Cde* and *cdE* and *CD^u^e* and *cD^u^E*. Only donors of type *cde/cde* are regarded as Rh-negative for the purpose of donation. The relatively more easily available mixtures of anti-D plus anti-C and anti-D plus anti-E should be used rather than pure anti-C and anti-E sera to group cells already known not to react with anti-D. In testing blood donors it is desirable, too, to employ the indirect antiglobulin method on all apparently Rh-negative samples, especially where the D^u antigen has a relatively high incidence as in blacks.

Grouping in antenatal work

Pregnant patients must be grouped for ABO and Rh and this should be done early in pregnancy as a routine. All Rh-negative patients and all those who give histories of having received a blood transfusion or histories suggestive of having had infants affected with haemolytic disease of the newborn (HDN) should have a specimen of their serum investigated for the presence of antibodies at regular intervals throughout pregnancy. This is particularly important in untransfused patients from the second pregnancy onwards and in transfused patients during the first pregnancy. By detecting antibodies during pregnancy an antenatal prediction of HDN can be made and appropriate steps can be taken in advance of delivery. All other patients should be screened at least once during the third trimester.

Ideally, the sera of all pregnant women, whether Rh-negative or Rh-positive, should be screened for antibodies engendered by the presence of the fetus, for these are not necessarily confined to anti-D. Indeed HDN has been described, albeit in some cases very rarely, as the result of incompatibilities in most, if not in all, of the other major blood-group systems. Of these, immunization against K is probably the commonest. Moreover, although HDN due to the formation of anti-D in Rh-negative women is by far the most important variety, it can occur, although not commonly, as the result of the formation of anti-c or anti-E in Rh-positive mothers.

In screening for antibodies in antenatal work it is best, therefore, not to confine the work to sera from Rh-negative mothers but to screen the sera of all patients. It may be impracticable to screen every patient for antibodies by the indirect antiglobulin method. A suitable compromise is to test all the sera with one sample of pooled enzyme-treated red cells made from a pool of not more than three group-O red-cell samples which between them possess all the antigens of all the common blood groups outside the ABO system. Suitable cells can be purchased commercially. The sera from all Rh-negative women and all women who have had previous transfusions or give a history suggestive of having had and infant affected with HDN are tested by the indirect antiglobulin method with the same cell samples (not enzyme-treated). If a positive result is obtained by any of these tests, the serum is investigated to ascertain the nature of the antibody present (see p. 373).

DETECTION OF ALLO-ANTIBODIES OTHER THAN ANTI-A AND ANTI-B

In parallel with determining the ABO and D groups of all blood samples sent to the blood transfusion laboratory it is ideal to screen all sera for the presence of antibodies other than anti-A and anti-B. This is essential in antenatal work, as already discussed, but it is of value, too, in detecting possible compatibility problems prior to blood being required for transfusion.

Screening tests

The tests should ideally include methods employing pooled group-O cells, enzyme-treated red cells and an indirect antiglobulin method. The test cells should be a pool of not more than three samples of group-O red cells that between them cover all the common red-cell antigens.

Method

Pooled group O cells. Add 1 volume (1–2 drops) of a 2% cell suspension in saline to 1 volume of serum placed in a tube set in a 37°C water-bath. Examine microscopically for agglutination after 1 h.

Indirect antiglobulin method. If a tile method is employed, use 5 drops of the patient's serum and add 1 drop of a 25% saline suspension of cells. Incubate for $1-1\frac{1}{2}$ h at 37°C and test for agglutinability by a broad-spectrum antiglobulin serum, as already described. Alternatively, a tube method can be used, in which case 2 drops of a 2–3% saline suspension of cells are added to 2 drops of serum.

IDENTIFICATION OF UNKNOWN ALLO-ANTIBODIES

As already mentioned, in carrying out screening tests for antibodies it is sufficient to use two or three cell samples (or a mixture of them) which collectively carry all the important blood-group antigens. If one (or all) of the cell samples is agglutinated, then the serum must be tested with a panel of cells of known but differing genotype. As a first step it is desirable to ascertain as far as is possible what is the genotype of the patient whose serum is being tested.

If, for instance, his Rh genotype is CDe/CDe (R^1R^1) the antibody might well be anti-E or anti-c; it could hardly be anti-C or anti-e (unless he had an auto-immune haemolytic anaemia): similarly, if he was Fy(a+) the antibody might be anti-Fy^b; it could hardly be anti-Fy^a. Again, the character of the antibody is a help: if this is clearly a cold antibody causing direct agglutination in saline at 20°C or 25°C but inactive at 37°C, it is not likely to be anti-D; but it might well be anti-P or anti-Le^a. The next practical step is therefore to set up the serum against a panel of cells of known genotype with particular reference to the antibody or antibodies which the patient appears most likely to have developed.

Table 22.3 illustrates the result of a typical investigation in a patient of Rh genotype CDe/CDe, who had received many transfusions and whose serum had been found to agglutinate a screening cell mixture.

The results of these tests suggest strongly a reaction with the E antigen common to cell samples 2, 3 and 4 and also with the K antigen (present in cells 4 and 6). The positive reaction obtained with cell sample 6 cannot be due to c or e because these antigens are present in cell sample 5, which was not agglutinated, or due to Le^b because this antigen is present in cell sample 1 which was also not agglutinated.

The finding of anti-E is not unexpected in a patient of genotype CDe/CDe and the probable presence of anti-K is consistent with the finding that the patient himself was K-negative. The next step, if it seems necessary to establish the identity of the antibodies beyond all possibility of doubt, is to test the serum with as many E+ K− and E− K+ cells as can be obtained. Without exception they should all give positive reactions.

THE COMPATIBILITY TEST IN BLOOD TRANSFUSION

It is essential to carry out a compatibility test between the serum of the recipient and the cells of the donor before every blood transfusion. Only if the degree of urgency is such that no delay at all is possible is it justifiable to break this rule (see later).

Table 22.3 Identification of unknown antibodies using a panel of red cells of known genotype

Cell sample		Genotypes and phenotypes							
1	O	CDe/CDe	MNS+	P+	Lu(a−)	K−	Le(a−b+)	Fy(a+)	Jk(a+)
2	O	CDe/cDE	MNS+	P−	Lu(a−)	K−	Le(a−b+)	Fy(a+)	Jk(a+)
3	O	cDE/cDE	NS+	P+	Lu(a+)	K−	Le(a+b−)	Fy(a−)	Jk(a+)
4	O	cde/cDE	NS−	P+	Lu(a−)	K+	Le(a+b−)	Fy(a−)	Jk(a−)
5	O	cde/cde	MNS−	P+	Lu(a−)	K−	Le(a−b−)	Fy(a+)	Jk(a+)
6	O	cde/cde	MS+	P−	Lu(a−)	K+	Le(a−b+)	Fy(a−)	Jk(a−)

Results

Cell sample	Agglutination* (20°C)	(37°C)	Indirect antiglobulin test (37°C)
1	−	−	−
2	−	−	+
3	−	−	+ +
4	−	−	+ +
5	−	−	−
6	−	−	+

+ and + + denote agglutination; − denotes absence of agglutination.
* The cells used were not enzyme-treated.

The compatibility test is carried out for two purposes:

1. To guard against a mistake in ABO grouping.
2. To demonstrate 'naturally-occurring' or immune antibodies in the patient's serum, active against the donor's cells, the presence of which could not be anticipated.

As no single test is capable of disclosing all types of incompatibility satisfactorily, four tests are recommended:

1. A 'saline' test carried out at room temperature (18–25°C).
2. A 'saline' test carried out at 28–30°C.
3. An 'albumin' test carried out at 37°C.
4. An indirect antiglobulin test (IAT), sensitizing the cells at 37°C.

Method

Patient's cells and serum

Obtain blood from the patient if possible a day or two before the transfusion is needed so that his or her cells may be grouped unhurriedly, with proper controls, and blood of corresponding ABO and Rh group obtained. Serum is preferred to plasma for matching purposes as strong rouleaux formation, which might be a source of confusion, is far less likely to occur. Keep the serum for 1–2 weeks at −20°C after the transfusion has been given.

Donor's blood

It is necessary to obtain a few drops of blood from the donor bag (or pilot bottle). The tubing which is attached to a donor bag may be in direct contact with the bag's contents or it may be sealed off from it by means of a clip. To obtain a blood sample when the tubing is sealed off from the bag, place another clip on the tubing c 1–2 cm from the distal end and cut off the segment beyond this seal. When the tubing has been left in direct contact with the bag, first empty the blood in the tubing into the bag by compressing it throughout its length firmly towards the bag. This is best done by using a 'tube-stripper' available commercially.* When the pressure is released the tubing will refill. Isolate a segment by doubling the tube over, invert the doubled portion into a 'hand-sealer clip', close the clip firmly, and cut off the segment. Wash the cells which

* Tube stripper, hand sealer clips and hand sealer can be obtained from Fenwall Division of Travenol Laboratories Ltd.

have been obtained in at least one change of saline and make a strong (25%) and a weak (2%) suspension in saline. Set up tests with these cells without delay.

Compatibility tests for non-urgent cases

Place 1 drop of the patient's serum in each of three 38 × 6.4 mm tubes and at least 5 volumes of the patient's serum in a large 65 × 10 mm tube. Add 1 volume of a 2% suspension of donor red cells to the serum in each of the small tubes and 1 volume of the 25% suspension of cells to the serum in the large tube. (For a spin IAT use 2 drops of serum and 2 drops of a 2% suspension of donor red cells.) Mix and place the large tube and one small tube at 37°C, one small tube at 28–30°C and one small tube at room temperature. After $1-1\frac{1}{2}$ h add 1 volume of 30% bovine albumin to the small tube kept at 37°C and incubate for a further 30 min.

Carry out an IAT on the cells in the large tube after $1-1\frac{1}{2}$ h at 37°C. Use a broad-spectrum antiglobulin reagent and control all negative tests by the subsequent addition of cells weakly sensitized with an IgG anti-D to the mixture of antiglobulin serum and donor cells on the tile or in the tube. The added cells should be agglutinated within 5 min.

Finally, examine the sedimented cells in the small tubes for agglutination microscopically.

The 'saline' test is carried out at room temperature, 20–25°C, rather than at 37°C because 'naturally-occurring' antibodies, including anti-A and anti-B, react better at room temperature. The agglutinin titre of anti-A and anti-B at 37°C is on the average about half that at 18°C.[13] If agglutination is observed at 20–25°C, the test at 28–30°C should be read and, provided there is no agglutination at this temperature and the results of the other tests are negative, the blood may be issued as compatible if it is needed in a hurry.

The test at 37°C employing albumin is included because it is a sensitive test which may sometimes detect incomplete antibodies missed by the indirect antiglobulin method.

Usually, however, such antibodies are best detected by the use of antiglobulin sera.

Difficulties: abnormal reactions not due to ABO or D incompatibility

Rouleaux. As the sera may be obtained from severely-ill patients, some rouleaux formation (associated with a raised serum globulin and / or fibrinogen) is not infrequent. Dextran given to a patient before his serum is taken for the compatibility test also causes exaggerated rouleaux formation. The differentiation of rouleaux formation from weak agglutination may not be easy, although experience helps to overcome the difficulty. If in doubt, the addition of 1 or 2 volumes of saline to the cell suspension on the slide aids differentiation by causing the rouleaux to break up to a greater or lesser extent. The difference between rouleaux formation and weak agglutination may be summarized as follows. *Rouleaux formation* affects nearly all the cells present; large clumps are not usually seen but the side-to-side adherence of the cells giving rise to many intermingling columns is a conspicuous feature. *Weak agglutination* affects only a small proportion of cells; large clumps are not formed but the small clumps that are present are widely separated in a field of free unagglutinated cells; the cells adhere to each other at all angles (Figs. 22.3 and 22.4).

Cold agglutinins. Not infrequently true agglutination is brought about by cold agglutinins. First, if agglutination is observed in the saline test, steps must be taken to make sure that there has been no mistake in ABO grouping by rechecking the groups of the donor and recipient. If ABO incompatibility is excluded, the likely cause of the agglutination — on the assumption that this does not occur at 37°C — is the presence of cold allo- or auto-agglutinins.

The temperature at which the compatibility tests are being carried out is important in the present context. They should not be carried out below 20°C for, if they are, incompatibility due to naturally-occurring antibodies of considerable frequency and normally of no clinical importance, such as anti-P_1, will be picked up, while if the temperature is 15°C or less agglutination due to anti-I cold agglutinins will be frequently encountered. Probably the best

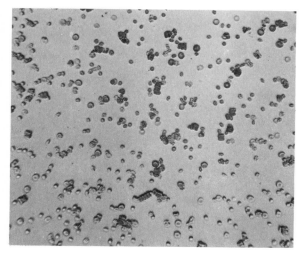

Fig. 22.3 Photomicrograph of a suspension of red cells in serum, showing a minor degree of rouleaux formation. ×300. The numerous small rouleaux are characteristically relatively evenly spaced throughout the field and do not vary greatly in size.

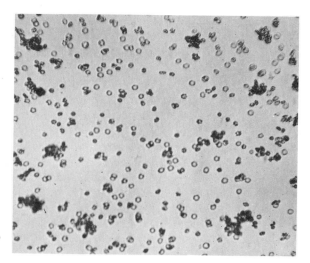

Fig. 22.4 Photomicrograph of a suspension of red cells in serum, showing weak agglutination. ×300. The small agglutinates are more irregularly distributed than rouleaux and vary more in size. There are also more free cells.

routine temperature is nearer 25°C than 20°C. If agglutination does occur at temperatures of 20°C or more it is important to establish that this does not happen at clinically important temperatures, i.e. 30°C or above. For this reason the 'saline' test at 28–30°C is carried out routinely.

If the transfusion is not urgently required, the cold antibody should be identified (see p. 395). If the transfusion cannot be delayed, the blood may be supplied if the test at 28–30°C is negative, for it is unlikely that an antibody which reacts at 20°C and not at 28–30°C will be of any clinical importance. When transfusing patients with auto-immune haemolytic anaemia due to cold antibodies it is advisable to set up, as an additional control, a suspension of the patient's own cells in his serum. If the donor's cells are not more strongly agglutinated at 28–30°C than are the patient's own cells, and if the IAT carried out strictly at 37°C is negative, the transfusion may go ahead without running any significant risks. The blood should be carefully warmed to 37°C and administered at this temperature.

Warm antibodies. Agglutinins other than anti-A, anti-B and anti-D which give rise to agglutination which persists at 37°C are not commonly met with. Other Rh antibodies, anti-M, anti-S, anti-Lu^a and anti-K are possible causes. An attempt should be made to identify the agglutinin by using a panel of cells of known genotype. It is more usual for the antibody to be of the IgG variety and to cause agglutination in albumin and not in saline and to give a positive IAT. Such antibodies should be always identified so that suitable blood can be obtained if further transfusions are necessary.

Use of enzyme-treated red cells in compatibility tests

A further alternative method is to carry out compatibility tests at 37°C using enzyme-treated donor red cells (see p. 346). This is a sensitive method of detecting some types of IgG and IgM antibodies, e.g. anti-Rh and anti-Lewis (not anti-Fy^a). It may usefully be used when the results of the IAT are doubtful or equivocal in patients suspected on clinical grounds of having formed immune antibodies. However, the method using Löw's papain is not more sensitive than the albumin-addition method. Pre-treatment of red cells with enzymes is too time-consuming for routine work and when done the increased sensitivity to relatively unimportant antibodies such as anti-I may invalidate the results.

COMPATIBILITY TESTS FOR URGENT TRANSFUSIONS

There seems to be no way of selecting compatible blood rapidly with perfect safety. However, ABO incompatibility and large (and consequently serious) amounts of 'incomplete' antibody, e.g. anti-Rh, can be detected by the above-described techniques if the cells and serum are allowed to stand in contact for as little as 15 min. In urgent cases it is recommended, therefore, that the same methods are employed as are used in non-urgent cases. After a minimum of 15 min the 37°C 'albumin' tube is centrifuged slowly at about 1000 rpm (150–200 g) for 1–2 min; 30% bovine albumin is then added to the 'albumin' tube which is incubated for another 15 min while the room temperature 'saline' test is read, also after having been centrifuged slowly for 1–2 min. If the red cells do not appear to be agglutinated, then at least no gross ABO incompatibility is present and if the clinician is demanding blood, it can be released. The IAT can now be read, the cells being washed as rapidly as possible, and by the time the blood has reached the patient the result of this test should be known. The albumin test should next be read and it is possible to complete the whole range of tests within about 30 min. It is usually possible to allow more time for compatibility tests on any subsequent bottles the patient is to receive.

The use of low ionic strength saline (LISS) in cross-matching is of particular value in an emergency since a short incubation period can be used while maintaining a high degree of sensitivity in the IAT.

If there is absolutely no time for a compatibility test, e.g. in a 'desperate' case, a unit of group-O Rh-negative blood should be issued if the patient is a woman. If a man, group-O Rh-positive blood can be given unless he is known to have been transfused previously when he should receive group-O Rh-negative blood, if this is available. If the patient's group is known with absolute certainty, he can be given blood of his own group. Any blood which has not been cross-matched must be grouped before issue.

It cannot be too strongly stressed that the laboratory staff should be given full particulars of the patients for whom they are asked to provide blood and that the patients' blood samples should be submitted at least 48 h before the blood is required, if this is at all possible. It is of the utmost importance that the staff be told the age and sex of the patient, the past history of transfusions and pregnancies, if any, and the urgency with which the blood is required. It is useful, in order to obtain this information, to issue a special laboratory form for blood transfusion requests. The form used at Hammersmith Hospital is reproduced in Fig. 22.5. Cases are divided into 'Desperate', 'Urgent' and 'Non-Urgent' categories.

SPECIAL PROBLEMS OF COMPATIBILITY

There are several situations in which the provision of compatible blood presents special problems: these are in patients undergoing extra-corporeal perfusion or other surgical procedures requiring massive transfusion, when the blood of many donors is mixed together, in newborn and unborn infants, in patients having repeated transfusions at short intervals, and in patients suffering from auto-immune haemolytic anaemia. These problems are considered briefly below.

Extra-corporeal perfusion

Here the problem is whether the large number of bottles of blood required (12 or more) should be matched one against the other, because of the possibility that one or more of the blood samples may contain immune antibodies capable of reacting against the cells of some of the others or of the recipient. This is a rather remote but not an impossible occurrence. In the United Kingdom, the plasma from all donor units is screened at the blood transfusion centre before issue. It goes without saying that the blood must all be of the same ABO group.

The compatibility tests are done in the usual way, and it is convenient to have previously screened the patient's serum for antibodies. If hypothermia is to be used, it is advisable to include another 'saline' test at 15°C. If the patient is group A, or AB the serum should also be tested with pooled A_1 cells to exclude the presence of anti-A. Any atypical antibodies demonstrated must be identified so that the appropriate blood may be obtained.

REQUEST FOR BLOOD GROUPING

Patient's blood (10 ml. Clotted) must accompany this form.

CASE No. _____

Patient's Name _____
(Surname first. Block Letters)

Sex _____ Age _____ Ward _____

Diagnosis _____

Consultant in Charge _____

- -

Houseman _____

Patient's group (if known) _____ Rhesus _____

Previous Transfusion(s) _____ Date (Year) _____

Reactions? _____

Pregnancies? _____

Haemolytic Disease of the Newborn _____

- -

REQUEST FOR TRANSFUSION

CASE No. _____

Patient's Name _____
(Surname first. Block letters)

Sex _____ Age _____ Ward _____

Diagnosis _____

Patient's group (if known) _____ Rhesus _____

Degree of Urgency (indicate thus: "X")

☐ (a) **Desperate** (blood needed at once without matching).

☐ (b) **Urgent** (blood needed as soon as matching can be done).

Note: In these circumstances the houseman *must* contact the Transfusion Laboratory (Tel. No. 379)

☐ (c) **Non-Urgent**

☐ (d) **Reserve for operations, etc.**

Number of bottles required Whole _____ Packed _____

Date and time required _____

Date _____ Signature _____

Note: Blood is reserved for 48 hrs. only

CROSS MATCHING REPORT FORM

LAB. No. _____

Patient's Blood Group _____ Rhesus _____

The following bottles are compatible with the patient's serum:

Bottle Number	Group	Expiry Date	Compatibility	Started Date & time	Dr's Initials

DATE OF TEST _____ Signed _____

CHECK NUMBERS AND GROUP AGAINST BOTTLE BEFORE TRANSFUSION AND INITIAL "GIVEN" COLUMN. BLOOD IS RESERVED FOR 48 HOURS ONLY.

TO BE RETAINED IN THE LABORATORY

NAME _____

CASE NO. _____ DATE _____

LAB. REF. BT ____ / ____ /

ACKNOWLEDGEMENT OF REQUEST FOR BLOOD GROUPING AND TRANSFUSION

LAB. No. BT ____ / ____ /

Blood Group _____ Rhesus _____

Serum has (has not) been reserved for two weeks.

_____ Bottle(s) of blood have been cross-matched for _____

_____ and will be kept for this patient until 9 a.m. on _____

Date _____ Signed _____

Fig. 22.5 Laboratory request form for blood grouping and transfusion, as used at Hammersmith Hospital, London.

Compatibility tests in newborn infants

In the newborn and during the first few weeks of life the only allo-antibodies present in the serum are those derived from the mother, and it has been argued that compatibility tests are hardly worth while if one can be sure that the infant is not suffering from HDN. It seems best, however, not to diverge from established routine. The simplest thing to do is to match the donor's cells with the mother's serum unless the child has a different ABO group from the mother, e.g. is group-A while the mother is group-O. Preferably, blood compatible with the serum of both mother and infant should be used. An antibody screen should always be carried out on the mother's serum.

Compatibility tests on infants before birth

Blood for an intra-uterine transfusion should be tested for compatibility with the mother's serum. It should be of the same group as the mother or group-O and always Rh-negative (except in the unusual circumstances in which the mother is Rh-positive and has made antibodies other than anti-D or anti-D mixtures). Compatibility tests for subsequent transfusions must be repeated every time using fresh serum, for the manipulations of intra-uterine transfusions are not uncommonly followed by the escape of fetal cells into the maternal circulation which could lead to the formation of antibodies of a new specificity. It is essential to test the mother's serum against a fully genotyped panel between each intra-uterine transfusion.

Compatibility tests in patients receiving transfusions at close intervals

Allo-antibodies may develop quickly following a transfusion early in a series. It is important, therefore, to obtain a fresh sample of serum from the recipient before each transfusion if they are separated by an interval of 2 days or longer; while, if the patient is receiving daily transfusion, only blood that is likely to be used in the 2 days following the collection of the serum should be matched. It is advisable to do a DAT on the patient's red cells each time his blood is sampled, as antibodies that have formed may be adsorbed to incompatible cells and not be present in the serum.

Compatibility tests in auto-immune haemolytic anaemia

The problem here is that all blood samples may be found to be incompatible with the patient's serum. Although it is true that Rh specificity can often be demonstrated, it is common for undefined 'non-specific' antibody components to be present alongside specific antibodies (see p. 385). If all the blood samples tested are incompatible, the best that can be done, if the patient must be transfused, is to select those samples which appear to be least incompatible. In practice, although the survival of the blood may well be very short, positive harm to the patient seldom follows. When free auto-antibody cannot be demonstrated in the patient's serum, or when auto-antibodies and allo-antibodies exist together, it is advantageous to test the donors' cells against an eluate made from the patient's cells as well as against his serum.

A clearer picture of the nature of the antibodies present and the possibility of avoiding incompatibility may be obtained in this way. It is helpful to know the patient's Rh genotype. The ABO groups of any unit to be transfused should be rechecked to avoid the possibility of ABO incompatibility being mistaken for a reaction with the patient's auto-antibody.

HAEMOLYTIC DISEASE OF THE NEWBORN

Haemolytic disease of the newborn (HDN) is the result of destruction of fetal red cells by maternal IgG antibody which has passed to the fetus transplacentally. It is most commonly brought about by IgG antibodies directed against ABO or Rh antigens. HDN due to anti-D is the most serious and best documented but other Rh antibodies, particularly anti-c, are sometimes involved; they have become relatively more common since the introduction of prophylactic immunization with anti-D immunoglobulin in the late 1960s.[12]

Rh HAEMOLYTIC DISEASE

Rhesus HDN is usually the result of the destruction of an infant's D-positive red cells by IgG anti-D antibodies produced by its D-negative (d/d) mother. Nowadays, maternal anti-D is generally the result of stimulation by *fetal* D-positive red cells which have crossed the placenta into her circulation at a previous delivery. In those cases where significant haemolysis occurs during the first pregnancy, it is thought that immunization may have occurred as a result of previous abortions, tubal pregnancies, amniocentesis or the accidental transfusion with Rh-positive blood. Transfusion of 1 unit of D-incompatible blood results in a 70% chance of immunization and is thus a potentially serious event.

Transplacental passage of fetal red cells is not such a potent stimulus as the transfusion of a large volume of D-positive blood. Even after five D-positive pregnancies only about 10% of mothers form anti-D. There are several reasons for this relative lack of stimulation. First, there is individual variation in the ability to produce antibodies. About 30% of Rh-negative subjects seem to be unable to respond by producing anti-D even though repeated injections of D-positive red cells are given.[15b] Secondly, there is the effect of ABO incompatibility of fetal red cells—it has been estimated that A incompatiblity gives 90% protection and B incompatiblity 53% protection against Rh-immunization.[19] Thirdly, the number of fetal red cells which get into the maternal circulation may be too small to initiate antibody formation. Large volumes of fetal blood (0.5 ml or more) are usually found only after delivery, and they are found more commonly in women who have had traumatic and manipulative procedures during labour and delivery such as manual removal of the placenta or Caesarean section—it is these women who are particularly likely to form Rh antibodies.[26] Fourthly, it is possible that the mother is partially tolerant to fetal antigens during pregnancy.

The initial maternal response to D-positive cells is the production of IgM anti-D and this is subsequently followed by the formation of IgG anti-D. It is this IgG anti-D which crosses the placenta and thus the level of IgG anti-D is an important factor in determining the severity of HDN.

Clinical features

Once a pregnant mother is found to have made anti-D, subsequent D-positive infants, whatever their ABO group, will require treatment in about 60% of cases.

Since the infant's *D* gene comes from the father his probable Rh genotype should be determined as far as possible. If he is homozygous for *D*, all his children will be affected; if he is heterozygous for *D* (*D/d*), some D-negative and therefore unaffected children can be expected.

Clinically, HDN may be mild, moderate or severe. Approximately 50% of infants have mild disease, with only moderate jaundice and no anaemia, and require no treatment. Approximately 25% will be severely affected, with severe jaundice and moderate anaemia, and kernicterus will develop if the infant is not treated. The remaining 25% are likely to be very severely affected and hydrops fetalis may develop before full term. Diagnostic and therapeutic measures carried out before the infant is born are designed to identify and treat this most severely affected group. Maternal sera should be examined for anti-Rh and other atypical red-cell antibodies when the mother first attends the antenatal clinic. It is important to test for the specificity of any antibodies detected using a panel of group-O red cells. Antibody titres are then followed at intervals during pregnancy. Knowledge of the titre helps in the selection of mothers who have a high risk of producing a severely affected infant and who are thus candidates for amniocentesis and plasmapheresis. A high antibody titre correlates with a bad prognosis, but criteria for amniocentesis based on titres vary from centre to centre. One recommendation is that amniocentesis is indicated if the IgG Rh antibody titre rises to above 16 by the albumin technique.[1] The first amniocentesis is carried out at 20–22 weeks.

The amount of anti-D present can now be estimated using a single-channel automated technique. Results are reported in iu/ml following the establishment of a WHO anti-D standard. A level greater than 2 iu/ml appears to be of significance and a rising level is of particular importance. A large series reported recently demonstrated that no fetal deaths occurred if the maternal antibody level was below 7 iu/ml.[24] However, at levels greater than this, the percentage of deaths increased progressively and reached 50% with an antibody concentration of 40 iu/ml.

A woman presenting with a raised antibody titre in early pregnancy and a history of a severely affected child, stillbirth or neonatal death will be a candidate for amniocentesis and plasmapheresis, especially if the husband is homozygous for the D antigen.

Amniocentesis

A more reliable indicator of fetal jeopardy than maternal anti-D levels is measurement of amniotic fluid bilirubin. When the absorbance of normal amniotic fluid is estimated at different wavelengths over the range of 350 nm to 700 nm and the curve is plotted on semi-logarithmic graph paper a smooth progression in absorbance from the lowest figure at 700 nm to the highest at 350 nm is obtained. Fluid from a pregnant woman severely affected by HDN causes a bulge in the curve with a peak at 450 nm. The magnitude of the increased absorption at 450 nm is related to the likely severity of haemolysis in the fetus.

Liley's original observations suggested that the results with amniotic fluid from affected fetuses could be divided into three groups on the basis of the increased absorbance at 450 nm.[14]

1. When there is only slight or no increase in absorbance the infant is not at risk.
2. When the increase is moderate the infant is only at low risk.
3. When the increase is marked the infant is usually seriously affected and at great risk of intra-uterine death. It is these babies that may require an intra-uterine transfusion if they are to survive. The

figures that constitute a moderate or marked increase vary with the length of gestation of the fetus.

If the fetus is found to be in the minimal risk group, amniocentesis should be repeated in 2 weeks. Once a high risk fetus is identified therapeutic intervention is required (see below).

TREATMENT

1. Plasmapheresis

Plasma exchange using a cell separator and starting early in pregnancy has been recommended as a non-hazardous form of treatment in the management of severe Rhesus HDN.[22] In Robinson and Tovey's series, a failure to maintain the anti-D level below 35 iu/ml was associated with a poor prognosis; they concluded that this was an indication for amniocentesis and intra-uterine transfusion.[22]

2. Intra-uterine transfusion

In experienced hands this has been successful in salvaging approximately 60% of severely affected fetuses. About 80–150 ml of Rh-negative blood is required and it should be taken and prepared as for exchange blood transfusions. One hazard may be the survival of lymphocytes which could lead to graft-versus-host disease. It may thus be advisable to use leucocyte-poor blood. The ABO group of the blood should be the same as the ABO group of the mother, or group O, and the blood must be carefully tested for compatibility with the mother's serum.

3. Assessment of the severity of the disease in the newborn infant in relation to exchange transfusion

The direct antiglobulin test (Coombs test) (DAT) should be done on every infant born to a Rh-negative mother. The blood should be taken with a dry syringe and needle from the cord while it is still pulsating. Two samples are necessary, a clotted sample and a sample taken into EDTA. In Rh HDN the DAT is almost always strongly positive in an infant that will require treatment (unless an intra-uterine transfusion has been done), and a weakly positive test usually means that the infant is only mildly affected. The infant's blood group

should be determined. If the DAT is strongly positive the infant may very occasionally appear to be Rh negative. This is due to so many receptors on the red cells being blocked by IgG anti-D that saline anti-D (IgM) cannot bring about agglutination. An in-albumin-acting anti-D should not be used for grouping as albumin alone may cause agglutination of the infant's cells if they are sensitized. The problem can usually be resolved by eluting some of the antibody by heating (see p. 397) and retesting the red cells with a saline anti-D. The best single criterion of severity is the cord haemoglobin concentration. The normal range is 13.6–19.6 g/dl. The criteria for treatment will vary in different hospitals.

Blood for exchange transfusions

There is continuing debate about the advisability of using heparinized blood as opposed to CPD blood for exchange transfusions. Rh-negative blood, not more than 4 days old and compatible with both mother and baby's ABO group, or compatible Rh-negative group-O blood, should be used. Heparinized blood can be prepared from CPD blood by adding 1500 iu of heparin and 4.0 ml of 100 g/l calcium gluconate to the bag (540 ml total volume). The bag is centrifuged and about half the plasma removed. Some authors recommend that 6 ml of 200 g/l THAM (trihydroxymethyl-aminomethane) should be added to neutralize the acidity of the blood. A compatibility test should be performed using the mother's serum before each exchange transfusion.

Prevention

In recent years it has been shown that the injection of IgG anti-D into an unsensitized Rh-negative woman immediately after the delivery of a Rh-positive infant can prevent the formation of Rh antibodies. The anti-D immunoglobulin should be given within 60 h of the birth of the child. The standard dose of IgG anti-D in the United Kingdom is 100 μg, which should be sufficient to protect against a bleed from fetus to mother of up to 4 ml of D-positive red cells. Less than 1% of mothers are likely to have more fetal red cells in their circulation at the time of delivery than are produced by a 4 ml bleed. In order to identify them a blood sample should be taken within 2 h of delivery and examined for the presence of fetal red cells by the Kleihauer method (p. 377).

Serological techniques for the prediction and diagnosis of Rh haemolytic disease of the newborn

Screening tests for maternal antibodies

As already discussed (p. 366), the sera of all ante-natal patients should be screened for atypical allo-antibodies and any such antibodies identified.

Titration of maternal antibodies

Rh antibodies may be titrated in several ways:

1. Using dilutions of the serum in saline and normal red cells.
2. Using dilutions of the serum in saline and normal red cells, adding 30% albumin.
3. Using the indirect antiglobulin test (IAT). If a single test is to be used, we recommend the IAT.

Titration in saline

Make doubling dilutions of the serum in saline using a marked Pasteur pipette calibrated to deliver about 0.05 ml volumes. It is convenient to use 38 × 6.4 mm tubes and to set them in a wooden block. Nine tubes, giving a range of serum dilutions from undiluted serum (1 in 1) to 1 in 256, are generally sufficient; a tenth tube to which saline alone is added serves as a control.

Add 0.05 ml of a 2% saline suspension of the selected red cells (e.g. group O, *CDe/cDE*) to each tube. After gently tapping the tubes to mix the cells in the serum, place the block of tubes at 37°C and leave undisturbed for 2 h. Determine the presence or absence of agglutination microscopically, as described on p. 348. If more than one type of cell is to be tested, make primary (or master) dilutions of serum in 65 × 10 mm tubes and deliver 0.02 or 0.05 ml sub-samples of each dilution into small tubes.

More often than not anti-D is present in the 'incomplete' form and little or no agglutination takes place even in the first tube. 'Incomplete' antibodies can be demonstrated by adding 1 drop of 30% bovine albumin to the settled red cells in each tube, re-incubating for a further 30 min and examining microscopically.

Titration in saline using enzyme-treated red cells

Exactly the same procedure is followed as that described in the previous section except that enzyme-treated red cells are substituted for the normal cells. However, care must be taken to ensure that the test is carried out strictly at 37°C to avoid possible agglutination by a cold antibody.

Titration using the albumin-addition method.

Make doubling dilutions of the serum in saline as for 'saline' titrations. Add an equal volume of a 2% saline suspension of red cells to each tube. After $1\frac{1}{2}$ h at 37°C, during which time the cells will sediment and adsorb any antibody present, add 1 volume of 30% bovine albumin carefully to each tube so that it runs under the serum-saline supernatant without disturbing the button of red cells. Look for agglutination microscopically after a further 30 min incubation.

Titration by the indirect antiglobulin method

Make doubling dilutions of the serum in saline as described on p. 353. Add 1 volume of a 25% saline suspension of red cells to 5 volumes of serum or serum dilution. Incubate the mixture at 37°C for $1\frac{1}{2}$ h. Then carry out an IAT on each dilution, as described on p. 350.

Relative value of methods using albumin, enzyme-treated red cells or indirect antiglobulin test (IAT)

The anti-D that passes the placental barrier and leads to haemolytic disease of the newborn is composed of IgG, and titrations employing the indirect antiglobulin method probably give the best estimation of the amount of IgG antibody present. Techniques using enzyme-treated red cells generally give tighter and more definite agglutination than techniques using albumin or the IAT and the agglutinin titres are likely to be higher. Occasionally, too, methods using enzyme-treated red cells demonstrate the presence of Rh antibodies that fail to cause agglutination in albumin or even by the indirect antiglobulin method. These, however, are not necessarily IgG antibodies, for enzyme-treatment of red cells also appears to potentiate their agglutinability by IgM antibodies.

AUTOMATED ANTIBODY SCREENING[2]

The development of machines such as the 15-channel AutoAnalyser (Technicon) and the Groupamatic 360 (Kontron Blood Bank Systems) has enabled much of the drudgery to be taken out of blood grouping when large numbers of blood samples have to be dealt with. However, they are not generally required in hospital practice and are not considered further here.

Single channel auto-analysers have been used in screening sera for allo-antibodies. A continous flow principle is used and the sera are aspirated in sequence. Two different methods have been used to provide sensitive conditions for antibody detection. In the first a protease is used together with a polymer, e.g. bromelin with polyvinylpyrrolidone (BPVP) or bromelin-methyl cellulose (BMC); in the second method a low ionic strength medium is used together with polybrene (LISP). The reaction mixture is pumped through mixing coils and may be warmed at 37°C or left at room temperature. The results are read, after the specific agglutinates have sedimented, by lysing the unagglutinated red cells and measuring the optical density of the haemolysate. The amount of antibody present is estimated by comparing the results with those given by sera containing known concentrations of anti-D (measured in ng/ml or as international units). Details of setting up a single channel auto-analyser system were reviewed by Ferrault and Hogman.[20]

An auto-analyser is capable of detecting extremely small amounts of anti-D. The lowest concentration detectable, using a low ionic strength polybrene method, is 0.2–0.4 ng/ml.[16,20] Mollison stated that the lowest concentrations of IgG anti-D detectable by a routine IAT were 10–200 ng/ml, by the agglutination of enzyme-treated cells 1–100 ng/ml, and by the Auto-Analyser 1–8 ng/ml.[15d]

ACID ELUTION METHOD FOR THE DETECTION OF FETAL RED CELLS (KLEIHAUER TEST)

The introduction of this cytochemical method provided a way of demonstrating the magnitude of any leak of fetal red cells into the maternal circulation at the time of delivery. The method, which is described on p. 111, depends upon the fetal cells containing Hb-F resisting acid-elution to a greater extent than do the maternal cells.

Interpretation

In a successful preparation, fetal red cells stain dark pink while the maternal cells appear as pale 'ghosts' (Fig. 6.14, p. 112). It is important to ascertain whether a transplacental haemorrhage (TPH) of more than 4 ml of fetal red cells has occurred, but for routine purposes it is not necessary to attempt to estimate the exact extent of any haemorrhage.

Using a 40 mm objective and ×10 eyepieces, at least 2400 red cells can be visualised in a single field of a well-spread blood film. If with such a film, four or less fetal cells can be seen, this means that no more than 4 ml of fetal red cells are present in the maternal circulation according to the formula:

$$\text{TPH (ml)} = \frac{1800}{\text{ratio adult:fetal red cells}} \times \frac{100}{90} \times \frac{120^\star}{100}.$$

The above calculation allows a margin of safety, but each laboratory should carefully determine the average number of red cells per low-power field, and high-power field, for the microscope used in

* This assumes that the average maternal total red-cell volume is 1800 ml, only 90% of the cord cells stain and the MCV of fetal cells is 20% greater than that of adult cells.[15c]

the investigation. If on scanning at low power more than 4 fetal red cells per low-power field are counted, then a more precise estimation of the number should be made based on the above formula. With this knowledge, an appropriate higher dose of Rh immunoglobulin can be administered.

ABO HAEMOLYTIC DISEASE OF THE NEWBORN

ABO HDN, severe enough to require treatment, is rare, even though about 20% of pregnancies in United Kingdom are associated with an ABO-incompatible fetus. There are several reasons for this: first, IgM antibody does not pass through the placenta; secondly, the A and B antigens are not fully developed at birth, and thirdly the antigens are present on cells other than red cells and also in plasma, so that extracorpuscular antigens help to neutralize the mother's antibodies.

HDN associated with ABO incompatibility is similar in its pathogenesis to Rh HDN in that maternal IgG antibodies enter the fetal circulation and react with A or B antigens on the erythrocytes. Most group-A and -B individuals form only IgM anti-A and anti-B. However, in group-O individuals, even before stimulation, some IgG anti-A and anti-B may be found in the serum and such antibodies are easily stimulated by the passage of A_1 or B antigens (on red cells or in solution) into the maternal circulation. Thus, the mothers of infants with ABO HDN are almost always group O.

For the diagnosis of ABO HDN, IgG anti-A or anti-B must be shown to be present in the mother's serum. IgM antibodies of the same specificity will also be present and they must be removed by treatment of the serum with 2-mercaptoethanol before the IgG antibodies can be demonstrated.

The infant must be group A or group B. The result of a DAT on the infant's red cells may not be helpful, for it may be negative or extremely weak even in proved cases. The cause of the weak or negative results is not clearly understood, for antibody can often be eluted from the red cells and will cause adult cells of the appropriate ABO group to be agglutinated by the same antiglobulin sera. In practice, antibody elution by Landsteiner and Miller's method (see p. 397) is the best method of establishing the diagnosis.

Free antibody capable of reacting with the appropriate adult cells can often be demonstrated in an affected infant's serum, either by using the indirect antiglobulin method or by using enzyme-treated adult cells. Antibody may, however, sometimes be demonstrated in clinically unaffected children.

The blood film of an affected child characteristically shows spherocytosis, and an increase in the osmotic fragility of the red cells can often be demonstrated. These features are less apparent in HDN due to Rh incompatibility.

SEROLOGICAL TESTS FOR THE DIAGNOSIS OF ABO HAEMOLYTIC DISEASE OF THE NEWBORN

As already mentioned above, the mother will almost always be group O and, to sustain the diagnosis, IgG anti-A or anti-B must be demonstrated in her serum. The IgG antibody will also be accompanied by an immune IgM antibody and both are powerfully lytic. A useful initial test is thus the demonstration of lysis. Provided the mother's serum contains an adequate concentration of complement, absence of lysis renders the diagnosis extremely unlikely.

Method

Demonstration of lysis by anti-A or anti-B in maternal serum

Suspend 1 volume of a 50% suspension of washed group-A_1 (or -B) red cells in 9 volumes of fresh patient's (maternal) anti-A (or -B) serum. Incubate the mixture at 37°C for 2 h, then centrifuge and inspect the supernatant for lysis. The serum should be tested within a day or so of collection.

Demonstration of IgG anti-A or anti-B in maternal serum

The best method of detecting IgG anti-A (or -B) is to treat the serum with 2-mercaptoethanol (see p. 403) and then to dilute the mixture 1 in 10 in saline and titrate it against A_1 (or B) cells, employing the indirect antiglobulin method. Agglutination to a titre of 40 or less is usually of no significance. Mothers of infants with ABO HDN generally have titres of IgG antibody that are at least 320 or more.

An alternative method of detecting IgG anti-A (or -B) is to neutralize the IgM antibody with A (or B) substance so that agglutination no longer occurs with A_1 (or B) cells. Saliva from a known secretor or commercially prepared AB substance must be tested to find the right amount to add. Too much A (or B) substance can neutralize IgG anti-A (or -B). The neutralized serum is then tested against A_1 (or B) cells using the indirect antiglobulin method.

Tests on the infant's blood

These have already been discussed (p. 375). Antibody can often be eluted off the cells in a positive case by Landsteiner and Miller's method (see p. 397). The stained blood film should show spherocytosis.

HAEMOLYTIC DISEASE OF THE NEWBORN DUE TO OTHER BLOOD-GROUP ANTIBODIES

With the introduction of prophylactic injections of anti-D immunoglobulin post partum, the incidence of HDN due to anti-D has declined sharply. However, as other antibodies, either within the Rh system, e.g. anti-c, or within other systems, e.g. Kell, Duffy or Kidd, may cause HDN, such antibodies are now assuming a relatively more important role in its causation. The serum of all pregnant mothers should thus be screened for atypical antibodies at the time of their first attendance at an antenatal clinic and at intervals during pregnancy. The management of patients in whom high titres of atypical antibodies are found is essentially similar to that outlined for Rh HDN.

COMPLICATIONS OF BLOOD TRANSFUSION AND THE INVESTIGATION OF TRANSFUSION REACTIONS

Blood transfusion is not without hazard however carefully the blood is typed and cross-matched. In addition to the haemolytic reactions brought about by serological incompatibility resulting in the destruction of the transfused red cells (or occasionally of the recipient's own red cells), transfusion may be accompanied or followed by a wide range of undesirable complications. The most important are listed below:

Sensitization to red-cell antigens, i.e. the production of antibodies against antigens in the transfused blood the patient himself lacks.

Problems associated with massive transfusions, e.g. 5 units or more of blood: haemorrhage due to lack of clotting factors in the transfused blood; antibodies in the transfused plasma which react against the patient's red-cell antigens; citrate toxicity; potassium toxicity or 2,3-DPG deficiency resulting from the transfusion of large volumes of stored blood.

Febrile reactions in a patient who has been transfused previously and has formed antibodies against leucocyte or platelet antigens or proteins in the transfused blood.

Febrile reactions due to pyrogens (proteins, dead bacteria etc.) in the anticoagulant solution or transfusion equipment. This is probably not a common cause of pyrexia now plastic equipment is so widely used.

Febrile and haemolytic reactions due to the transfusion of blood containing live microorganisms.

Transmission of infections, other than those occasioned by the contamination of blood after its withdrawal from the donor, e.g. hepatitis (B or non-A, non-B) cytomegalovirus infection, malaria, syphilis.

Urticarial reactions due to various allergies.

Fluid overload leading to heart failure and pulmonary oedema.

Air embolism, leading perhaps to sudden death.

Methods for the detection of antibodies against leucocytes and platelets are described on p. 412 and

p. 415, and a consideration of some of the other listed causes of reactions to, or complications of, transfusion are beyond the scope of this book. The laboratory worker is deeply concerned, however, in the investigation of reactions in order to establish, first, whether a particular reaction is due to serological incompatibility and, secondly, to find out how this has occurred.

Investigation of a transfusion reaction

The incident should be dealt with more or less as follows, depending upon the circumstances:

1. Stop the transfusion, or at least bring it almost to a standstill, as soon as there is a suspicion that there is anything wrong, and that this may be due to some kind of incompatibility leading to haemolysis.

2. Collect a sample of venous blood from a vein well away from the transfusion site. This blood should be withdrawn slowly into a dry syringe; deliver part into a bottle or tube containing heparin or a one-fifth volume of 32 g/l sodium citrate solution and part into a plain bottle or tube and allow it to clot. Every care should be taken to avoid haemolysis during collection. Instructions should be given that the next specimen of urine passed by the patient should be saved. The bag of blood which was being transfused at the time the reaction was suspected should be returned to the laboratory, with the giving set attached; and any bags that had been previously used should also be returned to the laboratory. Enquiry should be made as to how the blood had been treated; whether it had been warmed and how long it had been out of the refrigerator, etc.

3. On return to the laboratory immediately centrifuge part of the patient's heparinized or citrated blood and inspect the supernatant plasma. If there is no obvious naked-eye evidence of free haemoglobin or increase in bilirubin, it is not likely that there has been any serious degree of haemolysis. The presence or absence of oxyhaemoglobin, methaemalbumin or increased bilirubin in the plasma depends on the rate at which the blood was being transfused and the total volume transfused before the sample was taken and the rate of haemolysis.

Place a small drop of the recipient's blood on a slide and allow it to spread out under a cover-glass. If incompatible blood has been administered and not yet entirely destroyed, small clumps of agglutinated (donor) cells may be visible. Carry out a DAT on the recipient's blood. The test will probably be positive if incompatible donor cells are still circulating in relatively large numbers.

Centrifuge a sample of the donor's blood and inspect the supernatant plasma for haemolysis. Send samples of the blood used to the bacteriological laboratory if there is any suggestion that the blood was infected. Ascertain the age of the blood.

4. If it seems possible that the haemolysis was due to serological incompatibility, the next step is to ascertain the cause. This should be done in several stages:

a. Re-group the blood from the donor and the recipient and repeat the compatibility tests. The results may show straightaway that some gross error has been made. If the results of these tests are negative or doubtful, set up a compatibility test using enzyme-treated donor cells and incubate at 37°C.

Pre-transfusion serum from the patient should be used, if available. If serum withdrawn after transfusion is employed, incompatibility may be missed because the causal antibodies may have been completely absorbed in vivo by the donor's blood. Similarly, pre-transfusion red cells should be used for re-grouping the patient, if they are available. Confusion may arise if blood is used which has been withdrawn from the patient *after* an incompatible transfusion. Under these circumstances it is possible, for instance, for a group-A subject, transfused with group-B cells, to appear to belong to group AB, or a Rh-negative person, transfused with Rh-positive cells, to appear to be Rh-positive, because the recipient's and donor's cells may be present together.

b. If the compatibility tests fail to demonstrate any incompatibility, it is unlikely, although not impossible, that the haemolytic reaction is due to haemolysis of the donor's red cells. The next step is to consider the possibility that haemolysis of the patient's red cells has taken place, perhaps due to immune anti-A (or anti-B) being transfused in group-O blood given to a group-A (or -B) recipient. If group-O blood has been given, ascertain the agglutination and lysis titres of the anti-A and anti-B in the plasma. In paroxysmal nocturnal haemoglobinuria the patient's red cells are extraordinarily sensitive to lysis by complement-fixing allo-antibodies. Even small volumes of plasma may precipitate a haemolytic episode.[6]

If group-O blood has been given to a group-A or -B recipient, measure the osmotic fragility of the recipient's blood and stain blood films. An increase in osmotic fragility and the presence of spherocytes are pointers to the haemolytic reaction being due to the transfusion of immune anti-A or anti-B.[9]

c. If the patient is not seen until after the incident and if no donor blood is available, the cause of an incompatible transfusion may be revealed by an increase in titre of an allo-antibody present in the patient's serum; e.g. a many-fold rise in anti-A in a group-B subject, which reaches a peak 1–2 weeks after transfusion, is a clear indication that the recipient had received group-A blood.

The introduction of the technique of labelling red cells with ^{51}Cr has provided a valuable tool for the investigation of obscure transfusion reactions. In a patient who has recovered from a transfusion reaction, it is now possible to tag a few ml of the blood believed to be incompatible and to follow accurately (without harm to the patient) its survival after intravenous injection and thus to confirm or refute its incompatibility. Mollison gave extensive data on the survival and mode of destruction of incompatible red cells with particular reference to the nature of the antibody, to differences in behaviour between the various blood groups and to the effect of homozygosity or heterozygosity of the particular antigen concerned.[15e]

PREPARATION OF VARIOUS FRACTIONS OF BLOOD FOR TRANSFUSION PURPOSES

Leucocyte-poor blood

It may be necessary to remove the leucocytes as far as is possible from the blood that is to be transfused to patients who have high-titre leucocyte antibodies and have had severe transfusion reactions from this cause. Several methods can be used for this purpose:

Centrifugation of the inverted bag or bottle

This is a satisfactory practical method, in which the red cells are removed from the bottom leaving the topmost layer. According to Chaplin, Brittingham and Cassell, 90% of the leucocytes are removed if the top 20% of the red cells are left behind.[5] Aspiration of the buffy coat was found to be less satisfactory, as even when 20% of the red cells were removed, 20% of the leucocytes remained.

Sedimentation by high-molecular weight dextran

Cassell, Phillips and Chaplin described a method using Intradex (Glaxo), by which 95% of the leucocytes were removed by two sedimentations.[4]

Alternatively, Dextran 150 (Fison) may be used. The blood should be as fresh as possible, and in any case not more than 48 h old.

Microaggregate filters

A number of nylon filters are now available commercially which filter out particles as small as 30 μm. The filters fit into the giving system between the blood bag and standard giving set. Variable percentages of granulocytes are removed. The evidence so far available suggests that this technique may be useful in situations in which the removal of moderate numbers of granulocytes are required—for example, in patients experiencing febrile transfusion reactions and also in massive transfusions and in operations involving cardio-pulmonary bypass in which microaggregates of leucocytes have been implicated as a cause of pulmonary dysfunction.

The method is simple to use, relatively inexpensive and red-cell loss is minimal, although a potential disadvantage is that trapping of platelets on the surface of the filter may initiate clotting.[25b]

Cotton-wool filtration

There are now several commercially available cotton-wool filters which may be used for the preparation of leucocyte-poor blood. These filters (e.g. Immugard) remove virtually 100% of all leucocytes. When blood free of leucocytes is required, this appears to be an efficient method. As it is an open processing system, the filtration is performed immediately prior to the issue of the blood.

Washed red cells

Washing the red cells is a useful, if cumbersome, method of obtaining blood depleted of leucocytes and also free from plasma, e.g. in transfusing patients with paroxysmal nocturnal haemoglobinuria. The red cells should be washed in at least three changes of sterile saline. Automatic cell washers are available. The method does not, however, appear to be as effective as is cotton-wood filtration in providing leucocyte-free blood.

Frozen blood

Reconstituted blood which has been frozen and stored in liquid nitrogen is normally almost free of leucocytes. It may thus be useful for patients who react to leucocyte-poor blood when prepared by the methods described above.

Platelet-rich plasma and platelet concentrates

It is essential to use freshly collected blood, as platelets survive badly in stored blood. To prepare *platelet-rich plasma* the blood is col-

lected into a plastic double-bag which is then immediately centrifuged at c 250 *g* at room temperature for 30 min to sediment the red cells. The platelet-rich plasma is transferred to the second bag which is detached and centrifuged at 1200–1500 *g* at room temperature for a further 30 min to sediment the platelets.[18] Most of the supernatant plasma is then removed leaving a small volume behind in which to resuspend the platelets, which should then be given to the patient without delay.

In the United Kingdom, *platelet concentrates* are prepared by the National Blood Transfusion Service from fresh blood or by means of a cell separator deliberately taking platelets from the donor. Blood should be collected into a triple-pack donor bag (e.g. Fenwall). It is then centrifuged at c 250 *g* at room temperature for 30 min. The platelet-rich supernatant plasma is transferred to a second plastic bag. This should be clamped off from the first bag and the pack centrifuged at 1200–1500 *g* to sediment the platelets. The supernatant platelet-poor plasma is transferred to the third bag leaving about 30 ml of plasma behind in which to resuspend the platelets. The three components are then separated by clipping off each plastic bag. Thus from each unit of fresh blood, plasma-reduced whole blood, fresh plasma which can be rapidly frozen to produce fresh frozen plasma and a unit of platelet concentrate can be prepared.

If the patient requires red cells as well as platelets, it is preferable to transfuse fresh whole blood, as the highest yields of platelets are obtained in this way. If the volume given must be restricted, then either platelet-rich plasma or platelet concentrates can be used depending on the degree of volume restriction thought to be necessary. Recovery of transfused platelets corresponds to about one-third of the number transfused.[15a] To raise the platelet count of an adult from $12 \times 10^9/l$ to about $60 \times 10^9/l$ by transfusion of platelet concentrates requires the platelets from at least 5 units (2–2.5 l) of blood.[17,25a]

Cryoprecipitate

Although lyophilized factor VIII concentrates are now available commercially, factor VIII prepared as a cryoprecipitate from single units of donor plasma is still an important therapeutic substance for the treatment of haemophilia. Its preparation is based on the finding that factor VIII precipitates in the cold with the other cryoglobulins of fresh human plasma.[21] Donor blood is collected in the usual way into a double plastic bag set. The blood is then centrifuged at 1200–1500 **g** at 4°C and the plasma separated into the second (satellite) bag. The tubing between the two bags is then closed temporarily. The second bag is then frozen solid rapidly in a mixture of dry ice (solid CO_2) and ethanol. This can be prepared by adding dry ice to absolute ethanol in a wide-mouthed Thermos flask until the rapid bubbling ceases. Liquid nitrogen can be used as freezing agent when cryoprecipitate preparation is carried out on a large scale. Once the bag is frozen solid, which normally takes about 15–20 min, it can be left to thaw at 4°C still attached to its main bag. The thawing will take at least 24 h. Alternatively, the bag can be thawed in about $1\frac{1}{2}$ h at 8°C.[3] Thawing leaves behind a cold insoluble precipitate (cryoprecipitate). Both bags are then re-centrifuged at 4°C. The supernatant plasma in the satellite bag is transferred to the main bag leaving behind about 10 ml of plasma in which to resuspend the cryoprecipitate. The second bag is then detached and can be kept frozen at −20°C until required. Before use, the bag is thawed at 37°C, the cryoprecipitate resuspended and the contents are injected intravenously into the patient without delay by means of a syringe and needle.

In estimating the dosage of factor VIII to be given to a patient, the following formula may be used:[23]

$$\text{Units needed} = \% \text{ rise required} \times \text{body weight (kg)} \times R \text{ (Recovery factor)},$$

where R = 0.5 for factor VIII concentrates; 0.66

for cryoprecipitate. Cryoprecipitate contains approximately 60 units/bag.

The effect of various methods of preparation on the potency of factor VIII has been investigated by a working party of the Regional Transfusion Directors Committee.[11] Cryoprecipitate derived from group-A plasma was shown to have significantly higher activity than that from group-O plasma. The use of fresh plasma (frozen within 4 h after collection) and subsequent rapid thawing help to maintain the potency of the material.

Freeze-dried anti-haemophilic factor can be obtained commercially from a number of manufacturers. Each bottle contains c 250 iu of factor VIII. This is dissolved in sterile water before use. Instructions are given for its storage and administration and these should be followed carefully. The material is more stable on storage than cryoprecipitate; it is more convenient to prepare, and the exact number of units each bottle contains are known.

REFERENCES

[1] BOWMAN, J. M. (1975). Rh erythroblastosis fetalis. *Seminars in Hematology*, **12**, 189.

[2] BRODHEIM, E. and MOORE, B. P. L. (Eds.) (1981). Automation and data processing. *Vox Sanguinis (Basel)*, **40**, 133.

[3] BROWN, D. L., HARDISTY, R. M., KOSOY, M. H. and BRACKEN, C (1967). Antihaemophilic globulin: preparation by an improved cryoprecipitation method and clinical use. *British Medical Journal*, **ii**, 79.

[4] CASSELL, M., PHILLIPS, D. R. and CHAPLIN, H. Jnr (1962). Transfusion of buffy coat-poor red cell suspensions prepared by dextran sedimentation: description of newly-designed equipment and evaluation of its use. *Transfusion (Philadelphia)*, **2**, 216.

[5] CHAPLIN, H. Jnr, BRITTINGHAM, T. E. and CASSELL, M. (1959). Methods for preparation of suspensions of buffy coat-poor red cells for transfusion. *American Journal of Clinical Pathology*, **31**, 373.

[6] DACIE, J. V. (1948). Transfusion of saline-washed red cells in nocturnal haemoglobinuria (Marchiafava-Micheli disease). *Clinical Science*, **7**, 65.

[7] DAVIDSOHN, I. and TOHARSKY, B. (1940). The production of bacteriogenic hemagglutination. *Journal of Infectious Diseases*, **67**, 25.

[8] DUNSFORD, I. and BOWLEY, C. C. (1967). *Techniques in Blood Grouping*, 2nd edn., p 354. Oliver and Boyd, Edinburgh and London.

[9] ERVIN, D. M., CHRISTIAN, R. M. and YOUNG, L. E. (1950). Dangerous universal donors. II. Further observations on in vivo and in vitro behavior of isoantibodies of immune type present in group O blood. *Blood*, **5**, 553.

[10] GIBLETT, E. R. (1961). A critique of the theoretical hazard of inter *vs.* intraracial transfusion. *Transfusion (Philadelphia)*, **1**, 233.

[11] GUNSON, H. H., BIDWELL, E., LANE, R. S., WENSLEY, R. T. and SNAPE, T. J. (1978). Variables involved in cryoprecipitate production and their effect on Factor VIII activity: report of a working party of the Regional Transfusion Directors Committee. *British Journal of Haematology*, **43**, 287.

[12] HARDY, J. and NAPIER, J. A. F. (1981). Red cell antibodies detected in antenatal tests on rhesus positive women in South and Mid-Wales 1948–1978. *British Journal of Obstetrics and Gynaecology*, **88**, 91.

[13] JENNINGS, E. R. (1954). Tests for compatibility of blood. *American Journal of Clinical Pathology*, **24**, 381.

[14] LILEY, A. W. (1961). Liquor amnii analysis in management of pregnancy complicated by rhesus sensitization. *American Journal of Obstetrics and Gynecology*, **82**, 1359.

[15] MOLLISON, P. L. (1979). *Blood Transfusion in Clinical Medicine*, 6th edn., (a) p. 93; (b) p. 316; (c) p. 326; (d) p. 460; (e) p. 483. Blackwell Scientific Publications, Oxford and Edinburgh.

[16] MOORE, B. P. L. and PERRAULT, R. A. (1977). Automated techniques for antibody detection. In *Recent Advances in Haematology*, Vol 2, eds. A. V. Hoffbrand, M. C. Brain and J. Hirsh, p. 145. Churchill Livingstone, Edinburgh and London.

[17] MORRISON, F. S. (1966). Platelet transfusion: a brief review of practical aspects. *Vox Sanguinis (Basel)*, **11**, 656.

[18] MURPHY, S., SAYER, S. N. and GARDNER, F. H. (1970). Storage of platelet concentrates at 22°C. *Blood*, **35**, 549.

[19] MURRAY, S., KNOX, G. and WALKER, W. (1965). Haemolytic disease and the rhesus genotypes. *Vox Sanguinis (Basel)*, **10**, 257.

[20] PERRAULT, R. A. and HOGMAN, C. (1971). Automated red cell antibody analysis. A parallel study. I. Detection and quantitation. *Vox Sanguinis (Basel)*, **20**, 340.

[21] POOL, J. G. and SHANNON, A. E. (1965). Production of high-potency concentrates of antihemophilic globulin in a closed-bag system. Assay *in vitro* and *in vivo*. *New England Journal of Medicine*, **273**, 1443.

[22] ROBINSON, E. A. and TOVEY, L. A. D. (1980). Intensive plasma exchange in the management of severe Rh disease. *British Journal of Haematology*, **45**, 621.

[23] SMITH, J. K. and BIDWELL, E. (1979). Therapeutic materials used in the treatment of coagulation disorders. *Clinics in Haematology*, **8**, 183.

[24] TOMLINSON, J., JAMES, V. and WAGSTAFF, W. (1981). A survey of maternal anti-D levels related to haemolytic disease of the newborn. *British Journal of Haematology*, **49**, 130.

[25] WALLACE, J. (1977). *Blood Transfusion for Clinicians*. (a) p. 88; (b) p. 227. Churchill Livingstone, Edinburgh and London.

[26] ZIPURSKY, A., POLLOCK, J., CHOWN, B. and ISRAELS, L. G. (1963). Transplacental fetal haemorrhage after placental injury during delivery or aminocentesis. *Lancet*, **ii**, 493.

23

Serological investigation of the auto-immune haemolytic anaemias
(*Written in collaboration with P. Chipping and E. Lloyd*)

In many cases of acquired haemolytic anaemia the increased haemolysis is brought about by the production of auto-antibodies directed against the patient's own red cells. These are known as the auto-immune haemolytic anaemias (AIHA). They exist as disorders of as yet unknown origin—the 'idiopathic' type—and secondary or symptomatic types, which are mainly associated with malignant disease of the lympho-reticular system and systemic lupus erythematosus or may follow atypical (Mycoplasma) pneumonia and infectious mononucleosis. Paroxysmal cold haemoglobinuria, also, belongs to this group of disorders.

Occasionally, drugs may give rise to a haemolytic anaemia of immunological origin. The red cells of about 20% of patients on long-term α-methyldopa (Aldomet) treatment give a positive direct antiglobulin test (DAT) and these patients have auto-antibodies in their serum which will react with normal red cells, even though they often show no evidence of increased red-cell destruction. Other drugs such as penicillin, stibophen, phenacetin, quinidine, quinine, the sodium salt of *p*-aminosalicylic acid, salicylazosulphapyridine and insecticide preparations can also very rarely cause haemolytic anaemia by immunological mechanisms. With these drugs (with the exception of Aldomet) it is thought that the antibody is directed primarily against the drug and only secondarily involves the red cells (see p. 404).

TYPES OF AUTO-ANTIBODY

The diagnosis of an auto-immune haemolytic anaemia (AIHA) depends primarily upon the demonstration of auto-antibodies adsorbed to the patient's red cells; in addition, however, auto-antibodies free in the serum may be demonstrable. The auto-antibodies are of two kinds: warm antibodies, which will associate with the appropriate antigen more quickly at 37°C than at lower temperatures, and cold antibodies which typically do not associate with the appropriate antigen at 37°C although they do so as a rule readily at temperatures below 30–35°C.

Recently, a mixed picture has been described in a small percentage of patients, in whom both warm- and cold-reacting antibodies were demonstrated and the serological reactions were such that both types of antibody were considered capable of causing haemolysis. The affected patients mostly had markedly increased haemolysis and their illness ran a chronic intermittent course.[15]

The commonest type of warm auto-antibody is an immunoglobulin of the IgG class: these antibodies behave in vitro very similarly to Rh antibodies and, indeed, often seen to have Rh specificity; they are usually most readily detected in the serum by agglutination tests using enzyme-treated cells. In addition, they may also sensitize normal red cells to agglutination by antiglobulin sera.

Rarely, warm auto-antibodies of other immunoglobulin classes (IgM and IgA) are present on the red cells of the patient; they are usually more easily detected in the serum of such patients by the use of enzyme-treated red cells at 37°C. Quite frequently, patients who have a warm-antibody type of haemolytic anaemia have complement as well as IgG auto-antibody adsorbed to their red cells. The complement is probably, in most cases, not bound on by the IgG antibody and its presence may denote the simultaneous formation of subagglutinating amounts of IgM auto-antibody. Very

Table 23.1 Direct antiglobulin test in warm-antibody auto-immune haemolytic anaemia: incidence of different reactions to specific antiglobulin sera.[3]

Anti-IgG	Anti-IgA	Anti-IgM	Anti-C	No. of patients	%
+	–	–	–	43	36
–	+	–	–	3	2
+	+	–	–	4	3
+	–	–	+	52	43
+	–	+	+	6	5
–	–	–	+	13	11
				121	100

occasionally, patients are encountered in whom IgA alone is demonstrated on their red cells. Such IgA auto-antibodies do not bind complement and often show Rh-specificity. Sometimes patients with warm-antibody type haemolytic anemia may appear to have only complement on the red-cell surface. This is more difficult to interpret, as weak reactions of this type are not uncommon in patients with a variety of disorders in whom there is little evidence of increased red-cell destruction (see p. 393). In some patients this may be due to the binding to the red cells of circulating immune complexes. The frequency of these different patterns in a series of 121 patients is shown in Table 23.1.

When complement is detected by the direct antiglobulin test (DAT), the serum not infrequently contains an IgM auto-antibody which lyses enzyme-treated red cells at 37°C and does not seem to show any Rhesus specificity. Very occasionally, a similar antibody is present in the serum of normal persons or patients who do not have complement on the red-cell surface. The significance of such antibodies is not well understood.[3]

Cold auto-antibodies are nearly always IgM in type: such antibodies agglutinate normal red cells to high titres at 4°C, but the titre falls off markedly with rise of temperature and the antibodies do not usually react (with normal red cells) at temperatures over 32°C. In vivo, the antibodies can cause chronic intravascular haemolysis, the intensity of which is characteristically influenced by the ambient temperature. The resultant clinical picture is generally referred to as the cold-haemagglutinin syndrome. The haemolysis is due to destruction of the red cells by complement which is bound to the red-cell surface by the antigen–antibody reaction which takes place in the blood vessels of the exposed skin where the temperature is 28–32°C or less.

The red cells of patients suffering from the cold-haemagglutinin syndrome characteristically give positive antiglobulin reactions only with anti-complement (anti-C) sera. This is due to the presence of red cells which have irreversibly adsorbed sublytic amounts of complement; it is a sign, therefore, of an antigen–antibody reaction which has taken place at a temperature below 37°C. The complement component responsible for the reaction with anti-C sera is the C3d derivative of C3.

In vitro, a cold-type auto-antibody will often lyse normal red cells, especially if the cell-serum mixture is acidified to pH 6.5–7.0; it will usually lyse enzyme-treated red cells readily in unacidified serum, and agglutination and lysis of these cells may still be present at 37°C. Most of these cold-type auto-antibodies have anti-I specificity: i.e. they react strongly with the vast majority of adult red cells and only weakly with cord-blood red cells. A minority are anti-i and react strongly with cord-blood cells. Rarely, the antibodies have anti-Pr or anti-M specificity and react with antigens on the red-cell surface destroyed by enzyme treatment.

Another quite distinct, but rarely met with, type of cold antibody is the Donath-Landsteiner (DL) antibody. This is an IgG globulin and has anti-P specificity.[10] The clinical syndrome the antibody produces is aptly referred to as paroxysmal cold haemoglobinuria (PCH).

Some of the characteristics of IgG, IgM and IgA antibodies are illustrated in Table 23.2.

The clinical, haematological and serological aspects of the auto-immune haemolytic anaemias were extensively reviewed by Petz and Garratty,[12] Dacie,[3] Flaherty and Geary,[6] Pirofsky[13] and Sokol et al.[15]

SEROLOGICAL TECHNIQUES

Many of the methods used in the investigation of a patient suspected of suffering from AIHA have already been described in Chapter 22. Detailed description is given here of precautions to be taken when collecting blood samples from the patient and

Table 23.2 Main characteristics of IgG, IgM and IgA auto-antibodies

	IgG	IgM	IgA
Mol wt (daltons)	150 000	900 000*	160 000*
Sedimentation rate (s)	6.6	18	7
No. of heavy-chain subclasses	4	1	2
Cross placenta	Yes	No	No
Cause activation of complement	Yes	Yes	No
Cause monocyte/macrophage attachment	Yes	No	No
No. of antigen binding sites	2	5 or 10	2
Type of AIHA produced	Warm; PCH	Usually cold	Warm

* and multiples of this mol wt in polymers.

of methods of particular value in his or her investigation.

General technical methods

Collection of samples of blood and serum

It is convenient in dealing with a patient suspected of having AIHA to collect venous blood using a syringe and needle already warmed to 37°C and to deliver the blood (a) into a defibrinating container warmed in a water-bath at 37°C and (b) into ACD or CPD solution (1 ml of ACD or 0.5 ml of CPD is sufficient for 4 ml of whole blood).

Defibrination has an advantage over allowing blood to clot undisturbed in that large volumes of red cells are obtained as well as serum. In the first examination of a patient, it is desirable to carry out defibrination at 37°C rather than at room temperature so as to prevent adsorption of a cold auto-antibody should one be present. When defibrination is complete, the blood should be centrifuged to separate the serum in a 37°C centrifuge or in an ordinary centrifuge into the buckets in which water warmed to 37–40°C has been placed.

The red cells are available for antibody elution and the serum can be examined for free antibody or other abnormalities. The ACD or CPD sample is used for direct antiglobulin tests and other tests involving the patient's red cells. If the auto-antibody in a particular case is known to be warm in type, the blood may be defibrinated and separated at room temperature; otherwise, as already indicated, this should be carried out at 37°C. When samples are sent by post, it is best to send separately: (a) serum (separated at 37°C) and (b) whole blood added to ACD or CPD solution. Sterility must be maintained.

Storage of samples

Samples of patient's blood, while keeping quite well in ACD or CPD at 4°C, are more difficult to preserve than normal red cells (see p. 345 for methods of preservation of normal cells). In particular, if marked spherocytosis is present, considerable lysis develops on storage. However, satisfactory eluates can be made from washed red cells frozen at −20°C for weeks or months.

The patient's serum should be stored at −20°C or below in small (1–2 ml) volumes. If complement is to be titrated, the serum should be frozen as soon as practicable at −70°C or below if the titration is not performed immediately.

Scheme for the serological investigation of a patient suspected of suffering from a haemolytic anaemia of immunological origin

The problem arises as to which are the most profitable tests to carry out and the order in which they should be done. A suggested scheme covering the more important tests is given below. It has been set in the form of answers to questions; the recommended procedures are given in italics.

1. Are the patient's red cells 'coated' by immunoglobulins or complement (indicating antigen–antibody reaction)?

Direct antiglobulin test (DAT) using a potent 'broad-spectrum' antiserum at suitable dilutions (p. 350).

If negative, the diagnosis is unlikely to be an auto-immune haemolytic anaemia (AIHA).

a. If the test is positive, are immunoglobulins or complement adsorbed to the red cells?

Repeat the DAT using serial dilutions of polyspecific and monospecific sera (p. 390), i.e. broad-spectrum, anti-IgG, anti-IgM, anti-IgA and anti-C.

b. If immunoglobulins are present on the red cells, are they auto-antibodies?

Prepare eluates from the patient's red cells. Test these later (see 4a) (p. 396).

2. What are the patient's blood groups?

Determine the ABO group and other groups of the patient as far as possible: the probable Rh genotype is particularly important in warm-type AIHA; other groups must be determined if allo-antibodies are to be differentiated from auto-antibodies.

3. Is there free antibody in the serum? How does it react, at what temperatures and by what methods can it be demonstrated?

a. *Screen the serum with pooled adult red cells and pooled adult enzyme-treated red cells for agglutination and lysis by saline and antiglobulin methods at 20°C and 37°C (p. 394). (The red cells should be a pool of not more than three ABO-compatible samples which between them have the antigens of all the common blood-group systems. If these are not available, group O, R_1R_2 (CDe/cDE) cells may be used.)*

b. *Determine the agglutinin titre at 4°C with ABO-compatible pooled adult cells, pooled cord-blood cells and pooled adult enzyme-treated cells (p. 395).*

These tests will show whether cold or warm antibodies are present in the serum or a mixture of the two.

4. If the antibody is a *warm* one, proceed as follows:

a. What is the specificity of the antibody adsorbed to the red cells?

Test the eluate with a selected ABO-compatible panel of red cells of known blood groups by the antiglobulin method and by using enzyme-treated red cells (p. 398)

b. What is the specificity of any antibody detected in the serum? Is it an auto- or alloantibody?

Test the serum with the same panel of red cells by the methods that have given positive results in the screening test (3a).

c. What is the titre of the antibody?

Titrate in saline and/or in albumin using normal and enzyme-treated cells and the indirect antiglobulin method (p. 353).

d. If the antibody is lytic, proceed as follows:

Determine the lysis titre with enzyme-treated red cells (or PNH red cells) at 37°C, or with normal cells if these have been lysed in the screening test (3a).

5. If the antibody is a *cold* one, proceed as follows:

a. Has the antibody any specificity? Is it an auto-antibody or an allo-antibody? What is its titre?

Titrate at 4°C with ABO-compatible adult (I) cells, cord-blood (i) cells, the patient's cells, adult (i) cells (if possible) and enzyme-treated adult (I) cells (p. 395).

b. What is the thermal range of the antibody?

(i) *Determine the highest temperature at which auto-agglutination of the patient's whole blood takes place (p. 400).*

(ii) *Titrate the patient's serum at 20°C and 30°C with the panel of cells listed under 5a. (If there was any agglutination or lysis at 37°C in the screening test (3a), titrate with the appropriate cells at this temperature.)*

c. Has the antibody any lytic activity?

(i) *Titrate the antibody in fresh normal ABO-compatible serum with normal ABO-compatible I (or i) red cells and enzyme-treated I (or i) red cells at 20°C and (if necessary) 37°C (p. 400). (Paroxysmal nocturnal haemoglobinuria (PNH) red cells, if available, can be used as a valuable and sensitive reagent for detecting lytic activity.)*

(ii) *If PCH is suspected, carry out the direct and indirect Donath-Landsteiner tests (p. 402).*

6. Are drugs suspected as the cause of the haemolytic anaemia?

a. *If a penicillin is suspected, test for antibodies using cells pre-incubated with the appropriate drug (p. 404).*

b. *If other drugs are suspected, add the drug in solution to a mixture of the patient's serum, normal cells and fresh normal serum (p. 405). Look for agglutination of normal and enzyme-treated cells and use the indirect antiglobulin method.*

7. Are there any other serological abnormalities?

Consider carrying out the following tests: quantitative estimation of serum proteins; electrophoresis and quantitative estimation of immunoglobulins; complement level; tests for LE cells; tests for anti-nuclear factor (ANF); titration of heterophile (anti-sheep red-cell) antibodies; Wassermann and Kahn reactions; test for Mycoplasma antibodies.

The above scheme summarizes what may be done by way of serological investigation of a patient suspected of having AIHA. It is not suggested that every patient has to be investigated in such depth. However, there are other considerations than scientific interest and curiosity. For instance, not infrequently clinical diagnosis and prognosis depend on accurate investigation; and an exact knowledge of the specificity of an antibody may be of great importance in relation to blood transfusion. In some patients, too, quantitative measurements of antibody activity or immunoglobulin may provide valuable evidence of the efficacy of treatment. As in all spheres of laboratory medicine, a close collaboration between clinician and pathologist helps in deciding what tests should be done in any particular case.

Detection of incomplete antibodies by means of the direct antiglobulin (Coombs) test (DAT)

Principle. As already referred to (p. 349), the DAT involves testing the patient's cells without prior exposure to antibody in vitro. The anti-human-globulin serum normally used in routine screening and in the cross-match for blood transfusions is a broad-spectrum one (p. 349). However, for the investigation of cases of AIHA, antisera specific for IgG, IgM and IgA should be used. These valuable reagents are available from commercial sources. Antibodies specific for complement (anti-C) and for the complement components C4 and C3 and the breakdown product C3d can also be obtained.

Precautions

Certain precautions are necessary when investigating a patient with possible AIHA. The patient's red cells should be washed four times in a large volume of saline warmed to 37°C. The warm saline is used as a routine in order to wash off cold antibodies and obtain a smooth suspension of cells—there is no risk of washing off adsorbed complement components. However, the washing process should be accomplished as quickly as possible and the test should be set up immediately afterwards, for, occasionally, bound warm antibody elutes off the cells when they are washed and false negative results may be obtained. If for any reason the washing process has to be interrupted once it has begun, the cell suspension should be placed at 4°C to slow down the dissociation of the antibody. A tile method is particularly useful in the investigation of AIHA since it enables an estimation of the speed of agglutination as well as the final strength of the reaction.

Qualitative direct antiglobulin test

Prepare a 10–20% suspension of washed cells in saline. Pipette on to a flat opal tile:

1 drop of broad-spectrum serum at optimal dilution; 1 drop of anti-IgG serum at optimal dilution; 1 drop of anti-complement (anti-C) serum at optimal dilution; 1 drop of saline and, if available, 1 drop each of anti-IgA and anti-IgM sera at optimal dilution.

Add 1 drop of cell suspension to each drop of serum or saline, mix with a wooden swabstick and rock the tile gently from time to time and view over a light source at 1 min intervals. Read the results and if there is no agglutination, add the control cells as already described (p. 352). If the qualitative DAT is positive, a quantitative test should be carried out.

Quantitative direct antiglobulin test

The quantitative DAT gives an idea of the amount of antibody on the red-cell surface, i.e. the degree of sensitization.

Wash the cells as already described. Make four-fold dilutions of broad-spectrum, anti-IgG, and anti-C sera, ranging normally from a 1 in 4 dilution to 1 in 4096. Place 6 drops of saline in each of the master tubes to be used for preparing dilutions and add 2 drops of the appropriate neat antiserum to the first tube (1 in 4 dilution), dry the pipette carefully (see below), mix the diluted serum, place 1 drop on the tile and 2 drops in the next tube, and so on. The final layout is shown in Fig. 23.1. Care must be taken to minimize the carry over of more concentrated antiserum into the tubes destined to contain highly diluted serum. A simple way to minimize this is to wipe the sides and tip of the pipette with absorbent tissue between each dilution. For greater

accuracy (not required for routine purposes) separate pipettes should be used for each dilution. The effect of carry-over is illustrated in Table 23.3.

Anti-IgM and anti-IgA sera should also be used if they have given a positive reaction in the qualitative test.

As soon as possible after the dilutions of antiglobulin sera have been placed on the tile, add 1 drop of a 20% suspension of the patient's cells to each drop of diluted serum, mix using a wooden swab-stick, starting for each antiserum and cell sample with the saline control and finishing with the highest concentration of antiglobulin serum. Use a separate swab-stick for each series of serum dilutions. Rock gently and read the results at 15 min intervals, scoring as already described.

Normal unsensitized cells and control sensitized cells should be used to check the specificity and sensitivity of the antiglobulin sera (see p. 355)

Typical results in different types of quantitative DATs are shown in Table 23.4, which includes the reactions in undiluted serum; and the appearance of positive tests with cells coated with IgG and complement, respectively, are shown in Fig. 23.2.

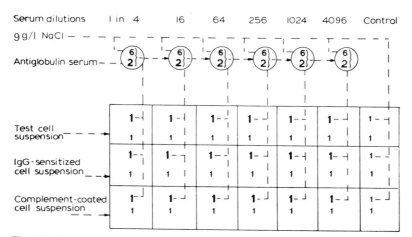

Fig. 23.1 Diagram illustrating method of dilution for the antiglobulin test. The figures represent drops. The circles indicate the tubes in which the dilutions are being made; the squares indicate the drops on a tile. The antiglobulin serum and its dilution are shown in large bold type.

Table 23.3 Comparison of titration end-points of a high-titre cold agglutinin using conventional doubling-diluting techniques with those obtained by making dilutions with separate pipettes

Final serum dilution		1 in 1024	1 in 4096	1 in 16 000	1 in 64 000	1 in 256 000	1 in 1 000 000	Control (saline)
1. Doubling dilutions using Pasteur pipette								
(a) no mixing in stem	macro	+	+	+	[+]	—	—	—
	micro	+	+	+	+	+	[+]	—
(b) with mixing in stem	macro	+	+	+	weak*	—	—	—
	micro	+	+	+	+	+	[+]	—
2. Doubling dilutions using glass automatic pipette	macro	+	+	+	[+]	(?)	—	—
	micro	+	+	+	+	+	[+]	—
3. Dilutions prepared using a separate pipette for each dilution	macro	+	+	[+]	(?)	—	—	—
	micro	+	+	+	[+]	—	—	—

* The titre read macroscopically was recorded as 32 000.
   Only the results of readings made on the last seven alternate tubes of the titrations are recorded. The doubling dilutions were prepared commencing with undiluted serum, and the separate dilutions (Series 3) were prepared from an initial serum dilution of 1 in 256.
   The titrations were carried out at room temperature (18°C) and the end-points of the titrations were determined macroscopically (macro) using a concave mirror, and also microscopically (micro). The end-points are indicated thus [+].
   The end-points determined *macroscopically* using the conventional doubling-diluting techniques give results which closely approximate to the truth, assuming that the correct titration figure is obtained when dilutions of serum are prepared using a separate pipette for each dilution and that the result is read microscopically.

Significance of positive direct antiglobulin test

A positive DAT does not necessarily mean that the patient has auto-immune haemolytic anaemia.[4,18] However, it certainly calls attention to this possibility. The causes of a positive test include the following:

1. An auto-antibody on the red-cell surface with or without haemolytic anaemia.

2. An allo-antibody on the red cell surface, as for example in haemolytic disease of the newborn or after an incompatible transfusion.

3. Antibodies provoked by drugs adsorbed to the red cell as the result of:

a. Drug adsorption as in penicillin-induced immune haemolysis.

b. Immune complex adsorption.

4. Normal globulins adsorbed to the red-cell surface as the result of damage by drugs, e.g. cephalothin.

5. Interaction between the antiglobulin sera and anti-T, as with polyagglutinable red cells.

6. Anti-albumin and anti-transferrin antibodies in antiglobulin sera giving rise to false-positive reactions.

7. Adsorption of immune complexes to the red-cell surface. This may be the mechanism of the (usually weak) reactions that are found in approximately 8% of hospital patients suffering from a wide variety of disorders.[4]

8. Sensitization in vitro. If for instance, clotted or defibrinated normal blood is allowed to stand in a refrigerator at 4°C, or even at room temperature, and the antiglobulin test is subsequently carried out, the reaction may be positive due to the adsorption of incomplete cold antibodies and complement from normal sera.[2c] Samples of blood taken into EDTA or ACD and subsequently chilled do not give this type of false-positive result as the anticoagulant inhibits the complement reaction.

9. It is not unknown for the DAT to be positive with the blood of apparently perfectly healthy individuals, e.g. blood donors. Such occurrences are rare and have not been satisfactorily explained; their incidence is probably less than 1 in 1000.[18] The possibility that α-methyldopa is being taken as an anti-hypertensive drug must not be overlooked: up to 20% of such patients on long-term therapy develop positive DATs—most show no signs of overt increased haemolysis.

Table 23.4 Patterns of agglutination by antiglobulin sera in the direct antiglobulin test using broad-spectrum and specific antiglobulin sera

IgG type

Reagent	Dilutions of antiglobulin sera							
	1 in 1	4	16	64	256	1024	4096	Saline
Broad-spectrum antiglobulin serum	1 +	2 +	3 +	4 +	4 +	3 +	2 +	0
Anti-IgG	1 +	2 +	3 +	4 +	4 +	3 +	2 +	0
Anti-C	0	0	0	0	0	0	0	0

IgG + C type

Reagent	Dilutions of antiglobulin sera							
	1 in 1	4	16	64	256	1024	4096	Saline
Broad-spectrum antiglobulin serum	3 +	3 +	3 +	2 +	2 +	1 +	0	0
Anti-IgG	0	1 +	1 +	2 +	2 +	1 +	0	0
Anti-C	3 +	3 +	2 +	1 +	0	0	0	0

C only type

Reagent	Dilutions of antiglobulin sera							
	1 in 1	4	16	64	256	1024	4096	Saline
Broad-spectrum antiglobulin serum	3 +	3 +	2 +	1 +	0	0	0	0
Anti-IgG	0	0	0	0	0	0	0	0
Anti-C	3 +	3 +	2 +	1 +	0	0	0	0

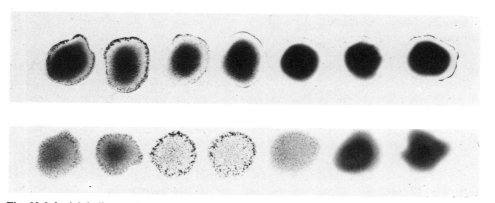

Fig. 23.2 Antiglobulin reactions carried out using various dilutions of an antiglobulin serum. *Upper series*: red cells coated by complement. *Lower series*: red cells sensitized with an IgG antibody. The dilutions of the antiglobulin serum ranged from 1 in 4 to 1 in 4096. The red-cell suspension on the extreme right is the control, with 9 g/l NaCl substituted for antiglobulin serum.

In connection with positive reactions given by nOrmal cells, it should be pointed out that slowly developing weak agglutination, occuring even in well diluted antiglobulin serum, is not uncommon. With suspensions on an opalescent tile, this is not, as a rule, evident to the naked eye under at least 5–7 min. However, this agglutination is probably real and appears to represent an interaction between globulins normally adsorbed to the red-cell surface and the antiglobulin serum. Tests should normally be read before this type of false-positive agglutination occurs.

Stratton and Renton emphasized yet another possible cause of false-positive agglutination.[16] This is due to a silica gel derived from glass, and it is most commonly produced by using sodium citrate solutions autoclaved in glass bottles or by scraping the surface of the glass tile in the course of mixing cells and serum with a corner of a microscope slide or glass rod.

False-negative antiglobulin reactions are mostly the consequence of poor technique, e.g. the result of:

1. Failure to wash the red cells properly—the antisera may then be neutralized by immunoglobulins or complement in the surrounding serum or plasma.

2. The use of impotent antisera so that weakly sensitized cells are not detected.

3. The use of incorrect dilutions of the antisera.

4. The use of antisera lacking the antibody corresponding to the subclass of immunoglobulin responsible for the red-cell sensitization.

5. The antibody being so readily dissociable that it is eluted in the washing process.

Unexpected negative reactions are sometimes encountered in patients who otherwise seem to be suffering from AIHA. In some of these patients auto-antibodies are being formed and have been demonstrated, e.g. by the use of radioisotope-labelled antiglobulin sera, but they are of such a nature or present in such small amounts that the routine tests that we have described fail to detect them. (The patients behave clinically as if they had warm-type AIHA and they usually respond to treatment with corticosteroids.)

Antiglobulin test titration scores give a good indication of the degree of sensitization of the red cells with IgG and complement without the necessity of performing sophisticated quantitative measurements. However, whilst a high titre (>1000) with anti-IgG is likely to be associated with haemolysis, titration scores cannot be used to determine whether or not increased haemolysis is occurring. Titres are, however, of value in the follow-up of the individual patient; e.g. a fall in titre is often associated with remission and a rising titre with relapse. In warm-type AIHA the presence of complement on the red-cell surface as well as IgG is more frequently associated with secondary than with 'idiopathic' AIHA. However, IgG without complement is typical of an α-methyldopa-induced positive DAT.

IgG subclasses

When the DAT is positive with anti-IgG, it is of interest to determine the subclass of IgG. The majority of IgG red-cell auto-antibodies are IgG1, sometimes in combination with IgG2 or IgG3. The formation of IgG3 (either alone or with IgG1) appears to be associated with active disease and marked haemolysis. Patients with IgG1 only on the red-cell surface may or may not have marked haemolysis, whilst IgG2 and IgG4 do not appear to be associated with any increased haemolysis.[5] Thus it is of value to know whether IgG3 is present since its presence indicates the likelihood of aggressive disease. The reactions with subclass antisera can be ascertained using 4-fold dilutions of the specific antisera exactly as has already been described. The sera are unfortunately difficult to prepare and are not readily available commercially.

Determination of the patient's blood group

ABO grouping

No difficulty should be encountered in ABO grouping patients with warm-type AIHA, but the presence of cold agglutinins may well cause difficulties. The cells should in all cases be washed in warm (37°C) saline. They should then be groupable without trouble; the reactions must, however, be controlled with normal AB serum. Serum grouping should be performed strictly at 37°C or, in an emergency, on a warmed tile. Warm the known A_1, B and O cells to 37°C before adding them to the patient's serum at 37°C. Read the results on microscope slides warmed to 37°C.

Rhesus grouping

When the DAT is strongly positive only antisera active in saline should be used, as the cells will spontaneously agglutinate in the presence of albumin. However, if the DAT is only weakly positive, antisera requiring albumin for agglutination can be be used provided the correct controls are included, namely: patient's cells + AB serum + albumin; patient's cells + AB serum.

DEMONSTRATION OF FREE ANTIBODY IN THE PATIENT'S SERUM

The sera of patients sufering from AIHA often contain free auto-antibodies. This is the rule in cold-haemagglutinin disease, but in the warm-antibody type of disease IgG antibodies detectable by the indirect antiglobulin test (IAT) are usually only found free in the serum of patients who are suffering from a moderate or marked degree of haemolysis. Free warm antibodies detectable by the use of enzyme-treated cells are, on the other hand, not infrequently found and they may often be detected in patients in clinical and haematological remission.

In investigating a patient's serum for auto-antibodies a comprehensive screening procedure should be followed. If positive results are obtained a more detailed quantitative assessment should be undertaken. If the results are negative no further tests need to be carried out.

Routine screening tests for auto- (and allo-) antibodies in serum

The patient's serum is tested under optimal conditions for agglutination and lysis and by the IAT using a pool of group-O adult red cells (chosen to possess between them all the common red-cell antigens) and the same cells enzyme-treated, e.g. pre-papainized.

The serum is tested undiluted and diluted 1 in 2 with fresh normal human ABO-compatible serum, both at the normal pH of the serum (pH 7.5–8.0) and acidified so that the pH of the cell-serum mixture is c 6.8. The pH of the serum should be checked before the cells are added; a pH of 6.0–6.5 is required.

Fresh serum is added because the sera of some patients with AIHA may be deficient in complement. Acid is added because the pH optimum for the lytic activity of some types of antibodies is 6.5–6.8. Tests are carried out strictly at 37°C and at 20°C, the cells and serum being allowed to come to the chosen temperature before they are mixed and being centrifuged subsequently at that temperature. In tests at 37°C the tubes should be spun either in a heated centrifuge or in a centrifuge the buckets of which are surrounded by water warmed to 37–40°C. For the IAT the cells should be washed in saline at the appropriate temperature.

The fresh normal serum used as complement must be tested against the same pool of test cells to ensure that it is free from antibody. Such sera should be separated immediately after collection and stored at −70°C or below.

Method

Set up a series of 30 tubes (65 × 10 mm) as illustrated in Fig. 23.3, the back row acting as master tubes. Pipette 9-drop samples from this row of tubes into the corresponding tubes of row B, C, D and E.

Place the tubes in rows B and D at 37°C and those in rows C and E at 20°C; add the pooled normal cells to the tubes in row B and C and the pre-papainized cells to the tubes in row D and E. Mix and allow to stand for 1–1½ h. Inspect all the tubes macroscopically for agglutination over a diffuse light source and then centrifuge at the temperature of the test and read for lysis by eye (see below). Wash the cells in row B in warm saline at 37°C four times and carry out an IAT using anti-IgG and anti-C sera at their optimal dilutions. If the DAT was positive with anti-IgM or anti-IgA sera, the cells should also be set up against the optimal dilution of the appropriate antiglobulin reagent.

Tube No.	A	B	C	D	E	F
Patient's serum	40	36	20	20	0	0
Fresh normal serum (complement)	0	0	20	16	40	36
0.2 mol/l HCl	0	4	0	4	0	4

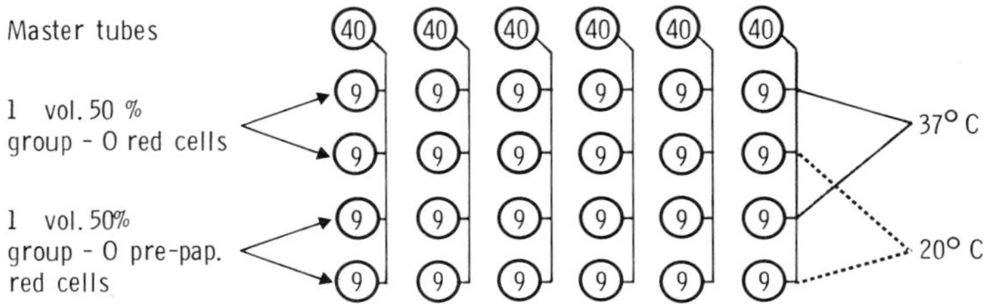

Master tubes

1 vol. 50 % group – O red cells

1 vol. 50% group – O pre-pap. red cells

37° C

20° C

Fig. 23.3 Suggested procedure for setting up a serum screening test for auto-immune haemolytic anaemia. The top row of circles represent the large master tubes in which the primary dilutions are made; the lower four rows of circles represent the tubes in which the tests are carried out. The figures represent drops or volumes.

Wash the cells in row C at room temperature and carry out an IAT as described above.

By using this technique the serum has been screened to see whether:

1. Free antibody is present which agglutinates normal group-O red cells at 37°C (row B) or at 20°C (row C).

2. Free antibody is present which agglutinates enzyme-treated group-O red cells at 37°C (row D) or at 20°C (row E).

3. Free antibody is present which reacts in the IAT with a pool of normal O cells (row B and C).

4. The pooled O or enzyme-treated pooled O cells are lysed and whether this shows pH dependence.

5. There is evidence of a lack of complement, lysis taking place in the presence of fresh normal serum but not without it (tubes 3 and 4, rows B and C).

If the screening test is positive, further tests are necessary to confirm the finding and demonstrate the antibody specificity.

Allo-antibodies will be detected by the screening procedure and will have to be carefully distinguished from auto-antibodies. Representative examples of results of the screening tests in the different types of AIHA are shown in Table 23.5.

Cold-agglutinin titre

While setting up screening procedures using serum, as described above, it is convenient to set up titrations for cold agglutinins in order to screen for their presence, and if present to obtain an indication of their specificity.

Prepare doubling dilutions of the serum in saline ranging from 1 in 1 to 1 in 512 and add 1 drop of each serum dilution into three series of small (e.g. 38 × 64 mm) tubes so that three replicate titrations can be made. Add 1 drop of a 2% suspension of saline-washed pooled adult group-O (I) cells to the first row, 1 drop of enzyme-treated pooled adult group-O cells to the second row and 1 drop of pooled cord-blood group-O (i) cells to the third row. Mix and incubate overnight at 4°C. Before reading place pipettes and a tray of slides at 4°C. Read microscopically at room temperature using the chilled slides.

Normal range. Using sera from normal Caucasians and normal adult I red cells, the cold-agglutinin titre at 4°C is from 1 to 32; using enzyme-treated I red cells the titre is from 1 to 64 and with cord-blood (i) cells 0 to 8. In cold-haemagglutinin disease (CHAD) the end-point may not have been reached at a

Table 23.5 (1) Antibody screening test: typical result with IgG antibody (direct antiglobulin test positive with anti-IgG serum only).

Method		Red cells	Temperature (°C)	S	AS	S + C	AS + C	C	AC
Indirect antiglobulin test	anti-IgG	N	37	3 +	4 +	2 +	3 +	—	—
	anti-C	N	37	—	—	—	—	—	—
	anti-IgG	N	20	2 +	3 +	1 +	2 +	—	—
	anti-C	N	20	—	—	—	—	—	—
Agglutination		N	37	—	—	—	—	—	—
		N	20	—	—	—	—	—	—
Lysis		N	37	—	—	—	—	—	—
		N	20	—	—	—	—	—	—
Agglutination		EN	37	3 +	3 +	3 +	3 +	—	—
		EN	20	2 +	2 +	2 +	2 +	—	—
Lysis		EN	37	—	—	—	—	—	—
		EN	20	—	—	—	—	—	—

Table 23.5 (2) Antibody screening test: typical result with antibody(ies) giving positive antiglobulin tests with anti-IgG and anti-C

Method		Red cells	Temperature (°C)	S	AS	S + C	AS + C	C	AC
Indirect antiglobulin test	anti-IgG	N	37	1 +	2 +	$\frac{1}{2}$ +	1 +	—	—
	anti-C	N	37	1 +	2 +	3 +	3 +	—	—
	anti-IgG	N	20	$\frac{1}{2}$ +	—	—	—	—	—
	anti-C	N	20	1 +	2 +	2 +	3 +	—	—
Agglutination		N	37	—	—	—	—	—	—
		N	20	1 +	1 +	—	—	—	—
Lysis		N	37	—	—	—	—	—	—
		N	20	—	—	—	—	—	—
Agglutination		EN	37	1 +	1 +	—	—	—	—
		EN	20	2 +	2 +	1 +	1 +	—	—
Lysis		EN	37	1 +	2 +	3 +	4 +	—	—
		EN	20	—	—	1 +	2 +	—	—

dilution of 1 in 512; if so, further dilutions should be prepared and tested.

If a cold agglutinin is present at a raised titre, the presence of a cold allo-antibody has to be excluded. In this case the patient's own red cells will be found to react *much* less strongly than do normal adult I red cells. It should be noted that in CHAD the patient's cells commonly react rather less strongly than do normal adult I cells (see Table 23.6).

Elution of antibodies from red cells

The preparation of potent antibody-containing eluates from the red cells of patients with AIHA is essential in determining the specificity of the antibody.

Several methods are available for the preparation of eluates; each has advantages and disadvantages. The first step is to wash the red cells at least four times in a large volume of saline. At the last washing, centrifuge for

Table 23.5 (3) Antibody screening test: typical result with warm antibody giving positive direct antiglobulin test with anti-C only

Method		Red cells	Temp- erature (°C)	S	AS	S + C	AS + C	C	AC
Indirect antiglobulin test	anti-IgG	N	37	—	—	—	—	—	—
	anti-C	N	37	2 +	3 +	2 +	2 +	—	—
	anti-IgG	N	20	—	—	—	—	—	—
	anti-C	N	20	2 +	3 +	1 +	2 +	—	—
Agglutination		N	37	—	—	—	—	—	—
		N	20	—	—	—	—	—	—
Lysis		N	37	—	—	—	—	—	—
		N	20	—	—	—	—	—	—
Agglutination		EN	37	—	—	1 +	1 +	—	—
		EN	20	1 +	1 +	2 +	2 +	—	—
Lysis		EN	37	3 +	4 +	1 +	2 +	—	—
		EN	20	1 +	2 +	—	—	—	—

Table 23.5 (4) Antibody screening test: typical result in the cold-haemagglutinin disease (direct antiglobulin test positive with anti-C only)

Method		Red cells	Temp- erature (°C)	S	AS	S + C	AS + C	C	C
Indirect antiglobulin test	anti-IgG	N	37	—	—	—	—	—	—
	anti-C	N	37	—	—	—	—	—	—
	anti-IgG	N	20	Cells too agglutinated to test					
	anti-C	N	20						
Agglutination		N	37	—	—	—	—	—	—
		N	20	4 +	4 +	4 +	2 +	—	—
Lysis		N	37	—	—	—	—	—	—
		N	20	—	—	—	2 +	—	—
Agglutination		EN	37	2 +	2 +	2 +	1 +	—	—
		EN	20	4 +	4 +	2 +	1 +	—	—
Lysis		EN	37	—	—	2 +	3 +	—	—
		EN	20	—	—	2 +	3 +	—	—

N = pooled normal adult group-O red cells; EN = the same cells pre-treated with the enzyme papain.
S = patient's undiluted serum; AS = patient's undiluted serum acidified to pH 6.0–6.5; C (complement) = fresh normal human compatible serum; AC = fresh normal human compatible serum acidified to pH 6.0–6.5.
S + C = equal volumes of patient's serum and complement.

10 min at 1200–1500 **g** and save the supernatant. Ideally 2–5 ml of packed red cells should be left at the end of this washing.

Landsteiner's method[9]

To the washed, packed cells add a suitable volume of saline containing 1% of human serum albumin or AB serum (see below). If the DAT gives a strong reaction (i.e. + + or

+ + +) add a volume of saline equal to the volume of the cells; if the reaction is a weak one (i.e. ± or +), add only half the volume. Mix and agitate continuously in a water-bath at 56°C for 5 min. Centrifuge rapidly while still hot and remove the cherry-red supernatant at once—this is the eluate.

Eluates made into saline must be tested at once; those made into albumin-saline or AB serum will keep quite well at −20°C, but the

Table 23.6 Agglutination titres using various types of cold auto-antibodies and normal adult and normal cord red cells, the patient's red cells and enzyme-treated (papainized) normal adult red cells

Patient	Agglutination titre (4°C)			
	Adult (I) cells	Cord (i) cells	Patient's cells	Papainized adult (I) cells
A.G.	4000	512	2000	8000
F.B.	512	32000	128	8000
A.R.	2000	2000	2000	16

A.G. This patient had the cold-haemagglutinin disease. The antibody was of the common anti-I type.

F.B. This patient had a terminal haemolytic anaemia associated with a lymphoma. The antibody was of the anti-i type.

A.R. This patient had the cold-haemagglutinin disease. The antibody was of the rare anti-Pr type.

AB serum must be known to be free of any antibody.

Rubin's modification[14] of Vos and Kelsall's method[17]

To washed packed red cells in a glass tube add a suitable volume of saline (see above); then add a volume of ether twice that of the packed red cells. Stopper loosely (e.g. with the thumb, allowing release of vapour frequently) and shake vigorously for 1 min. Place at 37°C for 30 min, mixing frequently; centrifuge at 1200–1500 *g* at 37°C for 10 min, after which, three layers will be found. The top layer is ether—this is discarded. The bottom haemoglobin-stained layer is the eluate. Collect this with a pipette passed through the middle layer of red-cell stroma. Free the eluate of residual ether by leaving it at 37°C for 30–60 min. The smell of ether should have vanished before the eluate is tested or frozen for testing at a later date. Eluates prepared by Rubin's method into saline keep well if stored at −20°C.

Hughes-Jones, Gardner and Telford[7] estimated that if the elution process is carried out as described above, 70% of antibody will be recovered, while the Landsteiner method yields only a third as much antibody from the same volume of cells. For this reason, and because of the ease with which eluates prepared by Rubin's method can be prepared and stored, this is the method we routinely use in the investigation of cases of AIHA.

Screening eluates

The eluate and the saline of the last wash (control) are first screened against pooled group-O cells to see if they contain any antibodies:

1. By titration against enzyme-treated pooled group-O cells. Prepare doubling dilutions of eluate and control in saline to give dilutions of 1 in 1 to 1 in 32. To 1 drop of eluate or dilution add 1 drop of 2% enzyme-treated cells. Incubate at 37°C for $1-1\frac{1}{2}$ h and read microscopically.

2. By the indirect antiglobulin test (IAT). To 10 drops of eluate or control add 1 drop of 50% pooled group-O cells. Incubate for $1-1\frac{1}{2}$ h at 37°C. Wash four times and, using optimal dilutions of anti-IgG (and of anti-IgM and anti-IgA if these sera gave positive reactions in the DAT), carry out the IAT by either the tile or tube method (p. 350).

If the control preparation gives positive reactions, the possibility that any eluted antibody contains or consists of serum antibody has to be considered.

DETERMINATION OF THE SPECIFICITY OF WARM AUTO-ANTIBODIES IN ELUATES AND SERUM

When tested against a fully genotyped panel, about two-thirds of auto-antibodies appear to have Rh specificity and in about half these cases specificity against a particular antigen can be demonstrated.

The other one-third of auto-antibodies may show specificity against other very high incidence antigens, for example, Wr^b and En^a, and rarely other blood-group specificities are involved. It is essential to differentiate between auto- and allo-antibodies, especially if transfusion is being considered. The presence of allo-antibodies in addition to auto-antibodies is suggested by any discrepancy between the serum and eluate results.

The ascertainment of specificity is not difficult but it is essential to have available a panel of normal red cells, the blood groups of which have been determined as completely as possible. Access to a source of $-D-/-D-$ or Rh^{null} cells is a great advantage. Within the Rhesus system anti-e is the commonest specificity. This will be shown by R_2R_2 cells reacting much more weakly than do cells of the other common Rh genotypes. So-called 'Rhesus-specificity' is demonstrated by Rh^{null} cells reacting very weakly or failing to react while all the other cells on the panel react strongly.

As already mentioned, the presence of allo-antibodies in a serum complicates the determination of the specificity of an auto-antibody, and it can be argued that it would be better to test only the eluted auto-antibody and to leave the serum strictly alone. However, only a small volume of an eluate may be available, especially in anaemic patients, and it is generally wise to test both serum and eluate. The procedure is the same for both.

Titration of antibody in eluate or serum

The methods used have already been described in Chapter 21, p. 353. The exact technique chosen, and the red cells used, should be those which have given the clearest results in the screening tests.

DEMONSTRATION OF LYSIS BY WARM AUTO-ANTIBODIES

Auto-antibodies in serum capable of bringing about lysis in vitro of normal red cells at 37°C ('warm haemolysins') have rarely been demonstrated in cases of AIHA. When present, the patients have usually been acutely ill.[2b] In contrast, it is not rare for warm antibodies—presumably of the IgM variety—to lyse in the presence of complement en-zyme-treated cells at 37°C, and it is significant that patients whose sera lyse these modified cells, but *not* normal cells, do not necessarily suffer from a serious degree of haemolysis.[1] PNH red cells, too, can be used, if available, as sensitive reagents for demonstrating the lytic potentiality of the antibodies (see p. 200).

Red cells which have been stored for several days at 4°C may occasionally undergo agglutination (or lysis) in certain pathological sera.[8] When this occurs at 37°C in the screening test, the preparation should be set up again with the same cells taken freshly from the donor. Not infrequently, lysis will not occur with perfectly fresh red cells even though sublytic amounts of complement may be bound. In all lysis tests using normal red cells the pH of the cell-serum mixtures should be adjusted to about 6.8, as this is the optimum pH for lysis. Adjustment of pH is less critical using enzyme-treated or PNH cells than when normal unmodified cells are used.[2a]

FURTHER INVESTIGATION OF COLD ANTIBODIES: TESTS FOR SPECIFICITY AND TITRATION

High-titre cold auto-antibodies have a well defined blood-group specificity which is almost invariably within the I/i system. Since the I antigen is poorly devloped in cord-blood red cells, whilst the i antigen is well developed (Fig. 23.4), group-O cord blood red cells should be included in the panel used to test for I/i specificity. Adult cells almost always have the I antigen but the strength of the antigen varies and it is of considerable advantage to have available adult cells known to possess strong I antigen. (The rare adult i cells, if available, are also a useful reagent.)

Cold agglutinin titration patterns

The presence of high-titre cold agglutinins in a patient's serum will be indicated by the screening procedure described above on p. 395. To demonstrate that the agglutinins are auto-antibodies, it is necessary to show that the patient's own cells are also agglutinated. It is interesting to note that the titre using the patient's cells is usually less (one-half

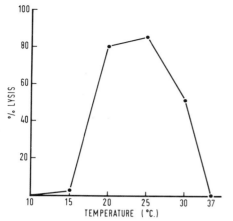

Fig. 23.4 Effect of temperature on lysis by a high-titre cold auto-antibody (anti-I). Chronic cold-haemagglutinin disease. Normal group O (I) red cells in patient's serum. The serum was diluted with an equal volume of fresh normal serum and acidified by the addition of a one-tenth volume of 0.2 mol/l HCl. Incubation was carried out for 10 min at each temperature.

or one-quarter) than that of control normal adult red cells (Table 23.6).

In cold-haemagglutinin disease, whether 'idopathic' or 'secondary' to Mycoplasma pneumonia or lymphoma, the auto-antibodies usually have anti-I specificity (Patient A.G. in Table 23.6).

In rare cases of haemolytic anaemia associated with infectious mononucleosis an auto-antibody of anti-i specificity has been demonstrated (Patient F.B. in Table 23.6), and this specificity, too, has been found in certain patients with lymphoma. Rarely, in chronic cold-haemagglutinin disease, the antibody has been shown to have anti-Pr or anti-M specificity; in either type of case the antigen is destroyed by enzyme treatment (Patient A.R. in Table 23.6).

Determination of the thermal amplitude of a cold auto-antibody

From a series of master doubling dilutions of serum in saline place 1 drop of serum or serum dilution into four rows of small (38 × 6.4 mm) agglutinin tubes. Set them up at 30°C, 25°C and 20°C and to each tube add 1 drop of a 2% saline suspension of the following cells:

1. Pooled normal adult group-O (I) red cells.

2. Pooled enzyme-treated (e.g. pre-papainized) normal adult group-O (I) red cells.
3. Pooled cord blood group-O (i) red cells.
4. Patient's red cells.

Titration should also be carried out at 37°C, if there had been agglutination at this temperature in the screening tests. After incubation at the appropriate temperature for $1\frac{1}{2}$–2 h, determine the presence or absence of agglutination macroscopically, using a concave mirror, as described on p. 349. It is hardly practical to read agglutination microscopically on slides warmed or cooled to the appropriate temperatures.

Alternatively, the thermal range of an antibody may be determined in the following simple way. Place three tubes each containing 10 drops of the patient's serum at 37°C. To each tube add 1 drop of a 50% saline suspension of pre-warmed red cells: to the first, pooled normal adult group-O (I) red cells; to the second, pooled normal cord-blood group-O (i) red cells, and to the third, the patient's own red cells. Mix the contents of each tube and allow the red cells to sediment for about 1 h in a water-bath at 37°C. After this time, transfer the tubes to a beaker containing water at 37°C which is allowed to cool slowly and in which a thermometer records the fall in temperature. Inspect the 3 tubes visually for agglutination at 37°C by tipping them gently and watching the behaviour of the red cells, and re-inspect each time the temperature falls by 1°C until agglutination is unmistakeable. Results typical of a case of chronic cold-haemagglutinin disease are given in Table 23.7.

Lysis by cold antibodies

If lysis is detected in the serum screening tests, the lysis titre and the thermal range for lysis should be determined and also the specificity of the antibody (anti-I, anti-i, anti-Pr or anti-M). To estimate the titre dilutions of the patient's serum are made in fresh normal serum to provide a source of complement. Typically, although not invariably, more lysis

Table 23.7 Macroscopic agglutination of various red-cell samples by the serum of a patient suffering from chronic cold-haemagglutinin disease

Cells	Temperature (°C)										
	30	29	28	27	26	25	24	23	22	21	20
Patient (I)	—	—	$\frac{1}{2}$ +	1 +	2 +	2 +	3 +	3 +	3 +	3 +	3 +
Normal adult (I)	—	$\frac{1}{2}$ +	1 +	1 +	2 +	3 +	3 +	3 +	3 +	3 +	3 +
Normal cord (i)	—	—	—	—	—	—	—	—	—	?	$\frac{1}{2}$ +

takes place if the serum-complement mixture is acidified.

Method

Prepare suitable dilutions of the patient's serum in fresh normal serum acidified to a pH of 6.0–6.5 (see p. 201). A series of master doubling dilutions should be set up initially. If a high lysis titre is anticipated, it is convenient to prepare a 1 in 10 dilution initially and then set up doubling dilutions (1 in 10, 1 in 20 etc. to a dilution of 1 in 640).

To 5 drops of each dilution add 1 drop of a 25% saline suspension of red cells. The cells used in the test should be:

1. Adult group-O cells known to possess a strong I antigen.
2. The same cells after enzyme-treatment.
3. Group-O (i) cord-blood cells.

Each test should be set up at 20°C, 30°C and 37°C, and it is most important that the cells and serum are brought to the correct temperature before they are mixed.

Optimum temperature for demonstrating lysis by a high-titre cold antibody

A temperature of 25°C is about optimum for the demonstration of lysis by high-titre (anti-I) antibodies. Below 15°C lysis will not take place because some complement components will not bind at a low temperature; above 30°C, depending on the thermal range of the antibody, lysis is prevented because antibody is not adsorbed. Lysis taking place in one phase at normal bench temperature without preliminary chilling has been referred to as monophasic (Fig. 23.4). This contrasts with lysis brought about by the Donath-Landsteiner (D-L) antibody which is typically described as biphasic.

Preliminary chilling below normal bench temperature is usually necessary to bring about binding on of the antibody, followed by warming for lysis to occur (see below). It should be noted that high-titre anti-I antibodies will often, too, bring about lysis when the red-cell-serum suspension is treated biphasically, i.e. give a type of positive D-L antibody test. Conversely, but rarely, genuine D-L antibodies, if active at a sufficiently high temperature, can also give rise to lysis monophasically, e.g. at 20°C. Anti-I antibodies can be distinguished from D-L antibodies by virtue of their remarkable agglutinating properties at low temperatures (and in other ways) even if they give a positive D-L test.

It is particularly important that the concentrated cell suspension be delivered directly into the serum dilution without running down the side of the tube, for tightly agglutinated cells lyse extremely easily under these conditions, even in the absence of complement. Lysis is usually read visually after the red cells have sedimented for 2 h, or, if practicable, after remixing and centrifuging at the appropriate temperature.

Enzyme-treated cells are typically much more sensitive to lysis by high-titre anti-I and anti-i antibodies than are normal red cells (Table 23.8) and they may even by lysed at 37°C. PNH cells are particularly easily lysed because of their remarkable sensitivity to complement (Table 23.8), and the lysis titre with these cells at 30°C is usually as great as or may exceed the agglutination titre. PNH cells can be used as a sensitive and reliable tool for the demonstration of the lytic potential of any antibody which fixes complement. However, when using PNH cells the serum must not be acidified, and the control tube, containing fresh normal serum but no patient's serum, must be carefully examined for lysis.

To ensure that lysis is easily visible a stronger cell-serum suspension should be used than that

Table 23.8 Relative sensitivity of red cells to lysis by a high-titre cold antibody at 20°C

Type of cell	pH	Dilutions of serum								Control (normal serum diluent)
		1 in 1	1 in 4	1 in 16	1 in 64	1 in 256	1 in 1024	1 in 4096	1 in 16 000	
Normal (I)	8.0	—	trace	—	—	—	—	—	—	—
Normal (I)	6.5	trace	+	(+)	trace	—	—	—	—	—
Trypsinized normal (I)	8.0	+	+ + +	+ +	+	(+)	—	—	—	—
PNH	8.0	+ + +	+ + +	+ + +	+ + +	+ + +	+ +	+ +	+	—

+ + + denotes marked lysis; + +, + and (+) denote lesser but definite degrees of lysis; — denotes no lysis.

used for agglutination tests. A final concentration of about 5% is suitable and this is attained by the method described above.

The lysis titre is given by the reciprocal of the highest serum dilution causing (+) lysis. It is convenient to score complete lysis as C. (+) represents definite but weak lysis compared with the colour of the supernatant of the control, while +, + + and + + + represent intermediate degrees of lysis.

Typical results obtained in a patient with chronic cold-haemagglutinin disease due to anti-I antibody are shown in Table 23.8.

DETECTION AND TITRATION OF A DONATH-LANDSTEINER ANTIBODY

The Donath-Landsteiner (D-L) antibody of paroxysmal cold haemoglobinuria differs from the high-titre cold antibodies referred to previously in that it is an IgG antibody and has a quite different specificity. It, too, is far more lytic to normal cells in relation to its titre than are anti-I or anti-i antibodies. Thus the lysis titre of a D-L antibody may be the same or greater than its agglutination titre. Almost maximal lysis develops in unacidified serum.

Direct Donath-Landsteiner test

Collect two samples of venous blood into glass tubes containing no anticoagulant, pre-viously warmed to 37°C. Incubate the first sample at 37°C for $1\frac{1}{2}$ h. Put the second sample in a beaker packed with ice and allow to stand for 1 h; then place the tube at 37°C for a further 20 min. Centrifuge both tubes at 37°C and examine the supernatant serum for lysis. A positive test is indicated by lysis in the sample which had been chilled.

Indirect Donath-Landsteiner test

Serum obtained from the patient's blood, which has been allowed to clot at 37°C is used for this test. Add 1 volume of a 50% suspension of washed normal group-O, P-positive red cells to 9 volumes of patient's unacidified serum in a glass tube. Chill the suspension in crushed ice at 0°C for 1 h, then place the tube at 37°C for 30 min. Centrifuge at 37°C and examine for lysis. Three controls should be set up at the same time:

1. A duplicate of the test cell-serum suspension, but kept strictly at 37°C for the duration of the test.

2. A duplicate of the test cell-serum suspension, except that an equal volume of ABO-compatible fresh normal serum is first added to the patient's serum as a source of complement. The same cells are added and the suspension is chilled and subsequently warmed in the same way as the test suspension. (This control excludes false-negative results due to the patient's serum being deficient in complement.)

3. A duplicate of the test cell-serum suspension, except that fresh normal serum is

used in place of the patient's serum. This control, too, is chilled and subsequently warmed.

A positive test will be indicated by lysis in the test suspension and in control No. 2. If ABO compatible *pp* cells are available they should be used in a duplicate set of tubes. No lysis will develop—confirming the P specificity of the antibody.

Titration of a Donath-Landsteiner antibody

Prepare doubling or four-fold dilutions of the patient's serum in fresh normal human serum. To each tube add a one-tenth volume of a 50% suspension of washed group-O P-positive red cells and immerse each of the tubes in crushed ice at 0°C. After 1 h place at 37°C and incubate for a further 30 min. Then centrifuge and inspect for lysis.

Detection of a Donath-Landsteiner antibody by the indirect antiglobulin test

Since the D-L antibody is an IgG antibody, it can be detected by the indirect antiglobulin test (IAT) using an *anti-IgG* serum if the cells which have been exposed to the antibody in the cold are washed in cold (4°C) saline. At this temperature the antibody will not be eluted during washing. It should be noted, however, that exposing normal red cells at 4°C to many fresh normal sera results in a positive IAT with broad-spectrum antiglobulin sera because of the adsorption of incomplete anti-H (a normally-occurring cold antibody) on to the red cells. At a low temperature, complement is bound, too, and it is its adsorption which gives rise to the positive tests with broad-spectrum sera. The adsorption of complement can be prevented by adding an anti-coagulant such as EDTA to the serum.

Method

Add a one-tenth volume of EDTA, buffered to pH 7.0 (see Appendix, p. 433) to the patient's serum. Prepare doubling dilutions in saline from 1 in 1 to 1 in 128. Add 1 volume (drop) of a 50% suspension of group-O, P-positive red cells to 10 volumes (drops) of each dilution. Mix and incubate at 4°C (preferably in a cold room). After 1 h wash the red cells four times in a large volume of cold (4°C) saline. Then carry out antiglobulin reactions using an anti-IgG serum, as described on p. 350, but with the title and serum previously chilled at 4°C. As controls, set up a series of tests using a serum known to contain a D-L antibody and a normal serum respectively. This technique is the most sensitive way of detecting, especially in stored sera, the D-L antibody present in an amount insufficient to bring about actual lysis.

Thermal range of a Donath-Landsteiner (D-L) antibody

The highest temperature at which D-L antibodies are usually adsorbed to red cells is about 18°C. Hence little or no lysis can be expected unless the cell-serum suspension is cooled below this temperature. Chilling in crushed ice results in maximum adsorption of the antibody and leads to the fixation of complement which brings about lysis when the cell suspension is subsequently warmed at 37°C. Hence the 'cold–warm' biphasic procedure necessary for lysis to be demonstrated by a typical D-L antibody.

Specificity of the Donath-Landsteiner antibody

The D-L antibody appears to have a well-defined specificity within the P blood-group system, namely, anti-P. However, in practice, almost all samples of red cells are acted upon, for the cells that will not react (P^k and *pp*) are extremely rare.[10,19] Cord-blood red cells are lysed to about the same extent as are adult P_1 and P_2 cells.

TREATMENT OF SERUM WITH 2-MERCAPTOETHANOL

Weak solutions of 2-mercaptoethanol destroy the inter-chain sulphydryl bonds of gamma globulins. IgM antibodies treated in this way lose their ability to agglutinate red cells while IgG antibodies do not.[31] IgA antibodies may or may not be inhibited depending upon whether or not they are made up of polymers of IgA globulin. Since almost all auto-antibodies are either IgM or IgG, treatment of serum or an eluate with 2-mercaptoethanol gives a reliable indication of the type of auto-antibody globulin under investigation.[11]

Method

To 1 volume of undiluted serum add 1 volume of 0.1 mol/l 2-mercaptoethanol in phosphate buffer, pH 7.2 (see p. 436). As a control, add a further volume of the serum to the phosphate buffer alone. Incubate both at 37°C for 2 h.

Then titrate the treated serum and its control with the appropriate red cells. If IgG antibody is present, the antibody titration in the control serum will be the same as that of the treated serum. However, if the antibody is IgM, the treated serum will fail to agglutinate the test cells or agglutinate them to a much lower titre compared with the control serum.

DRUG-INDUCED HAEMOLYTIC ANAEMIAS OF IMMUNOLOGICAL ORIGIN

As already mentioned (p. 385), acquired haemolytic anaemias may develop as the result of immunological reactions consequent on the administration of certain drugs. Clinically, they often closely mimic AIHA of 'idiopathic' origin and for this reason a careful enquiry into the taking of drugs is a necessary part of the interrogation of any patient suspected of having an acquired haemolytic anaemia. Two immunological mechanisms leading to a drug-induced haemolytic anaemia are recognized. These mechanisms are commonly referred to as 'immune' and 'auto-immune'.

Immune

In these cases antibodies are produced against a drug, and the drug is required in the in vitro system for the antibodies to be detected. The red cells become damaged by one or two mechanisms:

1. A drug–antibody immune-complex is adsorbed to the red-cell surface, as, for instance, happens with antibodies directed against quinine. In such cases the positive DAT is a reaction with adsorbed complement. The red cells in such cases have been referred to as 'innocent bystanders'.

2. The drug or a metabolite of the drug is firmly bound to the red-cell surface. IgG antibodies directed against the drug may then be bound to the red cells. The positive DAT is then usually due entirely to a reaction with bound IgG. Penicillin haemolytic anaemia is brought about in this way.

Auto-immune

In these cases the antibody is directed against the red cell, not the drug. The drug acts in some as yet ill-understood way to promote the development of anti-red-cell auto-antibodies which seem serologically identical to those of 'idiopathic' AIHA. Several drugs are known to act in this way (see p. 385). The great majority of cases have, however, followed the use of the anti-hypertension drug α-methyldopa (Aldomet). The red cells are coated with IgG and the serum contains auto-antibodies which characteristically have Rh specificity.

PENICILLIN-INDUCED HAEMOLYTIC ANAEMIA

The characteristic features are:

1. Haemolysis occurs only in patients receiving large doses of a penicillin.

2. The DAT is strongly positive with anti-IgG sera.

3. The patient's serum and antibody eluted from patient's red cells react only against penicillin-treated red cells—they do not react with normal untreated red cells.

Preparation of penicillin-treated red cells

Wash normal group-O red cells in 9 g/l NaCl (saline) and make up a c 15% suspension in saline to which a one-tenth volume of

0.14 mol/l barbitone buffer (pH 9.5) has been added. Add 2 ml of this suspension to 6 ml of buffered saline (pH 9.5) containing 0.4 g of penicillin G. Incubate for 1 h at 37°C, wash six times in saline and make up a 2% and a 50% saline suspension.

Detection of anti-penicillin antibodies

The antibodies can be detected by the IAT using a 50% saline suspension of penicillin-treated red cells. The tests are done in the usual way but three extra controls are necessary:

1. Red cells which have not been exposed to penicillin should be added to the patient's serum.

2. Penicillin-treated red cells should be added to two normal sera known not to contain anti-penicillin antibodies (negative controls).

3. Penicillin-treated red cells should be added to a serum (if one is available) known to contain anti-penicillin antibodies (positive control).

Cephalosporin can be used in a similar way to sensitize red cells. Control (2) is particularly important when penicillin derivatives such as cephalosporin are used, since over-exposure in vitro to these drugs can lead to positive results with normal sera.

High-titre IgG anti-penicillin antibodies often cause direct agglutination of penicillin-treated red cells in low dilutions of serum. The antibodies can be differentiated from IgM-agglutinating antibodies by treatment with 2-mercaptoethanol (see p. 403).

Detection of antibodies against drugs other than penicillin

In a patient with an immune haemolytic anaemia whose serum and red-cell eluate does *not* react with normal red cells and who is receiving a drug or drugs other than penicillin or a penicillin derivative, antibodies which react with red cells only in the presence of the suspect drugs or drugs should be looked for in the following way:

Table 23.9 Investigation of a suspected drug-induced haemolytic anaemia

Tube No.	1	2	3	4	5	6
Patient's serum volumes (drops)	10	10	5	5	0	0
Fresh normal serum volumes (drops)	0	0	5	5	10	10
Drug solution volumes (drops)	2	0	2	0	2	0
Saline volumes (drops)	0	2	0	2	0	2
50% normal group-O cells volumes (drops)	1	1	1	1	1	1

The patient's serum and red-cell eluates should be tested with normal and enzyme-treated group-O red cells, carrying out the tests with and without the drug that the patient is receiving. The approach is essentially empirical. A saturated solution of the drug should be prepared in saline and the pH adjusted to 6.5–7.0.

Set up six tubes containing the patient's serum and the drug solution in the proportions shown in Table 23.9, and add one drop of a 50% saline suspension of group-O cells to each tube.

Incubate at 37°C for 1 h and examine for agglutination and lysis. Wash the red cells four times in saline and carry out an IAT using a broad-spectrum antiglobulin serum or anti-IgG and anti-C sera separately.

REFERENCES

[1] BORNE, A. E. G. Kr. VON DEM, ENGELFRIET, C. P., BECKERS, D., KORT-HENKES, G. VAN DER, GIESSEN, M. VAN DER and VAN LOGHEM, J. J. (1969). Autoimmune haemolytic anaemia. II. Warm haemolysins—serological and immunochemical investigations and ^{51}Cr studies. *Clinical and Experimental Immunology*, **4**, 333.

[2] DACIE, J. V. (1962). *The Haemolytic Anaemias: Congenital and Acquired. Part II*: The Auto-Immune Haemolytic Anaemias, 2nd edn., (a) p. 437; (b) p. 439; (c) p. 461. Churchill, London.

[3] DACIE, J. V. (1975). Auto-immune hemolytic anemias. *Archives of Internal Medicine*, **135**, 1293.

[4] DACIE, J. V. and WORLEDGE, S. M. (1974). Auto-allergic blood diseases. In *Clinical Aspects of Immunology*. Eds. P. G. H. Gell and R. R. A. Coombs, 3rd edn., Blackwell Scientific Publications, Oxford.

[5] ENGELFRIET, C. P., BORNE, A. E. G. VON DEM, BECKERS, D. and VAN LOGHEM, J. J. (1974). Auto-immune haemolytic anaemia: serological and immunochemical characteristics of

the auto-antibodies: mechanisms of cell destruction. *Series Haematologica*, **VII**, 328.

[6] FLAHERTY, T. and GEARY, C. G. (1979). Auto-immune haemolytic anaemia. *British Journal of Hospital Medicine*, **22**, 334.

[7] HUGHES-JONES, N. C., GARDNER, B. and TELFORD, R. (1963). Comparison of various methods of dissociation of anti-D, using ^{131}I-labelled antibody. *Vox Sanguinis (Basel)*, **8**, 531.

[8] JENKINS, W. J. and MARSH, W. L. (1961). Autoimmune haemolytic anaemia. Three cases with antibodies specifically active against stored red cells. *Lancet*, **ii**, 16.

[9] LANDSTEINER, K. and MILLER, C. P. Jnr. (1925). Serological studies on the blood of primates. II. The blood groups in anthropoid apes. *Journal of Experimental Medicine*, **42**, 853.

[10] LEVINE, P., CELANO, M. J. and FALKOWSKI, F. (1963). The specificity of the antibody in paroxysmal cold haemoglobinuria (P.C.H.). *Transfusion (Philadelphia)*, **3**, 278.

[11] MOLLISON, P. L. (1979). *Blood Transfusion in Clinical Medicine*, 6th edn., p. 191. Blackwell Scientific Publications, Oxford.

[12] PETZ, L. D. and GARRATTY, G. (1980). *Acquired Immune Hemolytic Anemia*. Churchill Livingstone, New York, Edinburgh.

[13] PIROFSKY, B. (1976). Clinical aspects of auto-immune hemolytic anemia. *Seminars in Hematology*, **13**, 151.

[14] RUBIN, H. (1963). Antibody elution from red blood cells. *Journal of Clinical Pathology*, **16**, 70.

[15] SOKOL, R. J., JEWITT, S. and STAMPS, B. K. (1981). Autoimmune haemolysis: an 18 year study of 865 cases referred to a regional transfusion centre. *British Medical Journal*, **282**, 2023.

[16] STRATTON, F. and RENTON, P. H. (1955). Effect of crystalloid solutions prepared in glass bottles on human red cells. *Nature (London)*, **175**, 727.

[17] VOS, G. H. and KELSALL, G. A. (1956). A new elution technique for the preparation of specific immune anti-Rh serum. *British Journal of Haematology*, **2**, 342.

[18] WORLLEDGE, S. M. (1978). The interpretation of a positive direct antiglobulin test. *British Journal of Haematology*, **39**, 157.

[19] WORLLEDGE, S. M. and ROUSSO, C. (1965). Studies on the serology of paroxysmal cold haemoglobinuria (P.C.H.) with special reference to a relationship with the P blood group system. *Vox Sanguinis (Basel)*, **10**, 293.

24

Leucocyte and platelet antigens and antibodies
(By Sylvia D. Lawler[*])

THE HLA SYSTEM

The major histocompatibility system in man, which is called HLA, codes for cell membrane structures some of which occur on cells of most tissues of the body including leucocytes, both granulocytes and lymphocytes, and platelets.

Serology of the HLA system

The antigens that can be detected by serological techniques have been defined at a series of International Workshops.[13,14,15,16,17,18,19] Well-defined antigens assigned to a genetic locus, A, B or C are numbered, less well substantiated antigens have the additional prefix W. The specificities defined at the VIIIth Histocompatibility Workshop 1980[19] are listed in Table 24.1. The specificities of the DR locus, unlike those of A, B and C are found on B lymphocytes and activated T cells but not on other mature leucocytes or platelets. The D locus specifications are defined by the mixed lymphocyte culture technique (MLC). Splits of previously defined antigens are indicated by brackets and indentation. For example, both AW23 and AW24 have the broader specificity A9.

The main patterns of distribution of the antigens in different populations were established at the Fifth Histocompatibility Workshop 1972.[16] The frequencies of the antigens vary in different racial groups, some being found only in black populations, for example AW36 and AW43. The frequencies of the serologically defined antigens in Caucasians are given in Table 24.2.

[*] I should like to thank Dr. Elizabeth H. Jones, Mr. P. J. Dewar, Mr. A. Hockley and Miss S. Cleaver for their expert advice.

Table 24.1 The HLA specificities (WHO nomenclature 1980)

A locus	B locus	BW4 BW6	C locus	DR locus	D locus
A1	B5		CW1	DR1	DW1
A2	{ BW51		CW2	DR2	DW2
A3	{ BW52		CW3	DR3	DW3
A9	B7		CW4	DR4	DW4
{ AW23	B8		CW5	DR5	DW5
{ AW24	B12		CW6	DRW6	DW6
A10	{ BW44		CW7	DR7	DW7
{ A25	{ BW45		CW8	DRW8	DW8
{ A26	B13			DRW9	DW9
A11	B14			DRW10	DW10
A28	B15				DW11
AW19	{ BW62				DW12
{ A29	{ BW63				
{ AW30	BW16				
{ AW31	{ BW38				
{ AW32	{ BW39				
{ AW33	B17				
AW34	{ BW57				
AW36	{ BW58				
AW43	B18				
	BW21				
	{ BW49				
	{ BW50				
	BW22				
	{ BW54				
	{ BW55				
	{ BW56				
	B27				
	BW35				
	B37				
	B40				
	{ BW60				
	{ BW61				
	BW41				
	BW42				
	BW46				
	BW47				
	BW48				
	BW53				
	BW59				

Table 24.2 HLA per cent antigenic frequencies in European Caucasians (VIII Histocompatibility Workshop)[19]

A locus	%	%	B locus	%	%	C locus	%	DR locus	%
A2	45		B12	23		CW1	8	DR1	13
				BW44	21				
A1	28			BW45	2	CW2	10	DR2	25
AW19	31		B5	17		CW3	19	DR3	20
	A29	7		BW51	14	CW4	23	DR4	18
	AW32	9		BW52	3				
	AW31	6							
	AW30	5	B8	16		CW5	12	DR5	20
	AW33	4							
			B7	17		CW6	15	DRW6	4
A3	22		BW35	18					
						CW7	5	DR7	23
A9	23		B40	10		CW8	4	DRW8	5
	AW23	5		BW60	7				
	AW24	18		BW61	3			DRW9	2
			B15	12				DRW10	2
A11	12			BW62	11				
				BW63	1				
A10	11		B18	11					
	AW25	4							
	AW26	7	BW27	8					
A28	8		B17	8					
				BW57	6				
AW34	1			BW56	2				
			BW16	9					
				BW38	5				
				BW39	4				
			B14	6					
			B13	6					
			BW22	5					
				BW55	4				
				BW56	1				
			BW21	8					
				BW49	5				
				BW50	3				
			B37	3					
			BW41	2					
			BW53	2					
			BW47	1					
			BW48	1					
			BW59	1					
			BW42	<1					

The antigens A1 and B8 are predominantly characteristic of Caucasians, whilst the Caucasoid antigens A3 and B7 are also found in Negro and Oriental populations. The A2 antigen is spread throughout all populations but has the highest frequency in American Indians.

Genetics of the HLA system

The loci controlling the inheritance of the HLA system are located on the short arm of chromosome No. 6.[10] The control is mediated through four loci, A, B, C and D, each with multiple alleles, aligned

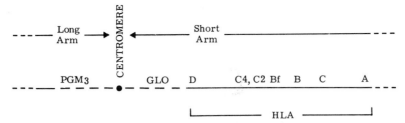

Fig. 24.1 Alignment of the HLA complex and other loci on chromosomes 6.
Key: PGM$_3$ = Phosphoglucomutase$_3$; GLO = Glyoxalase; C2 and C4 = components
of complement; Bf = Properdin factor B.

on the chromosome so that the C locus lies between
the A and B loci (Fig. 24.1). The precise relationship between the D locus, controlling the MLC
determinants, and the DR locus, determining
specificities on B lymphocytes, cannot as yet be
defined, although at the VIIth and VIIIth Histocompatibility Workshops, 1977 and 1980,[18,19] an
association with a high level of statistical significance was demonstrated between D specificities
and their correspondingly numbered DR specificities. The question whether more than one locus is
involved in the control of D and DR specificities
remains to be resolved.

As shown in Fig. 24.1, other genetic loci have
been assigned to chromosome 6, those controlling
the metabolic pathways of complement being in-
timately linked to the HLA loci. A close association
has been shown between complement components
and the blood-group systems Chido and Rodgers.[21]

Considering only the A and B loci, any individual
can express a maximum of four antigens, two
controlled by each locus, and such a phenotype is
described as a 'full house'. The contribution of
each parent, one allele from each locus, is called a
haplotype. The coupling between the alleles of the
A and B loci is not random and particular haplotype combinations of antigens are found in different races. This non-random association is termed
genetic disequilibrium. The commonest haplotypes
amongst Caucasians are HLA-A1,B8; A2,B12; and
A3,B7. The haplotypes of an individual can be
deduced when family studies are made as illustrated in Fig. 24.2. The A and B loci must be very
close together because the recombination frequency between them has been found to be 0.8%
by family studies. A family with a recombinant is
illustrated in Fig. 24.3. The second child has re-

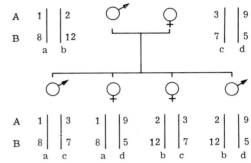

Fig. 24.2 HLA haplotypes. The paternal haplotypes are
labelled a and b, the maternal c and d. There are four possible
combinations amongst the off-spring.

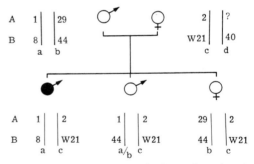

Fig. 24.3 HLA recombinant. The family was investigated to
find a donor for a patient (black circle).

ceived paternal A1 from the 'a' chromosome and
the BW44 from the 'b' chromosome.

The antigens of the B locus can be broadly
classified as W4 or W6 (Table 24.3). These two
antigens were originally defined by van Rood by
leucocyte agglutination reactions.[13] The BW4,
BW6 classification is useful in the definition of split
antigens; for example, BW16 can be split into
BW38 which is W4 associated and BW39 which is
W6 associated.

Table 24.3 Subdivision of HLA-B locus antigens

W4	W51(5), W52(5), W44(12), 13, W63(15), W38(16), W57(17), W58(17), W49(W21), 27, 37, W47, W53, W59.
W6	7, 8, W45(12), 14, W62(15), W39(16), 18, W50(W21), W54(W22), W55(W22), W56(W22), W35, W60(40), W61(40), W41, W42, W46, W48.

The main antigens to which the split antigens are related are shown in parenthesis.

Table 24.4. Red cell antigens on leucocytes and platelets

Leucocytes	
Definitely present	ABO, S, P(Tjª), I, i
Presence equivocal	M, N, Rh, P₁, Luª, Leª
Platelets	
Definitely present	ABO, P(Tjª), K, Fyª
Presence equivocal	M, N, Rh, P₁

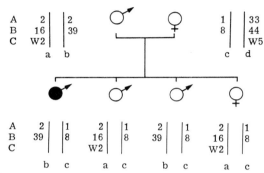

Fig. 24.4 HLA: the value of the C locus. The HLA identity of a patient (black circle) and the third child was confirmed by the C locus types.

The C locus antigens which show linkage disequilibrium with B locus antigens are sometimes useful in sorting out the haplotypes in a family. In the family illustrated in Fig. 24.4 the distribution of the paternal haplotypes amongst the children was confirmed by the C locus typing.

The mixed lymphocyte reaction (MLC)

This reaction is controlled by determinants at the D locus. In the absence of recombination the lymphocytes of an HLA identical sib give negative results in the MLC because they have the same D locus specificities. The D locus specificities are determined by using homozygous typing cells which preferably come from the offspring of first cousin marriages who have inherited an identical chromosome No. 6 from each of their parents.[17]

Non-HLA specificities

In addition to the determinants of the HLA system, leucocytes also carry species-specific antigens, tissue-specific antigens and some of the antigenic specificities that typify red cells. Examples of tissue-specific antigens are those peculiar to neutrophils that are not found on lymphocytes and the antigens that are confined to platelets. Some of the antigens detectable on red cells, the presence of which has been tested for on leucocytes and platelets, are listed in Table 24.4. There is only one defined serological system called 5, controlling antigens shared by lymphocytes and granulocytes, which is a separate entity from HLA.[31] The 5 system is not important in clinical practice. Two independent systems of granulocyte confined antigens have been described, the NA1 and 9 systems. The first anti-NA1 serum was found in a family in which an infant suffered from neonatal neutropenia.[20] The genetics of the 9 system have been investigated but as yet the system has not been shown to have clinical relevance.[14]

LEUCOCYTE ANTIBODIES

The first human leucocyte antigen was discovered in 1958 by Dausset using an antibody produced in a multi-transfused patient.[7] The antigen was then called Mac and it it now known to be the same as the antigen designated HLA-A2. The search for leucocyte antibodies in the sera of pregnant women was advocated by Payne[23] and van Rood.[32] During the late 1950s and early 1960s most of the work was done by leucocyte agglutination tests, and the chance of finding agglutinating antibodies was found to increase with the number of pregnancies. After the introduction of lymphocyte microcytotoxicity tests everyone opted to work with suspensions of lymphocytes. Like leuco-agglutinins, cytotoxic antibodies are also formed as the result of stimulation by pregnancy, transfusion or planned immunization. Unlike leuco-agglutinins, cytotoxic antibodies can be found in the sera of about 20% of primaparous women. The antibodies can be detected early in pregnancy but persistence after birth is very variable; they may disappear soon after parturition or be found in the serum of a non-transfused woman many years after the last birth. In a subject who has never been pregnant at least 4 l of blood are usually required to raised an antibody. The combined effect of pregnancy and transfusion is to evoke more antibody formation. Prolonged immunization tends to be associated with a broadening of the specificity of the antibody. In deliberately immunized donors the intradermal route is the most immunogenic.

Effects of leucocyte antibodies

Cytotoxic HLA antibodies do not harm the fetus in utero in spite of the fact that the antibodies can cross the placenta. On the other hand, neonatal neutropenia associated with an antibody specific for neutrophils was documented before the neutrophil-specific antigens were defined.[4] The presence of leucocyte antibodies should be sought for in patients with an unexplained transfusion reaction, and leucocyte-poor blood should be given to patients for whom sensitization to HLA antigens would constitute a risk. In order to ensure that a recipient does not receive transfusions of leucocytes carrying an antigen for which he or she may have an antibody, the serum of the recipient should be tested against donor cells, ideally with a range of samples collected from the recipient at different times.

TRANSPLANTATION

HLA typing has practical application in transplantation, and at present by far the most widely used application is in kidney transplantation. However, the precise value of matching recipient and donor for the serologically determined HLA antigens when cadaver transplants are used is as yet unsolved. If there is a match for all the A and B locus antigens the kidney is likely to survive well but the success with lesser degrees of matching is variable. The question has to be viewed against the background of data on the effects on graft survival of transfusions prior to transplantation.[29] It is not in doubt that in the presence of cytotoxic anti-bodies against A, B or C antigens present in the donor a kidney graft may undergo acute rejection but this is not necessarily the case with DR antibodies.[5] Also in the case of living donors, there is no doubt that an HLA identical sib, having inherited the same maternal and paternal haplotypes as the recipient, is the best donor.

Bone marrow

Due partly to improved histocompatibility matching during recent years, bone-marrow transplantation has come to play an increasingly important role in the treatment of certain potentially lethal blood disorders, notably severe aplastic anaemia, combined immunodeficiency diseases and leukaemia. The best donor for a patient with any of these conditions is a monozygotic twin, genetically identical with the recipient. Then neither host-versus-graft or graft-versus-host reactions need to be anticipated.

In the absence of an identical twin, the next donor in order of preference is an ABO-compatible sib with the same maternal and paternal HLA haplotypes. ABO incompatibility is not a contra-indication to transplantation but measures have to be taken to deal with anti-A or -B antibodies in the recipient directed against donor cells. An important test in donor selection is the MLC. A negligible reaction between the lymphocytes of donor and recipient is an essential prerequisite both in the one-way system, in which one population of cells acts as stimulator and the other as responder, and in the two-way system in which both populations are viable. Leukaemia patients should always be tested in remission because of the difficulties of interpreting MLC results in the leukaemic state. Family donors other than sibs and unrelated donors, particularly for patients with immune deficiency, are now being used. These may be selected on the basis of identity for the D locus determinants before proceeding to the MLC tests with recipient cells.

PLATELETS
Auto-antibodies

Auto-antibodies against platelets are probably responsible for most cases (at least) of idiopathic thrombocytopenic purpura (ITP) and transient thrombocytopenia has been observed in infants born to mothers with ITP, due probably to transplacental passage of anti-platelet antibodies. These antibodies have proved most difficult to demonstrate in vitro.[24]

Allo-antibodies

Allo-immune thrombocytopenia in the newborn due to the passage of anti-platelet IgG antibodies across the placenta occurs about once in every 10 000 births. The condition is usually benign and self-limiting but if the infant is severely affected, death can occur.[28]

Platelet antigens

Three diallelic systems have been discovered: Zw, Ko and Pl^E. The Zw system, described in the Netherlands,[30] was found by the exchange of sera to be the same as the Pl^A1 system described in America.[28] The antibody Zw^a (Pl^A1) was identified in the maternal serum in four out of six families with neonatal purpura of probable allo-immune aetiology.[30] Feto-maternal incompatibility is rare because the antigen Zw^a has a high incidence. The Ko system does not seem to have relevance in clinical practice.[13] The Pl^E system is also of more theoretical than practical interest because only one person, the patient who made the antibody, has ever been found to lack the Pl^E1 antigen.[28]

Most of the problems arising during platelet transfusions are likely to be due to HLA antibodies, and it is sometimes useful when finding donors for platelets to screen those who match the recipient for the BW4 or BW6 antigens. If fully typed panels of donors are available, then selection of donor according to HLA type is feasible; homozygous donors are most useful because they are more likely to be compatible with the recipient than 'full-house' donors.

Post-transfusion purpura

Post-transfusion purpura is a rare thrombocytopenic syndrome which develops about 1 week after transfusion in previously immunized patients. In every case the condition has been associated with the development of anti-Pl^A1.[11] Probably, the recipients' own platelets adhere to circulating platelet-antibody complexes. The syndrome could be avoided by cross-matching platelets, but since 97% of Caucasians are Pl^A1 positive it would be difficult to find a compatible donor.

Drug-induced thrombocytopenia

Drugs can cause thrombocytopenia in two ways: by a direct toxic effect on the bone-marrow, or, rarely, by a hypersensitivity reaction in which platelets are destroyed in the peripheral blood. Drugs known to have caused thrombocytopenia by the latter mechanism include, Sedormid, quinidine and quinine. The hypersensitivity mechanism can be demonstrated by in vitro tests. The patient's serum is capable of agglutinating platelets—either his or her own or those of a normal donor—in the presence of the drug. In Sedormid purpura the hypersensitivity can be diagnosed by the development of purpura under a skin patch test.

It was proposed by Ackroyd that drugs act as haptenes, combining with platelets and making them antigenic and capable of inducing antibody formation against the drug-platelet complex.[1] In Shulman's view the mechanism involves non-specific adsorption of antigen–antibody complexes on to platelets, with the platelets therefore participating as adsorbants rather than antigens.[27] According to this hypothesis the drug must also couple firmly with a macromolecule, probably a plasma protein, in order to become effectively antigenic.

GENERAL POINTS OF TECHNIQUE

Collection of blood samples

Blood collected for the preparation of leucocyte or platelet suspensions is taken into an anticoagulant, such as ACD or EDTA. The latter is the anticoagulant of choice for the separation of platelets but because of its anti-complementary activity it is not recommended for lymphocytes if these are to be tested by a cytotoxic method requiring complement. For leucocyte typing defibrinated blood has the advantage of freedom from platelets. Blood taken into heparin, free from preservative, is suitable for lymphocyte typing.

Separation of blood components

Leucocytes can be separated by sedimentation in the presence of high molecular weight dextran (6%), gelatin (3%), polyvinylpyrrolidone (PVP) or polybrene. Mix the anticoagulated blood thoroughly with the sedimentation agent in a siliconized tube. Then place this tube at 37°C at an angle of 45°C for about 30 min. Remove the upper two-thirds of the supernatant and count the leucocytes. Suspensions prepared in this way are suitable for agglutination tests if the WBC is $6-9 \times 10^9/l$.

Sera*

Separate the serum as quickly as possible, clear it by centrifugation, and store in small (e.g. 0.2 ml) volumes at ultra-low (e.g. $-70°C$) temperatures. To prepare DR antibodies free of ABC antibodies, sera may have to be absorbed with platelets.

Lymphocyte suspensions

To prepare suspensions of mixed T and B lymphocytes most workers use the method of Böyum[3] or a modification. Dilute anticoagulated blood 1 in 2 in 9 g/l NaCl (saline) and layer it over a mixture of Ficoll[†] and Triosil[‡] in a centrifuge tube. Centrifuge this tube at 400 **g** for 20 min. The lymphocytes (and platelets, too, when heparin is used) separate in a layer just below the interface of the plasma and Ficoll-Triosil layer. The red cells and most of the granulocytes sediment through the Ficoll-Triosil to the bottom of the tube.

Remove the lymphocyte layer with a pipette and wash the cells twice in Hanks balanced salt solution[§], spinning at 750 **g** for 1 minute. This method avoids gross contamination with platelets. Alternatively, the granulocytes can be removed by incubating the suspensions with carbonyl iron. The granulocytes ingest the particles which are then removed from the cell suspensions using a magnet.[6]

To prepare suspensions enriched with B lymphocytes for DR typing, remove the T cells from the mixture of T and B lymphocytes by rosetting the T lymphocytes on to sheep red blood cells. To make the rosettes as firm as possible, treat the sheep red cells with enzymes such as neuraminidase or papain before being mixed with the lymphocyte suspensions. After induction of rosette formation by centrifugation, separate the B cells from the T cells by the Ficoll-Triosil method and then wash them in a mixture of equal volumes of tris buffered saline and fetal calf serum.

Platelet suspensions

Prepare platelet suspensions from blood collected into EDTA. To obtain platelet-rich plasma centrifuge the blood at 4°C for 10 min at 200 **g**. Centrifuge the supernatant at 750 **g** for 30 min to obtain a button of platelets. Wash the platelets three times in saline and store at 4°C in saline containing 1 mg/ml sodium azide at an optimal concentration of $2 \times 10^{12}/l$.[25]

Storage of lymphocytes

Suspensions of lymphocytes can be posted round the world in transport medium[¶] and remain in a state suitable for HLA typing.[22] They can also be stored in ampoules in liquid nitrogen tanks. The freezing mixture must contain a cryo-protective agent, such as dimethyl sulphoxide (DMSO) or glycerol, and

---

* Hybridomas are now being used to produce monoclonal HLA antibodies.
† Ficoll powder: Pharmacia (G.B.), Paramount House, Uxbridge Road, London.
‡ Triosil: Vestric Ltd., Stonefield Way, Ruislip, Middx.

§ Flow Laboratories Ltd., Irvine, Scotland.
¶ McCoy's 5A Medium (Modified) or Medium 199, Gibco Bio-Cult Ltd.

an adequate amount of protein. Mixtures containing 10–20% DMSO in autologous plasma or AB serum are commonly used. The optimal rate of freezing lymphocytes that are to be stored and subsequently recovered for a lymphocytotoxicity test is 1°C/min. The freezing rate can be controlled by the use of a purpose built machine. A convenient and cheaper alternative is to place the ampoules containing the lymphocytes in the neck of the nitrogen tank within a plug that has been specially designed for the purpose.[26] After a few hours the ampoules can be transferred to the well of the liquid nitrogen tank.

Recovery of frozen lymphocytes

In order to obtain a good yield of cells for typing, their recovery must be carried out with care. Thaw the cells rapidly by warming the ampoules, with agitation, in a water-bath at 37°C. As soon as they are thawed—they must not be allowed to become warm—slowly suspend them to a concentration of c 3000/ml by drop by drop addition of the diluent. The condition of the cells can be checked by testing their capacity to exclude trypan blue, as for a cytotoxicity test it is necessary that the cells have functionally intact membranes. About 95% of the cells should remain unstained in a lymphocyte suspension that has been properly frozen and thawed.

If the purpose of storage is to maintain the capacity of the lymphocytes to respond to mitogens and allogeneic cells, then the freezing process has to be modified. A recommended procedure for optimal recovery of mitotic function of small volumes of lymphocytes in 5% DMSO is to interrupt rapid cooling with a timed exposure to a single sub-zero temperature. Hold the cells at −25 to −26°C for at least 5 min in a deep freeze before immersing them in liquid nitrogen.[9]

LYMPHOCYTE CYTOTOXICITY TESTS

The principle of the tests is the demonstration of a cytotoxic effect of antibody on lymphocytes in the presence of complement.[8,26] In most laboratories the tests are set up in Terasaki plates; these are plastic microplates, fitted with lids, and containing 60 wells. Single or multiple dispensing microlitre syringes are used for setting up the tests. Multiple dispensers are useful for setting up plates for typing or screening sera because the operation is speedier than with a single dispenser. Irrespective of the type of dispenser, great care must be exercised in order to avoid 'carry-over' of reagents from one well to another.

Lymphocytotoxic sera

Place the sera in wells under mineral oil. The plates can then be stored with lids on at −70°C until required.

Complement

Rabbit complement is an essential ingredient. Pool fresh sera from a number of rabbits, having ascertained that they are not individually cytotoxic in the absence of antibody before adding the sample to the pool. Store the sera at −70°C. Some workers also use complement-containing human AB serum as an ingredient of the medium for the lymphocyte suspensions. A pool of sera from male donors, each of which has been screened for the presence of cytotoxic antibodies, is the best source.

Cytotoxicity testing

The cytotoxicity of the serum is measured as a percent kill. Eosin (or trypan blue) can be used, in which case the dye is excluded from those cells that have not been affected by the antibody, the cell membrane remaining intact. Phase-contrast (or direct) illumination is used. Alternatively, the cells may be labelled with fluorescein salts; the label is retained by intact cells and lost by dead cells, which do not then fluoresce in UV or blue light. A two-colour fluorescence method for typing B lymphocytes has been described which has the advantage that no prior separation of the T and B lymphocytes is required.[33]

Official National Institutes of Health two-stage test used at international workshops

Each well of a Terasaki plate contains 1 μl of lymphocyte suspension containing 3000 cells per μl diluted with equal volumes of CFT buffer* or buffered saline, pH 7.2 (p. 436) and complement-containing AB serum.

Mix the serum and cells thoroughly in the wells with the tip of the needle of the dispenser. After agitation on a Vortex mixer let the suspension stand at 20°C for 30 min (A, B and C antigens) or at 37°C for 60 min (DR antigens). After the incubation, add 5 μl of rabbit complement to each well and mix the contents thoroughly; then let the plate stand for 60 min at 20°C (A, B and C antigens) or 120 min (DR antigens). Add 3 μl of 5% eosin and 3 μl of formalin to each well. Read the result under an inverted phase-contrast microscope at ×100 or ×250 magnification. Negative controls without antisera give the background of kill. This should not exceed 10%.

DR typing by the two-colour fluorescent method[33]

HLA-DR typing is normally performed on an enriched population of B lymphocytes and this requires a large initial volume of peripheral blood. The two-colour fluorescence method enables DR typing to be performed on small concentrations of lymphocytes (B and T), and B cell separation is not necessary.

Method

Incubate 10^7 lymphocytes in 0.5 ml of TC 199 medium (Wellcome), containing 10% of de-complemented fetal calf serum, with 0.05 ml of fluorescein isothiocyanate-conjugated sheep anti-human immunoglobulin. Incubate

* Complement Fixation Test Diluent Tablets (Oxoid Ltd.).

the cells at 37°C for 30 min, wash them three times with medium and resuspend at a concentration of 1×10^6 cells/ml.

Add 0.5 μl of the cell suspension to 0.5 μl of DR antiserum in flat bottom trays (Medicell) and incubate for 1 h in the dark. Add 2 μl of rabbit complement and continue the incubation for 2 h in the dark. Then add 0.5 μl of ethidium bromide and examine by means of a fluorescent microscope. Estimate the percentage of dead B cells; they are identified by their mixed green + red staining characteristics. Other cells stain only green or red or are unstained.

Comments on the lymphocytotoxicity test

When typing cells it is desirable to have three different antisera representing each specificity, but tests in triplicate may not be possible due to scarcity of antisera for certain specificities. Tissue typing antisera are supplied to bona fide users in the United Kingdom from the National Tissue Typing Reference Laboratory, South Western Regional Transfusion Centre, Bristol BS10 5ND (Director, Dr. B. A. Bradley).

A stored panel of lymphocytes well-characterized for the HLA antigens is necessary in order to screen sera for antibodies. As well as normal B lymphocytes, the lymphocytes from patients with chronic lymphocytic leukaemia can be used to screen for DR antibodies. If sensitivity is important, as, for example, in cross-matching recipients of kidney transplants, it is desirable to make the test as sensitive as possible and tests at different temperatures (20°C and 37°C) may reveal a wider spectrum of antibodies.

Lymphocytes suitable for typing can be obtained from lymph nodes as well as from the peripheral blood or spleen. Nodes are often an important source of donor material in cadavers.

TESTS FOR PLATELET ANTIBODIES

Allo-antibodies against platelets most frequently have HLA specificity. The method of typing platelets for HLA antigens and of demonstrating allo-antibodies is by complement fixation. The test can be done in Terasaki plates and serum placed under oil in the same way as for the lymphocyte cytotoxicity tests. The reagents required are human complement and sensitized sheep red cells (SSRC).[26]

Human complement

Obtain a pool of serum from five group-AB healthy, non transfused males who have fasted overnight. Allow their whole blood to clot at room temperature (18–25°C) for c 1 h, and then leave at 4°C for 2 h. Remove the serum aseptically and test a sample from each donor against SSRC in order to make sure that the complement is satisfactory. Pool the samples, freeze rapidly in 0.5 ml volumes and store at −70°C. Alternatively, the complement can be stored in a liquid nitrogen tank in ampoules such as are used for storing lymphocytes.

Haemolytic system

Commercially available sheep red cells are usually reliable although different batches vary in sensitivity. It is advisable to store the cells for about 7 days before use because fresh cells are resistant to the action of complement. (They will keep for several weeks in Alsever's solution if kept sterile.)

Wash the cells before use in CFT buffer (p. 415) and incubate at a concentration of c $0.4 \times 10^{12}/l$ with an equal volume of rabbit anti-sheep-red-cell haemolytic serum for 30 min at 37°C, at a final concentration of 4 minimal haemolytic units (MHU). The MHU is determined by preliminary titrations under test conditions. The sensitized cells can be kept at 4°C for up to 2 days.

Standardization of complement

Complement is standardized by testing serial doubling-diluted solutions of serum, prepared in bulk, in a Terasaki plate. Each well contains 4 μl of CFT buffer and 2 μl of serum dilution.

After agitation of the plate on a Vortex mixer, so that the contents of each well are thoroughly mixed, incubate the plate for 1 h at 37°C. Then add 2 μl of SSRC to each well and after a further 30 min at 37°C place the plate in a specially designed centrifuge head and then centrifuge at 300–700 g for 3 min. Read the degree of haemolysis with the naked eye.

The highest dilution of serum giving complete lysis is said to contain 1 H100 unit of complement, and as the amount of complement required in each complement fixation test is 2 H100 units, this is provided by twice the concentration of serum required for 1 H100 unit.

Complement fixation test

Each well of the plate contains: platelet suspension, $0.5 \times 10^6/\mu$l; serum or serum dilution, 2 μl; and 2 H100 units of complement in 2 μl. Mix the contents of the well by agitation on a Vortex mixer and incubate for 1 h at 37°C. Add 2 μl of SSRC ($0.2 \times 10^6/\mu$l) to each well and, after mixing, incubate the plate for 30 min at 37°C. Then gently centrifuge before reading. Sera being tested for complement-fixing antibodies must first be heated for 30 min at 56°C to inactivate any complement present. The test must be controlled for anti-complementary activity of the test serum or platelet suspension and for the potency of the complement. The test is very sensitive, and it is advisable to keep a separate microlitre syringe for dispensing complement.

Comments on complement fixation test

If a patient is being investigated for antibodies which might cause difficulties with platelet transfusions the specificity is most likely to correspond to HLA-A, B or C antigens. Therefore the specificity of the antibody can be found by using lymphocytes as indicator cells.

Platelet typing can provide additional information on HLA specificities if there are difficulties in obtaining adequate yields of normal lymphocytes. Useful platelet complement-fixing antibodies with

HLA specificities are not plentiful, and some specificities, for example A8 and B12, are difficult to determine by this method.

Platelet agglutination test

The test is done in plastic precipitin tubes using 0.1 ml of serum and 0.5 ml of a platelet suspension (0.2×10^9/ml). After incubation for 90 min transfer the deposited platelets to a microscope slide by means of a plastic pipette and look for agglutination under a low-power objective. Normal serum, a saline control, and a serum known to contain antibody must always be included with the test. The technique is relatively insensitive but useful and reproducible for the detection of rare agglutinins.[27]

Antiglobulin consumption test[12]

The direct antiglobulin test can be used to detect antibodies attached in vivo to platelets or leucocytes and the indirect antiglobulin consumption test can be used to detect free antibodies.

Wash the leucocytes (c 2×10^8) or platelets (c 2×10^9) six times in 9 g/l NaCl (saline), centrifuging at 900 g for 15 min in 75×8 mm plastic tubes. If leucocytes are the test cells, a tube containing as many red cells as are present as contaminants in the leucocyte suspension must be washed in the same way. After the final wash and removal of the supernatant, centrifuge the tubes again and remove any supernatant to ensure that the deposited leucocytes or platelets are as concentrated as possible. Then add 0.2 ml of diluted anti-human globulin (IgG) to each tube. (The antiglobulin serum used, when diluted a further 1 in 512 should just fail to agglutinate Rh-positive red cells sensitized with a strong anti-D antibody.)

Place each tube in a water-bath at 37°C for 6 min and then centrifuge at 1700 g for 15 min. Remove each supernatant and make ten doubling dilutions from it in saline. Add thoroughly washed strongly sensitised Rh-positive red cells in equal volumes to each dilution of antiglobulin on a tile. Then read agglutination as described on p. 350. For a positive result, i.e. antiglobulin has been consumed, the end point in the test must be at least two dilutions lower than that of the negative control.

In the indirect test, after the leucocyte or platelet suspensions have been prepared, add 0.3 ml of saline, normal serum, positive control serum or test serum to a series of cell deposits and mix the suspension well. After 90 min at 37°C, wash the leucocytes or the platelets six times. The procedure thereafter is the same as for the direct antiglobulin consumption test.

Comments on platelet antibodies

Although the complement fixation test and platelet agglutination tests are simple and suitable for detecting HLA antigens and platelet specific antigens, the tests cannot detect non-complement-binding and non-agglutinating antibodies.

Such antibodies can be detected by the antiglobulin consumption test, but this is a relatively insensitive method and depends on the quality of the antiglobulin serum used. The use of immunofluorescence tests on platelets had been limited by non-specific fluorescence caused by non-immunological binding of plasma proteins to the platelet membrane. Recently, fixation by paraformaldehyde has been recommended to overcome this problem (p. 256). Using this technique the detection of platelet-specific agglutinins, non-agglutinating platelet-specific antibodies, drug-dependent platelet antibodies, and HLA antibodies has been described.[2]

Mixed lymphocyte culture (MLC)

Preparation of lymphocytes

Sterility must be preserved throughout. Heparinized or defibrinated blood can be used. If heparin is used in the blood sample it should also be added to all the media at a concentration of 10 iu/ml. Dilute the blood sample with an equal volume of RPMI 1640 Medium* and separate the lymphocytes by sedimentation through sterile Ficoll-Triosil solution by centrifuging at 400 **g** for 20 min. Remove the lymphocytes from the interface, wash twice in RPMI 1640 and resuspend at 1×10^6/ml in a medium consisting of RPMI 1640 (80%), heat-inactivated pooled human AB serum (20%) and 2 mmol/l glutamine (Gibco), i.e. 1 ml of a 200 mmol/l solution per 100 ml.

Treatment of stimulator cells

A sample of lymphocytes from each person under test is treated so that the cells cannot respond to other lymphocytes but are able to stimulate untreated cells of a different DW type. This is done by irradiating the cells by c 4000 rads from a suitable source (X-Rays or γ-rays) or by treating them with mitomycin C. Add 0.625 ml (25 μg) of mitomycin C/1×10^6 lymphocytes (1 ml) and incubate the cell suspension at 37°C for 30 min. Then centrifuge the cells, wash three times in RPMI 1640 and finally resuspend in the culture medium containing the AB serum described above.

Setting-up cultures

Each individual one-way MLC test consists of 0.05 ml (5×10^4 cells) from a responder and an equal volume of stimulator cells. The two-way test consists of mixtures of the two cell populations, neither having been treated with X-Rays or mitomycin C. Each combination should be set up at least in triplicate and the experiments should include controls of responders plus mitomycin-treated stimulator cells from the same person. Each responder should be tested against an unrelated HLA-D different stimulator, preferably from a pool of donors covering as many HLA-DW specifici-

* Gibco Bio-Cult Ltd: Roswell Park Memorial Institute Medium.

ties as possible. Set up the MLCs in microtitre plates with U-shaped wells, and incubate at 37°C in an atmosphere of 5% CO_2 in air for 5 days. Then add 0.5 μCi of tritiated thymidine in a convenient volume, e.g. 50 μl, to each well and reincubate the cultures for a further 18 h.

Termination of cultures

Collect the cells using a cell harvester (several models of which are available commercially). The cells are washed from the micro plates and disrupted, and DNA is precipitated by washing with 50 g/l trichloroacetic acid, and collected on glass fibre sheets. The contents from each well form discrete areas on the glass fibre sheets. After drying the sheets, discs can be removed for scintillation counting. Place the glass fibre discs in counting vials, add a suitable phosphor and measure the activity in a liquid scintillation counter.

Record the results as counts per minute and calculate the mean of the triplicate sets of counts.

In family studies two indices are useful:

1. Stimulator index $= \dfrac{\text{cpm ABm}}{\text{cpm AAm}}$;

2. Relative response

$$= \frac{\text{cpm ABm} - \text{cpm AAm}}{\text{cpm AXm} - \text{cpm AAm}} \times 100,$$

where A and B are a sib pair and X is an unrelated control; m = mitomycin-treated.

An HLA identical pair should give a negative result in the two-way test, a stimulator index of <2.0 and a relative response of <4%. In HLA-DW typing using homozygous typing cells, a Double Normalization Value is determined.[19]

REFERENCES

[1] ACKROYD, J. F. (1955). Platelet agglutinins and lysins in the pathogenesis of thrombocytopenic purpura, with a note on platelet groups. *British Medical Bulletin*, **11**, 28.
[2] VON DEM BORNE, A. E. G. Kr., VERHEUGHT, F. W. A., OOSTERHOF, F., VON RIESZ, E., BRUTEL DE LA RIVIERE, A.

and ENGELFRIET, C. P. (1978). A simple immunofluorescence test for the detection of platelet antibodies. *British Journal of Haematology*, **39**, 195.

[3] BÖYUM, A. (1968). Separation of leukocytes from blood and bone marrow. *Scandinavian Journal of Clinical and Laboratory Investigation*, **21**, Suppl. 97.

[4] BRAUN, E. H., BUCKWOLD, A. E., EMSON, H. E. and RUSSELL, A. V. (1960). Familial neonatal neutropenia with maternal leukocyte antibodies. *Blood*, **16**, 1745.

[5] CARPENTER, C. B. and MORRIS, P. J. (1978). The detection and measurement of pretransplant sensitization. *Transplantation Proceedings*, **10**, 509.

[6] COULSON, A. S. and CHALMERS, D. C. (1964). Separation of viable lymphocytes from human blood. *Lancet*, **i**, 468.

[7] DAUSSET, J. (1958). Iso-leuco-anticorps. *Acta Haematologica*, **20**, 156.

[8] DICK, H. M. and CRICHTON, B. W. (1972). *Tissue Typing Techniques*. Churchill Livingstone, Edinburgh.

[9] FARRANT, J., KNIGHT, S. C., McGANN, L. E. and O'BRIEN, J. (1974). Optimal recovery of lymphocytes and tissues following rapid cooling. *Nature (London)*, **249**, 452.

[10] FRANCKE, U. and PELLEGRINO, M. A. (1977). Assignment of the major histocompatibility complex to a region of the short arm of human chromosome 6. *Proceedings of the National Academy of Sciences*, U.S.A., **74**, 1147.

[11] GOCKERMAN, J. P. and SHULMAN, N. R. (1973). Isoantibody specificity in post-transfusion purpura. *Blood*, **41**, 817.

[12] GOLDSMITH, K. L. G. and BRAZIER, D. M. (1974). *Techniques for the detection of leucocyte and platelet antibodies*. Laboratory protocol of the Blood Group Reference Laboratory, London.

[13] Histocompatibility testing, 1965 (1965). Munksgaard, Copenhagen.

[14] Histocompatibility testing, 1967 (1967). Munksgaard, Copenhagen.

[15] Histocompatibility testing, 1970 (1970). Munksgaard, Copenhagen.

[16] Histocompatibility testing, 1972 (1973). Munksgaard, Copenhagen.

[17] Histocompatibility testing, 1975 (1975). Munksgaard, Copenhagen.

[18] Histocompatibility testing, 1977 (1978). Munksgaard, Copenhagen.

[19] Histocompatibility testing, 1980 (1980). UCLA Tissue Typing Laboratory, Los Angeles, California.

[20] LALEZARI, P. and BERNARD, G. E. (1966). An isologous antigen–antibody reaction with human neutrophils, related to neonatal neutropenia. *Journal of Clinical Investigation*, **45**, 1741.

[21] O'NEILL, G. J., YANG, S. Y., TEGOLI, J., BERGER, R. and DUPONT, B. (1978). Chido and Rodgers blood groups are distinct antigenic components of human complement C4. *Nature (London)*, **273**, 668.

[22] PARK, M. S. and TERASAKI, P. I. (1974). Storage of human lymphocytes at room temperature. *Transplantation*, **18**, 520.

[23] PAYNE, R. and ROLFS, M. R. (1958). Fetomaternal leukocyte incompatibility. *Journal of Clinical Investigation*, **37**, 1756.

[24] PEARSON, H. A., SHULMAN, N. R., MARDER, V. J. and CONE, T. E. Jnr (1964). Isoimmune neonatal thrombocytopenic purpura: clinical and therapeutic considerations. *Blood*, **23**, 154.

[25] RACE, R. R. and SANGER, R. A. (1975). *Blood Groups in Man*, 6th. Ed., p. 42. Blackwell Scientific Publications, Oxford.

[26] RAY, J. G., HARE, D. B., KAYHOE, D. E., PEDERSON, P. D. and MULLALLY, D. I. (Eds.) (1976). *Manual of Tissue Typing Techniques*, DHEW Publication No. (NIH) 76 – 545.

[27] SHULMAN, N. R. (1964). A mechanism of cell destruction in individuals sensitized to foreign antigens and its implications in auto-immunity. *Annals of Internal Medicine*, **60**, 506.

[28] SHULMAN, N. R., MARDER, V. J., HILLER, M. C. and GOLLIER, E. M. (1964). Platelet and leukocyte isoantigens and their antibodies: serological, physiological and clinical studies. *Progress in Hematology*, **4**, 222.

[29] ULDALL, P. R., WILKINSON, R., DEWAR, P. J., MURRAY, S., MORLEY, A. R., BAXBY, K., HALL, R. R. and TAYLOR, R. M. R. (1977). Factors affecting the outcome of cadaver renal transplantation in Newcastle upon Tyne. *Lancet*, **ii**, 316.

[30] VAN DER WEERDT, Ch. M., VEENHOVEN-VON RIESZ, L. E., NIJENHUIS, L. E. and VAN LOGHEM, J. J. (1963). The Zw blood group system in platelets. *Vox Sanguinis (Basel)*, **8**, 513.

[31] VAN LEEUWEN, A., EERNISSE, J. G. and VAN ROOD, J. J. (1964). A new leucocyte group with two alleles: leucocyte Group Five. *Vox Sanguinis (Basel)*, **9**, 431.

[32] VAN ROOD, J. J., EERNISSE, J. G. and VAN LEEUWEN, A. (1958). Leucocyte antibodies in sera from pregnant women. *Nature (London)* **181**, 1735.

[33] VAN ROOD, J. J., VAN LEEUWEN, A. and PLOEM, J. S. (1976). Simultaneous detection of two cell populations by two-colour fluorescence and application to the recognition of B-cell determinants. *Nature (London)*, **262**, 795.

25

Miscellaneous tests

ESTIMATION OF THE ERYTHROCYTE SEDIMENTATION RATE (ESR)

Although an empirical test, the estimation of the erythrocyte sedimentation rate has been widely used in clinical medicine. Two methods have been commonly used for measuring the ESR—Wintrobe and Landsberg's method[63] in which the ESR is measured on undiluted blood in a haematocrit tube and Westergren's method[61] in which the blood is diluted and a much longer tube is used. The latter has been selected as a standard method by the International Committee for Standardization in Haematology[29] and also by various national organizations.[6,46]

Method of Westergren

The recommended tube is a straight glass tube 30 cm in length and 2.55 ($\pm$0.15) mm in diameter. The bore must be uniform to 0.05 mm throughout. A scale graduated in mm extends over the lower 20 cm.

Specially made racks with adjustable levelling screws are available for holding the sedimentation tubes firmly in an exactly vertical position. It is conventional to set up sedimentation-rate tests at room temperature (18–25°C). Sedimentation is normally accelerated as the temperature rises[40] and if the test is to be carried out at a higher ambient temperature, a normal range should be established for that temperature. Exceptionally, when high-thermal-amplitude cold agglutinins are present, sedimentation becomes noticeably less rapid as the temperature is raised towards 37°C.

109 mmol/l trisodium citrate (32 g/l $Na_3C_6H_5O_7.2H_2O$) is used as the anticoagulant diluent solution. It is filtered through a micropore filter (0.22 μm) into a sterile bottle. It can be stored for several months at 4°C but must be discarded if it becomes turbid through the growth of moulds. The test is performed on venous blood diluted accurately with the diluent in the proportion of 1 volume of citrate to 4 volumes of blood. The usual practice is to collect the blood directly into the citrate solution. This test can be carried out equally well on blood anticoagulated with EDTA, provided that 1 volume of 109 mmol/l (32 g/l) trisodium citrate or 9 g/l NaCl (saline) is added to 4 volumes of blood immediately before the test is performed. The test should be carried out within 2 h of collecting the blood, although a delay of up to 6 h is permissible provided that the blood is kept at 4°C.

Mix the blood sample thoroughly and then draw it up into the Westergren tube to the 200 mm mark by means of a teat or a mechanical device; mouth suction should never be used. Place the tube exactly vertical and leave undisturbed for 60 min, free from vibrations and draughts, and not exposed to direct sunlight. Read the height of the clear plasma above the upper limit of the column of sedimenting cells to the nearest mm. This measurement in mm is the ESR (Westergren 1 h). A poor delineation of the upper layer of red cells, so-called 'stratified sedimentation', has been attributed to the presence of many reticulocytes.[58]

Range in health

The ranges given in Table 25.1 are derived from several publications.[38] The values are means ±2SD.

Table 25.1 ESR ranges in health.

	ESR (mm/l h)	Upper limit (mm/l h)
Men aged (years)		
17–50	4 ± 3	10
51–60	6 ± 3	12
>60	6 ± 4	14
Women aged (years)		
17–50	6 ± 3	12
51–60	9 ± 5	19
>60	10 ± 5	20

In childhood and adolescence the ESR is the same as for normal men with no differences between boys and girls.[33]

Modified methods

Plastic tubes. A number of plastic materials—for example, polypropylene and polycarbonate—are possible substitutes for glass in the Westergren tube. Nevertheless, not all plastics have similar properties and it must be demonstrated by an adequate trial that tubes made from any such material give results that are reproducible and comparable to the standard method.

Length of tube. To comply with standard specifications the tube should extend 100 mm beyond the calibrated length. This ensures that it fits correctly into the commonly available holding rack. However, the overall length is not a critical dimension for the test itself, and if the tube is designed for use with some other form of holding device the uncalibrated component may be shorter provided all other specifications are met.

Capillary method. Narrow tubes result in slower sedimentation. Micro-methods have been devised but their comparability with the standard method has not been established.

Mechanism of erythrocyte sedimentation

The phenomenon of erythrocyte sedimentation has been exhaustively investigated.[19,23,56,59]

The rate of fall of the red cells is influenced by a number of inter-reacting factors. Basically, it depends upon the difference in specific gravity between red cells and plasma, but the actual rate of fall is influenced very greatly by the extent to which the red cells form rouleaux, which sediment more rapidly than single cells. Other factors which affect sedimentation include the ratio of red cells to plasma, i.e. the PCV, the plasma viscosity, the verticality or otherwise of the sedimentation tube, the bore of the tube and the dilution, if any, of the blood.

The all-important rouleaux formation is mainly controlled by the concentrations of fibrinogen and other acute-phase proteins; e.g. haptoglobin, ceruloplasmin, α_1 acid-glycoprotein, α_1 antitrypsin and c-reactive protein. Rouleaux formation is also enhanced by the immunoglobulins. It is retarded by albumin. Defibrinated blood sediments normally extremely slowly, not more than 1 mm in 1 h, unless the serum-globulin concentration is raised or there is an unusually high globulin: albumin ratio.

Anaemia, by altering the ratio of red cells to plasma, encourages rouleaux formation and accelerates sedimentation. In anaemia, too, cellular factors may affect sedimentation. Thus in iron-deficiency anaemia a reduction in the intrinsic ability of the red cells to sediment may compensate for the accelerating effect of an increased proportion of plasma.[50]

Sedimentation can be observed to take place in three stages: a preliminary stage of at least a few minutes during which time rouleaux form; then a period in which the sinking of the rouleaux takes place at approximately a constant speed, and finally a phase during which the rate of sedimentation slows as the rouleaux pack at the bottom of the tube. It is obvious that the longer the tube used the longer the second period can last and the greater the sedimentation rate may appear to be. This is an advantage of the Westergren tube. With a shorter tube, e.g. a Wintrobe tube, when there are rapidly sinking rouleaux, packing may start before an hour has elapsed. The relative merits of the Westergren and Wintrobe methods have been investigated by Bull and his colleagues.[5,44] They concluded that the Wintrobe method is more sensitive when the ESR is low, whereas, when the sedimentation rate is high, the Westergren method is a more reliable indication of the patient's clinical state. Adjusting the PCV to 0.35 makes the test more sensitive and more reproducible.[44] Such adjustment makes the test suitable as a reference method. However, this makes the test more laborious and the virtue of the ESR being a simple procedure is lost. Attempts have been made to correct for anaemia by means of a chart or normogram; the results are, however, unsatisfactory.

Significance of the measurement of the erythrocyte sedimentation rate in clinical medicine

Although the ESR is a non-specific phenomenon, it is clinically useful in disorders associated with an increased production of acute-phase proteins. In rheumatoid arthritis or tuberculosis it provides an index of progress of the disease, and it is also useful as a screening test in the routine examination of patients. A normal ESR cannot be taken to exclude organic disease, but the fact remains that the vast majority of acute or chronic infections and most neoplastic and degenerative diseases are associated with changes in the plasma proteins which lead to an acceleration of sedimentation. The ESR is increased in pregnancy from about the 3rd month and returns to normal by the 3rd–4th week post partum. The ESR is influenced by age, sex, menstrual cycle and drugs (e.g. corticosteroids, contraceptive pills); it is especially low (0–1 mm) in polycythaemia, hypofibrinogenaemia or congestive cardiac failure, and when there are abnormalities of the red cells such as poikilocytosis, spherocytosis or sickle cells.[38]

Zeta sedimentation rate (ZSR)[4]

In this method EDTA blood in a special capillary tube is centrifuged in a special apparatus (Zetafuge, Coulter Electronics) for four 45-second periods. After each 45-second period the tube is rotated 180° and the centrifuge reverses direction. In this sequential process of compaction and dispersion the red cells form rouleaux and travel down the tube under the force of gravity. The ratio of height of red cells to total height of the blood column is the zetacrit; the ratio of the true haematocrit to the zetacrit is the ZSR, which is expressed as a percentage. The normall range is 40–54% for both men and women[4,43] and a rise in ZSR is found in blood that shows a rise in ESR. The advantages of the ZSR are that it eliminates the effect of anaemia, takes less than five minutes, requires only 0.2 ml of blood and obviates the need for dilution. It is more sensitive than the Westergren ESR to minor rises in the acute-phase proteins.[44] But the need for special relatively expensive apparatus is a limitation, and the ZSR test has not replaced the universally used ESR in routine practice.

PLASMA VISCOSITY

Solutions of fibrinogen and other acute-phase proteins are more viscid than albumin which has a smaller molecular weight. The ESR and plasma viscosity in general increase in parallel. Viscosity is, however, not affected by anaemia and change in viscosity seems to reflect the clinical severity of disease more closely than does the ESR.[15,24] Also, changes in the ESR may lag behind changes in plasma viscosity by 24–48 h.[15]

Plasma viscosity can be measured by means of a capillary viscometer. The test is based on a comparison of the flow rate of plasma and distilled water under equal pressure and constant temperature through capillary tubes of equal bore (usually 0.3 mm) and length. The results are expressed as viscosity of plasma relative to that of water.

There are several types of suitable viscometer.[24] The Ostwald viscometer is a fairly simple piece of apparatus.[18] The Harkness viscometer (Coulter Electronics) is more elaborate but is more convenient to use in a routine laboratory and most reports of clinical studies have been based on it. It requires only 0.3–0.5 ml of plasma, obtained from EDTA blood. The test is reproducible with a CV of 1%. It is, however, very sensitive to changes in temperature. It is usually performed at 25°C although some workers recommend 37°C;[48] in either case the temperature should be closely controlled.

Precision is also affected by the way the plasma sample has been obtained and prepared. Venous blood should be collected with minimum stasis into EDTA (1.2 mg/ml) and, as soon as possible, centrifuge in a stoppered tube at 3000 g for 5 min to obtain clear plasma. After separation the plasma can be stored in a stoppered tube at room temperature (not in a refrigerator) for up to 1 week without change to its viscosity.

The technique of the test itself is described in the instruction manual for the instrument.

Reference values

Normal plasma from EDTA blood has a viscosity (at 25°C) of 1.61 centipoise (cP)*; SD ±0.05. At 37°C the normal range has been recorded as 1.26 cP ±0.05.[48] There are no significant differences in plasma viscosity between men and women, but it is affected by age (lower in infants; possibly slightly higher in old age), exercise and pregnancy. It is remarkably constant in health, with little or no diurnal variation, so that a change of only 0.03–0.05 cP in an individual will probably be clinically significant.

TESTS FOR HETEROPHILE ANTIBODIES IN HUMAN SERA: THE PAUL-BUNNELL TEST FOR THE DIAGNOSIS OF INFECTIOUS MONONUCLEOSIS

The presence of anti-sheep-cell haemagglutinins at unusually high titres in the sera of patients suffering from infectious mononucleosis (glandular fever) was described in 1932 by Paul and Bunnell[47] and the demonstration of these anti-bodies is still widely used as a confirmatory test—the Paul-Bunnell Test—for infectious mononucleosis. These (Paul-Bunnell) antibodies are apparently distinct from the Forssman type of anti-sheep red-cell antibodies which may develop in serum sickness. The Paul-Bunnell antibodies are, however, not

specific for sheep red cells. Thus, they react with horse red cells and ox red cells also; but they do not react with human red cells. They are known to be IgM (19S) globulins.[7,8,54]

For the diagnosis of infectious mononucleosis, it is necessary to demonstrate that the antibody present has the characters of the Paul-Bunnell antibody, i.e. it is absorbed by ox red cells but not by guinea-pig kidney. This is the basis of the absorption tests for infectious mononucleosis. Although sheep red cells have been widely used to demonstrate the Paul-Bunnell antibody, horse red cells give even better results.[35] Either type of cell, stabilized by formalin, can be used in screening tests;[25] however, the preserved cells are less able to detect low-titre antibodies than are fresh horse cells which have been collected in isotonic sodium citrate.[34,57] It is usual to carry out the tests on serum, but plasma can be used equally well.[14]

A slide screening test for infectious mononucleosis

Reagents*

Red-cell suspension. 20% suspension of horse blood in 109 mmol/l (32 g/l) trisodium citrate. Before use the suspension must be well mixed by repeated inversion. For the screening test it is unnecessary to wash the cells.

Guinea-pig kidney emulsion. See p. 426.

10% autoclaved ox red-cell suspension. See p. 426.

Method[34]

Place 1 large drop (approximately 30 μl) of guinea-pig kidney emulsion and 1 large drop of ox-cell suspension on two adjacent squares on an opal glass tile. Add 1 drop of test plasma or serum (fresh or heat-inactivated) adjacent to each. Deliver 10 μl of horse-blood suspension to the corner of each square, by means of a micropipette avoiding contact with the drops in the squares. With a wooden

---

* In SI units pressure is expressed in 'pascals' (Pa); 1 Pa = 1 newton per square metre. The unit of viscosity is 'poise' (P); 1 P (100 cP) = 0.1 Pa per second.

* Available commercially, e.g. Monospot Slide Test (Ortho).

applicator stick, mix the reagent (guinea-pig kidney emulsion or ox-cell suspension) and plasma or serum in each square. Then blend the blood in evenly so that the suspension covers the entire surface of the square. Leave the tile undisturbed for 1 min and then examine with the naked eye for agglutination, using oblique lighting over a dark background. Negative and positive serum controls should always be set up at the same time.

Interpretation

Positive. Agglutination stronger in square containing guinea-pig kidney emulsion.

Negative. Agglutination stronger in square containing ox red-cell suspension or absent in both squares.

Another slide screening test has been developed using aldehyde-treated horse red cells*.[45] It requires no absorption of serum. For the test 1 drop of serum and 1 drop of reagent are mixed on a slide with a rocking movement for 2 min. If agglutination occurs the test is positive. This test is said to have the same sensitivity and specificity as the Mono-spot slide test (Ortho).[45]

Quantitative Paul-Bunnell test

When the screening test is positive or doubtful a quantitative test with differential absorption should be carried out. The technique described below is based upon that of Barrett[2] and uses sheep red cells, but horse red cells, as recommended by Lee, Davidsohn and Slaby[35] can equally well be used.

Reagents

Patient's serum. 1 ml, previously inactivated by heating at 56°C for 30 min.

Guinea-pig kidney emulsion. See p. 426.

10% autoclaved ox red-cell suspension. See p. 426.

Sheep red cells. Prepare a 0.4% suspension in 9 g/l NaCl (saline). The sheep blood should preferably be not more than 7 days old. If

* Mono-Chek (Nyland).

stored horse red cells are used instead, they should be washed three times in saline immediately before the test.

Absorption of serum

Deliver three 0.25 ml volumes of patient's inactivated serum into three small glass or plastic tubes, A, B and C. Add 1.0 ml of saline to Tube A, 0.75 ml of saline and 0.3 ml of guinea-pig kidney emulsion to Tube B, and 0.75 ml of saline and 0.25 ml of 10% ox-cell suspension to Tube C. Mix the contents of the three tubes and place them at 4°C for at least 2 h or overnight. Then centrifuge the tubes and retain the supernatants. One in five dilutions in saline of unabsorbed serum and of the serum absorbed with guinea-pig kidney and ox red cells, respectively, are thus obtained.

Method

Make serial dilutions of the sera from Tubes A, B and C in saline. 0.15–0.2 ml volumes are suitable. Nine 75 × 8 mm tubes and a control tube to contain saline are usually sufficient. Add equal volumes of the 0.4% sheep (or horse) cell suspension to each tube, giving final serum dilutions of from 1 to 10 (Tube 1) to 1 in 2560 (Tube 9). After mixing their contents, incubate the tubes for 2 h at 37°C before reading the results. A standardized method of reading the end-point should be adopted. Macroscopic reading using a concave mirror is recommended (p. 349). Serum known to contain the Paul-Bunnell antibody should be absorbed and titrated to control the potency of the absorbents and the agglutinability of the red cells.

Interpretation

The following figures are given as examples of typical results with sheep cells:

1. Unabsorbed serum, end-point Tube 7; titre 640.

   Guinea-pig kidney absorbed serum, end-point Tube 7; titre 640.

Ox-cell absorbed serum, end-point Tube 4; titre 80.

Such a result would be positive for infectious mononucleosis, the antibody being *not* absorbed by guinea-pig kidney and significantly absorbed by ox cells. Naturally-occurring antibody is absorbed by guinea-pig kidney, but not by ox cells, and that of serum sickness is absorbed by both reagents.

2. Unabsorbed serum, end-point Tube 3; titre 40.
   Guinea-pig kidney absorbed serum, end-point Tube 3; titre 40.
   Ox-cell absorbed serum, no agglutination in Tube 1.

In spite of the low titre in the unabsorbed serum, this result would also be positive for infectious mononucleosis, the antibody *not* being absorbed by the guinea-pig kidney but absorbed by the ox cells.

3. Unabsorbed serum, end-point Tube 3; titre 40.
   Guinea-pig kidney absorbed serum, no agglutination in Tube 1.
   Ox-cell absorbed serum, end-point Tube 3; titre 40.

This is a normal result, and the screening test would have been negative. Caution is needed in interpreting the results when they are weakly positive or when there is only partial absorption by guinea-pig kidney.

Lack of complete absorption with guinea-pig kidney is not in itself diagnostic of infectious mononucleosis, as this may occasionally be observed with normal serum.[2] A positive test requires at least a two-tube difference in titre before and after absorption with ox cells.

The antibodies normally present in human sera which agglutinate sheep red cells are of the Forssman type, i.e. the antibodies react against an antigen widely spread in animal tissues. Antibodies of this type are formed by rabbits injected with an emulsion of guinea-pig kidney. The antibodies react with dog, cat and mouse tissues as well as with sheep and horse red cells, but not with the tissues of man, ox or rat.[62] The antibody formed in infectious mononucleosis is of a different nature and is not absorbed by red cells or tissues containing the Forssman antigen; hence the use, as absorbing agents, of guinea-pig kidney, rich in the antigen, and ox red cells, deficient in the antigen but capable of absorbing the Paul-Bunnell antibody.

The antibodies are lytic as well as agglutinating, and it is possible to read the results by recording lysis, if titrations are carried out in the presence of complement. Fresh ox red cells may be used instead of an autoclaved suspension, although less conveniently. It is remarkable that they may not be agglutinated although they absorb the antibody;[21] they will, however, regularly undergo lysis if complement is present. Leyton suggested that an ox red-cell lytic test might prove to be a satisfactory substitute for the orthodox Paul-Bunnell agglutination test.[39] He stated that lysins for ox red cells developed sooner and persisted longer than did the agglutinins for sheep red cells. Other workers have subsequently advocated the lytic test using ox red cells on the grounds of its greater sensitivity.[17,42] The use of horse kidney instead of guinea-pig kidney in the orthodox agglutination test has also been recommended because of the ease with which a large amount of a standard stable reagent can be prepared.[11]

The antigen on sheep red cells which reacts specifically with the Paul-Bunnell antibody is inactivated by papain and other proteolytic enzymes, and an enzyme test based on this has been proposed.[65] Davidsohn and Lee compared several serological tests and concluded that the differential absorption, enzyme and ox red-cell lysin tests were all equally valuable in the diagnosis of infectious mononucleosis.[12].

Technical factors affecting results

Temperature. The heterophile antibody of infectious mononucleosis reacts well at 37°C; agglutination is enhanced at lower temperatures and higher titres are obtained if Paul-Bunnell tests are carried out at 4°C. It is doubtful, however, whether this procedure increases the specificity of the test.[67] A cold agglutinin, anti-i, may appear transiently during the immunological reponse to infectious mononucleosis,[30,55] but as the antibody does not agglutinate sheep cells its presence does not affect the Paul-Bunnell test. It is usually present in a low titre but it may on rare occasions cause haemolytic anaemia.

Varying sensitivity of sheep red cells. A cause of difficulty in serial studies is the comparatively wide variation in sensitivity between one sample of sheep red cells and the next. Zarofonetis and Oster tested 24 sera with the red cells from 24 different sheep.[66] They found the titres given by the most sensitive cells to be from 4 to 16 times those given by the least sensitive cells. Comparable studies do not seem to have been carried out with horse red cells.

Clinical value of the Paul-Bunnell test

The Paul-Bunnell test is generally looked upon as a useful aid to the diagnosis of infectious mononucleosis, but like most tests it is not infallible. Most authors have reported 80–90% of positive results in patients thought to be suffering from infectious mononucleosis.[3,13,31] Antibodies are often present as early as the fourth to sixth day of the disease and are almost always found by the 21st day. They disappear as a rule within 4–5 months. There is no unanimity as to how frequently negative reactions are found in 'true' infectious mononucleosis. It has been shown that occasionally the characteristic antibodies develop very late in the course of the disease, perhaps weeks or even months after the patient becomes ill, and it is also known that a positive reaction may be transient and that the antibodies may be present at such low titres that they may be missed or may produce anomalous reactions when associated with the naturally-occurring antibody at similar titres. For all the above reasons it is difficult to state categorically that any particular patient has not or will not produce antibodies.

As far as false positive reactions are concerned, there is no substantial evidence that sera containing agglutinins in high concentration giving the typical reactions of infectious mononucleosis are ever found in other diseases uncomplicated by infectious mononucleosis. In particular, the heterophile-antibody titres in the lymphomas are similar to those found in unselected patients not suffering from infectious mononucleosis.[22] False positive Monospot tests have, however, been reported in malaria.[52] In virus hepatitis, although one-fifth of the patients in one series had antibody titres greater than normal, in only one patient did the result of absorption tests suggest the presence of the Paul-Bunnell antibody.[36]

Preparation of guinea-pig kidney suspension and heated ox red-cell suspension (after Barrett[2])

Guinea-pig kidney suspension

Strip the capsules and perirenal fat from at least two pairs of kidneys. Then wash them well in running water. Homogenize the tissue in 9 g/l NaCl (saline) in a blender for 2 min, sterilize it at 121°C (by autoclaving at 15 lb pressure for 20 min) and blend it again so as to obtain a fine suspension. Then centrifuge the suspension in saline and wash the deposit in two changes of saline. Finally, add to the deposit about four times its volume of 5 g/l phenol in saline. After resuspension, centrifuge the sample in a haematocrit tube in order to estimate its concentration. Then add sufficient phenol-saline to the remainder to produce a 1 in 6 suspension. Use it without further dilution. Its absorbing power must be tested with known positive and negative sera. The reagent will remain potent for at least 1 yr if stored at 4°C.

Ox red-cell suspension

Wash ox cells in several changes of 9 g/l NaCl (saline) and make a 30% suspension. Then sterilize it at 121°C (by autoclaving at 15 lb pressure for 20 min). When cool, adjust the PCV to 0.20 with saline and add an equal volume of 10 g/l phenol-saline to give a 10% suspension.

The ability of the suspension to absorb the infectious mononucleosis antibody must be tested with known positive sera. It should remain potent for several years if stored at 4°C.

DEMONSTRATION OF ANTINUCLEAR FACTORS

Antinuclear antibodies, or antinuclear factors (ANF), occur in the serum in a wide range of disorders, including systemic lupus erythematosus

(SLE), Sjögren's syndrome, rheumatoid arthritis, chronic hepatitis, thyroiditis, myasthenia gravis, pernicious anaemia, ulcerative colitis, red-cell aplasia and in a number of drug reactions. The antibodies may have specificity for DNA, soluble nucleoprotein or an extract of cell nuclei (Sm antigen). There are also antibodies which react with cytoplasmic antigens (Ro antigen), and mixed nuclear and cytoplasmic antigens (La antigen). Several techniques for demonstrating the antibodies in patients with SLE and other disorders have been described.[53]

Immunofluorescence provides a sensitive method.[10,20] For this, the serum under investigation is added to a section of tissue (e.g. rat liver). Uptake of antinuclear factor will be shown by fluorescence of cell nuclei when fluorescein-labelled rabbit anti-human-γ-globulin serum is subsequently added.[26] The hallmark of SLE is the presence of antibodies to double-stranded DNA (ds-DNA); they are detected and can be measured quantitatively by indirect immunofluorescence.[49]

Radioimmunoassay also provides a sensitive and specific method for the detection of anti-DNA antibodies. Isotope-labelled antigen is added to the serum and the resultant mixture is then treated with 50%-saturated ammonium sulphate in order to precipitate immunoglobulins; the precipitate will contain radioactivity only if an antigen–antibody reaction has occurred, and the amount of antibody can be estimated from the radioactivity in the antigen–antibody complex.[64] This test is of diagnostic value in SLE in which antibodies specific for ds-DNA are formed.[28]

A rapid and simple qualitative method for detecting the presence of antinuclear antibodies is based on the ability of the serum to aggregate polystyrene latex particles coated with the appropriate nuclear components. Thus, the LE factor can be demonstrated fairly reliably with a reagent comprising latex and desoxyribonucleoprotein obtained from calf thymus*.[51]

The antinucleoprotein antibody which occurs in the serum of patients with SLE is also detected by the LE-cell test (see below).

The LE factor is composed of 7S IgG. The LE factor has the property of causing in vitro lysis of the nuclei of neutrophil polymorphonuclears and subsequent phagocytosis of the lysed nuclei by other neutrophils. The test requires four components: the LE factor; nuclear protein material; complement, and actively phagocytic neutrophils. To provide access to the nuclear protein material the cell membranes must first be damaged by mechanical or chemical means.

DEMONSTRATION OF LE CELLS

In Romanowsky-stained preparations the LE cell appears as a neutrophil in the cytoplasm of which is a large spherical body (the LE body) which stains shades of pale purple. The nucleus of the ingesting leucocyte is usually displaced to one side and may appear to be wrapped around the ingested material (Fig. 25.1). The LE body, although derived from nuclear material, usually shows no evidence of nuclear structure and appears as an opaque homogeneous mass. The ingesting leucocyte is almost invariably and characteristically a neutrophil polymorphonuclear, very rarely a monocyte or eosinophil.

The 'Tart'* cell is a monocyte—rarely a neutrophil—which has phagocytosed another cell or the nucleus of another cell. The phagocytosed material most often resembles a lymphocyte nucleus, in which case a definite nuclear pattern can

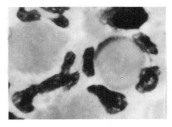

Fig. 25.1 Typical LE cell. The rounded amorphous LE body is well shown to the right of the picture with the segments of a neutrophil nucleus wrapped around it. Below and to the left is shown more amorphous nuclear material, but this is less obviously phagocytosed. ×1000.

---

* Available commercially as Hyland LE-test (Travenol Laboratoriess Ltd.).

* 'Tart' apparently refers to the name of the patient in whom cells of this type were first seen.

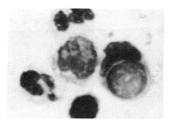

Fig. 25.2 'Tart' cell. A lymphocyte, with intact nuclear structure, has been engulfed by a monocyte, the nucleus of which has been compressed. ×1000.

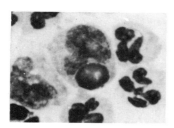

Fig. 25.3 'Tart' cell. A pyknotic (?) lymphocyte nucleus has been phagocytosed by a monocyte. ×1000.

be seen (Fig. 25.2); a common alternative form is a pyknotic nucleus smaller than an LE body and staining far more intensely (Fig. 25.3). Tart cells are often associated with leuco-agglutinins and may occur in drug reactions.[32] Such reactions have to be distinguished from the drug-induced lupus syndrome in which genuine LE cells occur.[16]

Many methods of demonstrating LE cells have been described. It seems clear that some degree of trauma to leucocytes is necessary for a successful preparation, for the LE factor does not appear to be capable of acting upon healthy living leucocytes. A good method of achieving the necessary degree of trauma is to rotate whole blood to which glass beads have been added before concentrating the leucocytes by centrifugation. The method described in the following section is based on that of Zinkham and Conley.[68]

1. Method using the patient's blood

Blood to which the minimum amount of heparin has been added should be used. Transfer 1 ml of the blood into a 75 × 12 mm glass test-tube; add four glass beads and seal the tube with a tightly fitting rubber bung. Rotate the preparation at c 33 rpm at c 20°C for 30 min; place it at 37°C for 10–15 min, and then transfer the contents of the tube to a Wintrobe haematocrit tube. Make buffy coat films after centrifuging for 10 min at 150–200 **g**. Allow the films to dry in the air, fix them in methanol and stain by a Romanowsky method in the usual way.

11. Method using the patient's serum and normal leucocytes

Patient's serum. Obtain this from blood allowed to clot undisturbed at room temperature or at 37°C or from defibrinated blood. It should be stored frozen at −20°C until used.

Normal leucocyte suspension. Deliver 5 ml of freshly drawn group-O blood into a container in which 1 mg of heparin has been dried. After mixing, centrifuge the blood at 1200–1500 **g** for 5 min. Remove the lower half of the column of packed red cells with a Pasteur pipette and discard it; remix the remaining red cells and the supernatant plasma, place in a tube of about 10 mm diameter and allow to sediment at 37°C. The removal of some of the red cells renders the blood anaemic and increases the rate of sedimentation.

Allow the blood to sediment until 1–2 ml of plasma are available. This usually takes 30–60 min. Place the supernatant plasma containing leucocytes, platelets and a small number of red cells in a 75 × 12 mm tube and wash once in 9 g/l NaCl (saline). It is important to centrifuge the leucocyte suspension at a slow speed (150–200 **g**) and for no longer than 5 min. Before the saline is added, it is essential to resuspend, by tapping the tube, the button of leucocytes in the small volume of fluid that remains after the supernatant fluid has been poured off. After washing, remove the supernatant by pipette as completely as possible. Resuspend the leucocyte button in the fluid remaining in the tube; it is then ready for use.

Technique of test

Mix equal volumes (5–10 drops) of leucocyte suspension and patient's serum in a 75 × 12 mm tube and add three small glass beads. Fit the tube with a rubber bung and rotate it at c 33 rpm for 30 min at c 20°C. Then incubate it for 30 min at 37°C, after which transfer its contents to a Wintrobe haematocrit tube. Make films of the deposited leucocytes after centrifuging at 150–200 *g* for 10 min. Dry them in the air, fix in methanol and stain by a Romanowsky dye.

Examination of films

Slides should be examined for at least 10 min before a negative report is given. With practice it is possible to recognise LE cells using a 16 mm objective. In addition to intracellular LE bodies, extracellular material may also be seen. This consists of basophilic aggregations, either amorphous or in the form of round bodies; they are homogeneous and have the same staining characteristics as typical LE bodies. Extracellular material may be seen in SLE, but it may also be found in rheumatoid arthritis, discoid LE, cirrhosis of the liver, myelomatosis and possibly even in normal subjects.[1] The material should not be considered of significance unless the characteristic LE cells are also seen.

Interpretation

The number of LE cells found in cases of SLE varies within wide limits. Occasionally, large numbers are present; not infrequently, particularly in patients who have received corticosteroid therapy, scattered cells are found only after a prolonged search. If sufficiently numerous, they may be reported as the number present per 1000 neutrophils. 'Tart' cells can usually be clearly differentiated from LE cells, but they are occasionally a source of difficulty, and, when LE cells are outnumbered by Tart cells, SLE should not be diagnosed.

Both the techniques described above are sensitive. That using the patient's whole blood is the simplest and should be used first, as positive results are more likely to be obtained in most instances than by the use of the patient's serum. The chief value of the indirect method is in the retrospective assessment of the effect of the treatment on the LE-cell-forming activity of a sample of the patient's serum, when a stored sample of the patient's serum can be used as a control.

The LE-cell phenomenon, its relationship to SLE and other auto-immune disorders, and methods for its demonstration, have a large literature.[41] A positive LE-cell test is very suggesting of SLE and LE-cell demonstration still holds an important place in diagnosis. However, the test is positive in only c 75% of patients with SLE,[28] and conversely, 'false' positive results have sometimes been found when immunofluorescence has failed to demonstrate antinuclear factor.[32] Moreover, clearly positive reactions have been reported in lupoid hepatitis, and in drug reactions.[9,16,60] Positive tests, too, have been found in 3.6% of patients with rheumatoid arthritis, especially when the disease is severe and highly active.[37]

REFERENCES

[1] ARTERBERRY, J. D., DREXLER, E. and DUBOIS, E. L. (1964). Significance of hematoxylin bodies in lupus erythematosus cell preparations. *Journal of the American Medical Association*, **187**, 389.

[2] BARRETT, A. M. (1941). The serological diagnosis of glandular fever (infectious mononucleosis): a new technique. *Journal of Hygiene (Cambridge)*, **41**, 330.

[3] BERNSTEIN, A. (1940). Infectious mononucleosis. *Medicine (Baltimore)*, **19**, 85.

[4] BULL, B. S. and BRAILSFORD, J. D. (1972). The zeta sedimentation ratio. *Blood*, **40**, 550.

[5] BULL, B. S. and BRECHER, G. (1974). An evaluation of the relative merits of the Wintrobe and Westergren sedimentation methods, including hematocrit correction. *American Journal of Clinical Pathology*, **62**, 502.

[6] British Standards Institution (1968). Specification for Westergren tube for measurement of erythrocyte sedimentation rate. BS 1554. BSI, London.

[7] CARTER, R. L. (1966). Antibody formation in infectious mononucleosis. I. Some immunochemical properties of the Paul-Bunnell antibody. *British Journal of Haematology*, **12**, 259.

[8] CARTER, R. L. (1966). Antibody formation in infectious mononucleosis. II. Other 19 S antibodies and false-positive serology. *British Journal of Haematology*, **12**, 268.

[9] CONDEMI, J. J., BLOMGREN, S. E. and VAUGHAN, J. H. (1970). The procainamide induced lupus syndrome. *Bulletin on the Rheumatic Diseases*, **20**, 604.

[10] COONS, A. H. and KAPLAN, M. H. (1950). Localization of antigen in tissue cells: II. Improvements in a method for the detection of antigen by means of fluorescent antibody. *Journal of Experimental Medicine*, **91**, 1.

[11] DAVIDSOHN, I. and GOLDIN, M. (1955). The use of horse kidney in the differential test for infectious mononucleosis. *Journal of Laboratory and Clinical Medicine*, **45**, 561.

[12] DAVIDSOHN, I. and LEE, C. L. (1964). Serologic diagnosis of infectious mononucleosis. A comparative study of five tests. *American Journal of Clinical Pathology*, **41**, 115.

[13] DAVIDSOHN, I., STERN, K. and KASHIWAGI, C. (1951). The differential test for infectious mononucleosis. *American Journal of Clinical Pathology*, **21**, 1101.

[14] DAVIDSON, R.J.L. and MAIN, S. R. (1971). Use of plasma instead of serum in laboratory tests for infectious mononucleosis. *Journal of Clinical Pathology*, **24**, 259.

[15] DINTENFASS, L. (1976). *Rheology of Blood in Diagnostic and Preventive Medicine*. Butterworth, London.

[16] DUBOIS, E. L. (1975). Serological abnormalities in spontaneous and drug-induced systemic lupus erythematosus. *Journal of Rheumatology*, **2**, 204.

[17] ERICSON, C. (1960). Sheep cell agglutinin and ox cell hemolysin in the serological diagnosis of mononucleosis infectiosa. *Acta Medica Scandinavica*, **166**, 225.

[18] FAHEY, J. L. (1963). Serum protein disorders causing clinical symptoms in malignant neoplastic disease. *Journal of Chronic Diseases*, **16**, 703.

[19] FISCHER, C. L., GILL, C., FORRESTER, M. C. and NAKAMURA, R. (1976). Quantitation of 'acute-phase proteins' postoperatively. *American Journal of Clinical Pathology*, **66**, 840.

[20] GELL, P. G. H. and COOMBS, R. R. A. (1975). Basic immunological methods. In *Clinical Aspects of Immunology* (ed. P. G. H. Gell, R. R. A. Coombs, and P. J. Lachmann), 3rd edn., p. 33. Blackwell Scientific Publications, Oxford.

[21] GLEESON-WHITE, M. H., HEARD, D. H., MYNORS, L. S. and COOMBS, R. R. A. (1950). Factors influencing the agglutinability of red cells: the demonstration of a variation in the susceptibility to agglutination exhibited by the red cells of individual oxen. *British Journal of Experimental Pathology*, **31**, 321.

[22] GOLDMAN, R., FISHKIN, B. G. and PETERSON, E. T. (1950). The value of the heterophile antibody reaction in the lymphomatous diseases. *Journal of Laboratory and Clinical Medicine*, **35**, 681.

[23] HARDWICKE, J. and SQUIRE, J. R. (1952). The basis of the erythrocyte sedimentation rate. *Clinical Science*, **11**, 333.

[24] HARKNESS, J. (1971). The viscosity of human blood plasma; its measurement in health and disease. *Biorheology*, **8**, 171.

[25] HOFF, G. and BAUER, S. (1965). A new rapid slide test for infectious mononucleosis. *Journal of the American Medical Association*, **194**, 351.

[26] HOLDBOROW, E. J., WEIR, D. M. and JOHNSON, G. D. (1957). A serum factor in lupus erythematosus with affinity for tissue nuclei. *British Medical Journal*, **ii**, 732.

[27] HOLMAN, H. and TOMASI, T. (1960). Lupoid hepatitis. *Medical Clinics of North America*, **44**, 633.

[28] HUGHES, G. R. V. (1973). The diagnosis of systemic lupus erythematosus (Annotation). *British Journal of Haematology*, **25**, 409.

[29] International Committee for Standardization in Haematology (1977). Recommendation for measurement of erythrocyte sedimentation rate of human blood. *American Journal of Clinical Pathology*, **68**, 505.

[30] JENKINS, W. J., KOSTER, H. G., MARSH, W. L. and CARTER, R. L. (1965). Infectious mononucleosis: an unsuspected source of anti-i. *British Journal of Haematology*, **11**, 480.

[31] KAUFMAN, R. E. (1944). Heterophile antibody in infectious mononucleosis. *Annals of Internal Medicine*, **21**, 230.

[32] KOLLER, S. R., JOHNSTON, C. L., MONCURE, C. W. and WALLER, M. V. (1976). Lupus erythematosus cell preparation-antinuclear factor incongruity. A review of diagnostic tests for systemic lupus erythematosus. *American Journal of Clinical Pathology*, **66**, 495.

[33] LASCARI, A. D. (1972). The erythrocyte sedimentation rate. *Pediatric Clinics of North America*, **19**, 1113.

[34] LEE, C. L., DAVIDSOHN, I. and PANCZYSZYN, O (1968). Horse agglutinins in infectious mononucleosis. II. The spot test. *American Journal of Clinical Pathology*, **49**, 12.

[35] LEE, C. L., DAVIDSOHN, I. and SLABY, R. (1968). Horse agglutinins in infectious mononucleosis. *American Journal of Clinical Pathology*, **49**, 3.

[36] LEIBOWITZ, S. (1951). Heterophile antibody in normal adults and in patients with virus hepatitis. *American Journal of Clinical Pathology*, **21**, 201.

[37] LENOCH, F. and VOJTÍŠEK, O. (1967). The prevalence of LE cells in 1000 consecutive patients with active rheumatoid arthritis. *Acta Rheumatologica Scandinavica*, **13**, 313.

[38] LEWIS, S. M. (1980). Erythrocyte sedimentation rate and plasma viscosity. *ACP Broadsheet No. 94*. BMA, London.

[39] LEYTON, G. B. (1952). Ox-cell haemolysins in human serum. *Journal of Clinical Pathology*, **5**, 324.

[40] MANLEY, R. W. (1957). The effect of room temperature on erythrocyte sedimentation rate and its correction. *Journal of Clinical Pathology*, **10**, 354.

[41] MIESCHER, P. W. and REITHMÜLLER, D. (1965). Diagnosis and treatment of systemic lupus erythematosus. *Seminars in Hematology*, **2**, 1.

[42] MIKKELSEN, W., TUPPER, C. J. and MURRAY, J. (1958). The ox cell hemolysin test as a diagnostic procedure in infectious mononucleosis. *Journal of Laboratory and Clinical Medicine*, **52**, 648.

[43] MORRIS, M. W., SKRODZSKI, Z. and NELSON, D. A. (1975). Zeta sedimentation rate (ZSR): a replacement for the erythrocyte sedimentation rate (ESR). *American Journal of Clinical Pathology*, **64**, 254.

[44] MOSELY, D. L. and BULL, B. S. (1981). A comparison of the Wintrobe, the Westergren and the ZSR erythrocyte sedimentation rate (ESR) methods to a candidate reference method. *Clinical and Laboratory Haematology*, **4**, 169.

[45] MYHRE, B. A. and NAKAYAMA, V. (1976). Serological evaluation of the Mono-Chek test. *American Journal of Clinical Pathology*, **65**, 987.

[46] National Committee for Clinical Laboratory Standards (1977). Standardized method for the human erythrocyte sedimentation rate (ESR) test (ASH-2). NCCLS, Villanova, Pa.

[47] PAUL, J. R. and BUNNELL, W. W. (1932). The presence of heterophile antibodies in infectious mononucleosis. *American Journal of Medical Sciences*, **183**, 90.

[48] PHILLIPS, M. J. and HARKNESS, J. (1981). A study of plasma viscosity-temperature relationships. *Bibliotheca Anatomica*, **20**, 215.

[49] PINCUS, T., SCHUR, P. H. and TALAL, N. (1968). A diagnostic test for systemic lupus erythematosus using a DNA binding assay. *Arthritis and Rheumatism*, **11**, 837.

[50] POOLE, J. C. F. and SUMMERS, G. A. C. (1952). Correction of E. S. R. in anaemia. Experimental study based on interchange of cells and plasma between normal and anaemic subjects. *British Medical Journal*, **i**, 353.

[51] PULLUM, C. and KEECH, M. K. (1964). Evaluation of the Hyland LE-Test. *Acta Rheumatologica Scandinavica*, **10**, 165.

[52] REED, R. E. (1974). False-positive monospot tests in malaria. *American Journal of Clinical Pathology*, **61**, 173.

[53] REICHLIN, M. (1981). Current perspectives on serological reactions in SLE patients. *Clinical and Experimental Immunology*, **44**, 1.

[54] ROSE, H. M., RAGAN, C., PEARCE, E. and LIPMAN, M. O. (1948). Differential agglutination of normal and sensitized sheep erythrocytes by sera of patients with rheumatoid arthritis. *Proceedings of the Society for Experimental Biology and Medicine*, **68**, 1.

[55] ROSENFELD, R. E., SCHMIDT, P. J., CALVO, R. C. and McGINNISS, M. H. (1965). Anti-i, a frequent cold agglutinin in infectious mononucleosis. *Vox Sanguinis*, **10**, 631.

[56] RUHENSTROTH-BAUER, G. (1961). Mechanism and significance of erythrocyte sedimentation rate. *British Medical Journal*, i, 1804.

[57] SCOTT, G. L. and PRIEST, C. J. (1972). An evaluation of the Monosticon rapid slide test diagnosis of infectious mononucleosis. *Journal of Clinical Pathology*, **25**, 783.

[58] STEPHENS, J. G. (1938). Stratified blood sedimentation—isolation of immature red cells. *Nature (London)*, **141**, 1058.

[59] THYGESEN, J. E. (1942). The mechanism of blood sedimentation. *Acta Medica Scandinavica*, Suppl. 134.

[60] WALSH, J. R. and ZIMMERMAN, H. J. (1953). The demonstration of the 'L.E.' phenomenon in patients with penicillin hypersensitivity. *Blood*, **8**, 65.

[61] WESTERGREN, A. (1921). Studies of the suspension stability of the blood in pulmonary tuberculosis. *Acta Medica Scandinavica*, **54**, 247.

[62] WILSON, C. S. and MILES, A. A. (1964). In *Topley and Wilson's Principles of Bacteriology and Immunity*, 5th edn., p. 1330. Arnold, London.

[63] WINTROBE, M. M. and LANDSBERG, J. W. (1935). A standardized technique for the blood sedimentation test. *American Journal of Medical Sciences*, **189**, 102.

[64] WOLD, R. T., YOUNG F. E., TAN, E. M. and FARR, R. S. (1968). Desoxyribonucleic acid antibody: a method to detect its primary interaction with desoxyribonucleic acid. *Science*, **161**, 806.

[65] WÖLLNER, D. (1956). Differenzierungsmethoden zur serologishen Diagnose der infektiösen Mononucleose. II. Die differential-Agglutination mit nativem und papainisierten Hammelerythrozyten nach Absorption mit Meeschweinchennierenzellen und papainisierten Hammelblut. *Zeitschrift für Immunitätsforschung und experimentelle Therapie*, **113**, 301.

[66] ZAROFONETIS, C. J. D. and OSTER, H. L. (1950). Heterophile agglutination variability of erythrocytes from different sheep. *Journal of Laboratory and Clinical Medicine*, **36**, 283.

[67] ZAROFONETIS, C. J. D., OSTER, H. L. and COLVILLE, V. F. (1953). Cold agglutination of sheep erythrocytes as a factor in false-positive heterophile agglutination tests. *Journal of Laboratory and Clinical Medicine*, **41**, 906.

[68] ZINKHAM, W. H. and CONLEY, C. L. (1956). Some factors influencing the formation of L.E. cells. A method for enhancing L.E. cell production. *Bulletin of the Johns Hopkins Hospital*, **98**, 102.

26

Appendices

1. PREPARATION OF CERTAIN REAGENTS, ANTICOAGULANTS AND PRESERVATIVE SOLUTIONS

Acid-citrate-dextrose (ACD) solution—'NIH-A'[11a]

Trisodium citrate, dihydrate (75 mmol/l)	22 g
Citric acid, monohydrate (42 mmol/l)	8 g
Dextrose (139 mmol/l)	25 g
Water	to 1 l.

Sterilize the solution by autoclaving at 126°C for 30 min. Its pH is 5.4. For use, add 10 volumes of blood to 1.5 volumes of solution.

Alsever's solution[8]

Dextrose (114 mmol/l)	20.5 g
Trisodium citrate, dihydrate (27 mmol/l)	8.0 g
Sodium chloride (72 mmol/l)	4.2 g
Water	to 1 l.

Adjust the pH to 6.1 with citric acid (c 0.5 g) and then sterilize the solution by micropore filtration (0.22 µm) or by autoclaving at 126°C for 30 min. For use, add 4 volumes of blood to 1 volume of solution.

Citrate-phosphate-dextrose (CPD) solution, pH 6.9[11b]

Trisodium citrate, dihydrate (102 mmol/l)	30 g
Sodium dihydrogen phosphate, monohydrate (1.08 mmol/l)	0.15 g
Dextrose (11 mmol/l)	2 g
Water	to 1 l.

Sterilize the solution by autoclaving at 126°C for 30 min. After cooling to c 20°C, it should have a brown tinge and its pH should be 6.9. For use in cell survival studies (see p. 298) add 1 volume of blood to 2 volumes of solution.

Citrate-phosphate-dextrose (CPD) solution, pH 5.6–5.8[11a]

Trisodium citrate, dihydrate (89 mmol/l)	26.30 g
Citric acid, monohydrate (17 mmol/l)	3.27 g
Sodium dihydrogen phosphate, monohydrate (16 mmol/l)	2.22 g
Dextrose (142 mmol/l)	25.50 g
Water	to 1 l.

Sterilize the solution by autoclaving at 126°C for 30 min. For use as an anticoagulant-preservative, add 7 volumes of blood to 1 volume of solution.

Low ionic strength solution[12]

Sodium chloride (NaCl) (30.8 mmol/l)	1.8 g
Disodium hydrogen phosphate (Na_2HPO_4) (1.5 mmol/l)	0.21 g
Sodium dihydrogen phosphate (NaH_2PO_4) (1.5 mmol/l)	0.18 g
Glycine (NH_2CH_2COOH) (240 mmol/l)	18.0 g
Water	to 1 l.

Dissolve the sodium chloride and the two phosphate salts in *c* 400 ml of water; dissolve the glycine separately in *c* 400 ml of water; adjust the pH of each solution to 6.7 with 1 mol/l NaOH. Add the two solutions together and make up to 1 l. Sterilize by Seitz filtration or autoclaving. The pH should be within the range 6.65–6.85, the osmolarity 270–285 mmol, and conductivity 3.5–3.8 mmho/cm at 23°C.

EDTA

Ethylenediamine tetra-acetic acid, dipotassium or disodium salt	100 g
Water	to 1 l.

Allow appropriate volumes to dry in bottles at *c* 20°C so as to give a concentration of 1.5 ± 0.25 mg/ml of blood.

Neutral EDTA, pH 7.0, 110 mmol/l

Ethylenediamine tetra-acetic acid, dipotassium salt	44.5 g
or disodium salt	41.0 g
1 mol/l NaOH	75 ml
Water	to 1 l.

Neutral buffered EDTA, pH 7.0

Ethylenediamine tetra-acetic acid, disodium salt (9 mmol/l)	3.35 g
Disodium hydrogen phosphate (Na_2HPO_4) (26.4 mmol/l)	3.75 g
Sodium chloride (NaCl) (140 mmol/l)	8.18 g
Water	to 1 l.

Trisodium citrate
($Na_3C_6H_5O_7 . 2H_2O$), 109 mmol/l

Dissolve 32 g in 1 l of water. Distribute convenient volumes (e.g. 10 ml) into small bottles and sterilize by autoclaving at 126°C for 30 min.

Heparin

Powdered heparin (lithium salt) is available with an activity of *c* 160 iu/mg. Dissolve it in water at a concentration of 4 mg/ml. Sodium heparin is available in 5 ml ampoules with an activity of 1000 iu/ml. Add appropriate volumes of either solution to a series of containers and allow to dry at *c* 20°C so as to give a concentration not exceeding 15–20 iu/ml of blood.

COAGULATION REAGENTS

Aluminium-hydroxide gel[2]

Dilute 50 ml of ammonia (sp gr 0.88) with 50 ml of water and then pour into 600 ml of water at 63°C containing 22 g of ammonium sulphate. Allow the temperature to fall rapidly to 58°C, stirring the mixture vigorously. Then pour it, in one lot, into a solution of 76.7 g of ammonium alum dissolved in 1 l of water at 58°C. The temperature rises to 61°C. Stir the mixture for 10 min; then separate the precipitate by centrifuging and wash five times with water, the first volume of washing water (300 ml) containing 0.44 ml of ammonia (sp gr 0.88) diluted 1 in 2 and the second volume of washing water containing 0.88 ml of the diluted ammonia; for the subsequent washings use plain water. After the washing has been completed, suspend the final precipitate in the least amount of water that is required to make a gelatinous suspension that can be pipetted.★

For use as an absorbent for prothrombin, etc. add 1 volume (drop) to 10 volumes of plasma. Incubate the mixture at 37°C for 2 min and then centrifuge for 8 min at 1200–1500 *g*. A one-stage prothrombin time carried out on the supernatant should exceed 60 s; if it is less than this, repeat the absorption.

Brain thromboplastin[17]

Acetone-dried brain. Strip a human brain fresh from the post-mortem room completely of its covering membranes, blood vessels and cerebellum. Then cut it into small pieces and macerate it in acetone in a mortar. Change the acetone several times, until a non-granular material remains. This is crude 'acetone-brain'.

Dry the granular material in an evacuated desiccator and when dry, place 0.3 g amounts in

★ A satisfactory commercial preparation is 1g of aluminium hydroxide moist gel (BDH Ltd) suspended in 4 ml of water.

75 × 12 mm glass tubes provided with cotton-wool plugs. Store these in an evacuated desiccator at 4°C until used. Under these circumstances they retain their potency for months. Each time that the desiccator is opened to remove a tube, re-evacuate it.

Saline extract of brain. Remove the membranes, blood vessels and cerebellum from a freshly obtained brain. Wash it free from blood. Then emulsify it in 9 g/l NaCl, either by grinding in a mortar or with the help of a blending machine. Incubate for 30 min at 37°C. Then leave for 24 h at 4°C and then centrifuge at *c* 700 g for 30 min. Discard the sediment and store the supernatant at 4°C for 2 weeks. Make dilutions of a small sample, up to 1 in 8 in saline, and choose the dilution which gives the shortest time in Quick's one-stage test. Dilute the remainder of the brain emulsion appropriately, using saline containing a one-tenth volume of barbitone buffer, pH 7.4. Distribute the extract in 5 ml volumes in small screw-capped vials and store at −20°C. They should retain their potency for months. Thaw a fresh vial for each batch of tests. A satisfactory extract should give a clotting time in the Quick test of 13–16 s with normal plasma.

Phenolized brain extract. Prepare as for the saline extract but emulsify in a mixture of 9 g/l NaCl and 5 g/l phenol which has been warmed at 45°C. Then continue as for the saline extract. After distribution of the suspension into vials, store at 4°C.

Inosithin. Crush 1 g of freeze-dried Inosithin (Uniscience Ltd.) with a pestle and mortar. Add 100 ml of 9 g/l NaCl (saline), prewarmed to *c* 40°C a little at a time, mixing well. Transfer the emulsion to a conical flask as it forms and add more saline until all the Inosithin has been emulsified. Leave the flask on a magnetic stirrer for *c* 2 h or longer until a smooth emulsion is obtained. Distribute into 3 ml volumes in screw-capped vials and store at −40°C. To obtain a 1% stock solution of Inosithin, thaw a vial and dilute the contents 1 in 20 with barbitone buffered saline, pH 7.4, before use.

Calcium chloride

Make a 25 mmol/l solution by dissolving 2.77 g of the anhydrous salt in 1 l of water.

Platelet substitute (Bell and Alton[1])

Take 1 g of acetone-dried human brain (see above) and carry out further extraction with 20 ml of acetone. Allow it to stand at room temperature for 2 h and then centrifuge the mixture. Discard the supernatant and dry the deposited brain tissue in an evacuated desiccator. Then extract the dried tissue at *c* 20°C with 20 ml of chloroform, shaking the mixture from time to time. Filter the mixture and evaporate the filtrate at 37°C in an evacuated desiccator. Then suspend the lipid residue in 10 ml of 9 g/l NaCl. Dilute the resultant saline emulsion to about 1 in 100 for use in the test, determining the optimum by trial.

Soy-bean phospholipid[13]

Prepare a stock solution by homogenizing soy-bean powder in barbitone-buffered saline, pH 7.4, at a concentration of 2 g/l. Store this stock at −20°C. For use, dilute it in buffered saline to obtain a clotting time of 10 s or less with normal plasma diluted 1 in 10.

HAEMOGLOBIN STANDARD

Gibson and Harrison's artificial haemoglobin standard

Chromium potassium sulphate $(CrK (SO_4)_2 . 12H_2O)$		11.61 g
Cobaltous sulphate (anhydrous) $(CoSO_4)$		13.1 g
Potassium dichromate $(K_2Cr_2O_7)$		0.69 g
Water	to	500 ml

Add 1.8 ml of 1 mol/l sulphuric acid to the dissolved salts and heat the mixture to boiling. After boiling for 1 min, cool the solution and make up the volume to 1 l with water.

The chromium potassium sulphate crystals must be free from any signs of whitening due to efflorescence. The cobaltous sulphate must be anhydrous. Heat *c* 30 g of $CoSO_4 . 7H_2O$ for *c* 2 h in a small porcelain dish placed in an oven at a temperature just below its melting point (96°C). Then heat the coarser particles overnight in an electric muffle furnace kept at 400°C. The product should be a uniform lilac powder. Transfer while still hot to a stoppered bottle. As soon as it has cooled, weigh out 13.1 g and dissolve in 80 ml of water with the aid of heat. As the anhydrous salt is hygroscopic, seal in glass tubes immediately after preparation.

The undiluted standard is equivalent to 160 ± 2 g Hb per l (based on iron determinations) when used as described on p. 31.

WATER

For most purposes still-prepared distilled water or deionized water is equally suitable. Throughout this text this is implied when 'water' is referred to. When doubly-distilled or glass-distilled water is required this has been specially indicated, and when tap-water is satisfactory or indicated, this, too, has been stated.

2. BUFFERS*

Barbitone buffer, pH 7.4

Sodium diethyl barbiturate ($C_8H_{11}O_3N_2Na$) (57 mmol/l)	11.74 g
Hydrochloric acid (HCl) (100 mmol/l)	430 ml

Barbitone buffered saline, pH 7.4

NaCl	5.67 g
Barbitone buffer, pH 7.4	1 l.

Before use, dilute with an equal volume of 9 g/l NaCl.

Barbitone-buffered saline, pH 9.5

Sodium diethyl barbiturate ($C_8H_{11}O_3N_2Na$) (98 mmol/l)	20.2 g
Hydrochloric acid (HCl) (100 mmol/l)	20 ml
NaCl	5.67 g

Before use, dilute the buffer with an equal volume of 9 g/l NaCl.

* Other buffers which are used for specific purposes are described under the appropriate tests.

Barbitone-bovine serum albumin (BSA) buffer, pH 9.8

Sodium diethyl barbiturate ($C_8H_{11}O_3N_2Na$) (54 mmol/l)	10.3 g
NaCl (102 mmol/l)	6.0 g
Sodium azide (31 mmol/l)	2.0 g
Bovine serum albumin (Sigma)	5.0 g
Water	to 1 l.

Dissolve the reagents in c 900 ml of water. Adjust the pH to 9.8 with 5 mol/l HCl. Make up the volume to 1 l with water. Store at 4°C.

Citrate-saline buffer

Trisodium citrate ($Na_3C_6H_5O_7 . 2H_2O$) (5 mmol/l)	1.5 g
NaCl (96 mmol/l)	5.6 g
Barbitone buffer, pH 7.4	200 ml
Water	800 ml

Glycine buffer, pH 3.0

Glycine (NH_2CH_2COOH) (82 mmol/l)	6.15 g
NaCl (82 mmol/l)	4.80 g
Water	820 ml
0.1 mol/l HCl	180 ml

HEPES buffer, pH 6.5

4-(2-hydroxyethyl)-1-piperazineethane sulphonic acid (100 mmol/l) 23.83 g.

Dissolve in c 100 ml of water. Add a sufficient volume of 1 mol/l NaOH (c 1 ml) to adjust the pH to 6.5. If the buffer is intended for use with Romanowsky staining (p. 54), then add 25 ml of dimethyl sulphoxide (DMSO). Make up the volume to 1 l with water.

Imidazole-buffered saline, pH 7.4

Imidazole (50 mmol/l)	3.4 g
NaCl (100 mmol/l)	5.85 g

Dissolve in c 500 ml of water. Add 18.6 ml of 1 mol/l HCl and make up the volume to 1 l with water. Store at room temperature (18–25°C).

Phosphate buffer, iso-osmotic

(A) $NaH_2PO_4 . 2H_2O$ (150 mmol/l)   23.4 g/l
(B) Na_2HPO_4 (150 mmol/l)   21.3 g/l

pH	Solution A	Solution B
7.0	32 ml	68 ml
7.2	24 ml	76 ml
7.4	18 ml	82 ml
7.6	13 ml	87 ml
7.7	9.5 ml	90.5 ml

Normal human serum has an osmolarity of 289 ± 4 mmol. Hendry recommended slightly different concentrations of the stock solution, namely, 25.05 g/l $NaH_2PO_4 . 2H_2O$ and 17.92 g/l Na_2HPO_4 for an iso-osmotic buffer.[5]

Phosphate-buffered saline

Equal volumes of iso-osmotic phosphate buffer and 9 g/l NaCl. For serological tests use a pH 7.0 buffer.

Phosphate buffer, Sörensen's

66 mmol/l stock solutions:

(A) KH_2PO_4 9.1 g/l
(B) Na_2HPO_4 9.5 g/l or
      $Na_2HPO_4 . 2H_2O$ 11.9 g/l

100 mmol/l and 150 mmol/l stock solutions may be similarly prepared. To obtain a solution of the required pH, add A and B in the indicated proportions:

pH	A	B
5.4	97.0	3.0
5.6	95.0	5.0
5.8	92.2	7.8
6.0	88.0	12.0
6.2	81.0	19.0
6.4	73.0	27.0
6.6	63.0	37.0
6.8	50.8	49.2
7.0	38.9	61.1
7.2	28.0	72.0
7.4	19.2	80.8
7.6	13.0	87.0
7.8	8.5	91.5
8.0	5.5	94.5

This buffer is not iso-osmotic with normal plasma (see above).

Tris-HCl buffer (200 mmol/l)

Tris (hydroxymethyl) aminomethane★
   (24.23 g/l)   250 ml

To obtain a solution of the required pH add the appropriate volume of 1 mol/l HCl and then make up the volume to 1 l with water:

pH	Volume
7.2	44.5 ml
7.4	42.0 ml
7.6	39.0 ml
7.8	33.5 ml
8.0	28.0 ml
8.2	23.0 ml
8.4	17.5 ml
8.6	13.0 ml
8.8	9.0 ml
9.0	5.0 ml

100 mmol/l, 150 mmol/l and 750 mmol/l stock solutions may be similarly prepared with an appropriate weight of tris and volume of acid.

Tris-HCl bovine serum albumin (BSA) buffer, pH 7.6, 20 mmol/l

Tris (hydroxymethyl) aminomethane (20 mmol/l)	2.42 g
EDTA, disodium salt (10 mmol/l)	3.72 g
NaCl (100 mmol/l)	5.85 g
Sodium azide (3 mmol/l)	0.2 g

Dissolve the reagents in c 800 ml of water. Adjust the pH to 7.6 with 10 mol/l HCl. Add 10 g of bovine serum albumin (Sigma) and make up to 1 l with water.

3. PREPARATION OF GLASSWARE

Flask for the defibrination of blood

Provide a 100 ml conical flask with a central glass rod to the bottom end of which are fused pieces of

★ 2-amino-2-(hydroxymethyl) propane-1,3-diol.

glass capillary (Fig. 1.1, p. 3). The rod is kept in position with a cotton-wool plug. Deliver 10–50 ml of blood into the flask and, after re-inserting the central rod, hold the flask by the neck and rotate it by hand. The blood is usually successfully defibrinated within 5 min, the fibrin forming on the glass rod, usually in one piece. Little or no lysis is caused, and the blood is as a rule completely free from small clots.

Siliconized glassware

Make a 10 ml/l solution of Siliclad (Clay-Adams Inc) in water. Immerse the clean glassware or syringes to be coated in the fluid and allow to drain dry. (It is advisable to wear rubber gloves and to prepare the apparatus in a fume cupboard provided with an exhaust fan.) Then rinse the coated glassware thoroughly in water, and allow to dry in an oven at 100°C for 10 min or overnight in an incubator.

4. METHODS OF CLEANING SLIDES AND APPARATUS

New slides

Place them in dichromate cleaning fluid for at least 48 h. (The cleaning fluid consists of potassium dichromate 20 g, dissolved in 100 ml of water, to which are then added 900 ml of concentrated sulphuric acid.)* Wash the treated slides well in running tap-water, rinse in water and store in 95% ethanol until used. Dry with a clean linen cloth and carefully wipe free from dust before they are used.

Dirty slides

When discarded, place in a detergent solution, heat to 60°C for 20 min and then wash in hot running tap-water. Finally, rinse in water before being dried with a clean linen cloth.

Chemical apparatus and glassware

Wash in running tap-water and then boil in a detergent solution, rinse in acid and wash in hot running tap-water, as described above. Alterna-

* For most purposes 2 mol/l HCL is a satisfactory alternative.

tively, the apparatus can be soaked in dichromate-sulphuric acid mixture or 2 mol/l HCL.

For the removal of deposits of protein and other organic matter, 'biodegradable' detergents are recommended. Decon 90 (Decon Laboratories Ltd., Portslade, Sussex), which is anionic, or Pyroneg (Diversey Ltd., Cockfosters, Barnet, Herts) is suitable.

5. SIZES OF TUBES

The sizes of tubes recommended in the text have been chosen as being appropriate for the tests described. The dimensions given are the length and external diameter (in mm). The equivalent in inches, as given in some catalogues, and certain corresponding internal diameters, are as follows:

75 × 10 mm (internal
    diameter 8 mm) $= 3 \times \frac{3}{8}''$
75 × 12 mm (internal
    diameter 10 mm) $= 3 \times \frac{1}{2}''$
65 × 10 mm $= 2\frac{1}{2} \times \frac{3}{8}''$
38 × 6·4 mm $= 1\frac{1}{2} \times \frac{1}{4}''$ ('precipitin
100 × 12 mm $= 4 \times \frac{1}{2}''$ tubes')
150 × 16 mm $= 6 \times \frac{5}{8}''$
150 × 19 mm $= 6 \times \frac{3}{4}''$

6. SPEED OF CENTRIFUGING

Throughout the book the unit given is the relative centrifugal force (g). Conversion of this figure to rpm depends upon the radius of the centrifuge; it can be calculated by reference to the nomogram illustrated in Fig. 26.1, or from the formula:
Relative centrifugal force (RCF)
$$= 118 \times 10^{-7} \times r \times N^2,$$

where r = radius (cm) and N = speed of rotation (rpm).

The following centrifugal forces are recommended:

'Low-spun' platelet-
   rich plasma   150–200 g (for 10–15
                            min).

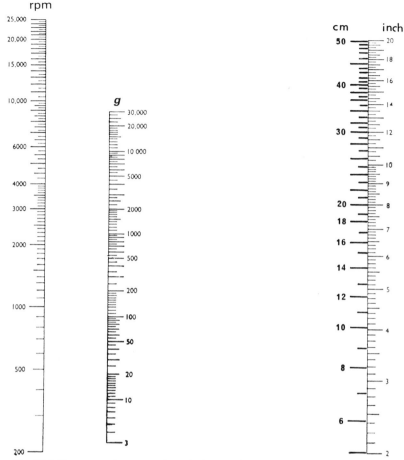

Fig. 26.1 Nomogram for computing relative centrifugal forces.
(By courtesy of MSE Ltd.)

'High-spun' plasma   1200–1500 *g* (for 15 min).
Packing of red cells   2000–2300 *g* (for 30 min).

7. UNITS OF WEIGHT AND MEASUREMENT IN COMMON USE IN HAEMATOLOGY

Throughout the book measurements have been expressed in SI units, in accordance with international recommendations.[18] These units are derived from the metric system. The base units are shown below and the abbreviated forms are indicated alongside.

Weight (unit: gram [g])
   $\times\ 10^3$ kilogram (kg)
   $\times\ 10^{-3}$ milligram (mg)
   $\times\ 10^{-6}$ microgram (μg) (formerly γ)
   $\times\ 10^{-9}$ nanogram (ng) (formerly μmg)
   $\times\ 10^{-12}$ picogram (pg) (formerly $\mu\mu$g)

Length (unit: metre [m])
   $\times\ 10^{-1}$ decimetre (dm)
   $\times\ 10^{-2}$ centimetre (cm)
   $\times\ 10^{-3}$ millimetre (mm)
   $\times\ 10^{-6}$ micrometre (μm) (formerly μ)
   $\times\ 10^{-9}$ nanometre (nm) (formerly mμ)

Volume (unit: litre [l] = dm^3)
   $\times\ 10^{-1}$ decilitre (dl) (formerly 100 ml)
   $\times\ 10^{-3}$ millilitre (ml) = cm^3 (formerly cc)
   $\times\ 10^{-6}$ microlitre (μl) = mm^3
   $\times\ 10^{-9}$ nanolitre (nl)
   $\times\ 10^{-12}$ picolitre (pl) (formerly $\mu\mu$l)
   $\times\ 10^{-15}$ femtolitre (fl) = μm^3

Amount of substance (unit: mole [mol])
  $\times\ 10^{-3}$ millimole (mmol)
  $\times\ 10^{-6}$ micromole (μmol)
Substance concentration (unit: moles per litre [mol/l]) (formerly M)
  $\times\ 10^{-3}$ millimole per litre (mmol/l)
  $\times\ 10^{-6}$ micromole per litre (μmol/l)
Mass concentration (unit: gram per litre [g/l])
  $\times\ 10^{-3}$ milligram per litre (mg/l)
  $\times\ 10^{-6}$ microgram per litre (μg/l)

When preparing a small amount of a reagent, it is more appropriate to express its concentration per ml or dl.

8. MICROSCOPE MAGNIFICATION

It has become customary for the objective lenses of microscopes to be marked with their magnifying power rather than their focal length. The approximate equivalents are as follows:

Focal length (mm)	Magnification
2	×100
4	×40
16	×10
40	×4

9. PREPARATION AND STANDARDIZATION OF ANTIGLOBULIN SERUM

Preparation of antiglobulin serum

Methods for the preparation of antiglobulin serum were given in the 4th edition of this book. Anti-IgG, anti-IgM, anti-IgA and anti-complement components sera as well as 'broad-spectrum' antiglobulin sera are now so widely available from many commercial firms that many hospital laboratories will find it more economical to buy the prepared reagents than to make them themselves. However, all these sera require careful standardization to determine their optimum dilution for use and to ensure that they contain all the wanted antibodies

and to check that they do not contain unwanted antibodies.

Absorption of antibodies reacting with unsensitized red cells

Antisera prepared for the antiglobulin test should have been absorbed free of antibodies reacting with unsensitized red cells, but antisera prepared for immuno-diffusion tests may not have been. It is important, therefore, at least to test serial dilutions of such sera with both fresh and stored washed, unsensitized A, B and O red cells. Completely negative results must be obtained with all the cells. If not, the serum must be absorbed with the appropriate cells and retested. It is very important that the cells used for absorption should be thoroughly washed so that all traces of human globulin are removed. At least six washes in a large volume of 9 g/l NaCl are needed and the last washing fluid should be tested subsequently with 25% sulphosalicylic acid to see if it contains any protein. If it does, adding a few drops of the sulphosalicylic acid will produce some turbidity. In this case further washing is necessary. The absorptions are carried out for 2 h or overnight at 4°C with an equal volume of washed packed cells.

Standardization of 'broad-spectrum' antiglobulin sera

A broad-spectrum antiglobulin serum must contain antibodies active against complement components as well as antibodies against IgG; it is, however, unnecessary for routine work for such a reagent to contain anti-IgM or anti-IgA antibodies.[7] The optimum dilution for each type of antibody present is obtained separately.

Prepare IgG-sensitized red cells using dilutions of a weak 'incomplete' anti-D, so that very weakly sensitized cells are obtained as well as comparatively strongly sensitized cells. Then test all of the cell samples with doubling dilutions of the antiglobulin serum (see p. 353). It is also important to test the serum with cells sensitized with IgG antibodies of specificities other than D as the optimum dilution of the antiserum may be slightly different for these antibodies. In the examples given on p. 356, cells sensitized with anti-Kell and anti-Jk^a were used, both of these sera having been treated with neutral

Table 26.1 Chequer-board titration of an antiglobulin serum using red cells (A) sensitized with IgG and (B) coated by complement

	Dilutions of antiglobulin serum								
	1 in 1	2	4	8	16	32	64	128	256
Cells sensitized with anti-D serum diluted:					Series A				
1 in 1	4+	4+	4+	4+	4+	4+	4+	4+	4+
1 in 2	3+	3+	3+	3+	3+	4+	4+	4+	3+
1 in 4	1+	2+	2+	3+	3+	3+	3+	3+	2+
1 in 8	—	—	1+	2+	2+	2+	2+	2+	2+
1 in 16	—	—	—	1+	1+	2+	2+	2+	2+
1 in 32	—	—	—	—	$\frac{1}{2}$+	1+	1+	1+	$\frac{1}{2}$+
1 in 64	—	—	—	—	—	$\frac{1}{2}$+	1+	$\frac{1}{2}$+	—
Cells sensitized with:									
anti-Kell ⎱ +EDTA	—	—	1+	2+	2+	2+	3+	2+	2+
anti-Jk^a ⎰	—	—	1+	2+	3+	3+	2+	1+	—
Cells sensitized with:					Series B				
Normal incomplete antibody	4+	4+	3+	3+	2+	2+	1+	$\frac{1}{2}$+	—
Anti-Le^a + complement	5+	5+	5+	4+	3+	3+	2+	2+	1+
Cells from patient with chronic cold-haemagglutinin disease	5+	5+	4+	4+	3+	2+	2+	1+	$\frac{1}{2}$+
Normal (not sensitized) red cells:					Controls				
Group A	—	—	—	—	—	—	—	—	—
Group B	—	—	—	—	—	—	—	—	—
Group O	—	—	—	—	—	—	—	—	—

EDTA (see p. 433) to ensure that the antibodies did not bind complement components.

Methods of preparing complement-coated red cells are outlined on p. 352. The proportions of the different complement components fixed to the red cells will vary according to the method used. Several methods should, therefore, be used, e.g. cells coated with normal incomplete cold antibody, cells from a patient with chronic cold haemagglutinin disease and cells coated with a weak IgM complement-binding antibody, for example anti-Lewis, in the presence of fresh serum. Each should be tested with serial dilutions of antiglobulin serum and the serum dilution giving good agglutination of each type of cells should be noted. It is wise also at the same time to test the antiglobulin serum once more with unsensitized A, B and O cells.

The titrations illustrated in Table 26.1 show that the optimum dilution of antiglobulin serum for agglutination of IgG-sensitized cells is likely to be different from that required for maximal agglutination of cells coated by complement components.

With a serum which reacted in the way shown in Table 26.1, it would be wise always to use it at two concentrations, namely, 1 in 2 and 1 in 50.

It is, however, convenient for routine work to have a reagent which can be used at one single dilution to detect both IgG and complement components. Sometimes this can be obtained by pooling several antisera with different titres of antibodies against IgG and complement. Usually such sera have to be diluted to a more than maximal dilution for complement components in order to detect IgG satisfactorily.

Standardization of anti-IgG, -IgM, -IgA and anti-complement sera

Specific antisera are standardized in the same way as 'broad-spectrum' sera. The antisera must react with the appropriately coated cells and must not react with cells heavily coated with inappropriate proteins. Unsensitized red cells must give negative results.

10. IMMUNO-DIFFUSION AND IMMUNO-ELECTROPHORESIS

The techniques of immuno-diffusion and immuno-electrophoresis have an important place in the study of proteins, including antibodies and complement components. They provide methods for the identification and quantitative estimation of specific serum or plasma proteins. In the investigation of haemolytic anaemias they have been used for identifying the chemical nature of antibodies present in serum or in eluates derived from antibody-coated red cells.

IMMUNO-DIFFUSION

Ouchterlony introduced the agar-gel plate method in which a thin layer of agar is allowed to set in a Petri dish, small holes are punched into the gel and a few drops of serum and antiserum, respectively, are placed in adjacent holes.[14] The proteins carrying antigens in the serum and the antibodies in the antiserum diffuse into the gel and precipitin lines slowly develop where an antigen comes in contact with its corresponding antibody. An illustrated review of the techniques and results of immuno-diffusion can be found in the monograph by Peetoom.[15]

Quantitative radial immuno-diffusion

This is a method by means of which the concentration of a specific protein in a purified form or in a mixture can be determined. The area enclosed by the precipitin ring formed by the contact of the protein with its specific antiserum is measured and compared with that produced by standards consisting of known concentrations of a purified preparation of the protein which are allowed to diffuse against the antiserum for the same length of time. When no purified preparation is available, pooled normal adult human serum can be used, the results then being expressed as a percentage of the mean normal.

The method of Mancini et al,[10] as modified by Hobbs,[6] is recommended. In the original method the test was run for at least 24–48 h, and washed for a further 3–4 days before being read. By the modified method, the concentration of IgG or IgA can be read after 18 h and that of IgM within 24 h.

IMMUNO-ELECTROPHORESIS

Immuno-electrophoresis was introduced by Grabar and Williams.[3,4] In this technique antigen–antibody precipitation in agar gel is combined with electrophoresis. A broad-spectrum antiserum, e.g. the serum of a rabbit immunized against whole human serum, is used for demonstrating the proteins present in a serum or the purity or identity of a serum fraction. Monospecific antisera, e.g. a serum prepared against the kappa light chains of human IgM can be used to type an immunoglobulin or protein fraction derived from it. The antisera, as usually prepared, are capable of detecting protein concentrations of 0.1–50 g/l.

The original method is only roughly quantitative. Laurell's 'rocket' electrophoresis is a modification which provides a more accurate method of measurement.[9] It is described on p. 00. A simple micromethod,[16] which is useful in clinical practice as a screening test, is described below.

Preparation of slides

Agar, 10 g/l. Add a 1-g tablet of I.D. Agar (Oxoid) to 100 ml of 50 mmol/l barbitone buffer, pH 8.6, at 100°C. As soon as the solution is clear, pour *c* 15 ml into each of two glass Petri dishes, 15 mm in diameter, placed on a level bench.

Slides. Spotlessly clean glass slides must be used. Place four slides on the solidified agar in the Petri dish and cover each lot with *c* 33 ml of hot 10 g/l agar, so as to cover them with agar of appropriate thickness (optimally 1.8 mm). After the added agar has solidified, the Petri dishes can be stored upside down at 4°C.

For use, cut the slides out of the agar using a scalpel and cut 4–5 mm of agar off the two ends of the slide. This enables the slides to be held by their ends without touching the agar. Particular care must be taken not to touch the working surface of the slides. Punch two wells, 2 mm in diameter, at a distance of 5 mm from the horizontal mid-line of each slide by means of the tip of a Pasteur pipette

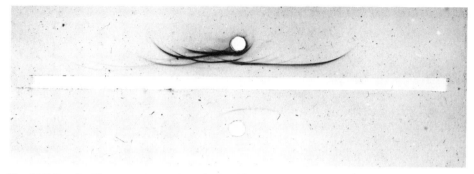

Fig. 26.2 Result of immuno-electrophoresis. Precipitation of whole human serum (top well) and IgM (bottom well) by a broad-spectrum anti-human antiserum (in trough). Electrophoresis was carried out for $1\frac{1}{2}$ h, and the subsequent diffusion for 24 h.

cut off vertically or, more easily, with a specially designed gel punch (e.g. LKB Instruments Ltd.).

Method

Fill the wells with the serum or antigen and place the slides in a slide frame which is then immediately fitted into an immuno-electrophoresis apparatus through which is passed a current not exceeding 10 mA per slide. Adequate separation occurs in about 1 h. Next, using a suitable knife blade, cut out troughs along the midline to the desired length; e.g. for γ-globulins only the cathode end need be cut. Then, with the slides placed level in a moist Petri dish, fill the troughs with antiserum and leave undisturbed at c 20°C for precipitation to occur. The time taken depends on the concentration of the proteins and also on the size of the molecules. Thus, Bence-Jones protein monomers develop a precipitin line in 1–2 h, IgG takes 2–4 h and IgM 6–24 h. A representative result is shown in Fig. 26.2.

Recording the results

The best way to obtain a permanent record is to photograph the slides (Fig. 26.2). As an alternative, the slides can be preserved by the following procedure. Wash them in three or four changes of 9 g/l NaCl (saline) over a 48 h period, and finally in water for 24 h. Shake off the excess water and dry the slides in the air. When dry, stain them with Ponceau S (2 g/l in 30 g/l trichloracetic acid) and then wash them in 50 ml/l acetic acid until no more

dye is eluted. Finally, rinse them in water and dry them in the air.

REFERENCES

1 BELL, W. N. and ALTON, H. G. S. (1954). A brain extract as a substitute for platelet suspensions in the thromboplastin generation test. *Nature (London)*, **174**, 880.
2 BIGGS, R. (Ed.) (1976). *Human Blood Coagulation, Haemostasis and Thrombosis*, 2nd edn., p. 658. Blackwell Scientific Publications, Oxford.
3 GRABAR, P. and WILLIAMS, C. A. Jnr (1953). Méthode permettant l'étude conjugée des propriétés électrophorétiques et immunochimiques d'un mélange de protéines. Application au sérum sanguin. *Biochimica et Biophysica Acta*, **10**, 193.
4 GRABAR, P. and WILLIAMS, C. A. Jnr (1953). Méthode immuno-électrophorétique d'analyse de mélanges de substances antigéniques. *Biochimica et Biophysica Acta*, **17**, 67.
5 HENDRY, E. B. (1961). Osmolarity of human serum and of chemical solutions of biological importance. *Clinical Chemistry*, **7**, 156.
6 HOBBS, J. R. (1970). Simplified radial immunodiffusion. *Association of Clinical Pathologists: Broadsheet No. 68.*
7 International Society of Blood Transfusion/International Committee for Standardization in Haematology (1980). Working party on the standardization of antiglobulin reagents of the expert panel of serology. *Vox Sanguinis* (Basel), **38**, 178.
8 KABAT, E. A. and MAYER, M. M. (1961). *Experimental Immunochemistry*, 2nd edn., p. 149. Thomas, Springfield, Ill.
9 LAURELL, C.-B. (1965). Antigen–antibody crossed electrophoresis. *Analytic Biochemistry*, **10**, 358.
10 MANCINI, G., CARBONARA, A. O. and HEREMANS, J. F. (1965). Immunochemical quantitation of antigens by single radial immunodiffusion. *Immunochemistry*, **2**, 235.
11 MOLLISON, P. L. (1979). *Blood Tranfusion in Clinical Medicine*, 6th edn., (a) p. 725, (b) p. 731. Blackwell Scientific Publications, Oxford.
12 MOORE, H. C. and MOLLISON, P. L. (1976). Use of a low-ionic-strength medium in manual tests for antibody detection. *Transfusion*, **16**, 291.
13 NEWLANDS, M. J. and WILD, F. (1955). Sources of platelet factor for the thromboplastin generation test. *Nature (London)*, **176**, 885.

[14] OUCHTERLONY, Ö. (1949). In vitro method for testing toxin-producing capacity of diphtheria bacteria. *Acta Pathologica et Microbiologica Scandinavica*, **26,** 507.

[15] PEETOOM, F. (1963). *The Agar Precipitation Technique and its Application as a Diagnostic and Analytic Method*. Oliver and Boyd, Edinburgh.

[16] SCHEIDEGGER, J. J. (1955). Une micro-méthode de l'immuno-electrophorése. *International Archives of Allergy*, **7,** 103.

[17] THOMSON, J. M. (1980). *Blood Coagulation and Haemostasis: A Practical Guide*, 2nd edn., p. 316. Churchill Livingstone, Edinburgh.

[18] World Health Organization (1977). The SI for the health professions. WHO, Geneva.

Index